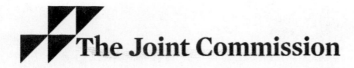

The Joint Commission

Official "Do Not Use" List[1]

Do Not Use	Potential Problem	Use Instead
U (unit)	Mistaken for "0" (zero), the number "4" (four) or "cc"	Write "unit"
IU (International Unit)	Mistaken for IV (intravenous) or the number 10 (ten)	Write "International Unit"
Q.D., QD, q.d., qd (daily)	Mistaken for each other	Write "daily"
Q.O.D., QOD, q.o.d, qod (every other day)	Period after the Q mistaken for "I" and the "O" mistaken for "I"	Write "every other day"
Trailing zero (X.0 mg)* Lack of leading zero (.X mg)	Decimal point is missed	Write X mg Write 0.X mg
MS	Can mean morphine sulfate or magnesium sulfate	Write "morphine sulfate" Write "magnesium sulfate"
MSO_4 and $MgSO_4$	Confused for one another	

[1] Applies to all orders and all medication-related documentation that is handwritten (including free-text computer entry) or on pre-printed forms.

*Exception: A "trailing zero" may be used only where required to demonstrate the level of precision of the value being reported, such as for laboratory results, imaging studies that report size of lesions, or catheter/tube sizes. It may not be used in medication orders or other medication-related documentation.

Additional Abbreviations, Acronyms and Symbols
(For <u>possible</u> future inclusion in the Official "Do Not Use" List)

Do Not Use	Potential Problem	Use Instead
> (greater than) < (less than)	Misinterpreted as the number "7" (seven) or the letter "L" Confused for one another	Write "greater than" Write "less than"
Abbreviations for drug names	Misinterpreted due to similar abbreviations for multiple drugs	Write drug names in full
Apothecary units	Unfamiliar to many practitioners Confused with metric units	Use metric units
@	Mistaken for the number "2" (two)	Write "at"
cc	Mistaken for U (units) when poorly written	Write "mL" or "ml" or "milliliters" ("mL" is preferred)
µg	Mistaken for mg (milligrams) resulting in one thousand-fold overdose	Write "mcg" or "micrograms"

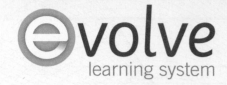
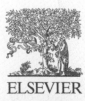

THE NURSE, THE MATH, THE MEDS

DRUG CALCULATIONS USING DIMENSIONAL ANALYSIS

Joyce M. Mulholland, RNP, Adult Nurse Practice

Nursing Education Consultant, Tucson, Arizona

M.S., California State University, Long Beach, California

M.A., Arizona State University, Tempe, Arizona

B.S., Fairleigh Dickinson College, Rutherford, New Jersey

SECOND EDITION

ELSEVIER
MOSBY

ELSEVIER
MOSBY

3251 Riverport Lane
St. Louis, Missouri 63043

THE NURSE, THE MATH, THE MEDS: DRUG CALCULATIONS   ISBN: 978-0-323-06904-5
USING DIMENSIONAL ANALYSIS

Notice

Knowledge and best practice in this field are constantly changing. As new research and experience broaden our understanding, changes in research methods, professional practices, or medical treatment may become necessary. Practitioners and researchers must always rely on their own experience and knowledge in evaluating and using any information, methods, compounds, or experiments described herein. In using such information or methods they should be mindful of their own safety and the safety of others, including parties for whom they have a professional responsibility.

With respect to any drug or pharmaceutical products identified, readers are advised to check the most current information provided (i) on procedures featured or (ii) by the manufacturer of each product to be administered, to verify the recommended dose or formula, the method and duration of administration, and contraindications. It is the responsibility of practitioners, relying on their own experience and knowledge of their patients, to make diagnoses, to determine dosages and the best treatment for each individual patient, and to take all appropriate safety precautions.

To the fullest extent of the law, neither the Publisher nor the authors, contributors, or editors, assume any liability for any injury and/or damage to persons or property as a matter of products liability, negligence or otherwise, or from any use or operation of any methods, products, instructions, or ideas contained in the material herein.

Library of Congress Cataloging-in-Publication Data

Mulholland, Joyce M.
  The nurse, the math, the meds : drug calculations using dimensional analysis / Joyce M. Mulholland.
-- 2nd ed.
    p. ; cm.
  Includes index.
  ISBN 978-0-323-06904-5 (pbk. : alk. paper)
  1. Pharmaceutical arithmetic--Problems, exercises, etc. I. Title.
  [DNLM: 1. Drug Prescriptions--nursing--Problems and Exercises. 2. Drug Prescriptions--nursing--Programmed Instruction. 3. Pharmaceutical Preparations--administration & dosage--Problems and Exercises. 4. Pharmaceutical Preparations--administration & dosage--Programmed Instruction. 5. Drug Administration Routes--Problems and Exercises. 6. Drug Administration Routes--Programmed Instruction. 7. Mathematics--Problems and Exercises. 8. Mathematics--Programmed Instruction. WY 18.2]
  RS57.M85 2011
  615'.1401513076--dc22

                                                         2010037138

Senior Editor: Yvonne Alexopoulos
Senior Developmental Editor: Danielle M. Frazier
Publishing Services Manager: Jeff Patterson
Senior Project Manager: Clay S. Broeker
Design Direction: Paula Catalano

Printed in the United States of America

Last digit is the print number: 9 8 7 6 5 4

Darlene Barnard-York, RN, MS
Instructor
College of Nursing
University of Oklahoma
Oklahoma City, Oklahoma

Donna Bowles, RN, MSN, EdD
Associate Professor
Indiana University Southeast
New Albany, Indiana

**W. Lawrence Daniels, PhD, RN,
 CPNP, NREMT-P**
Chairperson
Department of Graduate Nursing
 Education
Hampton University School of
 Nursing
Hampton, Virginia

Deborah Freyman, RN, MA, MSN
Nursing Faculty
National Park Community College
Hot Springs, Arkansas

April N. Hart, RN, MSN, FNP-BC, CNE
Assistant Professor and Nursing Lab
 Supervisor
Bethel College
Mishawaka, Indiana

Sophie Knab, MSN
Nursing Division
Niagara County Community College
Sanborn, New York

Kendra Seiler, MSN, RN
Associate Professor
Rio Hondo College
Whittier, California

Lori Stutte, MSN, RN
Assistant Professor
Ruth S. Coleman College of Nursing
Cardinal Stritch University
Milwaukee, Wisconsin

Ina E. Warboys, MS, RN
Clinical Assistant Professor and
 Director of Continuing Education
College of Nursing
University of Alabama
Huntsville, Alabama

Kathleen Weiss, MD
Assistant Professor of Biology
George Fox University
Newburg, Oregon
Medical Director
Friendsview Manor
Newberg, Oregon

To the Instructor

This second edition is designed for classroom and independent use by students at all levels in full-time, part-time, and accelerated nursing and physician assistant courses, as well as for those who are refreshing their profession. It has been updated for reader interest, clarity of equation format, currency of drugs and abbreviations, the nurse role, patient safety issues, and adverse drug events. Additional clinically relevant text box examples have been added. High-alert medications have been assigned special visual emphasis with the icon ▶. Worked-out answers are again provided in the answer keys as an obvious benefit to the student and instructor. Current TJC, ISMP and QSEN goals/competencies have been incorporated in the text. Several hundred questions have been added to the test bank.

As with the first edition, to avoid confusion only one method, dimensional analysis, is taught. It is introduced in Chapter 2 and used throughout to provide sufficient repetition for mastery of the method and the material for this typically brief course. Dimensional analysis has been documented to be a retained method of calculation and to reduce math calculation errors. It is easy to learn and apply to all the medication math problems. The method offers superior insight into the setup of problems, which is a most challenging area for students. Many students are already familiar with it because of prerequisite science courses.

Instructional design features, listed on the next page, are based upon adult learning theory and experience and evidence that drug calculations are best addressed as an integrated subject to make meaning out of the math. Medication math does not exist in a vacuum. Administering medications safely requires integration of a great deal of theory derived from several courses throughout the program of learning as well as clinical experience. Repetition and reinforcement enhance this approach. Brief questions and anecdotes tie the math to real-life situations to illustrate the comprehensive professional role needed for the complexities of safe medication administration, whether it's communication, math competence, medication-related assessments, or awareness of common errors. These features are particularly beneficial for those who are not yet in a classroom or clinical setting. Occasional departures from realistic problems are inserted to offer more math and metric practice and to test comprehension of medicated solutions usually prepared by a pharmacy

Chapters pertaining to two of the high-risk drug categories, **insulin** and **anticoagulants**, were selected for special emphasis to integrate the required broader background knowledge issues necessary for safe administration of high-alert medications. Hopefully mastery of these chapters will transfer into a broader realization of responsibilities related to other high-risk medications. Pediatric safety issues are addressed in a separate chapter.

It is strongly recommended that students demonstrate mastery of Chapter 1, which covers general math, before the first class session and Chapter 2, the introduction to dimensional analysis, before the first or second class session. There are questions covering each of these chapters in the online test bank. Use of a calculator is discouraged until the student has completed several chapters to ensure adequate analysis and understanding of the setup and the math.

A word about multiple-choice questions: The instructor always has the option of requiring for credit that students show all work. Guessing an answer is not recommended and is not the same as "estimation." The multiple-choice format adds another dimension to learning, a focus to distinguish correct from frequently encountered wrong answers. This kind of sorting clarifies understanding from a different perspective and can reduce errors.

The instructor resources contain teaching strategies of particular assistance to new instructors.

The author and the editors greatly appreciate feedback and suggestions for future printings and editions.

Instructional Design Features

- Selected **Essential Vocabulary** relevant to chapter content is provided for convenient reference at the beginning of each chapter.
- Frequent brief **five-question quizzes** that can be finished in one sitting provide quick content review.
- Selected **mnemonics** are supplied. These memory shortcuts conserve learning time.
- **Red arrow alerts** are included throughout to call attention to critical math and patient safety theory as well as issues related to practice.
- A **high-risk drug icon** ⚑ serves as a visual reminder of the high-risk drugs in the text.
- **FAQs and Answers** included in each chapter are derived from years of medication and math-related classroom questions compiled by the author. These break up the text, add to comprehension, and provide needed additional knowledge. FAQs enjoy high readership and are of particular benefit to students who are studying outside of a classroom environment.
- **Ask Yourself questions** within each chapter help students synthesize and check their broader comprehension of recent content.
- **Communication boxes** display brief sample nurse-patient or nurse-prescriber dialogues that help reduce medication errors. This increases motivation and interest in learning by relating the math to the medications and to clinical application.
- **Cultural boxes** describe selected math notation and medication-related cultural practices.
- **Clinical Relevance boxes** in each chapter offer additional information for integration of medication-related clinical practice concepts such as nursing practice, legal aspects, high-risk drugs, adverse drug events, and common errors.
- Answers to **quizzes** are worked out so that students can self-correct and have immediate feedback.
- Selected **references** are provided at the end of each chapter
- A sample shift communication hand-off report is provided as Appendix C to illustrate medication-related priorities to be reported.

Ancillaries

Instructor Resources for The Nurse, The Math, The Meds: Drug Calculations Using Dimensional Analysis, second edition are available to enhance student instruction. These resources correspond with the main book and include:
- Suggested teaching strategies
- Test bank
- PowerPoint slides

This resource is available online on the **Evolve** site at *http://evolve.elsevier.com/ Mulholland/themath/.*

NEW VERSION! *Romans & Daugherty Dosages and Solutions CTB, version 3.* This is a generic test bank available on Evolve at *http://evolve.elsevier.com/Mulholland/ themath/.* It contains over 700 questions on general mathematics, converting within the same system of measurements, converting between different systems of measurement, oral dosages, parenteral dosages, flow rates, pediatric dosages, IV calculations, and more.

Dimensional Analysis Companion for The Nurse, The Math, The Meds, second edition is an interactive student tutorial that includes an extensive menu of various topic areas within drug calculations, such as oral, parenteral, pediatric, and intravenous calculations to name a few. It includes animations and interactive exercises in which students can fill in syringes to answer problems. Covering the dimensional analysis method, this companion contains over 500 practice problems, including a comprehensive post-test.

The Nurse, The Math, The Meds: Drug Calculations Using Dimensional Analysis, second edition has been designed not only to teach you what you need to know but also to save your valuable time. Here are a few time-tested tips:

1 First, take an hour or so to review and master Chapters 1 and 2. They contain all the math and concepts of dimensional analysis you will need.

2 Set aside at least three study periods for each chapter—the first shortly after the initial presentation and the last shortly before the next class session or quiz. Working with a study buddy can help a lot. Working a practice problem or two each day will improve your retention.

3 Take the time to review Essential Vocabulary provided at the beginning of each chapter. This is a very useful reference as you proceed through each chapter.

4 Try to complete a topic and quiz in one sitting. The quizzes are brief.

5 The label on a bottle of aspirin would be very useful to have on hand for the topic of metric measurements and labels when it arises. Fifteen minutes spent studying medication labels in the over-the-counter drug section of a pharmacy will be of great help to clarify information needed about medication labels and drug measurements. If you have the opportunity, visit a laboratory setting on campus to view and handle the equipment that is mentioned in the chapters, such as syringes, calibrated medicine cups, and intravenous devices.

6 Be sure to estimate reasonable answers. Don't use your calculator until you get to very large numbers or the final chapters. The methods of solving the problems need to be fully understood before you try to use a calculator, and you need an independent method of calculation to verify answers. The discipline of writing out equations and solutions will make you competent quickly and help you avoid errors.

7 As you proceed through the text, some useful math operation shortcuts will occur to you. They have their place, but only after you are sure you understand what you are doing.

8 Write numbers as neatly as you can, using the metric notation guidelines. Sloppy writing of numbers, decimals, and commas contributes to major errors.

9 When you see a topic of interest, Google it for a quick read.

10 Be sure to review and refresh your memory after holidays and long breaks as well as before entering new clinical areas. And remember, think metric!

This text also offers key features to enhance your learning experience. Take a look at the following features so that you may familiarize yourself with this text and maximize its value.

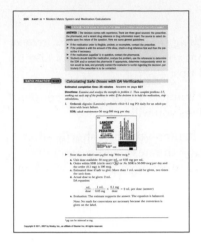

FAQ and Answers included in each chapter are derived from years of medication and math-related classroom questions compiled by the author. They break up text, add to comprehension, and provide needed additional knowledge

Ask Yourself questions within each chapter are based on content previously covered in the chapter to help you synthesize and reinforce comprehension of content.

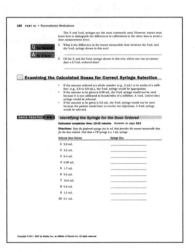

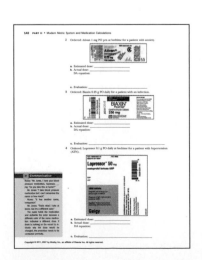

Communication boxes display sample nurse-patient and nurse-prescriber dialogues that can help reduce medication errors.

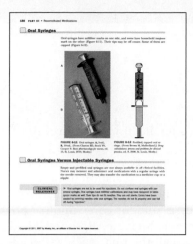

Clinical Relevance boxes in each chapter offer additional information for integration of medication-related clinical practice concepts such as nursing practice, legal aspects, high-risk drugs, and common errors.

High-risk drugs have been given special visual emphasis with this icon.

evolve

Look for this icon at the end of the chapters. It will refer you to the *Dimensional Analysis Companion for The Nurse, The Math, The Meds, second edition,* an interactive student tutorial that includes an extensive menu of various topic areas within drug calculations such as oral, parenteral, pediatric, and intravenous calculations to name a few. It includes animations and interactive exercises in which students can fill in syringes to answer problems. Covering the dimensional analysis method, this companion contains over 500 practice problems, including a comprehensive post-test and additional content information. This resource is located on Evolve at *http://evolve.elsevier.com/Mulholland/themath/.*

Best wishes. You've chosen a great profession!

Joyce M. Mulholland

Acknowledgments

I am very grateful to all those who gave suggestions for inclusions and revisions. Each suggestion was given serious consideration.

A special thanks to those reviewers who gave detailed recommendations. I incorporated as many of those ideas as was practicable. My appreciation to the ancillary writers Lisa Garsman, MS, FNP-BC, who wrote the PowerPoint slides, and Ann Tritak, RN, EdD, who revised the dimensional analysis student companion. Also, I'm very grateful to my friends Penny Lutsi, Maureen McLane, RN, and Shari Robinson, RN, for their assistance. My appreciation to all the pharmacists who answered questions about current prescribing at their respective agencies and to the drug and equipment manufacturers and their representatives who provided updated photos, charts, labels, and information.

At Elsevier, Yvonne Alexopoulos, Senior Editor, Danielle Frazier, Senior Developmental Editor, and Clay Broeker, Senior Project Manager, have been incredibly patient and supportive through several draft revisions and delays.

Contents in Brief

Detailed Contents

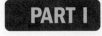

PART I

Essential Math Review For Medication Calculations

Estimated completion time: 30 minutes

Introduction

Time spent mastering any unfamiliar material in this basic review will be time very well spent. To increase your speed, this material is organized in a specific sequence, building on prior questions.

The basic mathematics in this review chapter is critical to subsequent medication calculations. Chapter 1 provides an essential math review for further study. Be able to define all the terms and do all of the operations in Chapter 1 with ease before proceeding to Chapter 2 or other chapters.

A calculator is not necessary for most medicine calculations. However, mental calculations and occasional quick use of pencil and paper are necessary for most medicine calculations. A calculator will be helpful later with more complex medication problems.

Directions: Answer all of the questions. Circle the problems that may need review. After you are finished, check your answers on p. 481. Review Chapter 1 for the areas needing further study.

Symbols (explanation on p. 6)

Write out the meaning of the following symbols:

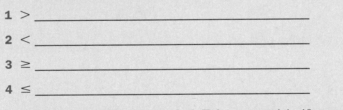

1 > _____

2 < _____

3 ≥ _____

4 ≤ _____

5 Fill in the appropriate symbol: Take two aspirin if your fever is _____ (greater than or equal to) 100 degrees F.

Whole Numbers (explanation on p. 8)

6 Write the whole number as a fraction without changing the value: 100 _____

7 Write the whole number *425* with a decimal point in the implied decimal place for whole numbers. _____

8 Edit the whole number to avoid misinterpretation: 125.000 _____

9 Use the whole number 256 to write a fraction that equals the number one (1). _____

Products, Factors, Multiples, Multipliers, and Common Factors (explanation on pp. 10-11)

10 Write the *product* of 10 and 9. _____

11 Write 5 *factors* of the number 16. _____

12 Write the *common factors* of the numbers 10 and 20. _____

13 Write the first 3 *multiples* of the number 15. _____

Squares, Square Roots, and Powers (explanation on pp. 12-14)

14 Write 10^3 out in the sequence, illustrating the process you would use to

calculate it. _____

15 Write the *square* of 3. _____

16 Write the *square root* of 25. _____

17 Which number is the *base?* 10^2 _____

18 Which number is the *exponent?* 10^8 _____

Fractions (explanation on pp. 23-33)

19 Write 2 divided by 3 as a fraction and label the numerator and denomenator.

20 Which is greater: a. $\frac{1}{10}$ or $\frac{1}{100}$? _____ b. $\frac{1}{4}$ or $\frac{1}{8}$? _____

21 Change the improper fraction $\frac{31}{6}$ to a whole number and a fraction. _____

22 Change the mixed fraction $7\frac{1}{5}$ to an improper fraction. _____

23 Find the lowest common denominator (LCD) in the pairs of fractions:

a. $\frac{1}{2}$ and $\frac{5}{8}$ _____   b. $\frac{2}{3}$ and $\frac{9}{10}$ _____

24 Find a common factor (if available) other than 1 for the numerator and denominator: $\frac{10}{15}$ _____

25 Reduce the fractions to lowest terms: a. $\frac{8}{10}$ _____   b. $\frac{4}{100}$ _____

26 Add the fractions: $\frac{3}{4} + \frac{2}{3}$ _____

27 Subtract the fractions: $\frac{5}{8} - \frac{1}{4}$ _____

28 Find the product and use cancellation to simplify:

a. $\frac{2}{3} \times \frac{6}{8}$ _____   b. $\frac{4}{5} \times \frac{3}{4}$ _____

29 Divide the fractions and use cancellation to simplify:

a. $\frac{1}{2} \div \frac{1}{9}$ _____   b. $2\frac{2}{3} \div \frac{1}{6}$ _____

30 Write each of the following expressions in fraction form:

a. 10 diapers *per* package _____   b. $2.00 *each* gallon _____
c. $30 *an* hour _____

Decimals (explanation on pp. 16-21)

31 Change the following fractions to a decimal and round to the nearest hundredth:

a. $\frac{1}{4}$ _____   b. $\frac{1}{8}$ _____

32 Write the following decimals in fraction form: a. 0.25 _____   b. 0.025 _____ (Do not reduce the result)

33 Round the following decimals to the nearest tenth: a. 0.54 _____ b. 0.08 _____

34 Round the decimals to the nearest hundredth: 1.344 _____

35 Round the decimals to the nearest thousandth: 0.23456 _____

36 Which is greater? 0.23 or 0.023 _____

37 Which is smaller? 0.15 or 0.1 _____

38 Change the following decimals to a fraction and reduce to lowest terms:

a. 0.3 _____   b. 0.5 _____   c. 0.125 _____

39 Multiply 0.4 by 1.2 and round to the nearest tenth. _____

40 Divide 0.5 by 0.125 _____

Percent (explanation on pp. 34-36)

41 What is the written spatial placement for a decimal point in this text: baseline or midline (e.g., 2.4 or 2 · 4)?

_____

42 How would you interpret a period inserted midway between numbers as illustrated below: *add* or *multiply*?

5 · 6 · 3 _____

43 Change the following decimals to a percent:

a. 0.1 _____   b. 0.75 _____   c. 0.075 _____

44 What is 25% of 200? _____

45 What is the numerical value of the *constant* used to convert hours to minutes? _____

Essential Math Review

OBJECTIVES

- Define and interpret the symbols and vocabulary of basic mathematics.
- Insert leading zeros and eliminate trailing zeros.
- Calculate sums, products, and multiples of numbers.
- Identify factors and multipliers.
- Calculate squares and square roots.
- Use mental arithmetic to calculate powers of base 10.
- Read, write, multiply, divide, and round decimal numbers.
- Add, subtract, multiply, cancel, divide, and reduce simple, mixed, and improper fractions.
- Compare fraction size by creating equivalent fractions.
- Convert fractions, decimal numbers, and percents.
- Solve basic equations.
- Estimate and evaluate answers.
- Calculate unit values.

Essential Prior Knowledge

- Basic addition, subtraction, division, and multiplication operations
- Multiplication tables

Essential Equipment

- No special equipment is needed for this chapter. It is recommended that this chapter be mastered using mental arithmetic and pencil and paper. You may wish to have a calculator on hand only for verification of paper and pencil calculations. There are two reasons for this suggestion: the underlying processes must be known in order to enter the data correctly in a calculator, and calculators may not always be available or function.

Estimated Time To Complete Chapter

- 1-2 hours (assuming some arithmetic background)

➤ Please do not skip this chapter if you missed questions on the Essential Math Self-Assessment.

Introduction

This chapter contains all of the mathematics needed for calculating medicine dosages. The math is basic. Being confident in one's own ability to understand and interpret basic arithmetic and do the basic math reduces chances of error.

Time is precious for students, staff nurses, and patients. Being skilled with the medication arithmetic frees up needed time for other aspects of nursing care. No one wants to wait a half-hour for a medication while the nurse laboriously attempts to calculate the dosage.

The short answers requested in writing are useful. Writing activity, even a very brief notation, will reinforce memory.

It is assumed that the reader has completed mathematics prerequisite courses and may only need occasional extra review and practice.

Directions

Set aside the time to complete this chapter in one sitting if you have a recent arithmetic background or in two or three sittings if you need a refresher.

- Skim the chapter objectives.
- Skim each topic in the chapter.
- When more review of a topic is needed, take the designated Rapid Practice quiz for that topic.
- The depth of your review depends on your assessment of your comprehension. A review *before* taking a test boosts scores.
- Be sure you can answer all of the questions provided.
- Revisit any content areas where questions are missed.
- When your review is completed, take the Multiple-Choice Review and the Chapter 1 Final Practice.
- Refer to a basic mathematics text if further explanation is needed.

➤ Remember: An investment of an hour or two in the basics will greatly accelerate your mastery of the rest of the text.

Essential Math Vocabulary and Concepts

Basic mathematical symbols are graphic representations of a mathematical expression. Many symbols such as $\div$, $\times$, and $\rightarrow$ are easily understood. Others may be misinterpreted and lead to errors. The first four symbols below are examples of symbols that are seen in patient-related records.

Read	Write	Example
$<$	Less than	The baby weighs $<$ 5 pounds.
$>$	Greater than	The total cholesterol was high ($>$ 200).
$\geq$	Greater than or equal to	Give the medications if the systolic blood pressure $\geq$ 160.
$\leq$	Less than or equal to	Hold the medication if his temperature is $\leq$ 100.
$\sqrt{\ }$	Square root	$\sqrt{16}$ means the square root of 16.

CLINICAL RELEVANCE

Keep in mind the potential effect on a patient receiving a medication that was supposed to be withheld for a pulse $<$50 because the nurse misinterpreted that symbol as "greater than." If this results in a patient medication error, remember that ignorance is not a defense.

✳ Mnemonic

Note the "L" in *less than* and *left.*
  The smaller end of the arrow *always* points to the *smaller* number:

5 is $>$ 3 but 5 is $<$ 10

The larger open end of the arrow always faces the *larger* number.

FAQ | *Are these symbols really seen much in medicine and nursing?*

ANSWER | Yes. These symbols are frequently seen in printed materials, such as drug and laboratory literature, medication references and medication orders. Misinterpretation has led to medication errors.

➤ Be able to read and interpret them. Do <u>not</u> write them. Write out the meaning. Refer to pp. 101-103 for The Joint Commission and Institute for Safe Medication Practices recommendations for writing out certain abbreviations that are frequently misinterpreted.

Interpreting Symbols

Estimated completion time: 5 minutes   Answers on page **481**

Directions: *Circle the correct definition for the symbols.*

TEST TIP: Keep the initial statement (stem) of the multiple-choice test questions in mind, and as you read each choice, say to yourself, "True or false."
   Put a mark to the right of the incorrect responses as you go through them. Marks on the right are suggested because if the answers are entered on a computer response sheet, any stray marks on the left or within the choices may cause the scanner to read them as a desired response. Eliminating wrong answer choices speeds a second review of the material if time is available.

1   A blood pressure goal for healthy adults is $\leq$120/80.
   1. less than
   2. greater than
   3. less than or equal to
   4. greater than or equal to

2   If the pulse is $<$50, notify the physician.
   1. less than
   2. greater than
   3. less than or equal to
   4. greater than or equal to

3   When a blood pressure is $\geq$120/80 in an otherwise healthy adult, lifestyle changes need to be instituted.
   1. less than
   2. greater than
   3. less than or equal to
   4. greater than or equal to

4   According to the Centers for Disease Control and Prevention (CDC), one of the characteristics of SARS disease is a temperature $>$100.4°F (38°C).
   1. less than
   2. greater than
   3. less than or equal to
   4. greater than or equal to

5   Identify the symbol used for square root.
   1. £
   2. ®
   3. $\sqrt{}$
   4. $\geq$

   The square root symbol does not appear in handwritten medical records. It appears in dosage formulas for body surface area.

Writing Math Symbols

Estimated completion time: 5 minutes   Answers on page **482**

Directions: *Write in the appropriate symbol in the space provided.*

TEST TIP: Writing a response is another way to reinforce memory and learning for visual and kinesthetic learners. It is emphasized that the nurse will write out the definition for the symbols in the nursing notations on the medical record to avoid misinterpretation.

1   Inject the medicine in the baby's thigh if he has walked _____ a year. (less than)

2   Give the patient 1 teaspoon of medicine if his age is _____ 5 years. (less than or equal to)

3   The risk of cancer from smoking is greatly accelerated when the patient has a history of smoking _____ 20 years. (greater than or equal to)

4   If the systolic blood pressure is _____ 180, notify the physician. (greater than)

5   The _____ symbol is used in medication math to determine body surface area for safe dosages for very powerful medicines. (square root)

Whole Numbers

A whole number is a number that is evenly divisible by the number 1.

Multiplying and dividing whole numbers by the number 1

Working with whole numbers is easier than working with fractions and decimals.

➤ Remember that a number divided by or multiplied by 1 will not change in value.

To write a whole number as a fraction, write the whole number as a numerator with the number 1 as the denominator.

The *numerator (N)*, the number above the dividing line, indicates the number of parts out of a total number of equal parts, the *denominator (D)*, designated below the dividing line.

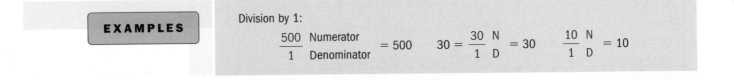

EXAMPLES

Division by 1:

$$\frac{500 \text{ Numerator}}{1 \text{ Denominator}} = 500 \qquad 30 = \frac{30}{1}\frac{N}{D} = 30 \qquad \frac{10}{1}\frac{N}{D} = 10$$

Implied Decimal Points and Trailing Zeros

A *whole* number has an *implied* decimal point immediately *following* the whole number (e.g., 1. and 20.).

➤ Do write 1 and 20; do *not* write 1. and 20.

Implied decimal points, if written, can be misread as commas, zeros, or the number one.

Zeros that follow the last number after a decimal point are called *trailing zeros*. Do write 1.3; do *not* write 1.30. Trailing zeros are only appropriate for printed laboratory reports and statistical reports.

➤ Avoid writing implied decimal points and trailing zeros.

EXAMPLES

Decimals can be mistaken for commas. Trailing zeros contribute to reading errors.

20.0   403.00   8.000   50.90   400.000   2.400

➤ Do *not* remove zeros that occur *within* a number. The number 3.08 would be read as 3.8 if this error was made, resulting in a tentimes error.

➤ Do not remove zeros that occur before a decimal point. They *alert* the reader to a decimal that follows the zero immediately:

0.04   0.4   0.004

➤ Always place a zero in front of a decimal point that is not preceded by a whole number.

➤ Always eliminate implied decimal points and trailing zeros that follow a whole number. Implied decimal points and trailing zeros do not change the value, but they do lead to reading errors and medication dosage errors.

Dividing a number or fraction by itself

A number or fraction divided by itself equals 1.
    A number or fraction divided by 1 equals itself.

Equals the number 1:	$\frac{500}{500} = 1$	$\frac{3}{3} = 1$	$\frac{10}{10} = 1$
Equals itself:	$\frac{500}{1} = 500$	$\frac{3}{1} = 3$	$\frac{10}{1} = 10$

EXAMPLES

Whole Numbers

RAPID PRACTICE   **1-3**

Estimated completion time: 5 minutes   Answers on page **482**

Directions: *Circle the correct equivalent for the whole number supplied.*

1   Identify the correct location of an implied decimal point for the *whole number* 10. _____

    1. 0.10   **3.** 1.0
    2. 100.   **4.** 10.

2   Identify the correct editing of decimals and trailing zeros for the number 350.000. _____

    1. 350,000   **3.** 350
    2. 3500   **4.** 35

3   When a whole number such as 30 is divided by itself, the numerical result is _____

    1. 1   **3.** 30
    2. 3   **4.** 900

4   Which fraction retains the value of the whole number 30? _____

    1. $\frac{30}{1}$ **3.** $\frac{30}{30}$
    2. $\frac{30}{10}$ **4.** $\frac{30}{1000}$

5   What is the numerical value of 50 multiplied or divided by 1? _____

    1. 1   **3.** 10
    2. 5   **4.** 50

Whole Numbers

RAPID PRACTICE   **1-4**

Estimated completion time: 5 minutes   Answers on page **482**

Directions: *Fill in the answers pertaining to whole numbers in the space provided.*

1   Write the whole number 100 as a fraction without changing the value of the whole number. _____

2   Write the whole number 100 with a decimal point in the implied decimal place. _____

3   Edit the number 125.50 to eliminate any trailing zeros. _____

4   Why is it necessary to remove decimals and trailing zeros after whole numbers? _____

5   Write a fraction that equals 1 with 100 in the numerator. _____

Sum

A sum is the result of *addition*.

EXAMPLES

The sum of 3 and 6 is 9.

The sum of 2 and 2 is 4.

Product

A product is the result of *multiplication* of numbers, decimals, fractions, and other numerical values.

EXAMPLES

The product of 3 and 6 is 18.

The product of $\frac{1}{3}$ and $\frac{1}{8}$ is $\frac{1}{24}$.

Factor

A factor is any whole number that can *divide another number evenly without* a *remainder*. For example, in addition to 1 and 18, the numbers 2, 3, 6, and 9 are factors of 18. Seventeen only has factors of 1 and 17. No other whole numbers divide 17.

EXAMPLES

3 has factors of 1 and 3.

25 has factors of 1, 5, and 25.

60 has factors of 1, 2, 3, 4, 5, 6, 10, 12, 15, 20, 30, and 60.

➤ A factor can only be less than or equal to a given whole number. One and the number itself are always factors. "Factoring" the number 9 gives you 1, 3, 9.

➤ *Factor* also has other meanings. It also can be used as a general term to describe relevant data. For example, "He examined all the factors in the case" or "A dimensional analysis equation permits all the factors to be entered in one equation."

Common Factors

A common factor is a whole number that divides every number in a pair or group of numbers evenly. The number 1 is always a common factor of whole numbers.

Common factors other than 1

EXAMPLES

5 and 10 have the common factor: 5. (It helps to see first whether the smaller or smallest number divides the other number or numbers evenly.)

4 and 16 have common factors of 4 and 2. (8 is not a common factor because the fraction $\frac{1}{2}$ will be the result of dividing 8 into 4 and the factor must be a whole number.)

12 and 8 have common factors of 2 and 4.

➤ A common factor can never be greater than the smallest number in the group. First, try to divide the numbers in the group by the smallest number. If that does not work, try to divide them by 2, 3, and so on.

Multiple

A multiple is the product of a *whole* number multiplied by two or more factors (*whole* numbers).

> Five *multiples* of the number 5 are 5 (5 × 1), 10 (5 × 2), 15 (5 × 3), 20 (5 × 4), and 25 (5 × 5).
>
> 50 is a multiple of factors 10 and 5, 25 and 2, and 50 and 1.

EXAMPLES

Factors Versus Multiples

> 5 has factors of 1 and 5. 5 has multiples of 5, 10, 15, . . .
>
> 8 has factors of 1, 2, 4, and 8. 8 has multiples of 8, 16, 24, . . .

EXAMPLES

Multiplier

A multiplier is the number used to multiply; it immediately follows the times sign.

> Right: The *multiplier* of 9 × 4 is 4.   Right: The *multiplier* of $10 \times \frac{1}{2}$ is $\frac{1}{2}$.

EXAMPLES

A multiplier does *not* need to be a whole number.

Multiplication Terms

RAPID PRACTICE `1-5`

Estimated completion time: 10 minutes   Answers on page 482

Directions: *Multiply or factor the numbers as requested.*

1 Write the product of 10 and 4. _____

2 Write four factors of the number 12 (excluding 1 and 12). _____

3 Write the two common factors of 8 and 12 (excluding 1). _____

4 Write the product of 3 and 4. _____

5 Write the first three multiples of the number 5. _____

Divisor, Dividend, Quotient, and Remainder

A *divisor* is the opposite of a multiplier. It is the number used to *divide* another number into smaller parts.

A **dividend** is the number being divided up, or the number the divisor is dividing.

A **quotient** is the result of division, or the answer.

The **remainder** is the amount left over in the answer when a divisor does not divide a dividend *evenly*.

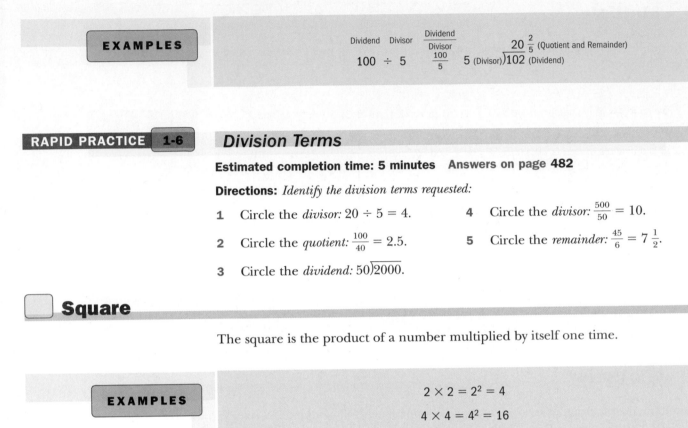

EXAMPLES

$$\text{Dividend} \quad \text{Divisor} \quad \frac{\text{Dividend}}{\text{Divisor}} \quad 20\tfrac{2}{5} \text{ (Quotient and Remainder)}$$

$$100 \div 5 \quad \frac{100}{5} \quad 5 \text{ (Divisor)}\overline{)102} \text{ (Dividend)}$$

RAPID PRACTICE **1-6**

Division Terms

Estimated completion time: 5 minutes **Answers on page 482**

Directions: *Identify the division terms requested:*

1 Circle the *divisor:* $20 \div 5 = 4$.

2 Circle the *quotient:* $\frac{100}{40} = 2.5$.

3 Circle the *dividend:* $50\overline{)2000}$.

4 Circle the *divisor:* $\frac{500}{50} = 10$.

5 Circle the *remainder:* $\frac{45}{6} = 7\frac{1}{2}$.

Square

The square is the product of a number multiplied by itself one time.

EXAMPLES

$$2 \times 2 = 2^2 = 4$$

$$4 \times 4 = 4^2 = 16$$

$$10 \times 10 = 10^2 = 100$$

Squares can also can be written and spoken as follows:

"4 squared (4^2) = 16; 16 is the square of 4."

"10 squared (10^2) = 100; 100 is the square of 10."

Think of the dimensions of a square box. To be a square, the sides must all be of equal size.

FAQ | When are squares used in medication administration?

ANSWER | Squares are used to denote square meters of body surface area (BSA). The most appropriate dosage for powerful drugs for pediatric and patients with cancer may be determined by milligrams per square meter (m^2) of body surface area rather than by weight. Nurses encounter the symbol when investigating the safe dosage ranges in a pharmacology reference. The symbol may also be on a record sent from the agency pharmacy on the patient's medical chart.

➤ Large medication errors may occur if the nurse does not understand the difference between m^2 and milligram (mg).

Square Root

The square root is the (root) number used to arrive at a square when multiplied *by itself*. It is the inverse of a square.

2 is the square *root* of 4.

10 is the square *root* of 100.

EXAMPLES

The square root symbol ($\sqrt{\ }$) is used to reduce writing and increase comprehension:

$$\sqrt{4} = 2, \sqrt{9} = 3, \sqrt{100} = 10$$

To obtain a square root on a calculator, enter the number followed by the square root symbol.

More Multiplication Terms

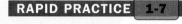

RAPID PRACTICE 1-7

Estimated completion time: 5 minutes   Answers on page 482

Directions: *Select the number of the correct answer. Narrow your choices by eliminating the obviously wrong answers with a lightly penciled mark on the right of the paper.*

TEST TIP: Create a different type of penciled reminder if you wish a reminder to revisit a question or response.

1   Which is a common factor of the numbers 8 and 10? _____
   1. $\frac{4}{5}$ **3.** 5
   2. 2   **4.** 80

2   Which is a multiple of 36? _____
   1. 6   **3.** 18
   2. 12   **4.** 72

3   What is the square of 4? _____
   1. 2   **3.** 8
   2. 4   **4.** 16

4   Which is the multiplier of $8 \times \frac{1}{4}$? _____
   1. $\frac{1}{4}$ **3.** 8
   2. 2   **4.** 32

5   What is the square root of 25? _____
   1. 2   **3.** 5
   2. 4   **4.** 625

Multiplication, Squares, and Division

RAPID PRACTICE 1-8

Estimated completion time: 5 minutes   Answers on page 482

Directions: *Fill in the answers to the multiplication and division problems in the space provided.*

1   Write the *product* of 3×4.   _____

2   Write the *square* of 7 (7^2).   _____

3   Write the *divisor* of $10 \div \frac{1}{2}$.   _____

4   Identify the *dividend* in 100 divided by 10. _____

5   Write the product of 3 and 5.   _____

Bases and Exponents

Bases and exponents are numbers written with two parts: $2^{3\leftarrow\text{exponent}}_{\uparrow\text{base}}$

The *base* is the number that must be multiplied by *itself*. The *exponent*, also known as *power*, is the small superscript number that indicates *how many times* the base must be multiplied *by itself*. Some examples were given in the section on squares. The expression 2^3 is a type of shorthand for $2 \times 2 \times 2$. Writing powers saves a lot of math time.

EXAMPLES

Examine the difference in the values for 3^2 and 2^3.

$$3^2 = 3 \times 3 = 9$$

$$2^3 = 2 \times 2 \times 2 = 8$$

$$4^5 = 4 \times 4 \times 4 \times 4 \times 4 = 1024$$

Multiply the base the *specified number of times* by *itself*.

Read and/or say 2^3 as, "2 to the third power" *or*, alternatively, "the third power of 2."
Note: The exponent is accompanied by the word "power".

Read or say

You would *say* or *read* 2^3 as, "2 to the third power" *or*, alternatively, "the third power of 2." The exponent is read as "power."

Powers of 10 Calculations

When working with powers of 10, such as $10^2, 10^3, 10^4$, and so on, note the number of zeros in the answers.

EXAMPLES

$$10^2 = 10 \times 10 = 100$$

$$10^3 = 10 \times 10 \times 10 = 1000$$

$$10^4 = 10 \times 10 \times 10 \times 10 = 10,000$$

The number of zeros in the result is equal to the number in the exponent.

FAQ | *How are powers and exponents used in medication administration?*

ANSWER | Using powers of 10 and exponents makes it much easier to understand decimals and metric system conversions. The metric system is a decimal system based on powers of 10. Most medications are delivered in milligrams and grams, which are converted using powers of 10. The nurse who understands these conversions will be less likely to make medication errors. It only takes a few minutes to comprehend powers and exponents of 10.

Powers

Estimated completion time: 5-10 minutes   **Answers on page 482**

Directions: *Use your understanding of powers and exponents to answer the following questions:*

1 Write 10^2 out in the sequence to illustrate the process you would use to arrive at the answer. _____

2 Write 2^5 out in the sequence to illustrate the process you would use to arrive at the answer. _____

3 Write in numerical shorthand: 10 to the eighth power. _____

4 Which number is the base in 10^4? _____

5 Which number is the exponent in 10^4? _____

Multiplying and Dividing by 10, 100, and 1000

Dividing and multiplying by a multiple of 10—such as 10, 100, and 1000—involves moving the decimal place to the left or right by a number of places that is *equal to the number of zeros* in the *divisor* or *multiplier*: 10, 100 or 1000, and so on. These three numbers are the most frequently used numbers in metric medication calculations. They are powers of 10: 10^1, 10^2, and 10^3.

- To divide, examine the *divisor*—10, 100, or 1000—for the number of zeros. In the dividend, move the decimal point (real or implied) to the left by a number of places that is equal to the number of zeros:

$$1000 \div 10 = 100$$

- To multiply, examine the *multiplier*—10, 100, or 1000—for the number of zeros. In the number being multiplied, move the decimal point to the right by a number of places that is equal to the number of zeros:

$$10 \times \underset{1\,2\,3}{1000} = 10,000$$

Verify your answer.

Whole Number × Multiplier = Answer			Whole Number ÷ Divisor = Answer		
50 × 10	= 500		500 ÷ 10	= 50.0̶ = 50	
400 × 100	= 40,000		40 ÷ 100	= .4̶0̶ = 0.4	
10 × 1000	= 10,000		4 ÷ 1000	= .004 = 0.004	

➤ Whenever there are more than four numbers in a group, insert a comma in front of every three digits from right to left to ease the reading: e.g., 1000000 becomes 1,000,000 (1 million), and 20000 becomes 20,000 (20 thousand).

Insert zeros in front of decimals, and avoid trailing zeros after whole numbers.

Multiplying and Dividing by 10, 100, and 100

Estimated completion time: 5-10 minutes   **Answers on page 483**

Directions: *Select the correct notation for multiplication and division using mental arithmetic and moving decimal places. Narrow the field of choices by quickly eliminating the obviously wrong answers.*

> **TEST TIP:** Since only the multiplier or divisor determines the number of places to move the decimal point, first identify the multiplier or divisor and the number of zeros in it. Then move the decimal point to the left or the right.

1 30 multiplied by 100 = _____.
   1. 300   **3.** 30,000
   2. 3000   **4.** 300,000

4 250 divided by 1000 = _____.
   1. 0.0025   **3.** 0.25
   2. 0.025   **4.** 2.55

2 0.4 multiplied by 1000 = _____.
   1. 0.004   **3.** 400
   2. 4   **4.** 4000

5 1500 divided by 100 = _____.
   1. 0.15   **3.** 15
   2. 1.5   **4.** 150

3 5000 divided by 100 = _____.
   1. 5   **3.** 100
   2. 50   **4.** 500

RAPID PRACTICE 1-11   *Multiplying and Dividing by 10, 100, and 1000*

Estimated completion time: 10 minutes   **Answers on page 483**

Directions: *Fill in the answer in the table by moving decimal points to the left for division and to the right for multiplication.*

Number	÷ 10	÷ 100	÷ 1000	Number	× 10	× 100	× 1000
1 50	_____	_____	_____	4 0.5	_____	_____	_____
2 125	_____	_____	_____	5 0.25	_____	_____	_____
3 10	_____	_____	_____				

Decimal Fractions

A decimal fraction is any fraction with a denominator that is a *power of 10*. It is easier to read and write decimal *fractions* in *abbreviated* form with a decimal point to replace the denominator, for example, 0.1 for $\frac{1}{10}$ and 0.06 for $\frac{6}{100}$. In this abbreviated form, these decimal fractions are called *decimals*. Our money system is based on decimals.

EXAMPLES

Decimal = Fraction	Decimal = Fraction
$0.1 = \frac{1}{10}$	$0.4 = \frac{4}{10}$
$0.05 = \frac{5}{100}$	$0.35 = \frac{35}{100}$
$0.005 = \frac{5}{1000}$	$0.025 = \frac{25}{1000}$
$0.0009 = \frac{9}{10,000}$	$0.0005 = \frac{5}{10,000}$

➤ Decimals replace the division bar and the denominator of a fraction with a decimal point in the specified place that identifies power of 10 in the denominator. Zeros are used to hold the place values.

FAQ | *How does the denominator of a decimal fraction differ from the denominators of other fractions?*

ANSWER | The decimal fraction has a denominator that is a power of 10. Other fractions, such as $\frac{2}{3}, \frac{5}{6}$, and $\frac{1}{5}$, do not have a power of 10 in the denominator.

Fractions with denominators other than powers of 10 are covered in more detail on p. 23.

Like other fractions, decimal fractions—or decimals—are numbers that indicate less than a whole unit.

Observe the number line below, which represents numbers as points on a line. The numbers to the *left* of the decimal point are whole numbers. The numbers to the *right* of the decimal point are decimal fractions.

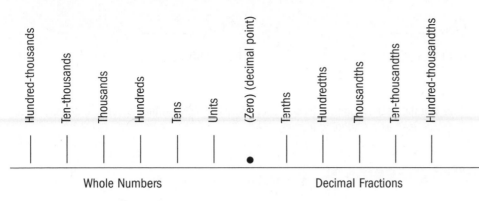

Read the number to the right of the decimal point as the numerator.

The number of places to the right of the decimal point determines the power of 10 in the denominator. One place denotes tenths, two places denote hundredths, three places denote thousandths, and so on.

1 Decimal Place	2 Decimal Places	3 Decimal Places	4 Decimal Places
0.5	0.12	0.375	0.0005
5 tenths	12 hundredths	375 thousandths	5 ten-thousandths

EXAMPLES

➤ A leading zero should always precede a decimal expression of less than 1 to alert the reader to the decimal.

Reading Numbers and Decimals

Decimals are read as fractions. Decimal points separate whole numbers from fractional parts of a number. The fractional part follows to the immediate *right* of the decimal point.

Read the number or numbers that appear to the left of the decimal point out loud.

Read the decimal *point* as "and" or "point."

Read the decimal in *fraction* form.

Written	Read and Spoken as a Fraction
0.5	"five tenths"
1.5	"one and 5 tenths" "or one point 5"
1.06	"one and 6 hundredths" or "one point zero 6"
42.005	"42 and 5 thousandths"
2.0008	"2 and 8 ten-thousandths" or "2 point zero, zero, zero, 8"

EXAMPLES

RAPID PRACTICE   1-12   *Reading Decimal Numbers*

Estimated completion time: 5 minutes   Answers on page 483

Directions: *Write the following decimals in fraction form.*

1 0.5 _____

2 0.003_____

3 0.25 _____

4 1.56 _____

5 2.0345_____

➤ Note that the decimal point is placed at the *baseline* between the numbers. If it is elevated, it may be read as a symbol to multiply.

Decimal Point Spatial Placement

| EXAMPLES | 1.4 is 1 and four *tenths*. | 1 · 4 is 1 times 4. |

Writing Decimals in Fraction Form

Write the number or numbers that appear to the right of the decimal point as the *numerator.*

Write the power of 10 (e.g., 10, 100, or 1000) according the decimal places in the *denominator.*

The number of zeros in the denominator is equal to the number of decimal places.

Eliminate the decimal point.

EXAMPLES

Decimal		Fraction Form	
0.5	5 "tenths"	$\frac{5}{10}$	One zero in the denominator because there is one place after the decimal point
0.05	5 "hundredths"	$\frac{5}{100}$	Two zeros in the denominator because there are two places after the decimal point
0.005	5 "thousandths"	$\frac{5}{1000}$	Three zeros in the denominator because there are three places after the decimal point

Be sure to include a zero for *each* decimal place, the *place value* of the decimal number (tenths, hundredths, thousandths, etc.), in the *denominator.*

➤ Insert leading zeros before decimal points and remove trailing zeros. Commas, decimal points, and the number 1 must be distinguished to avoid errors.

➤ To avoid 10-, 100-, and 1000-fold errors, the decimal point must be clearly identified and in the correct place:
0.5, *not* .5   0.025, *not* .025   625, *not* 625.00

Decimal	Fraction	Decimal	Fraction	Decimal	Fraction
0.5	$\frac{5}{10}$	0.01	$\frac{1}{100}$	0.025	$\frac{25}{1000}$

EXAMPLES

The decimal point replaces the division bar and the denominator of the decimal fraction.

Writing Decimal Fractions in Decimal Form

RAPID PRACTICE 1-13

Estimated completion time: 5-10 minutes   Answers on page 483

Directions: *Write the decimal fractions in decimal form. Place the decimal point at baseline.*

1 $\frac{25}{100}$ _____

2 $\frac{1}{10}$ _____

3 $\frac{25}{1000}$ _____

4 $\frac{4}{10}$ _____

5 $\frac{5}{100}$ _____

Reading and Writing Decimal Numbers in Fraction Form

RAPID PRACTICE 1-14

Estimated completion time: 5 minutes   Answers on page 483

Directions: *Write the decimal in fraction notation. Do not reduce to lowest terms.*

1 0.8 _____   4 0.25 _____

2 0.005 _____   5 0.015 _____

3 1.25 _____

➤ Tenths are the *largest* decimal fraction denominator. A tenth is 10 times larger than a hundredth.

☐ Comparing Decimals to See Which Is Larger

- Evaluate the *whole* number first. The higher number has the higher value (e.g., 1.21 < 2.21; 1.04 > 0.083).
- If the whole numbers are equal or there are no whole numbers, examine the *tenths* column for the higher number (e.g., 0.82 > 0.593; 0.632 < 0.71; 1.74 > 1.64).
- If the tenths columns are equal, examine the hundredths column (e.g., 0.883 > 0.87).

Comparing Decimal Values

RAPID PRACTICE 1-15

Estimated completion time: 5-10 minutes   Answers on page 483

Directions: *Circle the* larger-value *decimal in each* pair:

TEST TIP: Examine the place value of the denominators (e.g., tenths, hundredths, and thousandths), and read them as decimal fractions. Do not reduce to lowest terms.

1 0.1 and 0.5   4 0.01 and 0.005

2 0.3 and 0.03   5 0.6 and 0.16

3 1.24 and 1.32   6 0.5 and 0.25

7 0.0006 and 0.006   **9** 0.05 and 0.5

8 0.01 and 0.05   **10** 1.06 and 1.009

General Rules for Rounding Decimals and Whole Numbers to an Approximate Number*

1 Locate the *specified* place value (e.g., round to the nearest *tenth, hundredth, whole number,* etc.) in the quantity given.

2 If the number that immediately follows the *specified* unit *is 0 to 4,* leave the *specified* column *unchanged,* e.g., a quantity of 0.34 *rounded to nearest tenth is 0.3, unchanged.*

3 If the number that immediately follows the *specified* unit is 5 or greater, round the *specified* column number up by one (1).

*Refer to p. 17 for decimal place values.

EXAMPLES

Quantity	Nearest Tenth	Nearest Hundredth	Quantity	Nearest Whole Number
0.25	0.3	0.25	1.2	1
0.0539	0.1	0.05	15.5	16
2.687	2.7	2.69	2.687	3

FAQ | *Why do nurses need to learn how to round numbers?*

ANSWER | Rounding medicine doses will depend upon the equipment available. This will become more apparent as you view the medication cups, various size syringes, and IV equipment in later chapters. Volumes less than 1 mL (milliliter) usually are rounded to the *nearest hundredth of a mL,* and volumes greater than 1 mL are usually rounded to the *nearest tenth of a mL.* Some intravenous solutions are delivered in drops per minute. Drops cannot be split. They must be rounded to nearest whole number

RAPID PRACTICE **1-16**

Rounding Decimal Numbers

Estimated completion time: 5 minutes   Answers on page 484

Directions: *Round to the desired approximate value in the space provided:*

1 Round to the nearest *tenth.*

1. 0.34 _____
2. 1.27 _____
3. 0.788 _____
4. 1.92 _____
5. 0.06 _____

2 Round to the nearest *hundredth.*

1. 0.6892 _____
2. 3.752 _____
3. 0.888 _____
4. 2.376 _____
5. 0.051 _____

3 Round to the nearest *whole* number.

1. 2.38 _____
2. 10.643 _____
3. 0.9 _____
4. 1.52 _____
5. 3.47 _____

Adding and Subtracting Decimal Numbers

• To add and subtract decimal numbers, line them up in a column with the decimal points directly under each other. Add or subtract the columns, proceeding from right to left, as with whole numbers. Insert the decimal point in the answer directly under the decimal points in the problem.

Addition		Subtraction		
0.26	1.36	4.38	12.4	**EXAMPLES**
+1.44	+2.19	−1.99	−0.6	
1.70	3.55	2.39	11.8	

It is important to keep the decimal points aligned in addition, subtraction, and division.

Multiplying Decimals

- To multiply decimals, multiply the numbers as for any multiplication of whole numbers.
- Counting from *right* to *left*, insert the decimal point in the answer in the place equal to the *total number of decimal places* in the two numbers that are multiplied.

			EXAMPLES
1.2 1 Decimal Place	2.5 1 Decimal Place	3.4 1 Decimal Place	
×0.4 1 Decimal Place	×0.01 2 Decimal Places	×0.0001 4 Decimal Places	
0.48 2 Total Decimal Places	0.025 3 Total Decimal Places	0.00034 5 Total Decimal Places*	

- Insert a zero in front of the decimal point in the answer if the answer does not contain a value to the left of the decimal point. The decimal points in multiplication are *not* aligned with other decimal points in the problem, as in addition, subtraction, and division.
- Insert zeros in the answer to hold the place for the decimal point if there are insufficient digits in the answer.

Multiplying Decimals

RAPID PRACTICE 1-17

Estimated completion time: 10 minutes **Answers on page 484**

Directions: *Multiply the numbers. Count the total decimal places and insert the decimal point in the answer as needed.*

1	2	**3**	0.125	**5**	0.25
	× 0.4		× 2		× 2

2	1	**4**	1.5
	× 0.1		× 6

Dividing Decimals

Division of decimals is the same as division of whole numbers, with one exception: decimal point placement is emphasized.

Division of decimals when the divisor is a whole number

Examine the divisor. If it is a *whole* number, place the decimal point in the answer *directly above* the decimal point in the dividend, as shown in the examples that follow.

Proceed as with division for whole numbers.

EXAMPLES

A	B	C
2.6 Quotient	0.43 Answer	0.05 Answer
4 Divisor)‾10.4‾ Dividend	5)‾2.15‾	8)‾0.40‾

The alignment of decimal points must be exactly as shown in examples A, B, and C.

Insert a leading zero in front of a decimal that does not have an accompanying whole number, as shown in example B in red.

Add zeros if necessary to the dividend in order to arrive at a numerical answer, as shown in example C in red.

Division of decimals when divisor contains decimals

- If the divisor contains decimals, first change the divisor to a *whole* number by *moving* the real or implied decimal place in the dividend to the right by the number of decimal places *equal* to the decimal places in the *divisor.*
- *Place the decimal point in the answer directly* above the new decimal place in the dividend. Proceed with the division as for whole numbers.

EXAMPLES

A	B	C
45	5	2
0.4)‾18.0‾	0.5)‾2.5‾	1.25)‾2.50‾

- Add zeros if necessary as placeholders, as shown in example C.

Moving the decimal place an equal number of places in both the divisor and the dividend to make a whole number in the divisor is the equivalent of multiplying both figures by 10, 100, or 1000. The value of the answer will be *unchanged,* as seen in the following example.

EXAMPLES

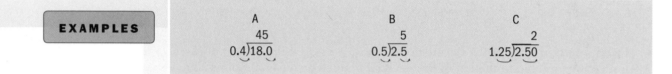

Dividend/Divisor = Quotient	Multiplying Divisor and Dividend × 10	Multiplying Divisor and Dividend × 100
$\frac{18}{0.4} = 45$	$\frac{180}{4} = 45$	$\frac{1800}{40} = 45$

FAQ | *Why do nurses need to understand division of decimals?*

ANSWER | Because medications may be ordered or supplied in decimal doses.

RAPID PRACTICE 1-18

Division of Decimals: Placing the Decimal Point

Estimated completion time: 10-15 minutes   Answers on page 484

Directions: *Move the decimal points in the divisor and dividend as necessary, in contrasting ink, to illustrate the correct placement of decimal points for division, as shown in the examples above. Place the decimal point prominently in the* answer *line in the correct place. Do* NOT *perform the math. Add zeros as necessary as placeholders in the dividend.*

1   0.1)‾0.5‾   3   3.05)‾20.32‾   5   1.2)‾5.06‾

2   0.025)‾0.1‾   4   0.25)‾1‾

Dividing Decimals

Estimated completion time: 10-15 minutes   Answers on page 484

Directions: *Perform the division. Do not use a calculator.*

TEST TIP: Move the decimal points and place the decimal point prominently in the answer *before* proceeding with the division.

1 $5\overline{)20.5}$

3 $0.02\overline{)0.03}$

5 $250\overline{)200}$

2 $0.5\overline{)2}$

4 $4\overline{)1}$

Fractions

A fraction is a number that describes the *parts* of a whole number. It is a form of division. A fraction has a numerator and a denominator. The numerator is the top number in the fraction and tells the number of parts in the fraction. The denominator is the bottom number in the fraction and tells the number of equal parts in which the whole number is divided. For math calculations or data entry on a calculator, the numerator is to be *divided by the denominator.*

➤ A denominator is the same as a divisor.

The fraction denotes two parts of a whole that is divided into three equal parts. The division line that divides the numerator and denominator, reading *top to bottom,* indicates "2 divided by 3."

$$\frac{2 \text{ (numerator)}}{3 \text{ (denominator, divisor)}} = 2 \div 3$$

※ Mnemonic

DDD: Denominator, divisor, down under or down below the *divide by* line

EXAMPLES

The whole pizza below is divided into six equal pieces (the denominator).

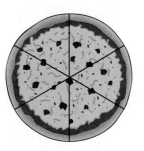

If you eat one piece of pizza, you have consumed $\frac{1}{6}$ of the pizza.

▲ Cultural Note

Placement of the decimal point according to usage in the country of employment, *baseline or midline,* is very important in avoiding errors. Many countries use a *baseline period for a decimal point* between the numbers (5.5). In these countries a *midline* dot *may* indicate *multiplication* (5 · 2 = 10). Several other countries use a *comma* to represent a decimal (5,5) and the period is placed *baseline or midline* between the numbers (2.2 = 4; 2 · 2 = 4) to denote multiplication.

The **baseline placement of the decimal point** will be used with this text.

$$\frac{1}{6} \begin{array}{l} \text{Numerator} \\ \text{Division Bar, Dividing Line} \\ \text{Denominator} \end{array} \quad \frac{1}{6} \begin{array}{l} \text{part} \\ \text{total number of equal parts} \end{array}$$

EXAMPLES

The denominator is a *divisor.*

Alternative Fraction Forms

The fraction $\frac{1}{2}$ can be expressed in the following forms:

1 decimal with a decimal point: 0.5 (numerator ÷ denominator, or 1 divided by 2)
2 percent with a percent sign: 50% (fraction × 100 with a percent sign added)

The forms above express one part of two equal parts.

Mixed Fractions

A fraction that consists of a *mixture* of a whole number and a fraction is called a *mixed fraction*.

EXAMPLES	$1\frac{2}{3}$, $41\frac{5}{6}$, $8\frac{1}{8}$

✳ Mnemonic

A mixed fraction represents a *mixture* of whole and part of a whole. An improper fraction is improper because it is top heavy.

Be sure to leave a space between the whole number and the fraction to avoid misinterpretation as a larger number.

Improper Fractions

A fraction that consists of a numerator that is *equal to* or *larger than* the denominator is called an improper fraction.

EXAMPLES	$\frac{10}{8}$, $\frac{12}{7}$, $\frac{4}{4}$

Converting Mixed and Improper Fractions

- To convert a mixed fraction to an improper fraction, *multiply* the denominator by the whole number and *add* it to the numerator.
- Place the new numerator over the original denominator of the fraction.

EXAMPLES	$3\frac{1}{2} = \frac{7}{2}$ (2 × 3 + 1), $4\frac{1}{3} = \frac{13}{3}$ (3 × 4 +1), $1\frac{1}{5} = \frac{6}{5}$ (5 × 1 +1)

Converting an Improper Fraction to a Mixed Fraction

- To convert an improper fraction to a mixed fraction, *divide* the numerator by the denominator to obtain a whole number and a remainder.
- Write the remainder as a fraction.

$$\frac{20}{6} = 3\frac{2}{6} \text{ or } 3\frac{1}{3} \qquad \frac{10}{8} = 1\frac{2}{8} \text{ or } 1\frac{1}{4} \qquad \frac{27}{23} = 1\frac{4}{23}$$

➤ Be careful when writing mixed fractions. Leave space between the whole number and the fraction. The mixed number $3\frac{1}{2}$ without adequate space could be misread as $\frac{31}{2}$ (thirty-one over two, or $15\frac{1}{2}$).

Basic Fraction Vocabulary

Estimated completion time: 5 minutes   Answers on page 484

Directions: *Identify the appropriate terms and forms for the fractions.*

1 Identify the numerator of $\frac{5}{8}$. _____

1. 1   **3.** 8
2. 5   **4.** 40

2 Identify the denominator of $\frac{2}{6}$. _____

1. 1   **3.** 3
2. 2   **4.** 6

3 Identify the improper fraction. _____

1. $\frac{1}{2}$ **3.** $10\frac{1}{2}$
2. $1\frac{1}{3}$ **4.** $\frac{11}{2}$

4 Identify the correct conversion of an improper fraction to a mixed fraction. _____

1. $\frac{1}{4} = \frac{4}{16}$ **3.** $\frac{21}{2} = 10\frac{1}{21}$
2. $\frac{4}{3} = 1\frac{1}{3}$ **4.** $\frac{11}{3} = 33\frac{1}{3}\%$

5 Identify the correct conversion of a mixed fraction to an improper fraction. _____

1. $\frac{1}{2} = \frac{4}{8}$ **3.** $2\frac{1}{4} = 2\frac{2}{8}$
2. $5\frac{1}{2} = \frac{11}{2}$ **4.** $\frac{1}{3} = 1{:}3$

Reducing Fractions

Reducing fractions to the lowest (simplest) terms simplifies the math. Reducing a fraction is usually requested for the final answer to a fraction problem, but this step can be performed at any point in calculations to make it easier.

✻ Mnemonic

The definition of the word *reduce* gives a clue to the operation.

- To reduce a fraction, divide the numerator and the denominator by the same (common) factor until it *cannot be divided* further into whole numbers.
- Try using the numerator as the common factor. Divide it directly into the denominator, as shown in the first example that follows.
- If that does not work, try dividing the numerator and denominator by 2.
- If the numerator and denominator are not divisible by 2, find all factors of the numerator and denominator. The common factors will divide both the numerator and the denominator evenly.

➤ A fraction *cannot* be further reduced if the numerator is 1 ($\frac{1}{2}$; $\frac{1}{280}$).

EXAMPLES

The numerator is the largest common factor.

Dividing the numerator and denominator by 100 reduces this fraction to its simplest terms.

$$\frac{\overset{1}{\cancel{100}}}{\underset{2}{\cancel{200}}} = \frac{1}{2}$$

Dividing the numerator and denomenator by the common factor, 2, reduces this fraction to its lowest terms.

$$\frac{\overset{3}{\cancel{6}}}{\underset{4}{\cancel{8}}} = \frac{3}{4}$$

Note that the value of the fraction is unchanged by reduction.

$\frac{1}{8}, \frac{1}{200},$ and $\frac{1}{9}$ cannot be reduced because a numerator of 1 or less is not a whole number. $\frac{3}{7}$ cannot be reduced because there are no common factors.

RAPID PRACTICE 1-21

Reducing Fractions

Estimated completion time: 5 minutes   Answers on page 484

Directions: *Identify the correctly reduced fraction.*

TEST TIP: Put a light "X" to the right to the obviously incorrect answers.

1   $\frac{4}{8}$ can be reduced to _____.

    1. $\frac{8}{4}$ **2.** $\frac{2}{3}$ **3.** $\frac{1}{2}$ **4.** $\frac{8}{16}$

2   $\frac{100}{500}$ can be reduced to _____.

    1. $\frac{100}{250}$ **2.** $\frac{10}{25}$ **3.** $\frac{2}{5}$ **4.** $\frac{1}{5}$

3   $\frac{25}{75}$ can be reduced to which lowest terms? _____

    1. $\frac{1}{4}$ **3.** $\frac{2}{3}$

    2. $\frac{1}{3}$ **4.** $\frac{5}{25}$

4   The lowest terms for the fraction $\frac{15}{26}$ are _____.

    1. $\frac{3}{13}$ **3.** $\frac{15}{26}$

    2. $\frac{5}{26}$ **4.** $\frac{30}{52}$

5   The lowest terms for the fraction $\frac{1}{12}$ are _____.

    1. $\frac{1}{12}$ **3.** $\frac{2}{24}$

    2. $\frac{2}{6}$ **4.** $\frac{3}{36}$

Common (Same) Denominator

Fractions are easier to compare and interpret if they have the *same* denominator.

EXAMPLES

Comparing the size of $\frac{8}{24}$ and $\frac{9}{24}$ is easier than comparing the size of $\frac{1}{3}$ and $\frac{3}{8}$ because you only have to compare the numerators when the denominators are equal.

Lowest Common Denominator (LCD)

Fractions can be added and subtracted if they share a common denominator. Finding the lowest common denominator simplifies the calculation.

Finding the lowest common denominator (LCD)

- To find the lowest common denominator (LCD), reduce fractions first where applicable.
- If the larger denominator can be divided by the other denominator or denominators with a whole-number result, the larger denominator will be the LCD.
- *Or*, if the denominators are low numbers, multiply the denominators by each other.
- *Or* test each multiple of the largest denominator, starting with $\times 1$, $\times 2$, and so on, until a common multiple is located.
- Reduce the answer to lowest terms.

> $\frac{1}{4}$ and $\frac{1}{8}$: 8 is the larger denominator. 4 will divide evenly into 8. $\frac{1}{4} = \frac{2}{8}$. 8 is the LCD.
>
> $\frac{1}{2}$ and $\frac{1}{3}$: 3 is the larger denominator. 2 will not divide evenly into 3. Multiply the denominators by each other. $3 \times 2 = 6$. 6 is the LCD.
>
> $\frac{1}{4}$ and $\frac{5}{6}$: 6 is the larger denominator. 4 will not divide evenly into 6. Try using multiples of 6. $6 \times 1 = 6$; $6 \times 2 = 12$. 12 is a multiple for both 4 and 6. 12 is the LCD.

EXAMPLES

Finding the Lowest Common Denominator (LCD)

RAPID PRACTICE 1-22

Estimated completion time: 15 minutes **Answers on page 484**

Directions: *Calculate the LCD for the fractions supplied.*

> **TEST TIP:** Since the LCD cannot be smaller than the largest denominator, start by examining the largest denominator to see if the smaller denominator or denominators divide the largest denominator evenly.

1 $\frac{1}{3}$, $\frac{1}{9}$, and $\frac{1}{18}$ _____

2 $\frac{1}{5}$ and $\frac{2}{6}$ _____

3 $\frac{1}{2}$, $\frac{1}{3}$, and $\frac{1}{4}$ _____

4 $\frac{1}{10}$ and $\frac{1}{25}$ _____

5 $\frac{1}{100}$, $\frac{1}{50}$, and $\frac{1}{200}$ _____

Equivalent Fractions

Equivalent fractions are fractions that have the same value.

- To create an equivalent fraction, multiply the denominator (D) and then the numerator (N) in that fraction by the *same factor*. The value will be *unchanged* because you are really multiplying by a fraction that equals 1 (e.g., $\frac{2}{2} = 1$)
- You can also divide the numerator and denominator by the same factor to arrive at smaller equivalent fractions.

Original Fraction	Factor 2	Equivalent Fraction	Original Fraction	Factor 3	Equivalent Fraction	Original Fraction	Factor 4	Equivalent Fraction
$\frac{5}{6}$	$\times \frac{2}{2}$	$= \frac{10}{12}$	$\frac{5}{6}$	$\times \frac{3}{3}$	$= \frac{15}{18}$	$\frac{5}{6}$	$\times \frac{4}{4}$	$= \frac{20}{24}$
$\frac{24}{36}$	$\div \frac{2}{2}$	$= \frac{12}{18}$	$\frac{24}{36}$	$\div \frac{3}{3}$	$= \frac{8}{12}$	$\frac{24}{36}$	$\div \frac{4}{4}$	$= \frac{6}{9}$

EXAMPLES

RAPID PRACTICE 1-23

Creating Equivalent Fractions

Estimated completion time: 5-10 minutes   **Answers on page 485**

Directions: *Using the common factor supplied, create an equivalent fraction.*

	Fraction	Common Factor	Equivalent Fraction
1	$\frac{1}{3}$	2	_____
2	$\frac{4}{5}$	3	_____
3	$\frac{1}{2}$	4	_____
4	$\frac{3}{4}$	2	_____
5	$\frac{3}{8}$	3	_____

Comparing Fractions

- To compare fractions with the *same denominator*, compare the numerators.

  Comparing $\frac{1}{8}$, $\frac{3}{8}$, and $\frac{7}{8}$, the largest is $\frac{7}{8}$ and the smallest is $\frac{1}{8}$.

  There are two ways to compare fractions when the denominators are *different*.

- The first way is to find the lowest common denominator and create equivalent fractions.
- The faster way to compare sizes of fractions is to multiply diagonally from the denominator of one fraction to the numerator of the next fraction. This is called *cross-multiplication*.
- The *numerator* of the fraction with the higher product indicates which is the larger fraction. Examine the example of cross-multiplication that follows.

EXAMPLES

Cross-multiply the *numerator* of each fraction by the *denominator* of the other.
If the products are equal, the fractions are equivalent.

Equivalent	Larger	Larger
40 40	12 15	200 100
$\frac{5}{10} \times \frac{4}{8}$	$\frac{2}{3} \times \frac{5}{6}$	$\frac{1}{100} \times \frac{1}{200}$
40 = 40	15 is the larger product.	200 is the larger product.
$\frac{5}{10} = \frac{4}{8}$	$\frac{5}{6}$ is the larger fraction.	$\frac{1}{100}$ is the larger fraction.

RAPID PRACTICE 1-24

Comparing Fraction Sizes

Estimated completion time: 5-10 minutes   **Answers on page 485**

Directions: *Circle the greater fraction in the pairs by calculating the LCD and creating equivalent fractions with common denominators.*

	Fractions	LCD	Equivalent Fractions	Result
1	$\frac{3}{7}$ and $\frac{1}{2}$	14	$\frac{6}{14}$ and $\frac{7}{14}$	$\frac{1}{2}$ is larger
2	$\frac{1}{8}$ and $\frac{2}{24}$	_____	_____	_____
3	$\frac{1}{100}$ and $\frac{1}{200}$	_____	_____	_____

4 $\frac{4}{5}$ and $\frac{5}{6}$ _____ _____ _____

5 $\frac{1}{250}$ and $\frac{4}{50}$ _____ _____ _____

Adding and Subtracting Fractions

- To add or subtract fractions that have the *same denominator,* just add or subtract the numerators.
- Place the result over the denominator. Reduce the answer to simplest terms.
- If the denominators are *not* the same, identify the LCD, create an equivalent fraction, and then use the numerators to add and subtract while retaining the new common denominator.

Denominators the same

$$\frac{2}{4} - \frac{1}{4} = \frac{1}{4} \qquad\qquad \frac{1}{8} + \frac{3}{8} + \frac{5}{8} = \frac{9}{8} = 1\frac{1}{8}$$

EXAMPLES

Denominators not the same

Fractions (LCD)	Equivalent Fractions with LCD	Solution
$\frac{2}{3}$	$\frac{8}{12}$	$\frac{8}{12}$
$+\frac{1}{4}$ (12)	$+\frac{3}{12}$	$+\frac{3}{12}$
		$\frac{11}{12}$
$1\frac{1}{4}$	$1\frac{2}{8}$	$1\frac{2}{8}$
$-\frac{1}{8}$ (8)	$-\frac{1}{8}$	$-\frac{1}{8}$
		$1\frac{1}{8}$

EXAMPLES

Adding Fractions

RAPID PRACTICE 1-25

Estimated completion time: 10 minutes   Answers on page 485

Directions: *Find the LCD, and create equivalent fractions if necessary. Add the fractions, as indicated. Reduce the answer to its lowest terms.*

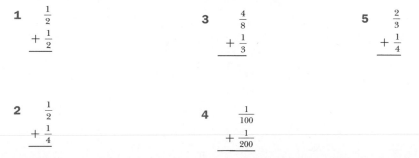

1 $\frac{1}{2}$
$+\frac{1}{2}$

3 $\frac{4}{8}$
$+\frac{1}{3}$

5 $\frac{2}{3}$
$+\frac{1}{4}$

2 $\frac{1}{2}$
$+\frac{1}{4}$

4 $\frac{1}{100}$
$+\frac{1}{200}$

Mixed fraction subtraction and borrowing

A mixed fraction consists of a whole number and a fraction (e.g., $1\frac{2}{3}$).

If the fractions have common denominators, subtract the numerator of the lower fraction from the numerator of the upper fraction and then subtract the whole numbers, if applicable (see Example A below).

If the lower fraction is larger than the upper one, *borrow* one whole number from the whole number accompanying the *upper* fraction and *add* it in *fraction form* to the upper fraction (see Example B below).

Subtract the numerators of the fractions. Reduce the answer (see Example B below).

Be sure the fractions have common denominators and that the upper fraction is larger than the lower fraction (see Examples A and B below).

EXAMPLES

A.
$$2\frac{3}{4}$$
$$-1\frac{1}{4}$$
$$\overline{1\frac{2}{4}} = 1\frac{1}{2}$$

The fractions have common denominators.

The upper fraction, $\frac{3}{4}$, is larger than the lower fraction, $\frac{1}{4}$.

Subtract the fraction numerators first. Then subtract the whole numbers.

B.
$$\begin{matrix} 1 \\ \cancel{2}\frac{1}{4} \end{matrix} \quad 1\frac{5}{4}$$
$$-1\frac{3}{4} \quad -1\frac{3}{4}$$
$$\overline{\frac{2}{4}} = \frac{1}{2}$$

The fractions have a common denominator: 4.

$\frac{3}{4}$ cannot be subtracted from $\frac{1}{4}$.

Borrow (subtract) 1 from 2, and convert it to a fraction: $\frac{4}{4}$.

Add it to $\frac{1}{4}$ to arrive at $\frac{5}{4}$. $\frac{5}{4}$ is equal to $1\frac{1}{4}$.

Subtract the fraction numerators: $\frac{5}{4} - \frac{3}{4}$.

Reduce the answer to its simplest terms.

RAPID PRACTICE 1-26

Subtracting Fractions

Estimated completion time: 15 minutes   **Answers on page 485**

Directions: *Identify the LCD. Create an equivalent fraction. Reduce the answer to its lowest terms.*

Fraction	LCD	Answer	Fraction	LCD	Answer
1 $1\frac{1}{2}$ $-\frac{1}{2}$			4 $10\frac{1}{4}$ $-4\frac{5}{8}$		
2 $\frac{3}{5}$ $-\frac{1}{2}$			5 $\frac{1}{8}$ $-\frac{1}{10}$		
3 $1\frac{1}{6}$ $-\frac{3}{4}$					

CHAPTER 1

Multiplying Fractions

- To multiply fractions, multiply the numerators straight across. Then multiply the denominators straight across.
- Reduce the answer to its simplest terms. The answer is the "product."

$$\frac{1}{2} \times \frac{1}{4} = \frac{1}{8} \qquad\qquad \frac{1}{4} \times \frac{1}{2} = \frac{1}{8}$$

$$\frac{1}{4} \times \frac{2}{3} = \frac{2}{12} = \frac{1}{6} \qquad\qquad \frac{2}{3} \times \frac{1}{4} = \frac{2}{12} = \frac{1}{6}$$

EXAMPLES

➤ The answer will be the same regardless of the order of the fractions.

Multiplying Fractions

RAPID PRACTICE 1-27

Estimated completion time 10-15 minutes   Answers on page 486

Directions: *Multiply the following fractions to find the product. Reduce the answer to its lowest terms.*

1 $\frac{1}{3} \times \frac{1}{9} =$ _____

2 $\frac{1}{2} \times \frac{3}{4} =$ _____

3 $\frac{2}{5} \times \frac{1}{6} =$ _____

4 $\frac{1}{2} \times \frac{1}{250} =$ _____

5 $\frac{9}{10} \times \frac{3}{5} =$ _____

▲ **Cultural Note**

In some countries, the word *of* is used instead of *time*s for multiplication of fractions. It might be simpler to understand multiplication of fractions by substituting the word *of* for *time*s. For example, $\frac{1}{2}$ of 4 is 2, $\frac{1}{2}$ of $\frac{1}{4}$ is $\frac{1}{8}$, and $\frac{1}{4}$ of $\frac{1}{2}$ is $\frac{1}{8}$.

Fraction Multiplication and Canceling Fractions

Simplification of fractions is very helpful in reducing math errors. Canceling fractions is a method of simplifying fraction *multiplication* by reducing numerators and denominators diagonally in *front* of the equals sign (the left side of the equation) by a common factor.

- *Diagonal reduction* can be done only *before* the equals sign, *not* after it.
- Cancellation must be on a one-for-one basis: one numerator for one denominator.

Canceling when the numerators and denominators are the same

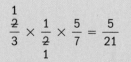

$$\frac{1}{\cancel{2}} \times \frac{1}{\cancel{2}} \times \frac{5}{7} = \frac{5}{21}$$

EXAMPLES

A numerator and denominator of 2 are the same. They cancel each other out.

Canceling when the numerators and denominators are not the same but have common factors

EXAMPLES

$$\frac{1}{\overset{}{\underset{5}{\cancel{15}}}} \times \frac{\overset{1}{\cancel{3}}}{6} = \frac{1}{30}$$

A common factor of 3 and 15 is 3.

Select only *one* numerator for *each* denominator.

In multiplication of fractions, cancel diagonally on the left side of the equation. Then reduce the answer (the product).

Examine the differences between reduction and cancellation of fractions in the examples that follow:

EXAMPLES

Reduction	Cancellation
$\dfrac{\overset{3}{\cancel{6}}}{\underset{4}{\cancel{8}}} = \dfrac{3}{4}$	$\dfrac{\overset{1}{\cancel{6}}}{\underset{2}{\cancel{8}}} \times \dfrac{\overset{1}{\cancel{4}}}{\underset{2}{\cancel{12}}} = \dfrac{1}{4}$

Cancellation is used to simplify math during *multiplication* of fraction forms. *Cancellation occurs diagonally* with two or more fractions on the *left* side of the equation.

Reduction is vertical. Reduction is used in addition, subtraction, and simplification of fractions in *multiplication*.

➤ Cancellation is used in all dimensional analysis equations to cancel units.

RAPID PRACTICE 1-28

Cancellation and Multiplication of Fractions

Estimated completion time: 10-15 minutes   **Answers on page 486**

Directions: *Multiply the following fractions. Use cancellations to simplify the process. Reduce the product.*

1 $\frac{1}{2} \times \frac{6}{8} =$ _____

2 $\frac{2}{3} \times \frac{3}{2} =$ _____

3 $\frac{3}{5} \times \frac{5}{6} =$ _____

4 $\frac{4}{5} \times \frac{10}{12} =$ _____

5 $\frac{100}{200} \times \frac{200}{250} =$ _____

Multiplication with Mixed Fractions

Before multiplying fractions that contain a mixed fraction, the mixed fraction must be changed to an *improper* fraction.

$$1\frac{1}{3} \times \frac{2}{5} = \frac{4}{3} \times \frac{2}{5} = \frac{8}{15}$$

$$2\frac{5}{8} \times 2\frac{1}{7} = \frac{\overset{3}{\cancel{21}}}{8} \times \frac{15}{\underset{1}{\cancel{7}}} = \frac{45}{8} = 5\frac{5}{8}$$

Use cancellation to simplify the improper form of the fraction.

Multiplication of Mixed Fractions

RAPID PRACTICE 1-29

Estimated completion time: 20 minutes **Answers on page 486**

Directions: *Multiply the fractions* after *changing mixed fractions in the equation to improper fractions. Cancel if appropriate. Reduce the answer to its lowest terms:*

1 $\frac{1}{4} \times 1\frac{1}{4} =$ _____

2 $3\frac{1}{6} \times 1\frac{1}{3} =$ _____

3 $2\frac{1}{2} \times \frac{1}{2} =$ _____

4 $\frac{1}{5} \times 4\frac{1}{3} =$ _____

5 $\frac{1}{6} \times 2\frac{1}{8} =$ _____

☐ Dividing Fractions

To divide fractions, invert the dividing fraction, as shown in red in the examples below.

Proceed as for multiplication of fractions, using cancellation to simplify before multiplying.

Reduce the answer.

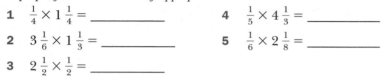

$$\frac{1}{3} \div \frac{1}{7} = \frac{1}{3} \times \frac{7}{1} = \frac{7}{3} = 2\frac{1}{3}$$

How many sevenths are there in $\frac{1}{3}$?

Answer: There are $2\frac{1}{3}$ sevenths in $\frac{1}{3}$.

$$\frac{1}{4} \div \frac{1}{8} = \frac{1}{4} \times \frac{8}{1} = \frac{2}{1} = 2$$

How many eighths are there in $\frac{1}{4}$?

Answer: There are 2 eighths in $\frac{1}{4}$.

➤ The most common error is to invert the dividend instead of the *dividing fraction,* the *divisor* (e.g., $\frac{1}{4} \div \frac{1}{8} = \frac{4}{1} \times \frac{1}{8} = \frac{1}{32}$).

Cancellation can be used to simplify during the multiplication process.

Division of Fractions

RAPID PRACTICE 1-30

Estimated completion time: 10 minutes **Answers on page 486**

Directions: *Divide the following fractions* after *converting any mixed fractions to improper fraction. Reduce the answer to its lowest terms.*

1 $\frac{1}{2} \div \frac{1}{6}$

2 $\frac{1}{3} \div \frac{1}{8}$

3 $\frac{2}{5} \div \frac{1}{4}$

4 $1\frac{1}{4} \div \frac{1}{4}$

5 $2\frac{1}{2} \div \frac{1}{2}$

Percentages

✴ **Mnemonic**

To remember the 100 divisor, it might be helpful to view a % as a "jumbled" 100.

Percent means parts per 100. Percentages reflect the numerator of a fraction that has a denominator of 100. A percentage is the ratio of a number to 100. For example, $50\% = \frac{50}{100}$ $(\frac{1}{2})$ or 50:100 or 0.5, and $2\% = \frac{2}{100}$ or 2:100 $(\frac{1}{50})$ or 0.02.

FAQ | *Why do nurses need to learn percentages?*

ANSWER | Percentages may appear in orders for dilution of nutritional formulas for babies and adults as well as solutions such as those used for wound irrigations.

Changing a Fraction to a Percentage

To change a *fraction* to a *percentage, multiply* the fraction by 100 and add a percent sign to the answer, as shown in the examples that follow.

It is helpful to remember one easy example, such as 50% and its fraction and decimal equivalents ($\frac{1}{2}$ and 0.5) when you work with other percentage conversions.

EXAMPLES

$$\frac{1}{2} \times 100 = \frac{100}{2} = 50\% \qquad \frac{2}{3} \times 100 = \frac{200}{3} = 66\frac{2}{3}\%$$

Changing a Percentage to a Fraction

To change a percentage to a fraction, *divide* the percentage by a denominator of 100. Reduce the fraction. Eliminate the percent sign.

EXAMPLES

$$50\% = 50 \div 100 \quad \frac{50}{100} = \frac{1}{2} \qquad\qquad 75\% = 75 \div 100 \quad \frac{75}{100} = \frac{3}{4}$$

➤ A percentage is just another form of a fraction. It has a denominator of 100.

RAPID PRACTICE **1-31**

Converting Fractions and Percentages

Estimated completion time: 15-20 minutes   **Answers on page 486**

Directions: *Change the fractions to percentages. Round the answer to the nearest tenth. Change the percentages to a fraction. Reduce the answer to its lowest terms.*

Fraction	Percentage	Percentage	Fraction
1 $\frac{1}{4}$	_____	6 10%	_____
2 $\frac{3}{4}$	_____	7 15%	_____
3 $\frac{1}{6}$	_____	8 50%	_____
4 $\frac{1}{3}$	_____	9 $12\frac{1}{2}\%$	_____
5 $\frac{5}{6}$	_____	10 25%	_____

☐ Changing a Decimal to a Percentage

- To change a decimal to a percentage, multiply the decimal by 100 by moving the decimal point two places to the right and adding a percent sign.
- Retain the leading zero and decimal point if there are numbers remaining after the decimal point (e.g., 0.003 = 0.3%). This lets the reader know a decimal will follow.
- Eliminate the decimal point and subsequent (trailing) zeros if there are no numbers higher than zero remaining after the decimal point (e.g., 0.590 = 59%). Examine the following examples. Note that the decimal point placement is the starting point when changing a decimal to a percentage.

0.3 = 30%	0.03 = 3%	0.003 = 0.3%	0.125 = 12½%	**EXAMPLES**

Remember: whenever percentages are involved, the number 100 is involved.

TEST TIP: If you know that 25% = 0.25, it will help apply the decimal movement and direction to any other decimal or percent.

Converting Decimals and Percentages by Moving Decimal Points

RAPID PRACTICE 1-32

Estimated completion time: 10 minutes **Answers on page 487**

Directions: *Calculate the decimal or percentage by moving the decimal points two places to the left or right as needed.*

Percentage	Decimal	Decimal	Percentage
1 1%	0.01	**6** 0.1	10%
2 35%	_____	**7** 0.05	_____
3 75%	_____	**8** 0.125	_____
4 5.5%	_____	**9** 0.0525	_____
5 200%	_____	**10** 0.5	_____

☐ Changing a Percentage to a Decimal

To change a percentage to a decimal, *divide* the percentage by 100 by moving the decimal point or implied decimal point two places to the left.

Insert zeros as placeholders and leading zeros where needed.

Remove the percent sign, and eliminate trailing zeros.

25% = 0.25	96% = 0.96	1.25% = 0.0125	5.9% = 0.059	**EXAMPLES**

Note that 0.059 has a leading zero in front of the decimal point and a zero placeholder after the decimal point.

RAPID PRACTICE `1-33`

Converting Fractions, Decimals, and Percentages

Estimated completion time: 15 minutes **Answers on page 487**

Directions: *Examine the example in the first row. Fill in the table with the requested numbers. Simplify by changing the fraction denominator to a multiple of 10.*

TEST TIP: Make equivalent fraction have a denominator with a power of ten.

	Fraction	Decimal	Percent
	$\frac{1}{4} = \frac{25}{100}$	0.25	25%
1	$\frac{3}{10}$	_____	_____
2	_____	1.5	_____
3	_____	_____	75%
4	$\frac{1}{5}$	_____	_____
5	_____	0.6	_____

Calculating the Percentage of a Whole Number

Change the percentage to a decimal (by dividing by 100) by moving the decimal point two places to the left. Then multiply the result by the number.

EXAMPLES

200% of 35   2.~~00~~ × 35 = 70 (no decimals in answer)

➤ Trailing zeros are eliminated after decimals.

EXAMPLES

%	% to Decimal		Number		Result
5% of 25	0.05	×	25	=	1.25
20% of 80	0.2	×	80	=	16.~~0~~
125% of 50	1.25	×	50	=	62.5~~0~~

Constants

A constant is a number or quantity that does *not* change. It can be used to simplify such calculations as intravenous flow rates.

EXAMPLES

To change minutes to hours, divide by the constant 60.

To change pounds to kilograms, divide by the constant 2.2.

Calculating percentages involves using the numerical constant 100.

CHAPTER 1

☐ Finding Unit Values and Totals

When performing calculations, comprehension is increased and the margin of error decreased if numbers can be *simplified*. If we buy more than one of something, we want to know the cost of each unit. Stores now assist us in comparing the value of similar products more quickly by posting the unit price on many items. If we pay $40 to fill our car's tank with gas, we usually are interested in the price *per* gallon: the unit price.

One of the common needs in medication math calculation is to find the value of *one part* of the whole of something. The math is very simple.

To find the unit value, divide the total by the number of units.

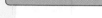

EXAMPLES

> What is the cost of *each tablet?*
>
> 10 tablets for 30 or 3 per unit (30 ÷ 10)
>
> How many dollars are earned *per hour?*
>
> $200 *every 8 hours* = $25.00 *each* hour ($200 ÷ 8)

TEST TIP: The unit and number in the question following "each" or "per" one unit become the *divisor*. The unit quantity in relation to another quantity expresses a *ratio* (e.g., $200 dollars per 8 hr; give 3 ounces each hr or per hr).

Drug concentrations are also expressed as ratios: for example, 100 milligrams per tablet, 10 grams per vial, or 15 milligrams per milliliter.

➤ Read slashes as per. Write "per." Do not handwrite slashes because they can be misread as a number one (1). Refer to the ISMP list of Error-Prone Abbreviations, Symbols, and Dose Designations on pp. 102-103.

☐ Finding the Total Value

Determine the unit value.

Multiply the unit value by the total quantity.

EXAMPLES

> Problem: 4 cups cost $1. How much will 16 cups cost?
> Solution: Each unit costs $0.25. 0.25 × 16 = $4.00 total cost.
>
> Problem: You earn $30 an hour. If you work 90 hr in two weeks, how much will you earn?
> Solution: $30 × 90 = $2700.

Finding Unit and Total Values

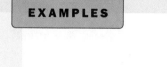

RAPID PRACTICE 1-34

Estimated completion time: 15 minutes   **Answers on page 487**

Directions: *Examine the worked-out first problem and calculate the unit values requested.*

1   You worked 20 hours this week. This week's gross paycheck is $600. How many *dollars per hour* did you earn?

Answer: $\frac{\$600}{20 \text{ hr}}$ = $30 per hour (the question asks for dollars *per hour*, which indicates that the divisor will be *20 hours*)

2 You are on a diet that is limited to 80 grams (g) of carbohydrate daily. This amounts to 320 calories of carbohydrates. How many *calories* are there in each gram of carbohydrate?

_____

3 Your car runs 300 miles on a tank of gas. The tank holds 12 gallons. How many miles per gallon does your car drive?

_____

4 Your computer has 6000 megabytes of memory storage. This equals 6 gigabytes. How many megabytes are there in 1 gigabyte?

_____

5 The patient has a water pitcher that contains 960 milliliters (mL) or 4 cups of water. How many mL of water per cup does the pitcher contain?

_____

Equations

Equations describe an *equal* relationship between two mathematical expressions. The expressions on both sides of the equals sign are equivalent when solved. The equation is said to be *balanced*.

EXAMPLES

$$1 + 1 = 2 \qquad 3 - 2 = 1 \qquad \frac{3}{1} = 3 \qquad 4 \times 5 = 20 \qquad \frac{1}{2} \times \frac{1}{4} = \frac{1}{8}$$

$$\frac{1}{2} \div \frac{1}{4} = \frac{1}{\cancel{2}} \times \frac{\cancel{4}}{1} = 2$$

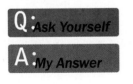
Q: Ask Yourself
A: My Answer

To further check comprehension, be sure that you can answer all of these medication math-related questions before taking the following chapter multiple choice review and final practice. Review Chapter 1 for explanations and answers if needed.

1 How will I remember the difference for *less than* and *greater than* when I read the symbols? Why should these symbols be written out? Why is being able to read and interpret symbols in printed medication-related materials important?

2 How might trailing zeros (e.g., 2.0) be misinterpreted and result in a medication math error? How does a zero before a decimal point help prevent a math error?

3 Does a whole number multiplied or divided by 1 change its value?

4 Can you write your age as a whole number in fraction form that will equal itself? Can you create a fraction using your age that will equal the number 1?

5 How will I distinguish the following terms: factors, multipliers, multiples, and products? Can I find some factors and multiples of my age? The product of my age times 2?

6 Which is the base and which is the exponent of 5^2? Does $5^2 = 2^5$? What is the difference in the results of these two calculations?

7 Which number will be smaller? The square or the square root of the number 9?

8 How do reduction and cancellation help prevent math errors?

9 Can I write the fraction ⅕ as a decimal and as a percent? Can I read 0.05 and write it as a fraction? What amount of error would result from misinterpreting 0.05 for 0.5 for a medication dose?

10 How can writing a slash for "per" result in a medication math error?

CHAPTER 1 MULTIPLE-CHOICE REVIEW

Estimated completion time: 15 minutes   Answers on page **487**

Directions: *Circle number of the correct answer.*

1 Interpret the symbol on a label of medicine in the following sentence: For children ≥ age 3 years, give 2 teaspoons of the medicine.

   1. less than
   2. greater than
   3. less than or equal to
   4. greater than or equal to

2 Identify the statement that describes a whole number that does not change in value.

   1. a whole number divided by itself
   2. a whole number divided or multiplied by 1
   3. a whole number multiplied by itself
   4. a whole number from which 1 is added or subtracted

3 Multiples of 50 are:

   1. 5, 10, 15
   2. 10, 20, 30, 40
   3. 5, 10, 20, 50
   4. 100, 150, 200

4 Factors of 30 include:

   1. 60, 90, 120
   2. 3, 5, 8
   3. 3 and 0
   4. 1, 10, 15

5 Common factors of 15 and 30 include:

   1. 1, 3, 5, 15
   2. 10, 15, 30
   3. 3, 6, 10
   4. 1, 2, 30

6 Five hundredths is written in decimal form as:

   1. 0.5
   2. 0.05
   3. 0.005
   4. 5.00

7 Identify 5% as a decimal.

   1. 0.0005
   2. 0.005
   3. 0.05
   4. 0.5

8 Identify 2.5% as a fraction.

TEST TIP: *Change the percentage to a decimal first.* Then "read" the decimal.

   1. $\frac{25}{100}$
   2. $\frac{25}{1000}$
   3. $\frac{2.5}{100}$
   4. $\frac{0.025}{1000}$

9 If you were going to give one tenth of 1 milliliter of a certain amount of medication, how much would you give?

   1. 0.001
   2. 0.01
   3. 0.1
   4. 1

10 A fraction equivalent to $\frac{6}{8}$ is:

  1. $\frac{2}{3}$ **3.** $\frac{8}{10}$

  2. $\frac{3}{4}$ **4.** $\frac{8}{16}$

11 Identify the improper fraction.

  1. $\frac{1}{8}$ **3.** $2\frac{1}{3}$

  2. $\frac{6}{5}$ **4.** $\frac{100}{200}$

12 The fraction $\frac{10}{15}$ can be reduced to which lowest terms?

  1. $\frac{2}{3}$ **3.** $\frac{24}{30}$

  2. $\frac{3}{5}$ **4.** $\frac{100}{150}$

13 Find the sum of $1\frac{1}{3}$ and $\frac{1}{5}$.

  1. $1\frac{1}{15}$ **3.** $1\frac{8}{15}$

  2. $2\frac{1}{8}$ **4.** $2\frac{2}{5}$

14 Identify the multiplier in the problem 5×100:

  1. 5   **3.** 100

  2. 20   **4.** 500

15 The product of $\frac{1}{2}$ and 3 is:

  1. $3\frac{1}{2}$ **3.** $1\frac{1}{2}$

  2. $\frac{1}{2}$ **4.** 10

16 $\frac{1}{8} \div \frac{1}{2} =$

  1. $\frac{1}{16}$ **3.** $\frac{2}{16}$

  2. $\frac{1}{4}$ **4.** $\frac{2}{8}$

17 Which is a definition of cancellation of fractions?

  1. Changing mixed whole numbers and fractions to improper fractions

  2. Reducing fraction answers to the lowest terms

  3. Diagonal reduction of fractions in fraction multiplication

  4. Converting fractions to percentages

18 The square of 4 is:

  1. 1   **3.** 4

  2. 2   **4.** 16

TEST TIP: Distinguish square root from square.

19 The sequence for writing out 10^3 would be:

  1. 10×3 **3.** $3 \times 3 \times 3$

  2. 3×10 **4.** $10 \times 10 \times 10$

20 If a package of medicine cups costing $20 contains 40 cups, what is the unit value per cup?

  1. $0.50   **3.** $20

  2. $2.00   **4.** $80

CHAPTER 1 FINAL PRACTICE

Estimated completion time: 20-30 minutes   **Answers on page 488**

Directions: *Supply the answer in the space provided.*

TEST TIP: Answer the easiest questions first. The easier questions will boost your confidence and, it is hoped, increase relaxation and jog memory for more complex processes.

1 The nurse looks up an unfamiliar medication in a current pharmacology reference. It says that, for children <2 years, the physician should be consulted for dosage. Write out the meaning of the symbol. _____

2 Formulas for medications based on body surface area require that a square root be obtained. Write out the symbol that illustrates the square root of 9. _____

3 Fill in the meaning of the symbol (noted in red) found in many laboratory reports indicating that a total cholesterol level ≥200 is abnormal. _____

4 Write the whole number 50 as a fraction *without* changing the value. _____

5 Write the whole number 85 with a decimal point in the *implied* decimal place for whole numbers. _____

6 Edit the trailing zeros in the following whole number to avoid misinterpretation: 500.00. _____

7 Use the whole number 500 to write a fraction that equals the number 1. _____

8 Write the *sum* of 8 and 7. _____

9 Write the *product* of 8 and 7. _____

10 Write all the *factors* of the number 12. _____

11 Write the *common factors* of the numbers 10 and 20. (Do not include 1.) _____

12 Write a multiple of both 4 and 3. _____

13 Write 3 *multiples* of the number 5. _____

14 Which number is the *multiplier* in $8 \times \frac{1}{2}$? _____

15 Write 10^4 out to illustrate the sequence you would use to calculate the result. _____

16 Write the *square* of 12. _____

17 Write the *square root* of 100. _____

18 Which number is the *base* in 10^8. _____

19 Which number is the exponent in 10^8? _____

20 Write *3 divided by 4* as a fraction. _____

21 Label the numerator and denominator in $\frac{7}{8}$ _____

22 Which is a decimal fraction: $\frac{1}{100}$ or $\frac{2}{3}$? _____

23 Which is larger: 0.089 or 0.42? _____

24 Divide 125.9 by 100 by moving the decimal place. _____

25 Multiply 8.03 by 1000 by moving the decimal place. _____

26 Round 0.893 to the *nearest* tenth. _____

27 Round 0.012 to the *nearest* hundredth. _____

28 Round 50.389 to the *nearest* whole number. _____

29 Write the decimal 0.5 as a fraction in simplest terms. _____

30 Change 0.025 to a fraction. _____

31 Change $\frac{5}{100}$ to a decimal. _____

32 Multiply 0.1×2.32. _____

33 Divide 20 by 5.9. _____

34 Which is greater: $\frac{1}{8}$ or $\frac{1}{10}$? _____

35 Which is smaller: $\frac{1}{12}$ or $\frac{1}{15}$? _____

36 Write the fraction $\frac{1}{100}$ as a percentage. _____

37 Change the improper fraction $\frac{25}{4}$ to a mixed fraction. _____

38 Change the mixed fraction $1\frac{1}{6}$ to an improper fraction. _____

39 Find the lowest common denominator (LCD) in the following group of fractions: $\frac{10}{12} + \frac{1}{3} + \frac{1}{4} =$ _____

40 Write two equivalent fractions for $\frac{2}{3}$. _____

41 The current pharmacology literature says, "Withhold the drug for a systolic blood pressure >180. Write out the meaning of the symbol. _____

42 Find the greatest common factor for the numerator and denominator: $\frac{12}{20}$. _____

43 Reduce the fraction to its lowest terms: $\frac{15}{60}$. _____

44 Add: $\frac{1}{2} + \frac{1}{6} + \frac{1}{8}$ _____

45 Subtract: $\frac{1}{5} - \frac{1}{8}$ _____

46 Find the product: $1\frac{1}{4} \times 2\frac{3}{7}$ _____

47 Divide: $\frac{2}{3} \div \frac{1}{6}$ _____

48 Change $\frac{1}{100}$ to a decimal and a percentage. _____

49 There are 50 syringes in a package that costs $75. What is the unit value of a syringe? _____

50 Write and solve an equation that reflects the product of 10 and 8. _____

Suggestions for Further Reading

www.aaamath.com/gwpg.html
www.math.com
www.mathworld.com
www.usp.org

℮volve   Additional information and practice can be found on the Student Companion on Evolve.

    Chapter 2 teaches the basic dimensional analysis style of solving equations. This method is used throughout the text to solve and verify medication dosage calculations.

Dimensional Analysis Calculations

OBJECTIVES

- Examine a problem to identify the desired units for the answer.
- Examine a problem to identify the quantity and units on hand that need to be converted.
- Select and orient appropriate conversion factors.
- Analyze the dimensional analysis (DA) setup to determine whether it will yield the desired answer units.
- Estimate answers.
- Solve basic arithmetic and simple metric medication equations using DA and units and number cancellation.
- Evaluate answers.

Essential Prior Knowledge

- Contents of Chapter 1

Essential Equipment

- No special equipment is needed for this chapter. Find a pencil and a quiet place.

Estimated Time To Complete Chapter

- 1 hour

Introduction

Derived from the sciences, Dimensional Analysis (DA) is a simple mathematical process. It begins with the identification of the desired answer. Equations are set up and solved in fraction multiplication format according to the *units* of measurement. The learner can see at a glance if the setup is incorrect. The math is as straightforward as simple multiplication of fractions. Other names for this method are *factor analysis, factor-label method,* and *unit-factor method,* reflecting the emphasis on factors, labels, and units of measurement, respectively.

It is important to have a solid foundation in basic arithmetic and equation solutions so that the focus in the clinical setting can be on the patient, the written order, the medication available, and safe administration in a timely manner. The nurse needs to know how to calculate independently and must have a thorough command of a method such as DA for verifying results and for more complex calculations.

Medication errors based on the wrong dosage can and do occur. Technical competence, including medication mathematics, is as important as communication skills when it comes to medications and treatments. The nurse cannot rely on colleagues and calculators for accuracy. The patient and employer cannot afford to wait a half-hour while the nurse refreshes math skills.

There are several advantages to learning the DA method of solving equations:

1 It is a simple, organized system for setting up problems.
2 Problems can be set up in one step.

3 It allows the nurse to easily identify incorrect setup before calculations are carried out; a key factor in accuracy and efficiency.

4 It can be used for all medication problems, which cannot be said for all medication calculation methods.

5 An incorrect answer resulting from incorrect setup can be immediately identified.

Once the method is mastered with simpler problems, it can easily be applied to more complex dosage problems. For students who have used DA in science courses, this chapter will require only a brief review.

ESSENTIAL *Vocabulary*

Conversion Factor	An expression of *equivalent* amounts for two entities, such as 12 inches = 1 foot, 3 feet = 1 yard, 5280 feet = 1 mile, 1000 mg = 1 g, 250 mg/1 tablet, $20/1 hr, and 5 mg/10 mL.
Dimensional Analysis	A practical scientific method used to solve mathematical equations with an emphasis on units of measurement to set up the equation. The method requires three elements: desired answer units, given quantity and units to convert, and conversion factors.
Dimension	Unit of mass (or weight), volume, length, time, and so on, such as milligram (mass or weight), teaspoon (volume), liter (volume), meter (length), and minute (time).
Equation	Expression of an equal relationship between mathematical expressions on both sides of an equals sign, such as $2x = 4$, $3 \times 2 = 6$, and $\frac{10}{2} = 5$. When an equation is solved, the values on both sides of the equals sign have equivalent value.
Factors	In DA, the data (numbers and units) that are entered in an equation in fraction form. In general, the word *factor* denotes anything that contributes to a result. The term has different meanings in different contexts.
Label	Descriptor of type, not necessarily a unit of dimension, such as 4 eggs, 4 dozen eggs, 1 tsp Benadryl, 100 mg tablets, 2 liters of 5% dextrose in water.
Numerical Orientation of a Fraction Form	Contents of the numerator (N) and denominator (D), such as $\frac{12 \text{ inches (N)}}{1 \text{ foot (D)}}$ and $\frac{1 \text{ foot (N)}}{12 \text{ inches (D)}}$.
Ratio	Relationship between two *different* entities, such as 10 mg per tablet, 1 g per capsule, and 2 boys for each 2 girls.
Unit*	Descriptor of *dimension,* such as length, weight, and volume, for example, 2 inches ointment, 3 m height, 1 qt water, 250 mg antibiotic, 2 tbs Milk of Magnesia, and 6 kg body weight. In the first example, 2 is a quantity and inches is the unit of dimension. In the last example, 6 is a quantity and kilograms is the unit of dimension.

*The word unit has different meanings in different contexts. Other definitions will be provided later in the text when relevant to the topic.

RAPID PRACTICE   **2-1**   *Essential Vocabulary Review*

Estimated completion time: 10 minutes   Answers on page 488

Directions: *Study the vocabulary to supply the requested information.*

1   What are the three required elements of a DA-style equation? _____

2   What is the difference between a quantity and a unit? _____

3 What is a conversion factor? _____

4 In the fraction $\frac{3}{4}$, what is the numerical orientation of 3? (Is it in the numerator or the denominator?) _____

5 In the fraction $\frac{1}{8}$, what is the numerical orientation of 8? (Is it in the numerator or the denominator?) _____

1 How will you remember the difference between a unit and a label when both appear?

_____

Q: *Ask Yourself*

A: *My Answer*

➤ Remember: The goal of a DA equation is to take a known quantity and multiply it by one or more conversion factors to solve an equation (find the desired answer).

Three Required Elements of a Dimensional Analysis Equation

- Desired answer units
- Given quantity and units to convert
- Conversion factor(s) (they will convert the given quantity and units to the desired answer units)

Setup of a Simple Equation Using Dimensional Analysis

After all of the required elements for the equation are *identified enter the factors in fraction form:*

1 Write the *desired answer* on the left as a reminder.
2 Enter a *factor in fraction form with a numerator* that contains the *desired answer units*. (This will be called the *starting factor* in the equation.)
3 Enter the given factor that needs to be converted, positioning it to be cancelled.
4 When all unwanted *units* are cancelled and only the desired answer units remain, estimate the size of the answer, then multiply.

Examine the setup and explanation in each of the following examples. Return to this page to review the steps if necessary. Notice that the setup is guided by the placement of the units, not the numbers.

These equations must always contain the desired answer units, the given quantity and units to be converted, and *one or more* conversion factors to get to the desired answer. The starting factor in a simple equation is often a conversion factor as shown.

EXAMPLES

How many inches are in 2 feet? Conversion factor: 12 inches = 1 foot.

Step 1	:	Step 2	×	Step 3	=	Answer
Desired Answer Units	:	Starting Factor	×	Given Quantity and Units	=	Estimate, Multiply, Evaluate
inches	:	$\dfrac{12 \text{ inches}}{1 \text{ } \cancel{\text{foot}}}$	×	$\dfrac{2 \text{ } \cancel{\text{feet}}}{1}$	=	24 inches

The final DA equation will be written like this:

$$\text{inches: } \frac{12 \text{ inches}}{1 \text{ } \cancel{\text{foot}}} \times \frac{2 \text{ } \cancel{\text{feet}}}{1} = 24 \text{ inches in 2 feet}$$

Continued

EXAMPLES

Analysis: For starting factor, we entered the entire conversion factor. It contains the desired answer units (inches). It is oriented so that inches are in the numerator *to match the desired answer position.*

The given factors that contain the unwanted units, *feet*, are placed in the next numerator and canceled diagonally.

A number 1 in the denominator of 2 feet helps maintain correct alignment for numerators and denominators to avoid errors during multiplication. It does not change the answer.

➤ *Before* multiplication, recheck the setup: After all unwanted units (feet) are canceled, only the desired answer units should remain. Estimate: the answer will be around 24 inches, larger than the given quantity of feet. These two checks help prevent setup and math errors.

Evaluation: All of the required elements appear in the equation. The answer gives only the desired answer units (inches). My estimate that the answer will be double the inches in 1 foot supports the answer. (Math check: $12 \times 2 = 24$). The answer is balanced.

➤ To reduce errors, please make it a habit to write the desired answer units on the left, analyze the setup *before* doing the math and evaluate the answer *after* doing the math. This will enhance your comprehension for longer or complex problems.

FAQ | *Why are the units canceled before multiplying?*

ANSWER | This ensures a correct setup of the equation. Incorrect math setups pose problems for some students. DA permits a fast check of setup to ensure that only the desired answer units will remain in the answer. Analyzing the setup before multiplying is a timesaver.

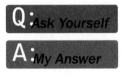

1 What are the three main elements of a DA equation that must be identified before the setup? *(Use brief phrases.)*

a. _____

b. _____

c. _____

➤ Remember: In DA, the placement of units, <u>not numbers</u>, guides the setup.

Examine the next example. The rest of the chapter will give brief practices for each phase of the setup.

EXAMPLES

How many ounces (oz) are in 5 pounds (lb)? Conversion factor: 16 oz = 1 lb

Step 1	:	Step 2	×	Step 3	=	Answer
Desired Answer Units	:	Starting Factor	×	Given Quantity and Units	=	Estimate, Multiply, Evaluate
ounces	:	$\dfrac{16 \text{ oz}}{1 \text{ lb}}$	×	$\dfrac{5 \text{ lb}}{1}$	=	80 oz

The final equation will be written like this:

$$\text{ounces: } \frac{16 \text{ oz}}{1 \text{ lb}} \times \frac{5 \text{ lb}}{1} = 80 \text{ oz in 5 lb}$$

Analysis: The required elements are highlighted and entered. The Starting Factor in this simple equation is the conversion factor with oz placed in the numerator to match the placement of oz in the desired answer units.

The given quantity and units to be converted appear in step 3. The number 1 is placed in the denominator under 5 lb to hold the 5 lb in the numerator position. This reduces chance of errors in multiplication.

A rough estimate is made that the answer in ounces will be much greater than 5. All the unwanted units (lb) can be canceled diagonally. The math is carried out last.

Evaluation: The answer gives only the desired answer units (ounces). My estimate that the answer will be several times larger than the given 5 lb is correct. (Math check: $16 \times 5 = 80$). The equation is balanced.

Take a second look at the setups. In order to cancel undesired units, each set of undesired units (pounds) must appear *twice* in the final equation. They must be in a denominator and a numerator in order to be canceled.

FAQ | *Does it matter in which order the data are entered in the equation?*

ANSWER | The order of data does not matter from a mathematical perspective. The data can be entered in any order as long as the desired answer units match up in numerical orientation and the undesired units cancel diagonally. However, the method shown is designed to reduce errors by providing a systematic approach, and many students find it easier to learn.

FAQ | *Which are the commonest types of errors?*

ANSWER | Math errors and incorrect setup of the units will result in the wrong answer.

➤ Even if the setup is correct and even if both sides of the equation are equal, the answer may be wrong. Wrong data entry and incorrect multiplication will yield a wrong answer. DA is one of the best methods of preventing a setup error, and the final math equality on both sides of the equation is very easy to prove. However, DA cannot prevent operator numerical entry errors and careless handwriting that can be misread.

How many yards are in 6 feet? Conversion factor: 3 feet = 1 yard.

EXAMPLES

Incorrect Setup

Step 1	:	Step 2	×	Step 3	=	Answer
Desired Answer Units	:	Starting Factor	×	Given Quantity and Units	=	Estimate, Multiply, Evaluate
yards	:	$\dfrac{3 \text{ feet}}{1 \text{ yard}}$	×	$\dfrac{6 \text{ feet}}{1}$	=	$\dfrac{18 \text{ feet squared}}{1 \text{ yard}}$

➤ Observe that this is an incorrect setup. The desired answer units (yards) should be in the numerator.

Analysis: A bad start. Because of the incorrect orientation of the starting factor, the unwanted feet cannot be canceled because they are both in a numerator. Incorrect orientation of units in the numerator or denominator leads to errors.

Evaluation: The answer doesn't make sense. If we had examined the units after cancelation, but before doing the math, we wouldn't have done the math. This is how you know to go back and check the setup.

Conversion Factor Review

Conversion factors:

1   Must contain a *quantity* and a *unit of measurement* and/or a *label* (e.g., 12 inches = 1 foot, 250 mg per 1 tablet, 10 employees per 1 supervisor).
2   Are equivalent.
3   Are inserted in an equation in fraction form.
4   Do not change the value of the other units in the equation because they equal the number 1. (Multiplying numbers by 1 does not alter the value.)
5   Must be positioned (oriented) to match the desired answer units and permit cancellation of the unwanted units.

Note that there are *three* methods of writing a conversion formula: an equation, fraction form orientation 1, and fraction form orientation 2. The three ways are equivalent. For DA equations, the fraction form of conversion formulas must be used in the correct orientation for the problem.

EXAMPLES

Conversion Factors	Fraction Form 1	Fraction Form 2
3 feet = 1 yard	$\dfrac{3 \text{ feet}}{1 \text{ yard}}$	$\dfrac{1 \text{ yard}}{3 \text{ feet}}$
1000 mg = 1 g	$\dfrac{1000 \text{ mg}}{1 \text{ g}}$	$\dfrac{1 \text{ g}}{1000 \text{ mg}}$
$5 per box	$\dfrac{\$5}{1 \text{ box}}$	$\dfrac{1 \text{ box}}{\$5}$
20 mg per capsule	$\dfrac{20 \text{ mg}}{1 \text{ capsule}}$	$\dfrac{1 \text{ capsule}}{20 \text{ mg}}$

➤ Write out and read "per" for slashes. Slashes are widely used in printed drug labels and references. However, they may be mistaken for the number one ("1").

RAPID PRACTICE   2-2

Selecting the Correct Starting Factor Orientation

Estimated completion time: 5 minutes   Answers on page 489

Directions: *Read the problem for the required elements. Place a circle around the correctly oriented starting factor (ensuring that numerator and denominator placement matches the desired answer units in the numerator and permits cancellation of the undesired units). Evaluate your setup. Review the previous examples if necessary.* **Do not** *carry out the math to solve the equation.*

1   How many eggs are in 10 dozen? Conversion factor: 12 eggs = 1 dozen.

Step 1: Desired Answer Units	:	Step 2: Starting Factor	Step 3: Given Quantity and Units
? eggs	:	$\dfrac{1 \text{ dozen}}{12 \text{ eggs}}$ *or* $\dfrac{12 \text{ eggs}}{1 \text{ dozen}}$	10 dozen

➤ Circle the correct conversion factor placement.

2 How many kilometers are in 5 miles? Conversion factor: 1 km = 0.6 mile.

Step 1: Desired Answer Units	:	Step 2: Starting Factor	Step 3: Given Quantity and Units
? km	:	$\dfrac{0.6 \text{ mile}}{1 \text{ km}}$ or $\dfrac{1 \text{ km}}{0.6 \text{ mile}}$	5 miles

➤ Circle the correct conversion factor placement.

3 How many quarts are in 10 gal? Conversion factor: 4 qt = 1 gal.

Step 1: Desired Answer Units	:	Step 2: Starting Factor	Step 3: Given Quantity and Units
? quarts	:	$\dfrac{4 \text{ qt}}{1 \text{ gal}}$ or $\dfrac{1 \text{ gal}}{4 \text{ qt}}$	10 gal

➤ Circle the correct conversion formula placement.

4 How many seconds are in 30 minutes? Conversion factor: 60 seconds = 1 minute.

Step 1: Desired Answer Units	:	Step 2: Starting Factor	Step 3: Given Quantity and Units
? seconds	:	$\dfrac{1 \text{ min}}{60 \text{ s}}$ or $\dfrac{60 \text{ s}}{1 \text{ min}}$	30 minutes

➤ Circle the correct conversion formula placement.

5 How many ounces are in 6 pounds? Conversion factor: 16 oz = 1 lb.

Step 1: Desired Answer Units	:	Step 2: Starting Factor	Step 3: Given Quantity and Units
? oz	:	$\dfrac{1 \text{ lb}}{16 \text{ ounces}}$ or $\dfrac{16 \text{ ounces}}{1 \text{ lb}}$	6 pounds

➤ Circle the correct conversion formula placement.

➤ Note that the correct abbreviation for seconds is the letter "s."

Identifying Desired Answer Units, Starting Factors, and Original Factors to Convert

RAPID PRACTICE 2-3

Estimated completion time: 10 minutes   Answers on page **489**

Directions: *Read the question, identify the required elements, and fill in the quantities and units in the space provided, as illustrated in problem 1. Select the correct conversion factor from the list provided as illustrated in problem.* **Do not** *solve the equation. Conversion factors: 3 feet = 1 yard, 4 cups = 1 quart, 1 yard = approximately 1 meter, 12 dozen = 1 gross, 1 eurodollar = approximately $1.40 U.S. dollars.*

1 How many feet are in 8 yards?

Step 1: Desired Answer Units	:	Step 2: Starting Factor (With Desired Answer in Numerator	×	Step 3: Given Quantity and Units
? feet	:	$\dfrac{3 \text{ feet}}{1 \text{ yard}}$	×	$\dfrac{8 \text{ yards}}{1}$

Since the step 2 denominator unit (yard) is repeated in the numerator in step 3 (yards), it can be canceled.

2 How many quarts are in 8 cups?

Step 1: Desired Answer Units	:	Step 2: Starting Factor	×	Step 3: Given Quantity and Units

Q: Ask Yourself

A: My Answer

1 How many times must an undesired unit be entered in order to cancel out?

_____

3 Approximately how many yards are in 50 meters?

Step 1: Desired Answer Units	:	Step 2: Starting Factor	×	Step 3: Given Quantity and Units

4 How many dozen are in 2 gross?

Step 1: Desired Answer Units	:	Step 2: Starting Factor	×	Step 3: Given Quantity and Units

5 If you have $500, how many eurodollars can you buy?

Step 1: Desired Answer Units	:	Step 2: Starting Factor	×	Step 3: Given Quantity and Units

Two Kinds of Conversions That Must Be Identified

Two kinds of conversions are commonly used for calculations:

1 Conversion factors within the same dimension, such as 12 eggs = 1 dozen (quantity), 4 qt = 1 gal (volume), or 1000 milligrams (mg) = 1 gram (g) (weight or mass)

2 Conversions factors within different dimensions (ratios), such as 10 pills per day (10 pills per 1 day), 250 mg per tablet (250 mg in 1 tablet), 1 g per capsule

(1 g in 1 capsule), 10 workers per 1 supervisor, $12 per hr, or 10 tickets per 2 free passes.

➤ These formulas are entered as conversion units in the same way, with the desired answer unit placed in the numerator of the starting factor.

Identifying Correct Equation Setup

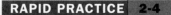

RAPID PRACTICE   2-4

Estimated completion time: 5-10 minutes   Answers on page 489

Directions: *Identify the required elements in the problem statement. Focus on the setup. Correct the incorrect setup. Do not solve the equation. You will see that you do not need to be familiar with the terminology to analyze these setups.*

1   If there are approximately 2.5 centimeters (cm) in 1 inch, how many centimeters are there in 50 inches?

Step 1: Desired Answer Units	:	Step 2: Starting Factor	×	Step 3: Given Quantity and Units
? cm	:	$\dfrac{2.5\ \text{cm}}{1\ \text{inch}}$	×	$\dfrac{50\ \text{inches}}{1}$

   a. Is the DA setup correct? _____
   b. If it is incorrect, correct it.

   c. Estimate: Will the numerical answer be larger or smaller than the units to be converted? _____

2   The average baby weighs 7 pounds (lb) at birth. There are 2.2 lb in 1 kg. How many kilograms does the average baby weigh? _____

Step 1: Desired Answer Units	:	Step 2: Starting Factor	×	Step 3: Given Quantity and Units
? kg	:	$\dfrac{2.2\ \text{lb}}{1\ \text{kg}}$	×	$\dfrac{7\ \text{lb}}{1}$

   a. Is the DA setup correct? _____
   b. If it is incorrect, correct it.

   c. Estimate: Will the numerical answer be larger or smaller than the units to be converted? _____

3   A bottle contains 2500 milliliters (mL) of fluid. There are 1000 mL in 1 liter (L). How many liters are in the bottle? _____

Step 1: Desired Answer Units	:	Step 2: Starting Factor	×	Step 3: Given Quantity and Units
? mL	:	$\dfrac{1000\ \text{mL}}{1\ \text{L}}$	×	$\dfrac{2500\ \text{mL}}{1}$

   a. Is the DA setup correct? _____
   b. If it is incorrect, correct it.

   c. Will the numerical answer be larger or smaller than the units to be converted? _____

4 There are 1000 milligrams (mg) in 1 gram (g). If you have 5.5 grams, how many milligrams do you have? _____

Step 1: Desired Answer Units	:	Step 2: Starting Factor(s)	×	Step 3: Given Quantity and Units
? mg	:	$\dfrac{1000 \text{ mg}}{1 \text{ g}}$	×	$\dfrac{5.5 \text{ g}}{1}$

a. Is the DA setup correct? _____
b. If it is incorrect, correct it.

c. Will the numerical answer be larger or smaller than the units to be converted? _____

5 The patient takes 10 pills per day. How many pills will the patient need for 7 days? _____

Step 1: Desired Answer Units	:	Step 2: Starting Factor(s)	×	Step 3: Given Quantity and Units
? pills	:	$\dfrac{10 \text{ pills}}{1 \text{ day}}$	×	$\dfrac{7 \text{ days}}{1}$

a. Is the DA setup correct? _____
b. If it is incorrect, correct it.

c. Will the answer be larger or smaller than the units to be converted? _____

FAQ | *Why practice the DA method with problems that can easily be calculated mentally?*

ANSWER | The goal is to practice the method to perfection with simple problems and to plant it in long-term memory so that the setup can be recalled when the solutions to more complex calculations are needed. Some problems call for more entries. If you can set up simple problems, you will be able to apply the technique to more complex problems.

CLINICAL RELEVANCE

Many medications ordered do not require calculations for administration, but some do. The nurse needs to know a calculation method very well. A calculation method is frequently needed with liquid oral doses or to determine whether an intravenous flow rate is delivering the correct amount of drug at the correct rate per hour.

➤ Even when a calculator is used, the nurse must understand the math process well enough to enter the data correctly. Frail and at-risk populations may require fractional doses, which involve calculations of a small dose from a large amount on hand. Almost all intravenous solutions require some calculations.

Solving Basic DA Equations

Estimated completion time: 20 minutes Answers on page **490**

Directions: *Set up equations 2-5 as shown in the first problem.*

Cancel undesired units. Check that only the desired answer units will remain. Estimate the answer, then solve the equation. Check answer with estimate.

Conversion factors: 32 ounces (oz) = 1 quart (qt); 1000 megabytes (Mb) = 1 gigabyte (GB); 4 liters (L) = approximately 1 gallon (gal), 5 CNAs per 2 LPNs, $20 = 1 hr pay.

1 You have 3 quarts of milk. How many ounces do you have?

Step 1:	Step 2:		Step 3:		Step 4:
Desired Answer Units:	Starting Factor	×	Given Quantity and Units	=	Answer

DA equation:

$$? \text{ oz}: \quad \frac{32 \text{ oz}}{1 \text{ q\!t}} \quad \times \quad \frac{3 \text{ q\!t}}{1} \quad = \quad 96 \text{ oz}$$

2 Your salary is $20 per hr. You earned $500. How many hours did you work?

Step 1:	Step 2:		Step 3:		Step 4:
Desired Answer Units:	Starting Factor	×	Given Quantity and Units	=	Answer

DA equation:

3 Your computer backup storage device holds 4 gigabytes (GB). How many megabytes (MB) is this?

Step 1:	Step 2:		Step 3:		Step 4:
Desired Answer Units:	Starting Factor	×	Given Quantity and Units	=	Answer

DA equation:

4 You buy 40 liters (L) of gas for your car in Mexico. About how many gallons (gal) did you buy?

Step 1:	Step 2:		Step 3:		Step 4:
Desired Answer Units:	Starting Factor	×	Given Quantity and Units	=	Answer

DA equation:

5 The hospital has 40 CNA employees. How many LPN slots are there?

Step 1:	Step 2:		Step 3:		Step 4:
Desired Answer Units:	Starting Factor	×	Given Quantity and Units	=	Answer

DA equation:

Problems That Call for More Than One Conversion Factor

The process is the same as for one conversion factor. Extra space is made after the starting factor to permit additional conversion factors.

EXAMPLES

How many seconds are in 5 hours?
Conversion factors: 60 seconds = 1 minute
60 minutes = 1 hour

Step 1	:	Step 2	×	Step 3	=	Answer
Desired Answer Units	:	Starting Factor	×	Given Quantity and Units and Conversion Factor(s)	=	Estimate, Multiply, Evaluate
seconds	:	$\dfrac{60 \text{ s}}{1 \text{ min}}$	×	$\dfrac{60 \text{ min}}{1 \text{ hr}} \times \dfrac{5 \text{ hr}}{1}$	=	18,000 seconds

Plan to cancel minutes, then hours

The final equation will be written like this:

$$\text{seconds} \quad : \quad \frac{60 \text{ s}}{1 \text{ min}} \times \frac{60 \text{ min}}{1 \text{ hr}} \times \frac{5 \text{ hr}}{1} = 18,000 \text{ seconds in 5 hr}$$

Analysis: There are two conversion factors to get from seconds to hours: one in the starting factor and the next one in step 3.

The selected starting factor is a conversion factor with seconds in the numerator accompanied by 1 min in the denominator. Positioning 60 *minutes* in the numerator of the next conversion factor permitted sequential cancelation of minutes. The additional conversion factor is placed in Step 3. There are *two* reasons 5 hr have to be in the next numerator: hr need to canceled diagonally and 5 hr needs to be treated like a whole number as <u>a numerator</u> with an implied denominator of 1.

Evaluation: Only seconds remain in the answer. An estimate of a very large number is supported by the answer (Math check: 60 × 60 × 5 = 18,000). The equation is balanced. If I used a calculator to multiply, I would enter the numbers twice to confirm the answer.

Note: You would probably use a calculator for large numbers. Be sure to estimate the size of the answer and enter the data twice.

EXAMPLES

How many seconds are in 30 days?
Conversion factors: 60 seconds (sec) = 1 minute (min)
60 min = 1 hour (hr)
24 hr = 1 day

Step 1	:	Step 2	×	Step 3	=	Answer
Desired Answer Units	:	Starting Factor	×	Given Quantity and Units and Conversion Factor(s)	=	Estimate, Multiply, Evaluate
seconds	:	$\dfrac{60 \text{ s}}{1 \text{ min}}$	×	$\dfrac{60 \text{ min}}{1 \text{ hr}} \times \dfrac{24 \text{ hr}}{1 \text{ day}} \times \dfrac{30 \text{ days}}{1}$	=	86,430 seconds

The final equation will be written like this:

$$\text{seconds:} \quad \frac{60 \text{ s}}{1 \text{ min}} \times \frac{60 \text{ min}}{1 \text{ hr}} \times \frac{24 \text{ hr}}{1 \text{ day}} \times \frac{30 \text{ days}}{1} = 86,430 \text{ seconds in 30 days}$$

Analysis: It takes four entries to convert days to seconds. After the Starting Factor was entered (a conversion factor), the remaining factors were entered in a diagonal sequence from left to right, permitting easy cancellation of min to min, hr to hr, and day to day. Sometimes factors cannot be entered in a "neat" sequence in complex equations, but as long as they are properly oriented in the numerator/denomination position, they can be canceled.

If I used a calculator to multiply, I would enter the numbers twice to confirm the answer.

Evaluation: Only seconds remain in the answer. The estimate of a very large number is supported by the answer (Math check: $60 \times 60 \times 24 \times 30 = 86{,}430$). The equation is balanced.

The following exercise will make the process of adding one more conversion factor easily understood.

DA Equations Using Two Conversion Factors

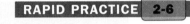

Estimated completion time: 25 minutes   Answers on page 490

Directions: *Circle A or B to indicate the correct setup of the equations for the following problems; then solve the equation using the correct setup as shown in Example 1. Label the answer. Remember to cancel all unwanted units before doing math.*

➤ Test principle: If *any part* of a solution is incorrect, the entire solution is incorrect.

1 How many cups in 5 qt? Conversion factors: 2 cups = 1 pt, and 2 pt = 1 qt.

Desired Answer Units	:		×		=	
A. ? cups	:	$\dfrac{2 \text{ cups}}{1 \text{pt}} \times \dfrac{2 \text{ pt}}{1 \text{ qt}}$	×	$\dfrac{5 \text{ quarts}}{1}$	=	20 cups
B. ? cups	:	$\dfrac{1 \text{ pt}}{2 \text{ cups}} \times \dfrac{2 \text{ pt}}{1 \text{ qt}}$	×	$\dfrac{5 \text{ quarts}}{1}$	=	

DA equation:

$$\text{cups}: \frac{2 \text{ cups}}{1 \text{ pint}} \times \frac{2 \cancel{\text{ pints}}}{1 \cancel{\text{ quart}}} \times 5 \cancel{\text{ quarts}} = 20 \text{ cups}$$

Evaluate your choice. Is the desired answer unit the only remaining unit? Did the setup permit sequential cancellation?

2 How many inches are in 20 yards? Conversion factors: 12 inches = 1 foot, and 3 feet = 1 yard.

Desired Answer Units	:		×		=	
A. ? inches	:	$\dfrac{1 \text{ yard}}{3 \text{ feet}} \times \dfrac{1 \text{ foot}}{12 \text{ inches}}$	×	$\dfrac{20 \text{ yards}}{1}$	=	Answer
B. ? inches	:	$\dfrac{12 \text{ inches}}{1 \text{ foot}} \times \dfrac{3 \text{ feet}}{1 \text{ yard}}$	×	$\dfrac{20 \text{ yards}}{1}$	=	Answer

DA equation:

Evaluate your choice. Is the desired answer unit the only remaining unit?

3 Approximately how many weeks are in 4 years? Conversion factors: 12 months = 1 year, and 4 weeks = 1 month.

Desired Answer Units :		×	=
A. ? weeks :	$\dfrac{4\ weeks}{1\ month} \times \dfrac{1\ year}{12\ months} \times$	$\dfrac{4\ years}{1}$	= Answer
B. ? weeks :	$\dfrac{4\ weeks}{1\ month} \times \dfrac{12\ months}{1\ year} \times$	$\dfrac{4\ years}{1}$	= Answer

DA equation:

Evaluate your choice. Is the desired answer unit the only remaining unit?

4 How many millimeters (mm) are in 10 inches? Conversion factors: 2.5 centimeters (cm) = 1 inch, and 10 mm = 1 cm.

Desired Answer Units :		×	=
A. ? millimeters :	$\dfrac{1\ cm}{10\ mm} \times \dfrac{1\ inch}{2.5\ cm} \times$	$\dfrac{10\ inches}{1}$	= Answer
B. ? millimeters :	$\dfrac{10\ mm}{1\ cm} \times \dfrac{2.5\ cm}{1\ inch} \times$	$\dfrac{10\ inches}{1}$	= Answer

DA equation:

Evaluate your choice. Is the desired answer unit the only remaining unit?

5 How many grams (g) are in 4000 micrograms (mcg)? Conversion factors: 1000 mg = 1 g, and 1000 mcg = 1 mg.

Desired Answer Units :		×	=
A. ? grams :	$\dfrac{1\ g}{1000\ mg} \times \dfrac{1000\ mcg}{1\ mg} \times$	$\dfrac{4000\ mcg}{1}$	= Answer
B. ? grams :	$\dfrac{1\ g}{1000\ mg} \times \dfrac{1\ mg}{1000\ mcg} \times$	$\dfrac{4000\ mcg}{1}$	= Answer

DA equation:

Evaluate your choice. Is the desired answer unit the only remaining unit or most common?

FAQ | *Which are the commonest errors when using two or more conversion factors?*

ANSWER | Assuming that the desired answer unit is entered correctly, the second conversion formula may be positioned incorrectly. The second conversion formula numerator must cancel the denominator of a previous conversion formula. Also, the numbers may be transposed if the writer is not focused. Finally, each *undesired unit* must be entered *two* times, once in a de-nominator and once in a numerator.

Solving DA Equations Using One or Two Conversion Factors

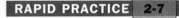

Estimated completion time: 20 minutes   **Answers on page 490**

Directions: *Identify the required elements. Solve the equations using the 4-column systematic approach presented in this chapter. Allow space for an extra conversion factor if needed. Evaluate your equation. Even if you can solve the equations mentally, the benefit of this practice is to reinforce a solid method of verification for more complex problems using DA.*

1   How many pounds (lb) are in 80 kilograms (kg)? Conversion factor:
    2.2 lb = 1 kg. _____

    DA equation:

2   How many pints are in 5 gallons (gal)? Conversion factors: 2 pt = 1 qt, and
    4 qt = 1 gal. _____

    DA equation:

3   How many inches are in 25 millimeters (mm)? Conversion factors:
    10 mm = 1 cm, and 2.5 cm = 1 inch. _____

    DA equation:

4   How many hours are in 7200 seconds? Conversion factors: 60 seconds =
    1 minute, and 60 minutes = 1 hour. _____

    DA equation:

5   A patient has to take 1 capsule 3 times a day. How many capsules will the
    patient need for a 2-week prescription. Conversion factors: 3 capsules = 1 day,
    and 7 days = 1 week. _____

    DA equation:

CHAPTER 2 MULTIPLE-CHOICE REVIEW

Estimated completion time: 20 minutes   **Answers on page 490**

Directions: *Circle the number of the correct choice.*

1 What is the *first* step in analyzing a problem to solve a DA equation? _____
   1. Identify the given units and quantities.
   2. Estimate the answer.
   3. Identify the desired answer units.
   4. Set up the equation.

2 Which of the following is a key process *that guides* the setup of DA equations? _____

  1. Placement of units   **3.** Multiplication of units
  2. Placement of numbers   **4.** Multiplication of numbers

3 Which of the following statements about DA setup is *incorrect?* _____

TEST TIP: Identify each statement as True or False. Select the false statement.

The given quantities tip: Identify each statement as True or False. Select the false statement.
1. The given quantities must always be accompanied by the unit of measure.
2. The units of measure are canceled after the numbers are multiplied.
3. More than one conversion factor may be needed to solve the equation.
4. Units of measure are addressed before quantities in solving DA equations.

4 Which conversion factor setup is correct for the following question?

Question: How many yards are in 72 inches?
Conversion factors: 12 inches = 1 foot, and 3 feet = 1 yard.
Circle the number of the correct choice.

TEST TIP: If the first or any entry is incorrect, the rest of that selection is incorrect.

1. ? yards $\dfrac{72 \text{ inches}}{1 \text{ foot}} \times \dfrac{3 \text{ feet}}{1 \text{ yard}} \times \dfrac{72 \text{ inches}}{1}$

2. ? yards $\dfrac{1 \text{ yard}}{3 \text{ feet}} \times \dfrac{1 \text{ foot}}{12 \text{ inches}} \times \dfrac{72 \text{ inches}}{1}$

3. ? yards $\dfrac{12 \text{ inches}}{1 \text{ foot}} \times \dfrac{3 \text{ feet}}{1 \text{ yard}} \times \dfrac{72 \text{ inches}}{1}$

4. ? yards $\dfrac{1 \text{ yard}}{72 \text{ inches}} \times \dfrac{3 \text{ feet}}{12 \text{ inches}} \times \dfrac{72 \text{ inches}}{1}$

5 Which DA equation is correct for solving the following question?

Question: How many kilobytes (KB) are in 2 gigabytes (GB)?
Conversion factors: 1000 kilobytes (KB) = 1 megabyte (MB), and 1000 MB = 1 GB.
Circle the number of the correct conversion formula.

1. ? kilobytes $\dfrac{1000 \text{ GB}}{1 \text{ MB}}$ $\dfrac{1 \text{ GB}}{1000 \text{ MB}} \times \dfrac{2 \text{ GB}}{1}$

2. ? kilobytes $\dfrac{1 \text{ MB}}{1000 \text{ KB}}$ $\dfrac{1 \text{ GB}}{1000 \text{ MB}} \times \dfrac{2 \text{ GB}}{1}$

3. ? kilobytes $\dfrac{1000 \text{ KB}}{1 \text{ MB}}$ $\dfrac{1000 \text{ MB}}{1 \text{ GB}} \times \dfrac{2 \text{ GB}}{1}$

4. ? kilobytes $\dfrac{1000 \text{ MB}}{1 \text{ GB}}$ $\dfrac{25000 \text{ KB}}{1 \text{ MB}} \times \dfrac{2 \text{ GB}}{1}$

6 Solving an equation using DA requires which of the following processes?
_____

  1. Cancellation of units followed by multiplication
  2. Multiplication of units followed by cancellation
  3. Cancellation of desired answer units
  4. Division of desired and undesired units

7 The analysis of the DA equation setup to ensure that all unwanted units are canceled should take place at which step of the process? _____

    1. After entering the first conversion fraction
    2. When entering the original factors
    3. After all the data are entered but before multiplication of quantities
    4. After all the data are entered and after the multiplication of quantities

8 Two types of conversion factors are as follows: _____

    1. Data and factors to be entered
    2. Units and fractions
    3. Those that contain the same dimensions and those that contain different dimensions
    4. Fraction equivalents and decimal equivalents

9 The *final* evaluation of a DA equation should include which of the following critical steps? _____

    1. Ensuring the desired answer units are the only remaining units
    2. Checking the conversion factor(s) for correct placement in the numerator and denominator
    3. Estimating the answer
    4. Identifying the known quantity

10 Which of the following choices reflects the *correct* setup for a DA equation? Circle the number of the correct choice.

    Question: How many micrograms are in 0.5 grams (g)? Conversion formulas: 1000 mcg = 1 mg, and 1000 mg = 1 g.

    1. ? grams   : $\dfrac{1000 \text{ mcg}}{1 \text{ mg}} \times \dfrac{0.5 \text{ g}}{1000 \text{ mg}} \times \dfrac{1000 \text{ mcg}}{1}$

    2. ? micrograms : $\dfrac{1 \text{ mg}}{1000 \text{ mcg}} \times \dfrac{1000 \text{ mg}}{0.5 \text{ g}} \times \dfrac{0.5 \text{ g}}{1}$

    3. ? milligrams : $\dfrac{0.5 \text{ g}}{1000 \text{ mg}} \times \dfrac{1 \text{ mg}}{1000 \text{ mcg}} \times \dfrac{0.5 \text{ g}}{1}$

    4. ? micrograms : $\dfrac{1000 \text{ mcg}}{1 \text{ mg}} \times \dfrac{1000 \text{ mg}}{1 \text{ g}} \times \dfrac{0.5 \text{ g}}{1}$

CHAPTER 2 FINAL PRACTICE

Estimated completion time: 1-2 hours   Answers on page **491**

Directions: *Set up and solve the following problems using the four-step DA method even if you can obtain the answer with mental arithmetic. Label all data. Evaluate your equations.*

1 Write the three required *elements* of dimensional style equations.

    a. _____
    b. _____
    c. _____

2 How many eggs are in 10 dozen? Conversion factor: 12 eggs = 1 dozen.

    _____

    DA equation:

3 How many meters are in 30 yards? Conversion factor: 1 m = 1.09 yards. Round to the nearest tenth. _____

DA equation:

4 How many pounds are in 60 kg? Conversion factor: 2.2 lb = 1 kg. _____

DA equation:

5 How many inches are in 50 yards? Conversion factors: 12 inches = 1 foot, and 3 feet = 1 yard. _____

DA equation:

6 How many millimeters are in 1 inch? Conversion factors: 10 mm = 1 cm, and 2.5 cm = 1 inch. _____

DA equation:

7 How many kilometers are in 50 miles to the nearest tenth? Conversion factor: 1 km = 0.6 mile. _____

DA equation:

8 How many DVDs can you buy for a gift certificate worth $100? How much money will you have left over? Conversion factor: $8 per DVD. _____

DA equation:

9 How many prescriptions (Rx) can be bought with an insurance policy that has a $2000 limit? Conversion factor: $50 average cost per prescription. _____

DA equation:

10 How many nurses per shift will be needed for a new 480-bed hospital? Conversion factor: 1 nurse per 12 beds per shift. Round answer to nearest whole number. _____

DA equation:

➤ Use two conversion factors in a DA-style equation for the next 10 questions.

11 How many liters are in 8 gal? Conversion factors: 1 L = 1 qt, and 4 qt = 1 gal. _____

DA equation:

12 How many inches are in 10 yards? Conversion factors: 12 inches = 1 foot, and 3 feet = 1 yard. _____

DA equation:

13 How many tablespoons are in a cup of fluid? Conversion factors: 2 tbs = 1 oz, and 8 oz = 1 cup. _____

DA equation:

14 How many cups are in 2 qt? Conversion factors: 2 cups = 1 pt, and 2 pt = 1 qt. _____

DA equation:

15 How many seconds are in 2 hours? Conversion factors: 60 seconds = 1 minute, and 60 minutes = 1 hour. _____

DA equation:

16 How many milliliters are in 3 tbs of milk? Conversion factors: 5 mL = 1 tsp, and 3 tsp = 1 tbs. _____

DA equation:

17 How many nurse assistants are needed for a 300-bed hospital? Conversion factors: 1 nurse per 10 beds per shift, and 2 nurse assistants for each nurse. _____

DA equation:

18 How many inches are in a meter (m)? Conversion factors: 2.5 cm = 1 inch, and 100 cm = 1 m. _____

DA equation:

19 How many centimeters are in a foot? Conversion factors: 2.5 cm = 1 inch, and 12 inches = 1 foot. _____

DA equation:

20 How many micrograms (mcg) are in 2 grams (g) of sugar? Conversion factors: 1000 mcg = 1 mg, and 1000 mg = 1 g. _____

DA equation:

Suggestions for Further Reading

www.cogsci.princeton.edu
www.mathforum.org
www.worldscinet.com
www.ncbi.nlm.nih.gov/pubmed/16496864

 Additional information and practice can be found on the Student Companion on Evolve.

   Chapter 3 focuses on the measurement units currently used for medications. Medications are primarily ordered and supplied in terms of metric system measurements, a system used in most parts of the world. DA-style equations are useful for verifying conversions and solving metric-equivalent medication dose problems.

PART II

Modern Metric System and Medication Calculations

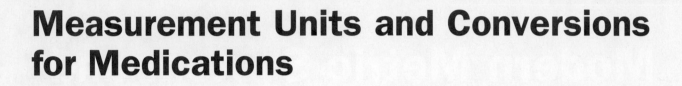
Measurement Units and Conversions for Medications

OBJECTIVES

- Memorize the units of metric measurement used in medication orders.
- State equivalent values of weight (mass) and volume used in metric dose calculations: micrograms, milligrams, grams, kilograms, milliliters, and liters.
- Distinguish milligram, milliliter, and milliequivalent.
- Define the uses of the term *Unit* related to measurements and medications.
- Calculate basic metric oral medication problems using mental arithmetic and decimal placement.
- Verify metric conversions using dimensional analysis.
- Use approved abbreviations for metric units.
- Distinguish metric and household measurements.

Essential Prior Knowledge

- Mastery of Chapters 1 and 2

Essential Equipment

- Yardstick measured in centimeters and meters or ruler measured in millimeters and centimeters
- Food package labels measured in grams
- Measuring cup illustrating ounces and milliliters
- 30-mL plastic medicine cup showing 1 and 2 tbs
- Several medication labels, prescription or over-the-counter

Estimated Time To Complete Chapter

- 2 hours

Introduction

Modern metric measurements have almost completely replaced an old English imprecise Apothecary system* in order to reduce medication errors. The modern metric system is logical, precise, and easy to work with because it's a standardized decimal measurement system using multiples (powers) of 10 similar to our monetary structure which is also based on a decimal structure. With a little practice and repetition, nurses will be very comfortable with it.

It has been adopted by most countries of the world for standardized weights and measurements. Known as the International System of Units (SI), it is the modern form of the former French metric system. It is required for admission to the European Union. Resistance to change and expense involved have slowed the U.S. "metrication" progress except in the scientific community.

This chapter focuses on understanding and interpreting the metric measurements used in medication orders and records, on medication labels, in laboratory reports, and nursing practice. It also includes examples of household measurements. Household measures are used for some medications taken at home, primarily liquids. Nurses need to know the metric-household equivalents for home care practice, for patient and family discharge and home-care teaching. Teaspoon A does not equal teaspoon B.

*Refer to Appendix A for the apothecary system.

ESSENTIAL *Vocabulary*

Base Units of Metric Measurement	Three base units are commonly used for metric measurement of medications to indicate weight (or mass), volume, and length: **gram** (g), **liter** (L), and **meter** (m). ➤ Memorize these base units of measurement. The abbreviation for *liter* is preferably capitalized, *L*, to avoid confusion with the number 1.
Household System of Measurement	Utensils used in the home, such as cups, teaspoons, tablespoons, droppers, etc. Their use can create a safety risk for measuring medication doses because of inconsistent capacities.
ISMP	Institute for Safe Medication Practices, a non-profit organization that educates the health care community and consumers about safe medication practices.
Modern Metric System	A popular name for the International System of Units (SI). Modified and adopted for uniform measurement in most countries, now recommended for all medication doses in the US by TJC and by ISMP.
SI Units	SI Units in the metric system refer to a dimension, such as weight (or mass), volume, and length. Examples of metric units of measurement include kilogram (kg), microgram (mcg), milligram (mg), gram (g), liter (L), and meter (m). ➤ Write out the words *unit* and *units;* do not use abbreviations such as U.
TJC	The Joint Commission, a national non-profit independent agency dedicated to improved quality of health care through the provision of accreditation and certification to health care organizations with an emphasis on high standards and patient safety including medication administration safety.

Vocabulary Review

RAPID PRACTICE   3-1

Estimated completion time: 10-15 minutes   Answers on page 492

Directions: *Study the vocabulary and write the answers in the space provided.*

1   What are the three base units of the metric system?
_____

2   Why is the symbol for liter capitalized? _____

3   What is one problem with using household utensils for medication doses?
_____

4   What system of measurement is currently used for most medication doses in the United States? _____

5   What are the abbreviations for two organizations which address safe medication practices? _____

Metric Equivalent Chart

Weight	Volume
1000 mcg (micrograms) = 1 mg (milligram)	1000 mL (milliliter) = 1 L (liter)
1000 mg = 1 g (gram)	
1000 g = 1 kg (kilogram)	
	Length
lb to kg conversion	10 mm (millimeters) = 1 centimeter (cm)
2.2 lb (pound) = 1 kg	100 cm = 1 meter (m)
inch to cm conversion	1000 mm = 1 meter (m)
1 inch = 2.5 cm (approximate)	

Metric Measurements: Base Units

Three *base* units are commonly used in the medical field. Two are used mainly for medication doses (gram and liter) and one (meter) is used occasionally for topical medications.

➤ Memorize these three base units.

Base Units

Dimension	Metric Base Unit	Approximate English System Equivalent
Weight (or mass)	gram (g)	About $\frac{1}{30}$ ounce dry weight
Volume	liter (L)	About 4 measuring cups, a little more than a quart
Length	meter (m)	About 39 inches, a little more than a yard

The abbreviation for the base unit liter is capitalized (L) to avoid misreading as the number 1. The base units abbreviations for gram (g) and meter (m) are written in lowercase letters. No other abbreviations are authorized.

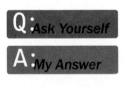

1 What are the three base units of metric measurement used for medications and their abbreviations?

Metric Units Number Line

The following metric units number line illustrates the relationship of the values for selected metric prefixes.

Prefix	Abbreviation		Value
kilo-	k		1000
hecto-	h		100
deka-	da		10
			0 (zero)
deci-	d		0.1
centi-	c		0.01
milli-	m		0.001
micro-	mc		0.000001

Metric Prefixes and Values

Four prefixes are commonly used for medication dose calculations:

- centi- (meaning hundredth)
- milli- (meaning thousandth)
- micro- (meaning millionth)
- kilo- (meaning a thousand times)
- A fifth prefix, deci- (meaning tenth), is used in laboratory reports.

➤ Memorize the prefixes and meanings.

Study Table 3-1, and note the numerical values and relationships. Metric prefixes are combined with bases to create new quantities, as shown in the examples in the table.

TABLE 3-1	Metric Measurements, Prefixes, Values, and Meaning				
Prefix	**Multiplier**	**Exponential Power of 10**	**Meaning**	**Examples**	**Meaning**
micro- (mc)	.000001	10^{-6}	millionth part of	microgram (mcg)	one millionth of a gram
milli- (m)	.001	10^{-3}	thousandth part of	milliliter (mL)	one thousandth of a liter
				milligram (mg)	one thousandth of a gram
centi- (c)	.01	10^{-2}	hundredth part of	centimeter (cm)	one hundredth of a meter
deci- (d)	.1	10^{-1}	tenth part of	deciliter (dL)	one tenth of a liter
kilo- (k)	1000	10^{3}	1000 times	kilogram (kg)	one thousand grams

Note: The prefix value never changes when combined with a base unit (e.g., the prefix *milli* [m] = .001).
1 mm = 0.001 (one thousandth of a meter).
1 mL = 0.001 (one thousandth of a liter).
1 mg = 0.001 (one thousandth of a gram).

1 What are the numerical values of the prefixes *m, c, d,* and *k*?

_____

- For review, write out the five prefixes and three base units used for medication administration. Learn them in preparation for analyzing medication orders.

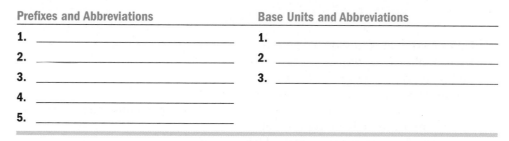

Prefixes and Abbreviations

1. _____
2. _____
3. _____
4. _____
5. _____

Base Units and Abbreviations

1. _____
2. _____
3. _____

➤ The abbreviation for the prefix micro- (mc) is preferred over the Greek letter mu (μ) in handwritten patient medical records. A handwritten μg (microgram) can be mistaken for mg (milligram).

It is very important to recognize the μ and distinguish it from zero and from mg. Either misinterpretation could lead to serious errors in medication dosage. The nurse should clarify the meaning of unfamiliar symbols and words with the prescriber.

CLINICAL RELEVANCE

Writing Metric Units and Abbreviations

Estimated completion time: 10 minutes **Answers on page 492**

Directions: *Study the metric units and abbreviations. Write the metric name and abbreviation in the space provided.*

1 Write the name and abbreviation for the prefix that means $\frac{1}{1000}$. _____

2 Write the name and abbreviation for the prefix that means $\frac{1}{100}$. _____

3 Write the name and abbreviation for the prefix that means $\frac{1}{1,000,000}$. _____

4 Write the name and abbreviation for the prefix that means $\frac{1}{10}$. _____

5 Write the name and abbreviation for the prefix that means 1000 times. _____

6 Write the name and abbreviation for the base unit of volume. _____

7 Write the name and abbreviation for the base unit of length. _____

8 Write the name and abbreviation for the base unit of weight, or mass. _____

9 Write the name for the base unit *m.* _____

10 Write the name for the prefix *m.* _____

Metric Notation

Writing metric unit combinations and equivalents

Study the example and note the correct order of writing as follows:

1 Numeral or numerals
2 Space
3 Prefix
4 Base unit

EXAMPLES

The following are examples of correctly written metric quantities: 100 mg, 1000 mL, 10 L, 250 cm, 2500 mcg, and 1,000,000 kg.

Do not write an *m* to look like a *w* or a *u.*
Do capitalize *L* for *liter.*
Metric abbreviations are case sensitive.
Do not close up a *c* so that *cm* looks like *am.*
Do use commas to group numbers with more than three consecutive zeros in groups of three from right to left.
Do not make up your own metric abbreviations
Do not pluralize metric abbreviations.

Guide to Metric Notation	Examples
Abbreviations are always used when accompanied by a number. The number, followed by a space, precedes the abbreviation.	10 mg, 2 g, 5 L Metric terms are written out when unaccompanied by a number, as illustrated in the following sentence: "Write out grams and milligrams."
When the number of units following the slash meaning *per* is 1, the number 1 may be omitted from the abbreviation. It is implied.	40 mg/ g (40 mg per 1 g)
Metric *abbreviations* are always singular. They are *not* pluralized.	*Milligrams* is abbreviated *mg*. *Liters* is abbreviated *L*. Write *mg*, not *mgs; g,* not *gs;* and *L,* not *Ls.*
There is no period after metric abbreviations except when they fall at the end of a sentence.	Give 2 mg, not 3 mg. He drank 2 L of water, followed by 1 L.

Slashes appear in many drug and laboratory references. The nurse must be able to interpret them. Do not write them. They have been mistaken for the number one (1). The word "per" is to be written out instead of a slash. Refer to the ISMP list of symbols that lead to medication errors on p. 103.

Writing Metric Measurements

RAPID PRACTICE 3-3

Estimated completion time: 5-10 minutes   **Answers on page 492**

Directions: *Write the metric measurement in the space provided.*

1 Write out the name and abbreviation for the base unit that is capitalized so that it will not be confused with the number 1. _____; _____

2 Which prefix shown in Table 3-1 equals 1000 times the base unit? _____

3 If a laboratory report indicated that a blood sugar level was 80 mg/dL, how would that quantity be written out and read aloud? _____

4 Which abbreviation is preferred over the Greek μ for micro? _____

5 Write the names and abbreviations for the three base units in the metric system. _____

Metric Abbreviations

RAPID PRACTICE 3-4

Estimated completion time: 3 minutes   **Answers on page 492**

Directions: *Circle the* recommended *abbreviation for the metric units of measurement:*

1 grams
   - **1.** gr
   - **2.** gms
   - **3.** G
   - **4.** g

2 milligrams
   - **1.** mgm
   - **2.** mg
   - **3.** Mgs
   - **4.** mcg

3 liters
   - **1.** L
   - **2.** l
   - **3.** ls
   - **4.** Ls

4 milliliters

1. m
2. mL

3. mg
4. mLs

5 microgram

1. μg
2. mg

3. mcg
4. mc

RAPID PRACTICE 3-5 *Combining Metric Measurements*

Estimated completion time: 5 minutes   **Answers on page 492**

Directions: *Write the recommended abbreviation for the metric unit combinations in the space provided:*

1 milligram _____

2 microgram _____

3 millimeter _____

4 milliliter _____

5 kilogram _____

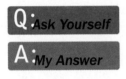

Q: Ask Yourself

A: My Answer

1 Are there 100 or 1000 cm in a meter?

_____

2 Are there 100 or 1000 mg in a gram?

_____

3 Are there 10 or 100 dL in a liter?

_____

RAPID PRACTICE 3-6 *Metric Base Units*

Estimated completion time: 5 minutes   **Answers on page 492**

Directions: *Write the requested metric base units in the correct form in the space provided.*

1 Which metric base unit abbreviation presented in this chapter must be capitalized? _____

2 Which metric base unit abbreviation would be added to the prefix *c* in a measurement of the length of a scar? _____

3 Which metric base unit abbreviation would be added to the prefix *m* in a measurement of fluids consumed? _____

4 Which metric base unit abbreviation would be added to the prefix *k* in a measurement of current weight? _____

5 Which metric base unit abbreviation would be added to the prefix *m* in a measurement of drug weight? _____

➤ To accelerate mastery of the metric system, begin to THINK METRIC.

Read the labels on food, beverages, medicines, and vitamins to speed learning of the uses of *g* and *mg*.

1 The average American consumes about 5 g of sodium per day. Intake should be restricted to about 2 g of sodium from *all* sources. 1 tsp of table salt (NaCl) contains 2300 mg of sodium. Approximately how many grams of sodium do you consume on an average day?

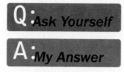

Q: *Ask Yourself*

A: *My Answer*

Equivalent Metric Measurements of Weight or Mass

Memorize:

1000 mcg = 1 mg   1000 mg = 1 g   1000 g = 1 kg

In clinical agencies, the kilogram is used for weight reporting and dose calculations. At birth the average baby weighs 3200 g, or 3.2 kg (approximately 7 lb). Low-birth-weight infants are those who weigh ≤2500 g (2.5 kg, or 5.5 lb) at birth. Many drug doses are ordered and adjusted on the basis of kilogram weight. Oral medications contain large ranges of doses in milligrams, such as 0.5 mg, 50 mg, 100 mg, 250 mg, or 500 mg. Doses of some oral medications are very small, such as those found in Synthroid (0.175 mg, or 175 mcg).

CLINICAL RELEVANCE

Metric Unit Identification

RAPID PRACTICE 3-7

Estimated completion time: 3 minutes   Answers on page **492**

Directions: *Place a circle around the metric unit(s) dose on the front of each of the labels, as shown in problem 1.*

1
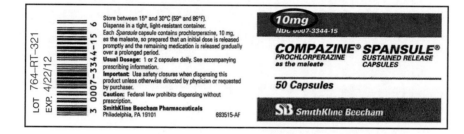

2
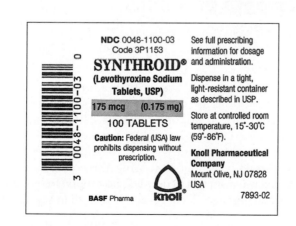

3

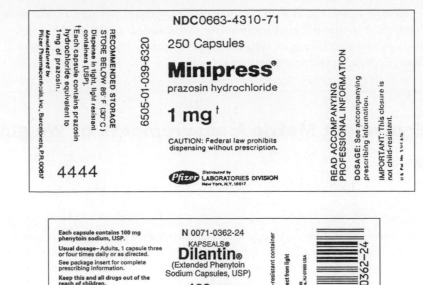

4

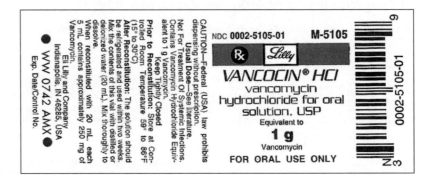

5 Some medications, particularly antibiotics, are supplied in grams.

Equivalent Metric Measurements of Volume

Memorize:

$$1000 \text{ mL} = 1 \text{ L}$$

The volume of a liter is slightly greater than a quart (1 L = 1.06 qt, 1 qt = 0.9 L). Many intravenous solutions are delivered in 1 L containers. Examine a water or soda bottle. Does it contain 750 mL or 1 L? Drink 240 mL of water several times a day instead of 8 ounces or 1 cup.

In many parts of the world, gasoline is purchased and paid for by the liter. If you normally buy 10 gal, you would buy about 40 L. While this conversion is not exact, using it when buying gas abroad will assist you in deciding how much to buy and give you an idea of what you will owe. Making a quick conversion is safer than saying, "Fill the tank."

➤ The abbreviation for cubic centimeter (cc) is often written to indicate milliliters (mL). The recommended and preferred abbreviation for milliliter is mL because cc has been misread as two zeros (00), resulting in medication errors.

➤ *Interpret* 1 cc as 1 mL. *Write* 1 mL.

In clinical agencies, liquids are usually ordered and supplied in milliliters and liters. When calculating liquid dose problems, the answer should be in milliliters. A special calibrated medicine teaspoon holds 5 mL of fluid. Plastic liquid medicine cups, referred to as *ounce cups,* hold 30 mL, which is approximately 1 oz. Think *30 mL* for an ounce. Intravenous medications are also supplied in milliliters and liters.

CLINICAL RELEVANCE

Equivalent Metric Measurements of Length

Memorize:

10 mm = 1 cm

100 cm = 1 meter

1000 mm = 1 meter

When you are assisting with cardiopulmonary resuscitation (CPR), it is helpful to know that fully dilated pupils (10 mm, or 1 cm) can indicate that the patient has been without oxygen for more than 4 minutes. Assessment of the pupils of the eye provides a clue as to a patient's response to CPR. The pinpoint pupil (1-2 mm) may be a reaction to strong light or to certain narcotics or other medications (Figure 3-1). Familiarity with millimeters and centimeters is also helpful in gauging the length of specified areas, such as wounds or scars, or in documenting the application of ointments in the clinical setting.

CLINICAL RELEVANCE

1 What is the width of a friend's, family member's, or friendly pet's eye pupil in millimeters? (Caution: Do not place the ruler on the eye or face.)

Q: *Ask Yourself*

A: *My Answer*

_____

2 Do you have any arm scars, freckles, or skin lesions you can measure in millimeters and/or centimeters? If so, what is the length?

_____

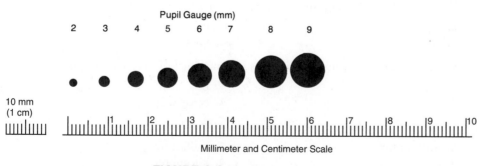

FIGURE 3-1 Pupil gauge (mm).

3 What is your height in centimeters? Multiply your height in inches by 2.5 (2.5 cm = approximately 1 inch).

_____

4 If you had to put 10 mm of ointment on a wound, how many centimeters would you need?

_____

CLINICAL RELEVANCE

Once you have established some personal landmarks in millimeters and centimeters, you can estimate the size of skin lesions at the bedside by comparing them with your own lesions without searching for a ruler. Topical prescription ointments usually supply paper tape rulers when exact measurements are needed. Note that some ointments may be prescribed and measured in inches.

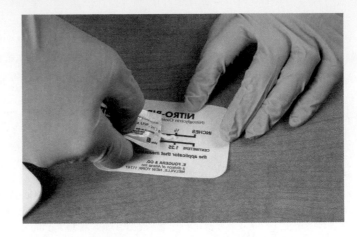

(From Perry AG, Potter PA: *Clinical nursing skills and techniques,* ed. 7, St. Louis, 2010, Mosby.)

RAPID PRACTICE 3-8

Metric Abbreviations Review

Estimated completion time: 5 minutes   Answers on page 493

Directions: *Identify the correct units of measurement.*

1 The three *base* units of measurement, noted correctly, in the metric system are: _____

   1. c, k, m   **3.** cm, mL, g
   2. g, l, m   **4.** g, L, m

2 Which of the following metric units is 0.001 of a liter? _____

   1. mL   **3.** mg
   2. kL   **4.** 1L

3 Which of the following metric units is a measure of liquid volume? _____

   1. mg   **3.** mL
   2. cm   **4.** mcg

4 Which of the following metric units is a measure of mass or weight? _____

   1. g   **3.** L
   2. m   **4.** cc or mL

5 Which of the following metric units is 0.001 of a meter? _____

   1. millimeter   **3.** milligram
   2. centimeter   **4.** kilometer

Q: Ask Yourself

A: My Answer

1 What are two abbreviations for the unit *microgram,* and which one is recommended for nurses to use? _____

➤ Metric measurements do *not* require *conversions* within the system. The prefixes *c, m,* and *k* denote the *equivalent* amount in powers of 10.

Metric Equivalents

Study the following major metric equivalents. The *values* are evident from the prefix and suffix combinations.

Weight, or Mass	Volume	Length
1000 mcg = 1 mg	1000 mL = 1 L	1000 mm = 1 m
1000 mg = 1 g		100 cm = 1 m
1000 g = 1 kg		10 mm = 1 cm

After you learn the major equivalent values, you can infer such values for quarters, halves, and one and a half. You find metric equivalents by moving the decimal place.

Sample Equivalent Metric Values

Row	Length	Volume	Volume	Weight	Weight	Weight	Weight	Weight	Weight
A	10 mm	500 mL	1000 mL	1000 mcg	250 mg	500 mg	1000 mg	1500 mg	1000 g
B	1 cm	0.5 L	1 L	1 mg	0.25 g	0.5 g	1 g	1.5 g	1 kg

➤ Do not confuse micrograms with milligrams. Note the difference in value between 1 mcg and 1 mg. The metric system uses only decimals for numbers less than 1. Note the leading zeros in front of decimals and the elimination of trailing zeros after numbers.

Use the examples in the table above to answer the following questions:

1 Can you identify the base unit in each abbreviation?

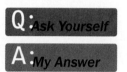

_____

2 Can you identify the numerical value (e.g., $\frac{1}{10}$ or $\frac{1}{1000}$) of the prefix (e.g., *milli-*, *centi-*, *micro-*, or *kilo-*) when you read them in an abbreviation?

_____

3 Can you distinguish when to read *m* as *meter* and when to read *m* as *milli-*? One is a prefix, and the other is a base. Which would be placed on the left and which would be placed on the right?

_____

4 Which dimension (weight or volume) does milliliter measure, as opposed to milligram?

_____

Finding Equivalents: Changing Milligrams to Grams and Grams to Milligrams

Grams and milligrams are the units most frequently encountered in the administration of tablets and capsules.

Equivalent amounts within units of the metric system are found by moving decimal places. Moving a decimal point three places to the right or left is needed to convert grams and milligrams.

Conversion factor: 1000 mg = 1 g.

Finding metric equivalents by moving decimals

➤ To change milligrams to grams, divide milligrams by 1000.

Divide milligrams by 1000 by moving the decimal place (implied or existing) three places to the left: 2500 mg = 2.5 g

➤ To change grams to milligrams, multiply grams by 1000.

Multiply grams by 1000 by moving the decimal place (implied or existing) three places to the right: 2.5 g = 2500 mg

---

EXAMPLES

How many milligrams are in 1.5 grams?
Conversion factor: 1000 mg = 1 g

Step 1	:	Step 2	×	Step 3	=	Answer
Desired Answer Units	:	Starting Factor	×	Given Quantity and and Conversion Factor(s)	=	Estimate, Multiply, Evaluate
mg	:	$\dfrac{1000 \text{ mg}}{1 \text{ g}}$	×	$\dfrac{1.5 \text{ g}}{1}$	=	1500 mg

Cancel units.
Stop and check setup.

The final equation will be written like this:

$$mg \quad : \quad \frac{1000 \text{ mg}}{1 \text{ g}} \quad \times \quad \frac{1.5 \text{ g}}{1} \quad = \quad 1500 \text{ mg in 1.5 g}$$

Analysis: The simple conversion equation contains the desired answer units and the given information. The selected Starting Factor, a conversion factor, is in the correct orientation. The given unwanted units, grams, are canceled. A number 1 is placed as a denominator under 1.5 g to hold the 1.5 g in the numerator position. This maintains alignment and helps prevent multiplication errors.

Evaluation: Only mg remain in the answer. My estimate that the number would be 1.5 times 1000 is supported by the answer. (Math check: $1000 \times 1.5 = 1500$). The equation is balanced.

See Chapter 2 for a more extensive review of DA equations.

FAQ | *How can I decide whether to divide or multiply in order to move the decimal point to the left or the right of a number for metric equivalents?*

ANSWER | The (memorized) conversion formula (e.g., 1000 mg = 1 g) reveals the direction in which to move the decimal point. Converting milligrams to grams requires division. Converting grams to milligrams requires multiplication. Write out the relevant conversion formulas when taking a test so that they are in front of you for reference until the conversions become automatic.

RAPID PRACTICE **3-9**

Milligram and Gram Equivalents

Estimated completion time: 10-20 minutes   **Answers on page 493**

Directions: *Fill in the equivalent amount. Insert leading zeros and eliminate trailing zeros when necessary. Label the answer using correct notation. It would be helpful to write out the relevant conversion formula.*

Milligrams	Grams		Grams	Milligrams
1. 500	_____		**6.** 0.25	_____
2. 2000	_____		**7.** 0.6	_____
3. 250	_____		**8.** 0.125	_____
4. 1500	_____		**9.** 0.04	_____
5. 60	_____		**10.** 2	_____

Basic Milligram-to-Gram Medication Conversions RAPID PRACTICE 3-10

Estimated completion time: 10-15 minutes   Answers on page 493

Directions: *Analyze the questions for the desired metric equivalent dose and move the decimal places accordingly to arrive at the correct equivalents. Insert leading zeros and remove trailing zeros from the answer. (Refer to p. 8 for a review of leading and trailing zeros.) Confirm your answer with a DA equation.*

1   The physician ordered 1.5 g of a medication. What is the equivalent dose in milligrams? _____

DA equation:

2   The physician ordered 0.15 g of a medication. What is the equivalent dose in milligrams? _____

DA equation:

3   The physician ordered 4 g of a medication. What is the equivalent dose in milligrams? _____

DA equation:

4   The physician ordered 500 mg of a medication. What is the equivalent dose in grams? _____

DA equation:

5   The physician ordered 60 mg of a medication. What is the equivalent dose in grams? _____

DA equation:

FAQ | *Why verify these decimal movements with a DA-style equation?*

ANSWER | Both methods require practice. Moving decimals gives an estimate. Mastery of a verification method for backup proof of any calculation is essential. If a nurse practices and masters DA with some simple equations, the more complex conversions requiring DA will be simple also.

RAPID PRACTICE 3-11

Identifying Metric Equivalents

Estimated completion time: 5 minutes   Answers on page 493

Directions: *Circle the correct metric equivalent for the amount presented:*

1   Ordered: 0.2 g
   1. 0.002 mg   **3.** 200 mg
   2. 0.02 mg   **4.** 2000 mg

2   Ordered: 400 mg
   1. 0.04 g   **3.** 40 g
   2. 0.4 g   **4.** 4000 g

3   Ordered: 1.6 g
   1. 1600 mg   **3.** 1.6 mg
   2. 160 mg   **4.** 0.016 mg

4   Ordered: 50 mg
   1. 0.05 g   **3.** 500 g
   2. 50 g   **4.** 5000 g

5   Ordered: 0.04 g
   1. 0.004 mg   **3.** 4 mg
   2. 0.04 mg   **4.** 40 mg

Examining Micrograms

Cultural Note

In some countries, such as the United States, a comma is used to separate groups of three numbers within large numbers, as in 20,000. In other countries, a *space is* used. Thus, 25,000 or 25 000 might be seen. In the past, the British used a comma to designate a *decimal point* between a whole number and a fraction: 5,5 would be read as 5.5. ("5 point 5" or "5 and 5 tenths"). This type of notation can still be seen in scientific math.

The metric equivalents of micrograms are as follows:

$$1000 \text{ mcg} = 1 \text{ mg}$$
$$1{,}000{,}000 \text{ mcg} = 1 \text{ g}$$

Milligrams and grams are among the commonest measurements in medications. Of the two, milligrams are used more frequently. In order to avoid errors, it is advisable to avoid using decimals and to select an equivalent that can be stated in whole numbers.

Micrograms are very small units. Microgram and milligram conversions are needed for intravenous calculations and occasionally for very small doses of powerful medications. Just as with milligrams and grams, it is helpful to examine the prefix to determine the equivalent units.

➤ To change micrograms to milligrams, divide micrograms by 1000.
➤ To change milligrams to micrograms, multiply milligrams by 1000.

RAPID PRACTICE 3-12

Mental Math: Micrograms to Milligrams, Milligrams to Micrograms, and Micrograms and Grams

Estimated completion time: 10 minutes   Answers on page 493

Directions: *Fill in the equivalent metric measure in the spaces provided by moving decimal points.*

Micrograms to Milligrams		Milligrams to Micrograms		Milligrams to Grams	
mcg	mg	mg	mcg	mg	g
1. 5000	_____	**6.** 2	_____	**11.** _____	0.001
2. 300	_____	**7.** 0.5	_____	**12.** 5000	_____
3. 1500	_____	**8.** 1.8	_____	**13.** _____	0.4
4. 20,000	_____	**9.** 0.15	_____	**14.** 600	_____
5. 2500	_____	**10.** 0.6	_____	**15.** _____	0.03

➤ Write numbers, commas, and decimals neatly and use the custom of the country where you work.

As with mastering arithmetic, mastery of the metric system frees precious time for other priorities, such as
· patient and medical record assessments
· patient and family communications
· medication preparation and administration
· clinical theory
· patient treatments
· documentation in the patient record

CLINICAL RELEVANCE

Review: Defining and Abbreviating Metric Units

RAPID PRACTICE 3-13

Estimated completion time: 10 minutes   **Answers on page 493**

Directions: *Fill in the full word or approved abbreviation for the metric units in the space provided:*

Full Word	Approved Abbreviation
1 cm _____	**6** liter _____
2 mL _____	**7** meter _____
3 mg _____	**8** kilogram _____
4 mm _____	**9** kilometer _____
5 mcg _____	**10** deciliter _____

Metric Equivalents Review

RAPID PRACTICE 3-14

Estimated completion time: 10 minutes   **Answers on page 494**

Directions: *Convert to equivalent metric units by moving decimal places.*

1 1 g = _____ mg		**6** 1 L = _____ mL	
2 1 kg = _____ g		**7** 2.5 g = _____ mg	
3 1 cm = _____ mm		**8** 500 mg = _____ g	
4 1 mg = _____ mcg		**9** 2500 mg = _____ g	
5 1 g = _____ mcg		**10** 500 mcg = _____ mg	

☐ Milliequivalents (mEq)

FAQ | *What is a milliequivalent (mEq), and what is the difference between a milliequivalent and a milligram (mg)?*

ANSWER | The milliequivalent is another way of expressing the contents of a medication in solution. A milliequivalent is the number of grams of solute in 1 mL of solution. It reflects the *chemical combining power* of the ingredients. Milligrams are a measure of *weight*.

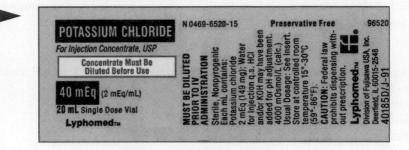

FIGURE 3-2 Potassium chloride label.

Solutions of electrolytes, such as potassium, sodium, and magnesium, are usually ordered and supplied in numbers of mEq/mL or mEq/L. The medication label may also state the amount of milligrams of drug contained in the product.

➤ Milligrams and milliequivalents are not equivalent.

CLINICAL RELEVANCE

Many intravenous solutions administered by nurses contain electrolytes. The sample medication label in Figure 3-2 includes both milliequivalents and milligrams. In small print, the label lists 2 mEq (149 mg).

➤ When interpreting the label shown in Figure 3-2, it is important for the nurse to recognize that 2 mEq *cannot be substituted for* 149 mg in dose calculations.

Other Medication Measurement Systems

Household measurements

Most people are familiar with household (kitchen) measurement terms. It is important to realize that household utensils are usually not calibrated precisely. There are small and large teaspoons and tablespoons, cups, and glasses. Medicines taken at home should be taken with specially calibrated droppers, measuring teaspoons, and cups. Patients and their families need instruction about the use of precisely calibrated household measuring devices before being discharged from the hospital. (Refer to Table 3-2.)

Apothecary system

The imprecise older apothecary system of weights and measures has been replaced in most health care agencies by the metric system for medication measurements. Refer to the Appendix for a brief explanation. Refer to The Joint Commission recommendations for apothecary units' possible future inclusion in the Official "Do Not Use" list on p. 101.

Compare the metric and household systems in Table 3-2.

TABLE 3-2	**Comparison of Metric and Household Liquid Measurements Used for Medications**
Metric	**Household**
1 mL	1 drop
5 mL	1 teaspoon (tsp)
15 mL	1 tablespoon (tbs) (½ oz)
30 mL	2 tablespoons (1 oz)
240 mL	1 measuring cup (8 oz)
500 mL	1 pint (16 oz)
1000 mL (1 L)	1 quart (32 oz)
4 L	1 gallon (gal) (4 quarts)

Note: All household equivalents are approximate.

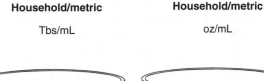

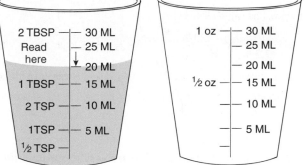

FIGURE 3-3 Household and metric measuring liquid containers. (From Brown M, Mulholland J: Drug calculations: process and problems for clinical practice, ed. 7, 2007, St. Louis, Mosby.)

Household and metric liquid measuring containers

➤ Syringes, calibrated medicine cups, and calibrated droppers are used in clinical practice to prepare small amounts of liquid doses (Figure 3-3).

1 If an order calls for 1 tsp of cough medicine, how many milliliters will the nurse prepare?

_____

2 If an order calls for 1 tbs of a laxative, how many calibrated teaspoons will the nurse prepare?

_____

3 If an order calls for $\frac{1}{2}$ oz of an antacid, how many milliliters will the nurse prepare?

_____

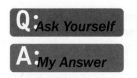

Q: *Ask Yourself*

A: *My Answer*

Converting pounds to kilograms

➤ Review the required elements of a DA equation

- Desired answer units
- Conversion factors
- Given quantity and units to be converted

To change pounds to kilograms, create a DA equation using the conversion factor 2.2 lb = 1 kg. Kilograms are metric units of measurement. Pounds are units used in the household systems of measurement. Medications are often ordered on basis of kilograms of a patient's body weight.

EXAMPLES

How many kilograms (kg) are equivalent to 120 pounds (lb)?
Conversion factor: 2.2 lb = 1 kg

Step 1	:	Step 2	×	Step 3	=	Answer
Desired Answer Units	:	Starting Factor	×	Given Quantity and and Conversion Factor(s)	=	Estimate, Multiply, Evaluate
kg	:	$\dfrac{1\ kg}{2.2\ \cancel{lb}}$	×	$\dfrac{120\ \cancel{lb}}{1}$	=	54.5 kg

The final equation will be written like this:

$$kg \quad : \quad \frac{1\ kg}{2.2\ \cancel{lb}} \times \frac{120\ \cancel{lb}}{1} \quad = \quad 54.5\ kg\ in\ 120\ lb$$

Analysis: This simple equivalent equation contains the required elements in the correct orientation.

Evaluation: My rough estimate of 60 lb (120 ÷ 2) is supported by the answer (Math check: 120 ÷ 2.2 = 54.5). The equation is balanced.

➤ Estimates can help prevent major math errors. The estimate needs verification.

1 A 150-lb adult weighs 68.2 kg (150 lb ÷ 2.2 rounded to the nearest tenth). What is your weight in kilograms to the nearest tenth? (Divide your weight in pounds by 2.2.)

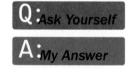
Q: *Ask Yourself*
A: *My Answer*

RAPID PRACTICE 3-15

Metric and Household Equivalents

Estimated completion time: 5 minutes   Answers on page 494

Directions: *Examine Table 3-2 and supply the correct approximate metric or household equivalent.*

1 How many milliliters are there in an 8 oz cup? _____

2 How many milliliters are in 2 tsp? _____

3 How many milliliters are in a tablespoon? _____

4 How many milliliters are in half an ounce? _____

5 How many mL are in 2 tbs? _____

➤ Use metric. Clarify any unclear orders with the prescribers and/or the pharmacist.
➤ Document the clarification in the medical record.

✳ Communication

A sample communication to clarify an order would be: "This is Bob Green, RN from fourth floor east. May I please speak to Dr. X? I have an order for patient Mary Smith for ferrous sulfate gr v̄ written by you. The medication label states 324 mg. Would you please clarify?" The nurse should document the response in the medication section of the medical administration records and in the nursing record. This is the safest action to take with rare or unfamiliar orders.

Key Points About the Measurement Systems

1 The metric system uses Arabic numerals and decimals.

2 The metric system basic unit for mass, or weight, is the gram.

3 Use only approved abbreviations to avoid misinterpretation.

4 The metric system measures *liquids* in milliliters and liters.

5 Household measurements have many implications for patient discharge teaching. Kitchen utensils are not calibrated for medicines.

6 A teaspoon order for medication doses must be calibrated for 5 mL capacity.

7 A tablespoon order is for 15 mL (3 calibrated tsp) or $\frac{1}{2}$ of a calibrated medication 30-mL cup.

8 An ounce is 30 mL (2 measuring tbs). Teach patients to use equipment supplied with the medication or calibrated ounce measurement cups at home. Do not substitute liquor "shot" glasses for ounce cups at home.

9 The milliliter is the preferred metric unit for liquid measurements. The abbreviation *mL* has been used interchangeably with *cc* (the abbreviation for cubic centimeters) by some prescribers. Write mL. Do not write cc.

10 A liter is a little more than a quart. Liters are used in clinical agencies. Quarts are not.

11 If the l in lb is written next to the number without a space (e.g., 2.2lb), it may be misread as the number 1.

12 Think metric but be prepared to see occasional unclear orders. Verify the equivalent measurement with pharmacy or the prescriber. Never guess.

➤ The nurse who confuses mg with mcg, or mL and mg with g or mEq, is at extreme risk for making grave medication dose errors.

Nurses must learn the metric system in order to read and interpret physicians' orders and medication labels. For the sake of patients' safety, nurses must master and become comfortable using all the metric units employed in medications. A nurse who has committed the relevant metric system terminology and values to memory and understands the system will never have to say, "I thought *mg* and *mcg* were the same thing," after administering a dosage that was a thousand-fold (thousand-times) error.

CLINICAL RELEVANCE

Examples of errors in the clinical setting include the following:
- Giving 10 mL of a liquid drug instead of 10 mg
- Converting 1 g to 100 mg instead of 1000 mg, a ten-fold error.
- Giving 20 mg instead of 200 mg for a 0.2 g order, a ten-fold error
- Reading 100U as 1000 because *units* was not spelled out or a space was not left between the number and the *U*, or the *U* was closed and looked like a zero, resulting in a ten-fold overdose
- Reading 7.5 mg as 75 mg because the decimal was not seen
- Reading 100 mEq as 100 mg, two very different measurements

➤ Knowing the value of the difference between a microgram, a milligram, and a gram is critical. Knowing that a milliequivalent is not a milligram is critical.

➤ Note that hospital policy may require that the prescriber be contacted for use of nonmetric terms and unapproved abbreviations.

➤ Table 3-3 lists some recommendations on how to avoid metric abbreviation errors.
➤ For the TJC "Do Not Use" list, refer to p. 101.
➤ Keep an eye out for TJC's "Do Not Use" abbreviations in the clinical setting and in written references. They are likely to cause errors.
➤ For the ISMP list of Error-Prone Abbreviations, Symbols, and Dose Designations, refer to pp. 102-103.

TABLE 3-3	**Metric Abbreviations That May Generate Errors**		
Unit	**Abbreviation to Use**	**Abbreviations to Avoid**	**Potential Errors**
milliliter(s)	mL	cc (cubic centimeter), ccs, mls	Misread when written poorly; *L* for *liter* capitalized to prevent misreading as the number 1; metric abbreviations not pluralized
gram(s)	g	gm, gms, gs, G, Gs	Misread when poorly written; should not be capitalized or pluralized
microgram(s)	mcg	μg, μgs, μ	Misread as *mg* (milligram) or zero (0)
milligram(s)	mg	mgm, mgms	Misread as microgram
Units	Write out Units (do not abbreviate)	U,* u*	Misread as zero (0)
International Units	Write out International Units (do not abbreviate)	IU*	Misread as the number 10

*Metric units included in TJC's "Do Not Use" list as of January 1, 2004. Their use has been banned in clinical agency handwritten medical records. Refer to pp. 101-103 for the complete TJC's "Do Not Use" list and the ISMP list of error-prone abbreviations.

CHAPTER 3 MULTIPLE-CHOICE REVIEW

Estimated completion time: 10-20 minutes **Answers on page 494**

Directions: *Circle the correct answer. Verify your math answers with a DA equation.*

1 The correct abbreviations for metric prefixes are
   1. L, m, g
   2. m, c, k, mc
   3. mg, mL, cc
   4. mm, cm, mg, kg

2 Select the correct equivalent for 0.003 g.
   1. 3 mcg
   2. 3 mg
   3. 30 mg
   4. 300 mg

3 Select the correct equivalent for 50 mg.
   1. 5 g
   2. 0.5 g
   3. 0.05 g
   4. 0.005 g

4 Select the correct equivalent for 3 kg.
   1. 1 g
   2. 3 g
   3. 3000 g
   4. 30,000 g

5 Which is the appropriate way to write *units* in the medical record?

1. Units
2. U
3. u
4. U's

6 Select the correct equivalent for 0.5 L.

1. 50 mL
2. 500 mL
3. 0.5 mL
4. 5000 mL

7 Select the correct equivalent for 0.2 g:

1. 2000 mg
2. 20 mg
3. 2 mg
4. 200 mg

8 Select the correct equivalent for 3500 g.

1. 3.5 kg
2. 350 kg
3. 3500 kg
4. 35 kg

9 Select the correct equivalent for 0.25 g.

1. 2500 mg
2. 250 mg
3. 25 mg
4. 2.5 mg

10 Select the correct equivalent for 100 mg.

1. 1 g
2. 10 g
3. 0.1 g
4. 0.05 g

CHAPTER 3 FINAL PRACTICE

Estimated completion time: 15-20 minutes   **Answers on page 494**

1 Write out the three approved base units and the five prefixes, as well as their abbreviations, covered in this chapter.

Base Unit	Abbreviation	Prefix	Abbreviation
a. _____	_____	d. _____	_____
b. _____	_____	e. _____	_____
c. _____	_____	f. _____	_____
		g. _____	_____
		h. _____	_____

2 The physician ordered 400 mg of a medication. How many grams would be the equivalent? _____ Use the DA method to back up your answer. Label all work.

DA equation:

3 The physician ordered 0.15 g of a medication. How many milligrams would be the equivalent? _____ Use the DA method to back up your answer. Label all work.

DA equation:

4 If you drank 0.25 L, how many milliliters would you have consumed? _____

DA equation:

5 How many milligrams are in a medication that contains 1500 mcg? _____

DA equation:

6 A baby weighs 1.5 kg. How many grams would be the equivalent? _____

DA equation:

7 The physician ordered 0.1 g of a medication. How many milligrams would be the equivalent? _____

DA equation:

8 If a scar measured 15 mm, how many centimeters would be the equivalent? _____ Use the appropriate conversion formula and DA style method to solve.

DA equation:

9 The physician ordered 0.2 mg of a medication. How many micrograms would be the equivalent? _____

DA equation:

10 How many grams are in 250,000 mcg? _____

DA equation:

11 If you were giving medications in home care, how many milliliters would you prepare for 3 tsp? _____

DA equation:

12 If 2 tbs were ordered for a home-care patient, how many milliliters would be prepared? _____

DA equation:

13 How many milliliters are in 1.5 oz of medication? _____

DA equation:

14 How many teaspoons are in a medication tablespoon? _____

DA equation:

15 How many medication tablespoons are in 2 ounces? _____

DA equation:

16 How many grams are in a kilogram? _____

17 How many pounds are in a kilogram? _____

18 How many milliliters are in a half-liter (0.5 L)? _____

19

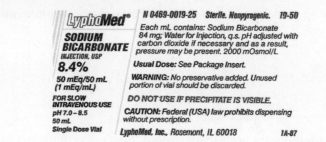

a. How many milligrams per milliliter of sodium bicarbonate are contained in the medication with the label shown above? _____

b. How many milliequivalents of sodium bicarbonate are contained in 1 milliliter? _____

20

 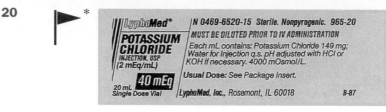

a. How many milligrams per milliliter of potassium chloride are noted on the label shown above? _____

b. How many milliequivalents per milliliter of potassium chloride are noted on the label? _____

---

*This red flag is a visual reminder that this drug is on the ISMP high-alert drug list, which means it has a heightened risk to cause harm when used in error. Refer to Appendix B.

Suggestions for Further Reading

www.ismp.org
www.jointcommission.org
http://lamar.colostate.edu/~hillger
www.mathforum.org/library
www.wordiq.com/definition/SI

⊖volve Additional information can be found in the Introducing Drug Measures section of the Student Companion on Evolve.

Chapter 4 incorporates the material that has been learned in Chapters 1 through 3—arithmetic, metric units, mental math, and dimensional analysis—and applies that knowledge to interpretation of medication orders, drug labels, and medication records.

"Perplexity is the beginning of knowledge."
—KHALIL GIBRAN

Patient Records, Medication Orders, and Labels

OBJECTIVES

- Interpret medication orders and labels.
- Identify abbreviations that cannot be used for handwritten medical records.
- Identify abbreviations that can lead to medication errors.
- Utilize TJC and ISMP medication-related recommendations
- Identify forms of medications.
- Read and write time using the 24-hour clock.
- Describe the data from the order and label that must be entered in all medication calculations.
- Interpret Medication Administration Records (MARs).
- Describe medication-related nurse actions that may lead to medication errors.
- Identify patients' rights.

Essential Prior Knowledge

- Mastery of Chapters 1-3

Essential Equipment

While not essential, the following items will be useful:
- Several medication labels (over-the-counter and/or prescription)
- 30-mL plastic medicine cup
- Glass measuring cup marked in ounces and milliliters

Estimated Time To Complete Chapter

- 1-2 hours

Introduction

Physicians and other prescribers enter medication and treatment orders on a computer or the patient's medical record on a page usually designated "Physician's Order Sheet" or "Doctor's Order Sheet." Several abbreviations are used to write medication orders, labels, and records.

The medication orders are sent to the pharmacy. The trend has been for the pharmacy to transfer the orders to their computerized forms. In most hospitals, medications are charged to the patient and delivered to the patient's area by the pharmacy in unit-dose (single-serving) packages labeled in metric system measurements. The medications may be stocked in a locked cabinet or in drawers of a locked medication cart until needed and restocked periodically by the pharmacy, usually every 24 hours.

The nurse must check the complete written order against the label on the medication supplied. If there is any discrepancy, the physician or pharmacist, whoever is more appropriate for the situation, must be contacted. If the amount of the dose is ordered based on the patient's weight or the amount of drug on hand is not identical to the amount ordered, a calculation may be needed. Usually, such calculations can be performed mentally, but sometimes written mathematics or a calculator is needed.

There is potential for error in each step of the written process, including the order, the medication administration record, the supplied medication and its label, and the preparation and administration. The nurse who administers the medication is legally responsible for the medications given even if the order was wrong or the medication and/or dose supplied by the pharmacy was in error. The nurse provides the final protection for patients in the medication chain.

This chapter focuses on reading and interpreting medication dose orders, labels, and abbreviations within the context of patients' safety. Abbreviations and measurements learned in earlier chapters are incorporated.

ESSENTIAL *Vocabulary*

Adverse Drug Event (ADE)	A medication-related event that causes harm to a patient. Can be caused by improper label, prescription, dispensing, administration, among other factors. Refer to http://www.psqh.com/novdec06/librarian.html.
Drug Form	The composition of a drug: liquid or solid; tablet, capsule, or suppository, etc.
Drug Route	The body location where the drug will be administered, e.g., mouth, nasogastric (nose to stomach), vein, muscle, subcutaneous tissue, rectum, or vagina.
FDA	Food and Drug Administration, the federal agency responsible for approving tested drugs for consumer use in the United States.
Generic Drug	*Official* name used for a drug by all companies that produce it. For example, there are many brands and trade names for *acetaminophen,* the *generic* name for Tylenol. *Acetaminophen* is the official name. Tylenol is a brand name.
	Generic drugs are identical or bioequivalent to brand-name drugs in dosage form, safety, strength, route of administration, quality, performance, and intended use.
High-Alert Medications	High-alert medications are medications that have been identified by ISMP as those that can cause significant harm to patients when used in error. The icon is a visual reminder to help you become familiar with some of these medications. Refer to the ISMP's list of high-alert medications in Appendix B as you work through the text and prepare patient care plans.
MAR	Medication Administration Record, the official record of all medications ordered for and received by each patient during an inpatient visit. It is maintained by nurses. Each page may reflect one or more hospital days.
ISMP	Institute for Safe Medication Practices.
NF	National Formulary, the official resource for the contents of generic drugs. *NF* is occasionally seen on medication labels.
NKA	No known allergies.
NKDA	No known drug allergies.
OTC Drug	Drug sold and purchased "over the counter" in drugstores, grocery stores, and health food stores without a prescription. Some were formerly required to be dispensed only by prescription and have been released from that requirement by the FDA.
Patent	Official permission from the U.S. Patent Trade Office to market a drug exclusively for 20 years from the time of application. The patent period compensates the first company to market a drug for the costs of drug research and development.
	After the patent period expires, other manufacturers may apply to sell the generic form of the drug and must meet the same standards as the original company.
Sentinel Event	An unexpected occurrence involving death or serious physical or psychological injury, or the risk thereof. Includes among other, severe adverse drug events (ADE). Refer to www.jointcommission.org/SentinelEvents.

TJC	The Joint Commission.
Trade Name	Name assigned to a product by its manufacturer. The symbol ® written as a superscript after a trade name indicates that the manufacturer has officially registered that name for the product with the U.S. Patent Trade Office.
24-Hour Clock	System for telling time that begins with 0001 (1 minute after midnight) and ends with 2400 (midnight). Also known as the international clock or military time.
	The 24-hour clock system is used internationally and has been adopted in the United States by many agencies to avoid potential confusion caused by duplication of AM and PM hours (a 12-hour clock).
Unit Dose	Single serving size of a drug (e.g., 250 mg per tablet, 250 mg per 5 mL).
Unit-Dose Packaging	Unit-dose packaging of single servings functions as a safety net. It helps limit the amount of overdose and/or waste that might occur. Refer to Figure 4-3.
USP	United States Pharmacopoeia, the official drug reference that lists all FDA-approved generic drugs. *USP* can be seen next to the generic name on some drug labels.
Usual Dose	Manufacturer's recommendation for the average dose strength (concentration) that usually achieves the desired therapeutic effect for the target population (e.g., "for adults with fever, 1-2 tablets every 4-6 hours, not to exceed 6 tablets in 24 hours").
	Based on clinical trials, the usual dose is often specified by the patient's weight and occasionally by body surface area or age.

1 What is the difference between a trade-name product and a generic product and why must the nurse know the difference?

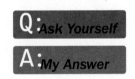

_____

2 What are some examples of drug forms?

_____

3 How may unit-dose packaging help prevent a medication error?

_____

4 What is the abbreviation for the daily medication record maintained by the nurses?

_____

Essential Vocabulary

RAPID PRACTICE 4-1

Estimated completion time: 5 minutes **Answers on page 495**

Directions: *Circle the correct answer.*

1 The term that describes the difference between a medication capsule, suppository, tablet, or liquid solution is

   1. form   **3.** trade

   2. generic   **4.** OTC

2 Medications, vitamins, and minerals that can be purchased without a prescription are designated

1. generic
2. trade
3. OTC
4. Unit Dose

3 The official organization that approves the sales of new drugs for consumers based on laboratory and clinical testing is

1. USP
2. FDA
3. NF
4. PTO

4 The abbreviation for a medication error that harms a patient

1. TJC
2. ADE
3. NKDA
4. NKA

5 The name for a drug that can be sold under a variety of trade names by a variety of manufacturers after the original patent has expired is

1. proprietary
2. generic/official
3. over-the-counter
4. USP

Medication Storage and Security

Medications for institutional use are stored in locked cabinets, carts, and drawers (Figure 4-1).

Bar codes are increasingly used to reduce medication errors. The pharmacy enters the patients' drug information, records, and medication orders into a computer. Each dose is bar-coded in the pharmacy. The nurse uses a hand-held scanner to scan the drug and the patient's wrist bracelet (Figure 4-2). The computer checks that it is the right medication for the right patient. Unit-dose medications supplied by the pharmacy also reduce medication errors.

Controlled (scheduled) drugs such as narcotics, opiates, and some non-narcotic drugs such as tranquilizers and anti-anxiety agents, have special locked storage, dispensing, disposal, and documentation requirements because of potential risk for abuse. They are placed in **schedules** by the Federal Drug Administration (DEA). Schedule C I (Control I) refers to drugs at the highest risk for abuse, such as crack cocaine and heroin, Schedules C II through C V drugs, which are prescribed for medical purposes, are labeled as such, with Schedule C V having least potential for abuse. Note the C II classification for morphine on the label below.

➤ Check your agency storage, disposal, and documentation policies for these medications.

Refer to Essential Vocabulary in this chapter and Appendix B for a list of high-alert medications.

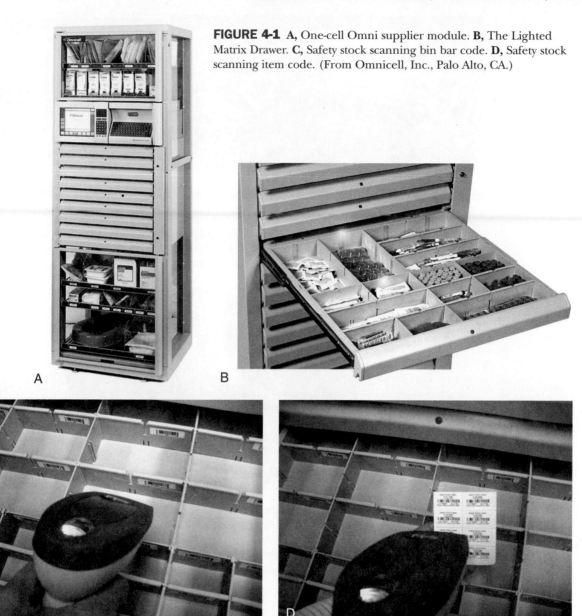

FIGURE 4-1 **A,** One-cell Omni supplier module. **B,** The Lighted Matrix Drawer. **C,** Safety stock scanning bin bar code. **D,** Safety stock scanning item code. (From Omnicell, Inc., Palo Alto, CA.)

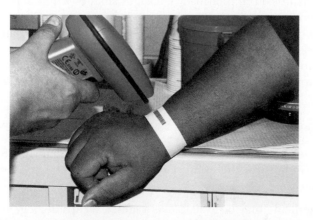

FIGURE 4-2 Bar code reader. (From Kee JL, Marshall SM: *Clinical calculations: with applications to general and specialty areas,* ed. 6, St. Louis, 2009, Saunders.)

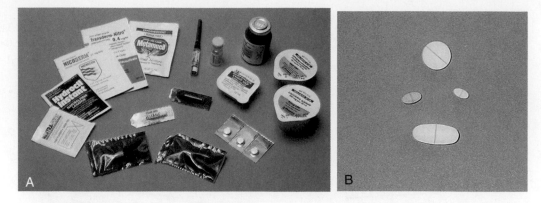

FIGURE 4-3 **A,** Unit dose packages. **B,** Scored tablets: they can be cut in half if needed. (**A,** From Clayton BD, Stock YN, Cooper S: *Basic pharmacology for nurses,* ed. 15, St. Louis, 2010, Mosby. **B,** In Brown M, Mulholland J: *Drug calculations: process and problems for clinical practice,* ed. 8, St. Louis, 2008, Mosby. Courtesy Amanda Politte, St. Louis, MO.)

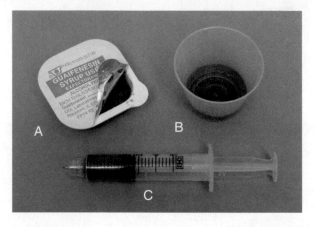

FIGURE 4-4 **A,** Liquid medication in single-dose package. **B,** Liquid measured in medicine cup. **C,** Oral liquid medicine in syringe. (From Potter PA, Perry AG: *Fundamentals of nursing,* ed. 7, St. Louis, 2009, Mosby.)

Medication Forms and Packaging

Medications are supplied in a variety of solid and liquid forms, including granules, tablets, capsules, suppositories, and various liquid preparations. The physician's order must specify the form of the medication. A single medication may be prepared in several forms and marketed and packaged in several single and/or multidose sizes. Multidose sizes are convenient for pharmacy and home use (Figure 4-3). At most clinical facilities, the pharmacy packages smaller single-serving-size amounts from the multidose containers to reduce medication errors (Figure 4-4).

Since medications are supplied in a variety of forms to meet patients' needs, it is important to select the form that matches the physician's order. This is done by matching the order to the medication label. The orders for medication forms are abbreviated. There is a trend to reduce and or eliminate abbreviations in medical records.

Solid Drug Forms

Table 4-1 lists solid medication abbreviations, terms, and forms. Since the nurse must be able to interpret the abbreviations and terms, the contents of Table 4-1 should be memorized.

➤ A single medicine may be available as a tablet, a capsule, a gel cap, and an enteric-coated tablet. When there is a choice, the prescriber offers the one that is best for the patient.

TABLE 4-1	Solid Medication Forms
Abbreviation or Term	**Description**
cap: capsule	Medication covered in hard or soft gelatin. They are supplied in various sizes. The entire contents may be sprinkled in food such as applesauce or a liquid if the physician so specifies. Capsules should never be cut or divided into partial amounts.
caplet	Smooth, lightly coated, small oval tablet. The name is derived from capsule and tablet. It may or may not be scored.
compound	Medication consisting of a combination of two or more drugs. Each ingredient may be available in one or more strengths. The order will specify the number of tablets. If there is more than one strength, the order will specify the strength.
enteric-coated tablet (Always write out.)	Tablet containing potentially irritating substances and covered with a coating that delays absorption until it reaches the intestine. This protects the oral, esophageal, and gastric mucosa. Should not be crushed, cut, or chewed. *Enteric* should be written out to avoid misunderstanding.
gelcap, soft-gel	Capsule cover made of a soft gelatin for ease of swallowing.
Oral dissolving tablet (ODT)	Tablet that dissolves in the mouth and does not need to be taken with water.
powders and granules	Pulverized fragments of solid medication, to be measured and sprinkled in a liquid or a food such as applesauce or cereal.
scored tablet	Tablets scored with a dividing line that may be cut in half.
supp: suppository	Medication distributed in a glycerin-based vehicle for insertion into the rectum, vagina, or urethra and absorbed systemically.
tab: tablet	Medication combined with a powder compressed into small round and other shapes.
ung: ointment	Medication contained within a semisolid petroleum or cream base.
CD: controlled-dose (sustained action)	Terms reflecting the use of various processing methods to extend or delay the release and absorption of the medication. They need to be differentiated from a regular form of the same medicine.
DS: double-strength* LA: long-acting SR: slow-release XL: extra-long-acting XR: extended-release	A regular medication may be ordered, for example, every 4 hours. An XR version may be given only every 12 or 24 hours. Some medications, such as Celexa, are marketed in both SR and XL forms.

*Does not mean long-acting or extended-release. However, a DS pill probably will be given less frequently than a "regular" counterpart.

➤ Never crush gelcaps, enteric-coated or other long-acting or slow release medications. Only scored tablets should be cut.

1   How is DS different from medications marked XL, XR, CD, and LA?

_____

Q: *Ask Yourself*

A: *My Answer*

Abbreviations and Terms for Solid Medication Forms

RAPID PRACTICE   4-2

Estimated completion time: 5-10 minutes   Answers on page 495

Directions: *Study the abbreviations in Table 4-1. Supply the abbreviation that may be seen in the prescriber's orders for the following types of medication:*

1 capsule _____   6 long-acting _____

2 double-strength _____   7 extra-long-acting _____

3 extended-release _____   8 enteric _____

4 suppository _____   9 controlled dose (sustained action) _____

5 tablet _____   10 ointment _____

Solid Medication Forms

Estimated completion time 5-10 minutes   Answers on page 495

Directions: *Study the abbreviations in Table 4-1. Give the requested information pertaining to oral medication forms. Use brief phrases.*

1   Name the only oral medication form that may be *cut* in order to give a half-serving. _____

2   What is the abbreviation for the kind of oral medication that is packaged in a soft or hard gelatin covering? _____

3   Name two solid medication forms that should never be crushed or cut.
_____

4   What is the name for a medication that contains more than one drug, will be ordered by the *quantity* to be given, and may include the strength of each medication within the form supplied? _____

5   Give five abbreviations for *longer-acting* oral medications that would be given less often than a regular medication. _____

Liquid Drug Forms

Liquid drug forms are packaged in small prefilled unit-dose-serving containers and larger stock bottles, such as the containers seen for multidose home prescriptions. The liquids are supplied and administered through a variety of routes to the patient in an amount of *milliliters.*

Liquid drug forms are administered using specially calibrated equipment: cups; teaspoons; needles attached to tubing; syringes with needles; needle-less syringes; droppers for the mouth, eye, or ear; or tubes for the stomach and intestine. See Figures 4-5 and 4-6 for some examples of oral liquid medication equipment.

Doses of oral liquid medications such as milk of magnesia (MOM) can be supplied in small single-dose packages or larger multidose bottles. As stated in Chapter 3, 5 mL and 15 mL are the equivalents of 1 calibrated teaspoon and 1 calibrated tablespoon, respectively. The manufacturer attempts to provide the usual drug dose for the target population within those two measurements because they are reasonable volumes to swallow.

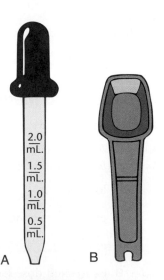

FIGURE 4-5 A, Medicine dropper. **B,** Measuring teaspoon. (From Clayton BD, Stock YN, Cooper S: *Basic pharmacology for nurses,* ed. 15, St. Louis, 2010, Mosby.)

Abbreviations appear in most patients' orders and medication records. They may be handwritten or printed. Memorize the abbreviations in Table 4-2.

➤ Manufacturer-supplied equipment provides precise dose measurement.

TABLE 4-2	Liquid Medication Forms
Abbreviation: Term	**Form**
aq: aqueous	Medication supplied in a water-based solution
elix: elixir	Liquid medication sweetened with alcohol, e.g., elixir terpin hydrate (ETH), a cough medicine
emul: emulsion	A mixture of two liquids, such as oil and water, that normally do not mix
fld: fluid	Of liquid composition
gtt	gtt is an old abbreviation derived from Latin meaning drop. Recognize it but do not write it. Write out "drop(s)."
mixt: mixture	Compound medicine consisting of more than one liquid medication
sol: solution	Water-based liquid medication
susp: suspension	Solid particles mixed in liquid that must be gently but thoroughly mixed immediately before administration; should not be shaken vigorously

➤ Liquid forms such as elixirs and suspensions cannot be distinguished without reading the label.

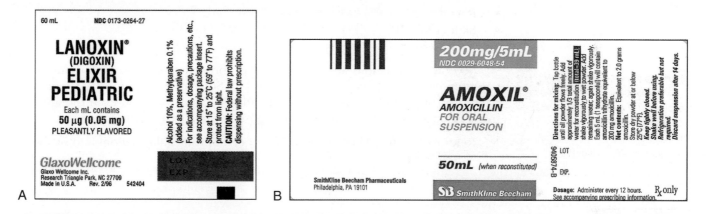

Liquid Medication Abbreviations

RAPID PRACTICE 4-4

Estimated completion time: 5-10 minutes **Answers on page 496**

Directions: *Study Table 4-2 and supply the abbreviations requested if approved. If recommended, write out the term.*

Liquid Type	Abbreviation
1 Suspension	_____
2 Mixture	_____
3 Solution	_____
4 Elixir	_____
5 Aqueous	_____

1 Which of the oral liquid drug forms contains alcohol?

_____

Q: *Ask Yourself*

A: *My Answer*

2   Which of the liquid drug forms must be gently and thoroughly mixed before administration?

_____

Medication Routes

Medication routes can be divided into two types:

*   Nonparenteral (noninjectable)
*   Parenteral (injectable)

➤   The nurse may *not* substitute a different route for the one ordered. Only the prescriber can write and change the medication order.

Nonparenteral routes through which medications are delivered include the following:

*   Oral
    *   Mouth
    *   Buccal and sublingual
*   Nasogastric
*   Enteric (intestinal)
*   Eye and ear
*   Gastric
*   Rectal
*   Skin (topical)
*   Vaginal

Several abbreviations are used in medication orders to describe specific nonparenteral routes of administration (Table 4-3). Some of these abbreviations are derived from Latin and Greek. The abbreviations must be learned even though the trend is to write more of them out in English to avoid misinterpretation.

➤   Refer to pp. 102-103 for the ISMP list of error-prone abbreviations and symbols.

<table>
<tr><td>✳ **Mnemonic**</td></tr>
<tr><td>Associate *O* with *oral* and *N* with *nothing* or *no*. (*NPO* is the abbreviation for the Latin phrase *non per os*, meaning "*nothing by mouth*.")</td></tr>
</table>

TABLE 4-3	Nonparenteral Medication Routes
Abbreviation or Term	**Route**
Ear and eye (write out)	Right ear or eye
Ear and eye (write out)	Left ear or eye
Ear and eye (write out)	Both ears or eyes
buccal (bucc)	To be dissolved in the cheek, not swallowed
enteric (write out)	Administered through a tube or port to the small intestine
GT	Gastrostomy tube; given through a tube or port directly to the stomach
MDI	Metered dose inhaler
NG (T)	Nasogastric; given through a tube inserted in the nose to the stomach
NPO	Nothing by mouth
PO	Given by mouth
Rectal	Write "per rectum"; do not write "PR"
SL, subl	Sublingual, meaning "under the tongue"; to be dissolved, not swallowed
Top	Topical, meaning "applied to the skin" (e.g., ointments and lotions)
Vag	Given per vagina

1   What is the difference between NPO and PO?

_____

2   What is the difference between the buccal and sublingual routes?

_____

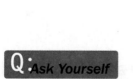

> **FAQ** | _What is an example of the kind of error that can occur from administering medication via the wrong route?_
>
> **ANSWER** | A student nurse did not interpret the route GT for a medication. The patient was acutely ill and had a gastric tube as well as a tracheotomy tube. The student administered the medication without supervision into the tracheotomy tube. The tracheotomy tube is an airway tube, and the liquid medication went into the patient's lungs.

Nonparenteral Routes

RAPID PRACTICE **4-5**

Estimated completion time: 5-10 minutes   Answers on page 496

Directions: _Study the nonparenteral routes. Supply the abbreviation for the route in the space provided. If an abbreviation is not recommended, write out the term._

1   cheek _____

2   sublingual _____

3   nasogastric _____

4   left ear _____

5   gastric tube _____

6   topical _____

7   by mouth _____

8   metered dose inhaler _____

9   vaginal _____

10   nothing by mouth _____

1   What cue will help you remember that _PO_ means "by mouth"?

_____

2   How will you distinguish _subl_ and _subcut_?

_____

3   How will you distinguish _GT_ and _NGT_?

_____

The routes listed in Table 4-4 are for parenteral, or injectable, medications. Parenteral medications are administered under the skin into soft tissue, muscle, vein, or spinal cord. Memorize the abbreviations and terms in the table.

4   Why should the route for rectal medications be spelled out rather than abbreviated with the letter _R_?

_____

5   How will you distinguish _IV, IVP,_ and _IVPB_?

_____

6   What is the abbreviation for the intramuscular route?

_____

TABLE 4-4	Parenteral Medication Routes
Abbreviation or Term	**Route**
epidural	Injected into the epidural space, usually in the lumbar region
hypo	Hypodermic; injected under the skin; refers to subcutaneous and intramuscular routes
ID	Intradermal; given under the skin in the layer just below epidermis (e.g., skin test)*
IM	Intramuscular, intramuscularly; given into the muscle layer, usually the gluteal muscles, the thigh, or the deltoid
intrathecal	Given into the spinal canal
IV	Intravenous, intravenously; given into vein
IVPB	Intravenous piggyback; given into vein via a small container attached to an established intravenous line.
subcut†	Subcutaneous, subcutaneously; given beneath the skin, usually into the fat layer of abdomen, upper arm, or thigh
PN	Parenteral nutrition; nutritional feedings per intravenous line into a large vein

*Do not confuse ID route with the word "identify."
†Do not write SC or Subc for subcutaneous.

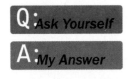

7 What is the abbreviation for the intradermal route?

_____

8 What is the abbreviation for metered dose *inhaler?*

_____

9 What kind of solution is PN?

_____

Frequency and Times of Medication

> **Mnemonic**
>
> tid (three times daily)—"tricycle"
> bid (two times daily)—"bicycle"

Table 4-5 lists abbreviations for terms that denote the frequency and times of medication administration. Memorize the abbreviations in the table.

➤ "Give with food" and "Give after meals" are usually orders for medications that irritate the gastric mucosa.

Refer to the TJC "Do Not Use" list on p. 101.
Refer to the ISMP List of Error-Prone Abbreviations, Symbols, and Dose Designations on pp. 102-103.

➤ "Give 1 hour before meals" and "Give 2 hours after meals" are orders for medications that have reduced absorption if given with food.

1 How will you remember to distinguish the abbreviations for *before* and *after* meals?

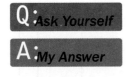

_____

TABLE 4-5 Medication Frequency and Time

Abbreviation or Term	Meaning
ā or a	Before
p̄	After
c̄	With (e.g., with meals)
s̄	Without
ac	Before meals
pc	After meals
ad lib	Give as desired; pertains to fluids and activity, *not* to medication
bid	Two times a day
tid	Three times a day
qid	Four times a day
on call	Give the medication when the x-ray department or the operating room (OR) calls for the patient
prn	As needed
q	Each, every
qh	Every hour
q2h	Every 2 hours
q4h	Every 4 hours
q6h	Every 6 hours
q8h	Every 8 hours
q12h	Every 12 hours
qhs	Every night at bedtime
stat	Immediately and only one dose

TABLE 4-6 The Joint Commission Official "Do Not Use" List

Do Not Use	Potential Problem	Use Instead
U (unit)	Mistaken for "O" (zero), the number "4" (four) or "cc"	Write "unit"
IU (International Unit)	Mistaken for IV (intravenous) or the number 10 (ten)	Write "International Unit"
Q.D., QD, q.d., qd (daily)	Mistaken for each other	Write "daily"
Q.O.D., QOD, q.o.d., qod (every other day)	Period after the Q mistaken for "I" and the "O" mistaken for "I"	Write "every other day"
Trailing zero (X.0 mg)†	Decimal point is missed	Write X mg
Lack of leading zero (.X mg)		Write 0.X mg
MS	Can mean morphine sulfate or magnesium sulfate	Write "morphine sulfate"
MSO_4 and $MgSO_4$	Confused for one another	Write "magnesium sulfate"

Additional Abbreviations, Acronyms and Symbols
(For possible future inclusion in the Official "Do Not Use" List)

Do Not Use	Potential Problem	Use Instead
> (greater than)	Misinterpreted as the number "7" (seven) or the letter "L"	Write "greater than"
< (less than)	Confused for one another	Write "less than"
Abbreviations for drug names	Misinterpreted due to similar abbreviations for multiple drugs	Write drug names in full
Apothecary units	Unfamiliar to many practitioners. Confused with metric units	Use metric units
@	Mistaken for the number "2" (two)	Write "at"
cc	Mistaken for U (units) when poorly written	Write "mL" or "ml" or "milliliters" ("mL" is preferred)
μg	Mistaken for mg (milligrams) resulting in one thousand-fold overdose	Write "mcg" or "micrograms"

Copyright The Joint Commission, 2010. Reprinted with permission.
*Applies to all orders and all medication-related documentation that is handwritten (including free-text computer entry) or on pre-printed forms.
†Exception: A "trailing zero" may be used only where required to demonstrate the level of precision of the value being reported, such as for laboratory results, imaging studies that report size of lesions, or catheter/tube sizes. It may not be used in medication orders or other medication-related documentation.

| TABLE 4-7 | ISMP's List of Error-Prone Abbreviations, Symbols, and Dose Designations |

Dose Designations and Other Information	Intended Meaning	Misinterpretation	Correction
Drug name and dose run together (especially problematic for drug names that end in "l" such as Inderal40 mg; Tegretol300 mg)	Inderal 40 mg Tegretol 300 mg	Mistaken as Inderal 140 mg Mistaken as Tegretol 1300 mg	Place adequate space between the drug name, dose, and unit of measure
Numerical dose and unit of measure run together (e.g., 10mg, 100mL)	10 mg 100 mL	The "m" is sometimes mistaken as a zero or two zeros, risking a 10- to 100-fold overdose	Place adequate space between the dose and unit of measure
Abbreviations such as mg. or mL. with a period following the abbreviation	mg mL	The period is unnecessary and could be mistaken as the number 1 if written poorly	Use mg, mL, etc. without a terminal period
Large doses without properly placed commas (e.g., 100000 units; 1000000 units)	100,000 units 1,000,000 units	100000 has been mistaken as 10,000 or 1,000,000; 1000000 has been mistaken as 100,000	Use commas for dosing units at or above 1,000, or use words such as 100 "thousand" or 1 "million" to improve readability

Drug Name Abbreviations	Intended Meaning	Misinterpretation	Correction
ARA A	vidarabine	Mistaken as cytarabine (ARA C)	Use complete drug name
AZT	zidovudine (Retrovir)	Mistaken as azathioprine or aztreonam	Use complete drug name
CPZ	Compazine (prochlorperazine)	Mistaken as chlorpromazine	Use complete drug name
DPT	Demerol-Phenergan-Thorazine	Mistaken as diphtheria-pertussis-tetanus (vaccine)	Use complete drug name
DTO	Diluted tincture of opium, or deodorized tincture of opium (Paregoric)	Mistaken as tincture of opium	Use complete drug name
HCl	hydrochloric acid or hydrochloride	Mistaken as potassium chloride (The "H" is misinterpreted as "K")	Use complete drug name unless expressed as a salt of a drug
HCT	hydrocortisone	Mistaken as hydrochlorothiazide	Use complete drug name
HCTZ	hydrochlorothiazide	Mistaken as hydrocortisone (seen as HCT250 mg)	Use complete drug name
MgSO4*	magnesium sulfate	Mistaken as morphine sulfate	Use complete drug name
MS, MSO4*	morphine sulfate	Mistaken as magnesium sulfate	Use complete drug name
MTX	methotrexate	Mistaken as mitoxantrone	Use complete drug name
PCA	procainamide	Mistaken as patient controlled analgesia	Use complete drug name
PTU	propylthiouracil	Mistaken as mercaptopurine	Use complete drug name
T3	Tylenol with codeine No. 3	Mistaken as liothyronine	Use complete drug name
TAC	triamcinolone	Mistaken as tetracaine, Adrenalin, cocaine	Use complete drug name
TNK	TNKase	Mistaken as "TPA"	Use complete drug name
ZnSO4	zinc sulfate	Mistaken as morphine sulfate	Use complete drug name

Used with permission, Institute for Safe Medication Practice (ISMP), www.ismp.org.
*These abbreviations are included on The Joint Commission's "minimum list" of dangerous abbreviations, acronyms, and symbols that must be included on an organization's "Do Not Use" list, effective January 1, 2004. Visit www.jcaho.org for more information about this Joint Commission requirement.
Permission is granted to reproduce material for internal newsletters or communications with proper attribution. Other reproduction is prohibited without written permission. Unless noted, reports were received through the ISMP Medication Errors Reporting Program (MERP). Report actual and potential medication errors to the MERP via the web at www.ismp.org or by calling 1-800-FAIL-SAF(E). ISMP guarantees the confidentiality of information received and respects reporters' wishes as to the level of detail included in publications.

TABLE 4-7	ISMP's List of Error-Prone Abbreviations, Symbols, and Dose Designations—cont'd		
Stemmed Drug Names	**Intended Meaning**	**Misinterpretation**	**Correction**
"Nitro" drip	nitroglycerin infusion	Mistaken as sodium nitroprusside infusion	Use complete drug name
"Norflox"	norfloxacin	Mistaken as Norflex	Use complete drug name
"IV Vanc"	intravenous vancomycin	Mistaken as Invanz	Use complete drug name
Symbols	**Intended Meaning**	**Misinterpretation**	**Correction**
ʒ	Dram	Symbol for dram mistaken as "3"	Use the metric system
♍	Minim	Symbol for minim mistaken as "mL"	Use the metric system
x3d	For three days	Mistaken as "3 doses"	Use "for three days"
> and <	Greater than and less than	Mistaken as opposite of intended; mistakenly use incorrect symbol; "< 10" mistaken as "40"	Use "greater than" or "less than"
/ (slash mark)	Separates two doses or indicates "per"	Mistaken as the number 1 (e.g., "25 units/10 units" misread as "25 units and 110" units)	Use "per" rather than a slash mark to separate doses
@	At	Mistaken as "2"	Use "at"
&	And	Mistaken as "2"	Use "and"
+	Plus or and	Mistaken as "4"	Use "and"
°	Hour	Mistaken as a zero (e.g., q2° seen as q 20)	Use "hr," "h," or "hour"

1 What is the error on the TJC list, Table 4-6 that can occur with abbreviations beginning with a "Q"?

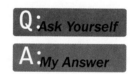

<table><tr><td>Q:</td><td>*Ask Yourself*</td></tr><tr><td>A:</td><td>*My Answer*</td></tr></table>

_____

2 What is the error that can occur with the abbreviation for International Unit?

_____

3 To which kind of specific orders and documentation must the TJC official "Do Not Use" list apply?

_____

4 What does the ISMP List, Table 4-7, recommend about writing of drug names and doses? Numerical doses and unit of measure?

_____

5 What does the ISMP list state about periods following mg or mL abbreviations?

_____

➤ If a medication order contains an abbreviation that has been banned or may be misinterpreted, clarify it with the prescriber. Refer to TJC "Do Not Use" list on p. 101 and the ISMP list of error-prone abbreviations on pp. 102-103.

RAPID PRACTICE **4-6**

Abbreviations for Time and Frequency

Estimated completion time: 10-15 minutes   **Answers on page 496**

Directions: *Study the terms and abbreviations for time and frequency on p. 101. Write in the term or abbreviation requested in the space provided. If an abbreviation is listed as not recommended, write out the term.*

1 pc _____

2 bid _____

3 prn _____

4 s̄ _____

5 stat _____

6 q4h _____

7 NPO _____

8 ac _____

9 c̄ _____

10 ad lib _____

11 with _____

12 as needed _____

13 subcutaneously _____

14 three times daily _____

15 before meals _____

16 each, every _____

17 four times a day _____

18 every 2 hours _____

19 without _____

20 every 12 hours _____

RAPID PRACTICE **4-7**

Terms and Abbreviations for Time and Frequency

Estimated completion time: 5 minutes   **Answers on page 496**

Directions: *Answer the following questions pertaining to abbreviations for times of medication administration in brief phrases.*

1 What commonly used words that begin with *t* and *b* will you use to distinguish the abbreviations for three times a day (tid) and two times a day (bid)? _____

2 What abbreviation would be used if the physician's order indicated to take acetaminophen only *when needed?* _____

3 What would be the *total times* a day a patient would receive a medication q4h? _____

4 How would you interpret the following orders?

   a. Give Tears No More 2 drops in each eye bid prn itching or burning.

   _____

   b. Give antacid Mylanta 1 oz. tid ac. _____

   _____

   c. Whom would you consult if you were unfamiliar with these abbreviations?

   _____

5 If you were going to administer two medications, one four times a day (within 12 hours) and the other q4h (within 24 hours), how many doses would you give of each? four times a day: _____ q4h: _____

△ Cultural Note

Note that there are significant differences in the way abbreviations are used in different countries. In the United Kingdom, *QD* means "four times day." In the United States, *qid* or *QID* means "four times a day."

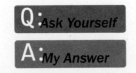

1 Why would it be very important for the nurse to differentiate the meaning of *ad lib* and *prn* in medication orders?

_____

FAQ | *Why are orders written for four times a day versus q6h?*

ANSWER | Many medications, such as a cough medicine, may be given totally within waking hours, such as 0900, 1300, 1700, and 2100. The patient will not have to be disturbed during sleep. Other medications, such as some antibiotics, need to have a more stable blood level concentration to be effective and/or safe and are ordered at equal intervals around the clock, such as q6h, q4h, or q8h.

Abbreviations for Form, Route, and Times

RAPID PRACTICE 4-8

Estimated completion time: 10 minutes **Answers on page 497**

Directions: *Write the medical abbreviation in the space provided.*

1 suspension _____

2 elixir _____

3 solution _____

4 fluid _____

5 fluid extract _____

6 as needed _____

7 nothing by mouth _____

8 intramuscular _____

9 immediately _____

10 apply to the skin _____

Directions: *Write the meaning in the space provided.*

11 bucc _____

12 ad lib _____

13 MDI _____

14 bid _____

15 ID _____

16 prn _____

17 NPO _____

18 IVPB _____

19 on call x-ray _____

20 q6h _____

➤ Look up unfamiliar abbreviations. Contact the prescriber when a banned or unclear abbreviation is used. Do not guess. Document the clarification.

Abbreviations Review

RAPID PRACTICE 4-9

Estimated completion time: 5-10 minutes **Answers on page 497**

Directions: *Write the correct term in the space provided.*

1 SL _____

2 sol _____

3 IM _____

4 DS _____

5 qh _____

6 elix _____

7 q6h _____

8 NGT _____

9 q4h _____

10 NPO _____

11 PO _____

12 GT _____

13 ac _____

14 qhs _____

15 pc _____

16 prn _____

17 bid _____

18 q8h _____

19 tid _____

20 stat _____

➤ Memorize these two important abbreviations seen on medication records:

- NKDA, no known *drug* allergies
- NKA, no known allergies

➤ These are not interchangeable.

The 24-Hour Clock

Most health care agencies use the 24-hour clock. The 24-hour clock runs sequentially from 0001, one minute after midnight, to 2400, midnight. Each hour is written in increments of 100. It is written with four digits, the first two for hours and the second two for minutes.* No number is repeated.

The system is computer compatible and helps avoid the confusion of duplication of numbers (e.g., 1 AM, 1 PM, 12 AM, 12 PM, etc.) in the traditional AM/PM time.

- At 2400 hours, midnight, the clock is reset to 0000 for counting purposes only so that 0001 will be 1 minute after midnight. Examine the preceding illustration of the clock at midnight.
- The AM clock begins at midnight, 2400 hours (12:00 AM), and ends at 1159 hours (11:59 AM).
- The PM clock begins at noon, 1200 hours (12:00 PM), and ends at 2359 hours (11:59 PM).
- Observe the chart again: The major difference from traditional time begins at 1300 hours, or 1 PM. This is when duplication is avoided. Focus on the PM hours.

---

*Seconds may be designated as follows: 1830:20 (6:30 PM and 20 seconds).

12-hr Clock	24-hr Clock	12-hr Clock	24-hr Clock
Midnight 12:00 AM	2400	Noon 12:00 PM	1200
1:00 AM	0100	1:00 PM	1300
2:00 AM	0200	2:00 PM	1400
3:00 AM	0300	3:00 PM	1500
4:00 AM	0400	4:00 PM	1600
5:00 AM	0500	5:00 PM	1700
6:00 AM	0600	6:00 PM	1800
7:00 AM	0700	7:00 PM	1900
8:00 AM	0800	8:00 PM	2000
9:00 AM	0900	9:00 PM	2100
10:00 AM	1000	10:00 PM	2200
11:00 AM	1100	11:00 PM	2300

FIGURE 4-6 Comparison of the 12-hr clock and the 24-hr clock. The 24-hour clock does not use colons or AM and PM. Adding or subtracting 1200 is the constant that converts PM hours between the two systems.

Note: 24-hour time is always stated in hundreds (e.g., "twelve hundred"). Do not say "one thousand two hundred."

1 Can you describe an acute problem that might arise if there was confusion about carrying out an urgent order at "2" as opposed to the clarity of 1400 or 0200 hours?

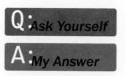

_____

2 If you were going to set your timer for a TV show at noon, would you set it for 12:00 AM or 12:00 PM? Would 1200 or 2400 hours be more helpful?

_____

Remember:

PM Hours	AM Hours
12:00 PM = noon = 1200 hours	12:00 AM = *midnight* = *2400* hours and resets to 0000 hours
1:00 PM = 1300 hours	1:00 AM = 0100 hours

The 24-Hour Clock

RAPID PRACTICE 4-10

Estimated completion time: 10-20 minutes   Answers on page 497

Directions: *Analyze the question to determine whether AM or PM hours are to be identified. Calculate the time using mental arithmetic. Circle the correct answer.*

1 Which is the correct 24-hour clock designation for 1:10 AM?
   1. 0100   **3.** 0110
   2. 1000   **4.** 2110

2 The maximum hour for the 24-hour clock is
   1. 1200   **3.** 2400
   2. 0001   **4.** 2459

3 A medication given at 1:30 AM would be written in the medication administration record (MAR) as
   1. 1300   **3.** 1030
   2. 0130   **4.** 01:30

4 A medication given at 1 PM would be charted in international time as
   1. 1300   **3.** 0001
   2. 1000   **4.** 0100

5 A change of shift at 4 PM would be noted on the MAR as
   1. 0400   **3.** 1400
   2. 4000   **4.** 1600

1 At what time, in 24-hour terms, do you usually wake up, eat dinner, and go to bed?

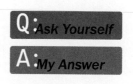

_____

Write all your appointments from now on in 24-hour clock terms, and in a couple of days the time will be automatic for you.

Medication Orders

The following terms and abbreviations may be seen in medication orders and prescriptions:

Abbreviation	Meaning	Example
Rx	Prescription	Rx Sig aspirin 325 mg q4h prn
Sig	Take	Sig aspirin 325 mg q4h prn
TO	Telephone order	TO Dr. Smith
VO	Verbal order	VO Dr Smith

Complete medication orders

In order to be *complete*, a medication order *must be legible* and contain the following elements:

- Patient's name
- Date and time ordered
- Medication name
- Form
- Total amount in strength to be given
- Route
- Frequency schedule
- Additional instructions if needed
- Signature

Sample physician's order sheet

Directions: *See if you can read and translate the orders. Check your interpretation on the next page.*

John Q. Smith   Hospital # _____   **Allergies: NKDA**

Male 45

1/05/11   0900   Ampicillin cap 250 mg PO q6h × 5d
1/05/11   0900   ASA tab 325 mg ent tab PO q4h prn headache $\bar{c}$ food
1/05/11   0900   Compazine SR cap 10 mg PO q12h prn nausea
1/05/11   0900   MOM 15 mL PO hs prn
           1/05/11 William Smith, MD

1/07/11   1000   DC ampicillin
1/07/11   1000   Bactrim DS 1 cap PO stat and daily × 3d
           1/7/11 William Smith, MD

1/09/11   1800   NPO $\bar{p}$ midnight TO Dr. Smith, Jan Brown, RN

1/10/11   0700   Atropine 0.4 mg IM on call OR TO Dr. Smith, Cal Pearce, RN

| Interpretation | No known drug allergies. |

Ampicillin 250-milligram capsule by mouth every 6 hours for 5 days.

Aspirin 325-milligram enteric-coated tablet by mouth every 4 hours as needed for headache. Give with food.

Compazine sustained-release capsule 10 milligrams by mouth every 12 hours as needed for nausea.

Milk of magnesia 15 mL by mouth at bedtime when needed.

Discontinue ampicillin.

Bactrim double-strength capsule by mouth immediately and daily for 3 days.

Nothing by mouth after midnight, telephone order Dr Smith, Jan Brown, RN

Atropine 0.4 milligram intramuscular route when receive call from operating room, telephone order Dr Smith, Cal Pearce, RN

➤ Consult a current drug reference text, glossary, or the pharmacy for interpretation of unfamiliar abbreviations such as ASA (aspirin) or MOM (milk of magnesia).

➤ The nurse cannot give medications more often or earlier than ordered. The prescriber must always be contacted if there is a need to revise the order, such as a need for a prn pain or nausea medication before the prescribed interval.

➤ When orders are handwritten, capitalization, periods, and decimal guidelines are often obscured or ignored. Be very careful with interpretation of handwritten orders.

Interpreting Labels and Orders

Medication labels must be read carefully and compared with the prescriber's order before preparing a medication. Many drug names look and sound alike, for example, Flonase and FluMist; dopamine and dobutamine, prednisone and prednisolone; digoxin and digitoxin; phentermine and phentolamine; and Norcet and Nordette, to name a few. Analyze the contents, abbreviations, and *differences* among the labels for solid and liquid medications shown in this section.

Most of the information on a medication label is self-explanatory if one understands metric measurements and abbreviations. The unit dose concentration is usually specified in milligrams per tablet or capsule for *solid* forms and micrograms or milligrams per milliliter(s) for *liquid* forms.

➤ Key pieces of information are used in all medication calculations:

1 Ordered dose

2 Drug concentration (on the label)

➤ Misreading a label usually results in a medication error. Accurate medication administration is the responsibility of the nurse.

The nurse focuses on the order in the medical record and on the label. For example,

Order: Principen 250 mg cap PO tid

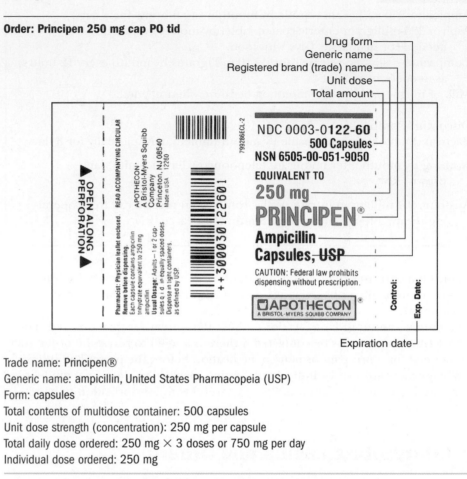

Trade name: Principen®
Generic name: ampicillin, United States Pharmacopeia (USP)
Form: capsules
Total contents of multidose container: 500 capsules
Unit dose strength (concentration): 250 mg per capsule
Total daily dose ordered: 250 mg × 3 doses or 750 mg per day
Individual dose ordered: 250 mg

Note that the drug is contained in capsules. Oral solid drugs are usually placed in some type of *capsule* or *tablet*. Read the cautions; the expiration date; the usual dose, if mentioned; and storage directions, if any. The nurse seldom has access to the multidose container in large institutions. The pharmacy dispenses the individual doses from the multidose containers. The *label* must match the medication *order,* either the trade name or the generic name.

FAQ | *What should the nurse do if the name of the drug on the order is not the same as the name on the label?*

ANSWER | Check carefully to see whether the ordered name is the generic equivalent of the name on the label. The order may be written with either the trade or the generic name. Look in a drug reference. Then call the pharmacy if you are uncertain.

Order: Tegretol susp 100 mg PO bid c̄ food for a patient with seizures

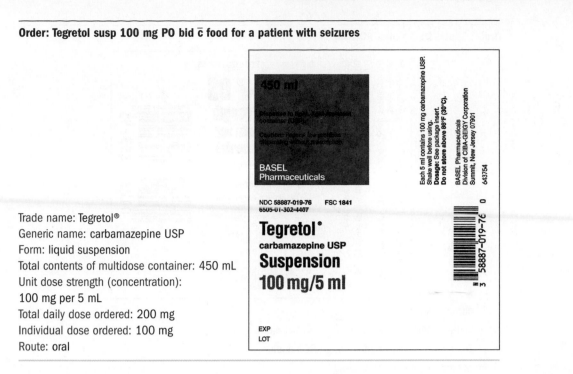

Trade name: Tegretol®

Generic name: carbamazepine USP

Form: liquid suspension

Total contents of multidose container: 450 mL

Unit dose strength (concentration):

100 mg per 5 mL

Total daily dose ordered: 200 mg

Individual dose ordered: 100 mg

Route: oral

1 How large an error would a nurse make who did not read the entire label, assumed that it was a single-dose container instead of a multidose container, and administered the entire contents of 450 mL to the patient?

Q: *Ask Yourself*

A: *My Answer*

Order: ferrous sulfate 648 mg PO bid pc

Trade name: none

Generic name: ferrous sulfate (USP)

Form: tablets

Total contents of multidose container: 100 tablets

Total daily dose ordered: 1296 mg

Individual dose ordered: 648 mg

Unit dose strength (concentration): 324 mg per tablet. Note the apothecary measurement of grains (5 gr). Focus on the metric measurement (mg). Do not use the apothecary measurement.

Order: Septra DS 1 tablet PO daily

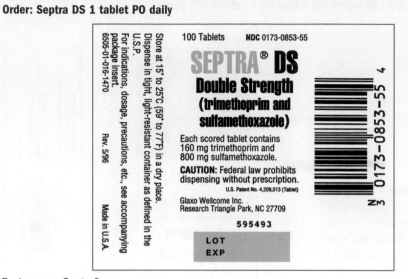

Trade name: Septra®

Generic name: trimethoprim and sulfamethoxazole

Total contents of multidose container: 100 tablets

Form: scored tablet compound drug

Unit dose strength (concentration): double-strength (DS) compound containing two drugs; 800 mg trimethoprim and 160 mg sulfamethoxazole (If a medication has *DS* on the label, it is available in at least one other strength: regular. It is important to read the order and label carefully to find a match for dosage in a regular-strength or a DS order.)

Route: oral*

* When the route is not mentioned on the label of an unfamiliar medication, check the route with a current reference or pharmacy.

Compound medications can be ordered by the quantity (i.e., the number of tablets or capsules, e.g., Septra DS 1 capsule daily). Compound medications are combined in one capsule.

➤ Tablets can be administered through various routes.

Order: Nitrostat 0.6 mg SL q 5 min × 3 prn angina (chest pain). Call MD if relief is not obtained.

Trade name: Nitrostat®
Generic name: nitroglycerin
Total contents of multidose container: 100 tablets
Form: tablet
Unit dose strength (concentration): 0.6 mg per tablet
Route: sublingual SL (or subl)

➤ Sublingual (SL) tablets must be held under the tongue until they are absorbed. They are not to be swallowed nor crushed.

1 What are the key differences among the following terms: total contents, total daily dose, dose ordered, unit dose, and usual dose? (Give brief answers.)

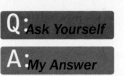

Q: Ask Yourself

A: My Answer

_____

Interpreting Labels

RAPID PRACTICE 4-11

Estimated completion time: 10-20 minutes   **Answers on page 497**

Directions: *Examine the labels provided, and write the requested information.*

1

| DU PONT PHARMA | DUPONT PHARMA **SINEMET®** (CARBIDOPA-LEVODOPA) | 10-100 | NDC 0056-0647-68 3346/7826602 7784/HC |

100 TABLETS

Lot

Exp.

Each tablet contains:
Carbidopa _____ 10 mg*
*(Anhydrous equivalent)
Levodopa _____ 100 mg
Marketed by:
DuPont Pharma
Wilmington, DE 19880
Manufactured by:
MERCK & CO., INC.
WEST POINT, PA 19486, USA

USUAL ADULT DOSAGE: See accompanying circular.

PROTECT FROM LIGHT. Dispense in a well-closed, light-resistant container. This is a bulk package and not intended for dispensing.

CAUTION: Federal (USA) law prohibits dispensing without prescription.

SINEMET is a registered trademark of MERCK & CO., INC.

a. Trade name: _____
b. Number of drugs contained in the tablet: _____
c. Generic names and doses within the compound: _____

2

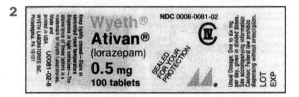

a. Generic name: _____
b. Total number of tablets in container: _____
c. Unit dose concentration per tablet: _____

3

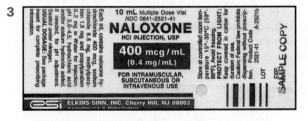

a. Single- or multiple-dose vial? _____
b. Unit dose concentration in micrograms: _____
c. Unit dose concentration equivalent in milligrams: _____

4
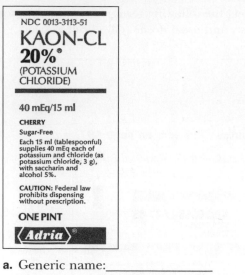

a. Generic name:_____

b. Unit dose concentration:_____

5
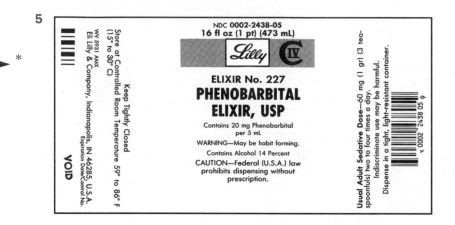

*High alert if prescribed for a pediatric patient.

a. Form of medication: _____

b. Unit dose concentration: _____

c. What percent alcohol is contained in this medicine? _____

Note: The red flag icon used throughout this text is a visual reminder of high-alert medications that may cause significant harm if used in error. See Appendix B.

Q: Ask Yourself

A: My Answer

1   What is the *amount* of difference between a microgram and a milligram?

_____

Calculating Dose Based on Label and Order Information

Interpreting orders and labels provides the information for dose calculation, mental arithmetic, and/or DA equations.

Remember:

The prescribed dose ordered (a given quantity) and the unit dose concentration on the label are two factors that must be entered in *every medication dose* calculation. Other entries in the calculation are conversion factors as needed.

- The desired answer unit will almost always contain tablets, capsules, or milliliters.
- The drug concentration, often will be placed in the first conversion formula, step 2, in fraction form, just as were entered in fraction form in earlier DA-style equations.
- The given factors to be converted will be the prescriber's original ordered drug and quantity.

EXAMPLES

Ordered: (a dose) of aspirin (ASA) 0.65 g q 4 h prn headache.
Available: Unit dose concentration on label: 325 mg per tablet (1 tablet = 325 mg)
How many tablets will you give (per dose)?
Conversion factor: 1000 mg = 1 g.

Step 1	:	Step 2	×	Step 3		=	Answer
Desired Answer Units	:	Starting Factor	×	Given Quantity and Conversion Factor(s)		=	Estimate, Multiply, Evaluate

$$\frac{\text{tablets}}{\text{dose}} : \frac{1 \text{ tab}}{325 \text{ mg}} \times \frac{1000 \text{ mg}}{1 \text{ g}} \times \frac{0.65 \text{ g}}{\text{dose}} = \frac{650 \text{ tabs}}{325} = 2 \text{ tabs per dose}$$

Answer: 2 tabs per dose

The final equation will be written like this:

$$\frac{\text{tablets}}{\text{dose}} : \frac{1 \text{ tab}}{325 \text{ mg}} \times \frac{1000 \text{ mg}}{1 \text{ g}} \times \frac{0.65 \text{ g}}{\text{dose}} = \frac{650 \text{ tabs}}{325} = 2 \text{ tabs of aspirin per dose}$$

Analysis: The starting factor must contain "tablets in the numerator." This will be found on the medication label (see below) as will the concentration (325 mg) per tablet. The accompanying 325 mg concentration must be entered in the denominator as shown. They "go together."

The rest of the desired answer "per dose" will need to appear in a later denominator to match the desired answer position.

The ordered units (g) do not match the units in the container on hand (mg). A conversion factor changes grams to milligrams (1000 mg = 1 g).

➤ The medication may be ordered every 4 hours but you only give one dose at a time!

Evaluation: Only tablets per dose remain. The estimate of two tablets supports the answer (Math check: 100 × 0.65 ÷ 325 = 2). The equation is balanced.

Note: Equations for medications need to differentiate orders per dose, per day, per hr, etc.

Note: The equation entry pattern from left to right—the label concentration, conversion factor if needed, and the order—works well with oral and injectable medication orders.

Reminder: The goal of DA is to multiply a known quantity (the ordered dose) by one or more conversion factors to solve an equation.

1 What are the additional factors that may need to be added if the units ordered and supplied do not match?

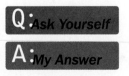

Q: Ask Yourself

A: My Answer

_____

CLINICAL
RELEVANCE

Some unofficial abbreviations for medications will be seen with clinical experience, for example:

Aspirin (ASA for its chemical name: acetylsalicylic acid)

Penicillin (PCN)

Codeine (Cod)

➤ These are given so often that they are abbreviated. There have been recommendations to ban the use of abbreviations for names of medicines.

FAQ | *Why isn't the medication administered in milligrams?*

ANSWER | When all the calculations are completed, the correct amount of medication is given in the form of solids or liquids (e.g., 1 or 2 tablets or capsules or a number of milliliters).

Drug/Form	Drug/Form	Drug/Form	Drug/Form
1 mg/1 tablet	1 mg/2 capsules	1 mg/1 suppository	1 mg/1000 mL

RAPID PRACTICE 4-12

Order and Label Interpretation for DA Equations

Estimated completion time: 20-30 minutes **Answers on page 498**

Directions: *Examine the example shown in problem 1. Read the order and the label to obtain the answers. Be sure you can read the abbreviations in the order.*

1 Ordered: aspirin tab 0.65 g tid and at bedtime for a patient with joint pain.

N 0047-0606-32

6505-00-153-8750   325 mg.

Aspirin Tablets, USP

Analgesic (Pain Reliever)/ Antipyretic (Fever Reducer)

Directions—Adults: Oral dosage is 1 tablet every three hours; or 1 to 2 tablets every four hours; or 2 to 3 tablets every six hours, while symptoms persist, not to exceed 12 tablets in any 24-hour period, or as directed by a doctor. Drink a full glass of water with each dose. Children under 12 years of age: Consult a doctor.

Indications—For the temporary relief of minor aches and pains and to reduce fever.

Quality Sealed for your protection*

*Do not use if the innerseal over the opening of the bottle printed "SEALED for YOUR PROTECTION" is broken or missing.

1000 Tablets
325 mg (5 grains) each

WARNER CHILCOTT

WARNER CHILCOTT LABS ©1991
Div of Warner-Lambert Co   0606/G022
Morris Plains, NJ 07950 USA

SPECIMEN

a. Identify desired answer units: <u>tablet</u>

b. Identify the unit dose metric concentration : <u>325 mg per tablet</u>.

c. Identify the factor(s) to be converted: <u>0.65 g</u>

d. State the given conversion factor needed: <u>1000 mg = 1 g</u>

e. How often should the medication be administered? <u>3 times a day and at bedtime</u>

f. What is the ordered dose equivalent in mg? <u>650 mg</u>

2 Ordered: cephalexin cap 0.5 g PO q8h × 5 days for a patient with an infection.

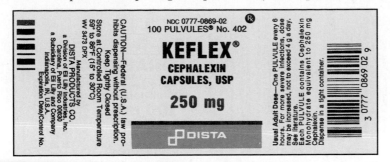

    a. Identify desired answer units._____

    b. Identify the unit-dose concentration to be entered in a DA equation._____

    c. Identify the given factors to be converted. _____

    d. State the conversion factor needed. _____

    e. What is the total daily dose ordered? _____

    f. What is the ordered dose equivalent in milligrams? _____

3 Ordered: cephalexin susp 0.25 g PO q6h × 10 days for a child discharged with an infection

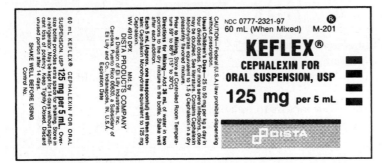

    a. Identify the desired answer units. _____

    b. Identify the unit dose concentration to be entered in a DA equation._____

    c. Identify the given factors to be converted. _____

    d. State the given conversion factor needed. _____

    e. What is the total daily dose ordered? _____

    f. What is the ordered dose equivalent in milligrams? _____

4 Ordered: morphine sulfate 15 mg IM stat for pain.

    a. Identify desired answer units. _____

    b. Identify the unit dose concentration to be entered in a DA equation._____

    c. What is the route ordered? _____

    d. When is the drug to be administered? _____

    e. Three routes by which the label states the drug can be administered:

    _____

5 Ordered: loracarbef susp 0.2 g PO q12h for a patient with a skin infection.

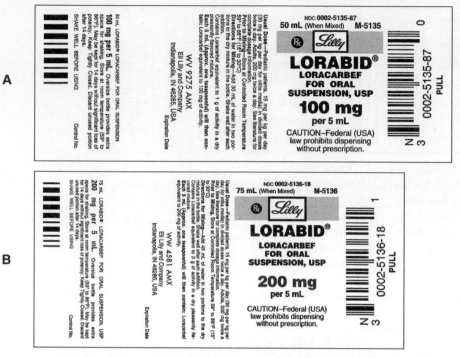

a. What is the generic name? _____

b. What is the form? _____

c. What is the unit dose strength of the medication you would select? _____

d. What are the given factors to be converted? _____

e. What conversion factor would convert the given quantity to the dose supplied?_____

➤ Morphine (see #4) has a C II (Class 2) printed on the label. This means that it is regulated under the Controlled Substances Act, which is enforced by the Drug Enforcement Agency (DEA). There are five classifications or schedules for these drugs. C II drugs have a high potential for abuse but are permitted by prescription for medical use. C II drugs include barbiturates, Percodan, and methylphenidate (Ritalin) as well as other medications.

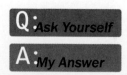

1 Morphine is a powerful opioid narcotic. What would probably happen to a patient if the nurse gave the total contents instead of the unit dose strength?

_____

➤ Do not abbreviate morphine sulfate as MS. It has been mistaken for magnesium sulfate.

➤ Remember that liquid medications are delivered in milliliters. Solid drugs are supplied in many forms, including tablets, capsules, powders, and suppositories.

For reinforcement, the next time you are in a pharmacy section of a store, spend 5 or 10 minutes browsing the cold, cough, and headache medication section and examine the labels. Note the variety of forms and strengths on the labels. Look for the registered sign ®, the generic name, the total dose, and the unit dose on the container. Stores sell drugs in multidose containers so that the customer does not have to return hourly or daily for refills.

Q: Ask Yourself
A: My Answer

1 What are the *sources* of the two key pieces of information that must be entered in all DA equations for medications?

_____

Orders for Two or More Medications to Be Combined

Examine this sample order:

9/9/11 1800	{ morphine 10 mg Vistaril 25 mg }	IM stat and q4h prn pain TO Dr. John Smith, Jane Nurse, RN

Translation:
9/9/11, 6 PM. Give morphine 10 mg and Vistaril 25 mg together, intramuscular route, immediately and every 4 hours as needed for pain, telephone order, Dr. John Smith per Jane Nurse, RN.

Telephone and Verbal Orders

➤ Telephone and verbal orders are reserved for urgent situations and must be countersigned at the next visit or within 24 hours by the person who gave the order. They are strict. Some agencies forbid verbal medication orders.

TJC recommends that telephone orders be written or entered in a computer and then read again to the person who gave the order. Be sure to write the name of the person giving the order. Check TJC and agency policies regarding telephone orders.

> **✳ Communication**
>
> ➤ It is safer to read back and re-state numbers individually, such as "three five zero milligrams" as opposed to "350 mg."

Examples of Orders That Must Be Clarified

Order: Tylenol (acetaminophen) 650 mg PO 2 tablets q4h fever over 38˚C.

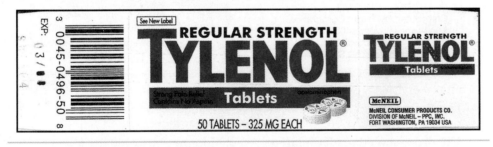

➤ The prescriber wrote "2 tablets." The medication is supplied as 325 mg per tablet. Does the order mean 2 tablets of 650 mg, 2 tablets of 325 mg, or 4 tablets of 325 mg? Guidelines require the total dose to be written. This order is confusing and could result in a toxic overdose. Most medicines are supplied in more than one strength. The prescriber cannot second guess which strength the pharmacy will supply. The nurse cannot guess what dose the prescriber meant.

➤ Clarify unclear dose orders, such as total dose desired, with the *prescriber*.

The order should read: Tylenol (acetaminophen) tab 650 mg PO q4h fever over 38˚ C. The nurse will calculate the number of tablets to give depending on the strength supplied.

Order: Children's Tylenol 1 tsp q4h.

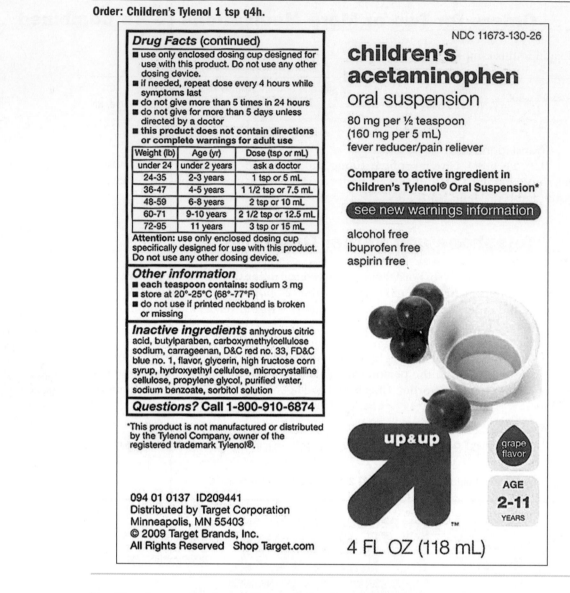

Drug Facts (continued)
- use only enclosed dosing cup designed for use with this product. Do not use any other dosing device.
- if needed, repeat dose every 4 hours while symptoms last
- do not give more than 5 times in 24 hours
- do not give for more than 5 days unless directed by a doctor
- this product does not contain directions or complete warnings for adult use

Weight (lb)	Age (yr)	Dose (tsp or mL)
under 24	under 2 years	ask a doctor
24-35	2-3 years	1 tsp or 5 mL
36-47	4-5 years	1 1/2 tsp or 7.5 mL
48-59	6-8 years	2 tsp or 10 mL
60-71	9-10 years	2 1/2 tsp or 12.5 mL
72-95	11 years	3 tsp or 15 mL

Attention: use only enclosed dosing cup specifically designed for use with this product. Do not use any other dosing device.

Other information
- each teaspoon contains: sodium 3 mg
- store at 20°-25°C (68°-77°F)
- do not use if printed neckband is broken or missing

Inactive ingredients anhydrous citric acid, butylparaben, carboxymethylcellulose sodium, carrageenan, D&C red no. 33, FD&C blue no. 1, flavor, glycerin, high fructose corn syrup, hydroxyethyl cellulose, microcrystalline cellulose, propylene glycol, purified water, sodium benzoate, sorbitol solution

Questions? Call 1-800-910-6874

*This product is not manufactured or distributed by the Tylenol Company, owner of the registered trademark Tylenol®.

094 01 0137 ID209441
Distributed by Target Corporation
Minneapolis, MN 55403
© 2009 Target Brands, Inc.
All Rights Reserved Shop Target.com

NDC 11673-130-26

children's acetaminophen
oral suspension

80 mg per ½ teaspoon
(160 mg per 5 mL)
fever reducer/pain reliever

Compare to active ingredient in
Children's Tylenol® Oral Suspension*

see new warnings information

alcohol free
ibuprofen free
aspirin free

up&up

grape flavor

AGE
2-11
YEARS

4 FL OZ (118 mL)

➤ The dose strength and form need to be specified.

The order should read: Children's Acetaminophen susp 160 mg PO q4h.

RAPID PRACTICE **4-13**

Review of Abbreviations Used for Medication Orders

Estimated completion time: 15 minutes **Answers on page 498**

Directions: *Use brief phrases to describe the hazards of the following types of abbreviations.*

1 How will you distinguish the Latin-derived abbreviation for the word *with* from the abbreviation for *without?*

_____

2 With whom will you consult if the order contains unapproved or questionable unclear abbreviations?

_____

3 What do you think may be some of the safety hazards of TO and VO?

_____

4 If a medication order appeared as follows, would the medications be given separately or together?

[Morphine sulfate 10 mg] ⎫
[Atropine 0.4 mg] ⎭ IM stat

5 How can handwritten abbreviations, numbers, decimals, and slashes result in medication errors?

➤ Do not attempt to interpret incorrectly written or confusing orders. Contact the prescriber promptly.

FAQ | *How do I go about questioning orders?*

ANSWER | ➤ Keep in mind that *only* the prescriber or designated physician can change the order.
There are a few ground rules:

➤ Illegible or incomplete order: be prepared to contact the prescriber.
➤ Questionable dose or total dose unspecified: contact the prescriber.
➤ Form or dose supplied is a mismatch with the order: contact the pharmacy.

An experienced nurse may not find the order illegible or incomplete. Verify all questions with your instructor after investigation. Students need to review the prescriber's recent progress notes, check a current drug reference, and then clarify with the instructor.

➤ Just because someone else has been giving this medication on earlier shifts does not mean that it is right. Decide whether the pharmacy or the prescriber is the appropriate first contact.

➤ Document all clarifications in the patient's record.

✳ Communication

"This is Rose Quartz, RN at General Hospital, Unit 4 A. I'm calling Dr. Doe to clarify a medication order written by Dr. John Doe for patient Mark Smith, aged 60, admitted with appendicitis in room 222." (Read the whole order.) "Please confirm the order for _____ (dose, medication, route, times, etc.). The telephone number here is _____." One more sentence may be added regarding the reason for clarification, for example, "The patient is allergic to _____," "The patient is having difficulty swallowing solids," or "The patient had only been receiving half that dose in the past," and so on.

Medication Administration Records

The MAR is the official record of all the medications given to the patient. It is maintained by the nurses. The forms are usually computerized in large agencies, but some smaller agencies may use handwritten records (Figures 4-7 and 4-8). The MAR must match the original medication orders.

The nurse enters data as *soon as possible* after administering medications so that no other personnel will mistakenly think a medication was not given and give it again. A medication that is ordered but not given for any reason, including refusal by patient, must also be noted on the MAR. The codes for abbreviations on the MAR differ among departments and agencies, but they are similar enough that they are self-explanatory or can be understood after only a few minutes of consultation with the staff.

Mary Laura	GENERAL HOSPITAL	Allergies
ID 13254444		*Penicillin (PCN); Aspirin (ASA)*
Age: 49 Rm 250-B		
Adm. 06/01/11		Today's Date: *6/03/11*

Date Ordered	Medication Dose Rte, Freq	Start Date	Stop Date	1st shift 2400–0659	2nd shift 0700–1459	3rd shift 1500–2359
6/01/11	*Lasix 20mg po daily AM*	*6/01*			(0930) *Xray JP*	
6/01/11	*Humalog 75/25 mix 20 units subcut daily 15 min before bkst*	*6/01*		*0630 MS RA*		
6/01/11	*Digoxin 0.25mg PO daily*	*6/01*			*P=76 0930 JP*	
6/01/11	*Minocin 100mg PO q12h*	*6/01*	*6/05*	*0600 MS*		*1800 LG*

Handwritten MARs may be seen in smaller clinical agencies. They also may be seen on admission until pharmacy computerizes the admission orders. The information contained in MARs is fairly similar. Check agency protocols for data entry requirements. Medications that are withheld typically have the time due encircled with a brief reason for the omission such as NPO, Xray, Lab, or See notes. Some medications such as antibiotics and control drugs have an automatic stop date. Agency policies must to be consulted for those automatic expirations. Take special care with interpretation of handwritten medications and numbers, decimal points and zeros. Also be aware that these records have been hand-copied from prescriber order sheets. Any copying increases risk for error.

PRN and ONE TIME ONLY MEDICATIONS

6/01/11	*Morphine 10mg IM q4h prn pain*	*1400 LJ JP*			

Signature	Init.	Signature	Init.
Mary Smith, RN	*MS*		
John Pauli, RN	*JP*		
Louise Gray, RN	*LG*		

FIGURE 4-7 Example of a handwritten medical administration record for 24 hours day of admission.

| Patient ID stamp
John Douglas
523469
Room 569-A | MEDICATION
ADMINISTRATION
RECORD

GENERAL HOSPITAL | ALLERGIES:

NKDA | |

DATE START STOP	MEDICATION DOSAGE, ROUTE ADMINISTRATION TIME	First Shift 07:00 to 14:59	Second Shift 15:00 to 22:59	Third Shift 23:00 to 06:59
	Ord. 08-01-11 5% Lactated Ringer's Sol. 1000 mL IV TKO at 20 mL/hour continuous			
	Ord. 08-01-11 losartan (Cozaar) tablet 50 mg once daily AM and HS Hold for systolic BP less than 130. Call MD.			
	Ord. 08-01-11 Insulin glargine (Lantus) 20 units subcut. daily at 8 AM Give on time. Record on insulin MAR. Do not mix with other insulins or medications.			
	Ord. 08-02-11 norfloxacin (Noroxin) 400 mg q12h × 3 days STOP 8-05-11 after 6 doses Take with glass water 1 hr before or 2 hr after meals			

This type of a 24-hour printed MAR for routine scheduled medications can be computer or pharmacy generated. It mentions some administration priorities and includes both the generic and the trade name to reduce chance of error. Separate MARs may be used for one-time-only and prn orders (refer to p.138) and certain drugs such as heparin and insulin, which require coagulation or blood glucose assessment prior to administration.

SIGNATURES (FIRST & LAST NAME)	INITIALS	SIGNATURES (FIRST & LAST NAME)	INITIALS	SITE CODES	MEDICATIONS NOT GIVEN
				LU - L Gluteus RU - R Gluteus LT - L Thigh RT - R Thigh LA - L Abdomen RA - R Abdomen LV - L Ventrogluteal RV - R Ventrogluteal LM - L Arm RM - R Arm LD - L Deltoid RD - R Deltoid	NPO - NPO RF - Refused WH - Withheld

A

FIGURE 4-8 **A,** Example of a computerized medical administration record. *Continued*

1   Refer to the ISMP's list of high-alert medications in Appendix B. Are there any drugs there that you recognize? How many on the list pertain to oral drugs?

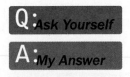

_____

2   What are some of the recommendations made at the top of the list for reducing errors with these medications?

_____

▢ PRN Medication Administration Record

```
                **** PRN ****
     ACETAMINOPHEN 650MG SUPP
   650 MG PR    Q4H PRN PAIN DOC
  DO NOT GIVE > 4000 MG APAP/24H
       * AS NEEDED FOR TEMP
 Start: 9/23      Stop:

        50% INJ 50ML*
     MP   IV   PRN
     PRN BS <70

 Start: 9/23      Stop:

 PURALUBE NP OPTH OINT (LACRI-LUBE) UD
    1.00  OU    BID PRN
       FOR THE EYE

 Start: 9/23      Stop:

 POTASSIUM CL 10MEQ ER TAB (KLOR-CON) UD
    20 MEQ PO    PRN
      MAY GIVE Q8H X 3 FOR K=3-3.4
       OR Q12H X 2 FOR K=3.5-3.8
 Start: 9/23      Stop:
```

RN/LPN SIGNATURE & INIT: _____

Note: The third order states "OU" for route. This is an old abbreviation for "both eyes." Do not use it.
Write "both eyes."
Call pharmacy for clarification of unfamiliar abbreviations.

B

FIGURE 4-8, cont'd **B,** Example of computer-generated medication administration record for PRN medications. (*Example of an unclear order that must be clarified with the prescriber and/or pharmacy.)

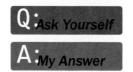

Q: Ask Yourself

A: My Answer

1 What form of medication is the first order? What form of tablet (ER) is the potassium CL in the last order?

_____

Spaces in rows are avoided as each medication order is entered to prevent overlooked medication order errors.

RAPID PRACTICE 4-14

Interpreting MARs

Estimated completion time: 10-15 minutes   Answers on page 498

Directions: *Refer to handwritten MAR in Figure 4-7 to answer these questions.*

1 What are the patient's medication allergies? _____

2 When is the next dose of meperidine for pain available for the patient if needed? _____

3 Which medication must be given before breakfast? _____

4 Which drug was withheld because the patient was in x-ray? _____

5 At what time will a new MAR be used? _____

Directions: *Read the computerized MARs in Figure 4-8, A and B, and answer the following questions.*

6 Does the patient have medication allergies? (See Figure 4-8, A.) _____

7 Which medication order for a tablet is based on a bedside physical assessment? (See Figure 4-8, A.) _____

8 Which prn medication is given per rectum? (See Figure 4-8, B.) _____

9 The prn ophthalmic ointment route uses a "Do Not Use" abbreviation: OU. What action would you take about an unfamiliar or prohibited abbreviation? _____

10 How often may the patient have acetaminophen if needed? _____

You must witness patients taking their medications in order to document on the MAR that they were administered. Often, when administration is unsupervised, medications have been found in the bedding or have gone back to the kitchen on a food tray. Check your agency's policies for any exceptions to this rule.

CLINICAL RELEVANCE

Patients' Rights

Meeting the patient's basic rights makes sense to everyone and is an accreditation requirement of TJC. The process of guaranteeing them involves several steps that must be followed consistently to be permanently embedded in practice. The means to ensure each of these rights and many other rights are addressed throughout the text. Think of *yourself* as a patient as you read the patient's rights regarding medications.

Seven Basic Rights

Right patient	Right route
Right drug	Right documentation
Right dose	Right to refuse treatment
Right time	

Right Patient TJC requires that two methods be used to identify the patient for medications and treatments. Identify the patient by checking the wristband identification number or birth date and asking for the patient's full name. A patient who is hard of hearing may respond to a wrong name. A room number or bed number does not constitute a valid identification. Medication errors have occurred from relying on room and bed numbers as means of identifying patients. The trend is to scan the patient's ID bracelet with a barcode scanner.

Right Drug Name the drug and dose you are administering. Ask the patient and family about allergies or problems with medications. The stress on admission may cause patients to forget some of these details. Mention the class and purpose of the drug. Many patients do not know their medications by name.

> ✳ *Communication*
>
> "What is your name?" is best. Asking, "Are you Mr. Smith?" may yield a "Yes" answer from a confused or hard-of-hearing patient. You need to check the full first and last names.

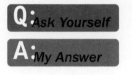

Q: Ask Yourself

A: My Answer

1   Do you think that giving a "look-alike" drug to a patient instead of the ordered drug because the spelling was very similar would constitute a valid legal defense (e.g., AndroGel, which is testosterone, for Amphojel, an antacid)?

Right Dose The dose prepared must be the same as the *ordered* dose. The ordered dose may involve giving 1 to 2 tablets or 1 to 2 unit-dose servings of an injectable or oral liquid. When the dose to be administered exceeds 1 to 2 portions of the unit-dose serving, withhold the medication and promptly recheck the order. Clarify the order with the prescriber. Remember that the unit dose is the usual average dose ordered.

➤   Beware of decimal-reading errors, and look up unfamiliar drugs and doses in current drug references.

Right Time Medications generally should be given within 30 minutes of the designated time. Check your agency policies. The need to give medications on time can present delivery difficulties if the institution schedules all daytime medications at the same time for all patients, for example, at 0900, 1300, 1700, and 2100.

➤   Some priority medications must be given very promptly:

  •   Stat and emergency medications
  •   Medications for acute pain or nausea and powerful intravenous medications
  •   Medications to be taken with meals or before or after meals, such as insulin and other antidiabetic agents

If the nurse is delivering many medications to a group of patients, the delivery schedule must be prioritized. Safe prioritization can be achieved through experience and study. Students need to consult with an instructor and/or clinical mentors.

➤   Ask for help when the medication work load is too heavy to deliver medications in a timely manner.

Right Route Many medications are packaged in several forms: solids and liquid, oral and injectable, or for intravenous or intramuscular injection. The name will be the same, but the forms and routes may differ.

Compare the ordered route with the fine print on the label. Students in particular need to ask for help from the appropriate source when they meet the unfamiliar.

The *route* was not specified in the order. Occasionally, the physician may omit writing the PO route when the medication is a tablet or capsule. That is an error. The front of labels specifies tablets or capsules, but the oral route is not always mentioned on the label. All other routes are specified on the label. Suppository labels contain the words *suppository* and *the route*. It is understandable that some very large pills and capsules might seem too large to swallow, but giving them rectally would not be effective or wise. The form (suppository) of a drug and the route (rectal) must be specified in the order and on the label.

Store refrigerated between 2°-8° C (36°-46° F)
Dispense in well-closed container

NDC 0008-0498-01
6505-01-153-4128   12 Rectal Suppositories

Phenergan®
(promethazine HCl)

12.5 mg

Caution: Federal law prohibits
dispensing without prescription.

W Wyeth Laboratories Inc.
A Wyeth-Ayerst Company

Right Documentation Prompt documentation on the correct MAR prevents duplication errors. Such errors can occur when another nurse gives the medication again because the first nurse did not record it in the right record or in a timely manner.

➤ Document soon *after* medication is given, never *before* it is given. Include drugs that had to be held or omitted.
➤ Remember the cliché, "If it wasn't documented, it wasn't done."

Right to Refuse Treatment Promptly report and document the refusal and the reason given for it. Be sure to include an assessment of the patient's mental status.

Identifying Patients' Basic Rights

RAPID PRACTICE 4-15

Estimated completion time: 5-10 minutes   Answers on page 498

Directions: *Match the nurse action to the letter that corresponds to the appropriate basic patient right:*

Patient's Basic Rights

a. Right patient	**e.** Right time
b. Right drug	**f.** Right documentation
c. Right dose	**g.** Right to refuse
d. Right route	

1 Instruct the patient to hold a sublingual tablet under the tongue until dissolved. _____

2 Check wrist identification band with full written name. _____

3 Give the stat medication within 10 minutes after order is received. _____

4 Compare the order and name of the drug on the label three times before administering it. _____

5 Recalculate and question an order that exceeds 2 times the unit dose supplied by the manufacturer and pharmacy. _____

6 The patient refuses to swallow the ordered medications. _____

7 Record medication administration promptly on the MAR. _____

➤ Write out the seven basic patient's rights in abbreviated form.

_____

_____

CHAPTER 4 MULTIPLE-CHOICE REVIEW

Estimated completion time: 10-15 minutes   Answers on page 499

Direction: *Circle the correct answer. Consult Chapter 2 if necessary.*

1 Which is the correct interpretation for the following physician's order: Amphojel antacid 15 mL tid pc and hs?

1. Amphojel 15 mL 3 times a day after meals and at bedtime
2. Amphojel 15 mg twice a day before meals and at bedtime
3. Amphojel 15 mL twice a day before meals and at bedtime
4. Amphojel 15 mL 4 times a day after meals and at bedtime

2 Which is the correct interpretation for the following physician's order: ampicillin 500 mg IM stat and q8h?

1. Ampicillin 500 mg intramuscular whenever necessary and three times a day
2. Ampicillin 0.5 g intramuscular immediately and every 8 hours
3. Ampicillin 500 mg intravenously and every 8 hours
4. Ampicillin 500 mg intramuscularly at discharge and every 8 hours

3 What is the correct interpretation for the following abbreviations: *tid ac*?

1. Twice a day after meals and periodically
2. Twice a day before meals and periodically
3. Three times a day before meals
4. Three times a day after meals

4 What would be the appropriate interpretation for the following order: morphine sulfate 10 mg IM stat?

1. Give morphine sulfate 10 mg IM when needed
2. Give morphine sulfate 10 mg IM as desired
3. Give morphine sulfate 10 mg on call to x-ray
4. Give morphine sulfate 10 mg IM immediately

5 How would you interpret the following order: NPO p midnight?

1. May not eat after 1200
2. Nothing by mouth after 2400 hours
3. No physical activity after midnight
4. Do not wake after midnight

6 What would be an appropriate schedule for the following order: 8 oz H_2O q6h?

   1. 0800, 1400, 2000, and 0200
   2. 0900, 1300, 1700, and 2100
   3. 0900, 1300, 1700, 2100, 0100, and 0500
   4. 0800, 1200, 1800, and 2400

7 How would you interpret the following 24-hour time in standard time: 0001 and 1425?

   1. 1 AM and 4:25 PM
   2. 1 PM and 2:25 AM
   3. 12:01 AM and 2:25 PM
   4. 12:01 PM and 2:25 AM

8 How many times a day is a q4h medicine given?

   1. 4
   2. 6
   3. 8
   4. 12

9 How should a suspension be prepared for administration?

   1. Shake well until completely dissolved.
   2. Shake vigorously until completely dissolved.
   3. Administer as supplied without shaking.
   4. Shake gently until completely dissolved.

10 If a medicine was ordered PO and the patient had a GT, what action would the nurse take?

   1. Mix the PO medicine with liquid and place in the gastric tube.
   2. Clarify the route with the physician who wrote the order.
   3. Give the medicine PO as ordered.
   4. Clarify the route with another, more experienced nurse on duty.

Directions: *For problems 11-20, read the labels supplied to obtain the answer. Use mental arithmetic to calculate a dose if requested. Circle the correct answer.*

11 Ordered: Synthroid 0.05 mg for a patient with hypothyroidism.

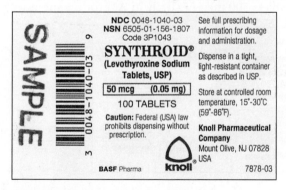

The unit dose concentration is

   1. 100 tablets
   2. 50 mcg per tab
   3. 0.5 mg per tab
   4. 50 mg per tab

12 Ordered: Lanoxin (digoxin) 62.5 mcg for a child with heart failure.

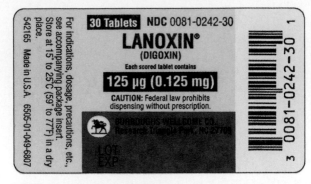

1. You would give 1 tablet
2. You would give $\frac{1}{2}$ tablet
3. You would hold this tablet and clarify with the physician
4. You would give two tablets

13 Ordered: Ery-tab 250 mg q8h PO for a patient with an infection.

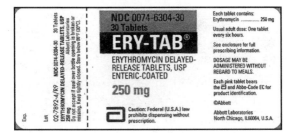

What is the form of this drug?

1. Milligrams
2. Enteric-coated tablets
3. Capsules
4. Double-strength tablets

14 Ordered: Dexamethasone tablets 500 mcg PO daily in AM for a patient with an inflammatory disorder.

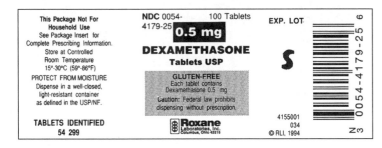

The nurse would administer (use mental arithmetic)

1. 1 tablet
2. 2 tablets
3. 3 tablets
4. 5 tablets

15 Ordered: Percodan 1 tab q4h PO prn severe pain for a patient who is allergic to aspirin.

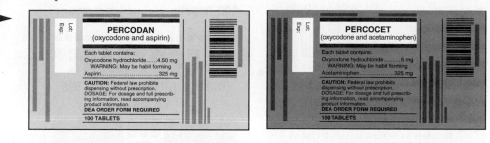

Which action should the nurse take?

1. Give the Percodan as ordered by the prescriber.
2. Give the Percocet because the patient is allergic to aspirin.
3. Withhold the medication and contact the prescriber.
4. Withhold the medication until the prescriber visits the patient.

---

*Always check doses for compound medications such as Percocet and Percodan. They may be offered in different strengths.

16 Ordered: Cimetidine 0.8 g at bedtime daily for an adult with a gastric ulcer.

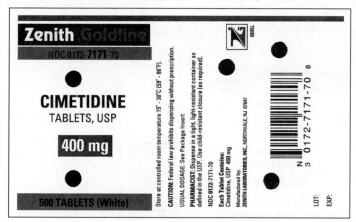

What would be the appropriate complete nurse interpretation?

1. Give 1 tablet daily at bedtime.
2. Give 2 tablets daily at bedtime.
3. Give $\frac{1}{2}$ tablet daily at bedtime.
4. Hold the medication and notify the prescriber.

17 Ordered: epinephrine 1:1000 0.5 mg IM stat for a patient who is having a severe allergic reaction.

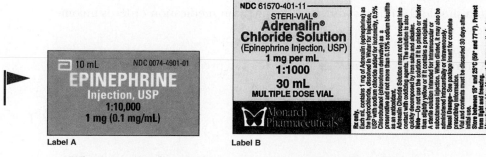

Label A   Label B

Which medication and dose would you select and prepare?

1. Label A and 5 mL   **3.** Label A and 0.5 mL
2. Label B and 0.5 mL   **4.** Label B and 5 mL

18 Ordered: Glucophage 1 g bid with meals for a patient with Type 2 diabetes.

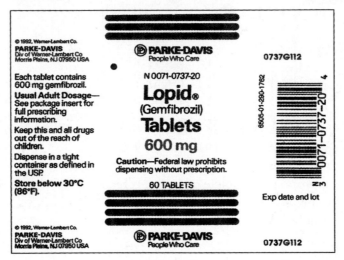

What is the information from the label that would need to be entered in a complete DA equation to calculate the dose?

1. The total amount supplied in the container, the unit dose supplied, and a conversion formula

2. The generic name of the drug

3. The unit dose concentration supplied

4. The ordered dose

19 Ordered: Lopid 0.6 g bid 30 minutes ac for a patient with hypercholesterolemia.

How many tablets would the nurse administer to the patient?

1. 1 tablet   **3.** $\frac{1}{2}$ tablet

2. 2 tablets   **4.** 0.3 g

20 Whom should the nurse consult if a handwritten medication order is incomplete or unclear?

1. The prescriber

2. A nurse who gave the medication during the preceding shift

3. A drug reference

4. The pharmacy

CHAPTER 4 FINAL PRACTICE

Estimated completion time: 10-20 minutes **Answers on page 499**

Directions: *As you read the following paragraph, write out the definition of each italicized abbreviation in the space provided. Reread the paragraph as often as necessary to become comfortable with the abbreviations.*

A patient was admitted to the hospital in a diabetic coma. X-rays and laboratory tests were ordered **1** _____ *(stat)*. The vital signs were assessed **2** _____ *(qh)* and **3** _____ *(prn)*. All of the medications were given **4** _____ *(IV)* because the patient was **5** _____ *(NPO)*. Patients who are in a coma cannot swallow **6** _____ *(PO)* medications. Oral medications and feedings may go into their airways. The patient's mental status was slow to respond to treatment. Feedings were administered via **7** _____ *(PN)* with a tube inserted into the subclavian vein. Later, as the patient began to be more alert, an **8** _____ *(NG)* tube was inserted to deliver liquid food and medications with the patient in an upright position. Insulin was discontinued **9** _____ *(IV)* and given **10** _____ *(subcut)*. The patient still had difficulty swallowing for a while but eventually graduated to sips and chips: sips of water and chips of ice. Because that was tolerated well, the **11** _____ *(NG)*. tube was removed and small **12** _____ *(PO)* soft feedings were introduced **13** _____ *(q2h)* during the daytime hours and fluids **14** _____ *(ad lib)*. The nurse always assessed the patient's mental status and ability to swallow before giving a feeding. Medications for pain were given **15** _____ *(IM q4h prn)*. Rectal **16** _____ *(supp)* were given for complaints of nausea. Medications for coexisting problems were now given **17** _____ *(po)*, such as **18** _____ *(elix* and *susp bid)* because they were easy to swallow **19** _____ *(s̄)* choking incidents. The patient had a history of angina and chest pain attacks and now was able to take nitroglycerine pills **20** _____ *(subl)*. The nurse checked at each visit to find out how many the patient had taken because the physician needed to be called if more than a maximum of 3 tablets, 5 minutes apart, did not provide relief. The nurse knew that all chest pain signals a heart attack unless proven otherwise. The patient did not suffer any adverse drug events (ADE) during hospitalization and was discharged in 10 days.

Directions: *For questions 21-27, state the seven patient's basic rights.*

21 _____

22 _____

23 _____

24 _____

25 _____

26 _____

27 _____

28 Ordered: 0.1 g PO daily of a medication. It is supplied in 50-mg capsules.

How many capsules will you give? _____

29 a. Write the two required pieces of information from the medication order and the label which must be entered in all medication dose calculations.

_____

_____

b. Write the variable piece or pieces of information that may need to be entered in medication dose calculations. _____

30 Ordered: erythromycin 0.5 g enteric coated, delayed-release c̄ food bid for a patient with an infection.

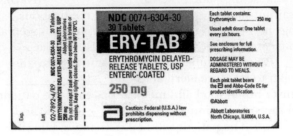

a. What is the trade name of this medication? _____
b. What is the total daily dose in grams and milligrams? _____
c. What is the unit dose concentration? _____
d. How many tablets will you give per dose? _____

Suggestions for Further Reading

Lilley LL, Collins SR, Harrington S, Snyder JS: _Pharmacology and the nursing process,_ ed. 6, St. Louis, 2011, Mosby.

www.usdoj.gov/dea/pubs/csa.html
www.fda.gov/cder
www.health.rutgers.edu/quality.htm
www.ismp.org
www.jointcommission.org/PatientSafety
www.fda.gov/Safety/MedWatch

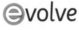volve   Additional information can be found in the Safety in Medication Administration section of the Student Companion on Evolve.

Chapter 5 introduces a large variety of metric medication problems using dimensional analysis to calculate and verify results.

"Perseverance is not a long race. It is many short races one after the other."
—WALTER ELLIOT

5

Solid and Liquid Oral Dose Calculations

OBJECTIVES

- Estimate, calculate, and evaluate a variety of solid and liquid medication doses.
- Calculate dosages for liquid medications to the nearest tenth of a milliliter.
- Measure oral liquids in a calibrated measuring cup.
- Measure syringe volumes in 3- and 5-mL syringes.
- Calculate and evaluate safe dose ranges (SDRs) for medication doses.

Essential Prior Knowledge

- Mastery of Chapters 1-4

Essential Equipment

- Calculator for converting pounds to kilograms and calculating SDR

Estimated Time To Complete Chapter

- 2 hours

Introduction

This chapter builds on prior knowledge to solve many basic and complex medication dose problems using DA, with an emphasis on estimation and evaluation of the answer. Calculations based on weight are included.

Assessments and safety checks are critical before, during, and after medication administration.

It is always helpful to have a simple example in mind to build on for more complex equations. This chapter covers situations involving a variety of orders, medications, and metric units of measurement. Analysis, repetition, and practice are the keys to ease of problem solving.

ESSENTIAL *Vocabulary*

Calibration	Set of graduations that indicate capacity or size in standard units of measure. Measuring devices for precise doses of medications have calibrations, such as the lines on a measuring cup or a syringe.
Concentration, Liquid	Ratio of a specific amount of drug in a specified amount of solution; for example, 10 mg per mL or 5 mg per 5 mL.
Concentration, Solid	Ratio of a specific amount of drug contained in the solid drug form supplied; for example, 50 mg per cap. The concentration of a medication, solid or liquid, is always found on the label.
Divided Doses	Total dose for the day divided by a frequency schedule.

Continued

ESSENTIAL *Vocabulary*

Precise	Having sharply defined, accurate limits based on a standard. For example, syringes, special medication droppers, and teaspoons have precise capacities. Household equipment does not.
Ratio	The relationship between two quantities.
Safe Dose Range (SDR)	Manufacturer's dosage guidelines for minimum and maximum safe medication doses based on laboratory and clinical trials of therapeutic effectiveness. For example, the SDR for aspirin for adults is 325 to 650 mg q4h.

RAPID PRACTICE 5-1

Vocabulary Review

Estimated completion time: 5-10 minutes   Answers on page 500

Directions: *Indicate whether the statement is true or false.*

1 When a reference states that a drug must be given in divided doses, the total dose must be administered in parts at specified intervals during the 24-hour period. _____

2 50 mg per mL refers to the concentration of a drug in solution. _____

3 An SDR specifies the safe minimum and maximum dose for patients. _____

4 The concentration of a liquid is the amount of solution in the liquid. _____

5 The concentration of a medication is always found on the label. _____

RAPID PRACTICE 5-2

Metric Solid Oral Dose Calculations and Review

Estimated completion time 10-20 minutes   Answers on page 500

Directions: *Convert the dose ordered to the desired dose using estimation and mental arithmetic. Verify your answer with calculations.*

Ordered	Dose Concentration Supplied	Amount to Give
1 0.25 mg	0.125 mg per tab scored	_____
2 150 mg	0.1 g per tab scored	_____
3 0.5 mg	0.25 mg per cap	_____
4 125 mg	250 mg per tab scored	_____
5 350 mcg	0.175 mg per tab scored	_____
6 0.5 mg	0.25 mg per tab scored	_____
7 0.1 mg	0.2 mg per tab scored	_____
8 1 g	500 mg per cap	_____
9 2.5 g	1000 mg per tab scored	_____
10 250 mg	0.5 g per tab scored	_____

Only cut scored tablets. Cutting unscored tablets can result in uneven distribution of drug amounts. (In Brown M, Mulholland J: *Drug calculations: process and problems for clinical practice,* ed. 8, St. Louis, 2008, Mosby. Courtesy Amanda Politte, St. Louis, MO.)

➤ To avoid major math errors, make it a habit to estimate the approximate dose before calculations. Recheck orders that exceed one to two times the unit dose supplied.

Ordered: 250 mg.

Available: dose concentration 125 mg per cap.

The nurse can see at a glance that the order is about *twice* the amount on hand. If the numbers do not divide evenly, an *approximate* amount of the unit dose is estimated.

EXAMPLES

Metric Oral Solid Dose Calculations Using Estimation and DA Equations

RAPID PRACTICE 5-3

Estimated completion time: 30-60 minutes   Answers on page 500

Directions: *Review the metric equivalents in Chapter 4. Study worked-out problem 1, and solve problems 2-5. Estimate answers by moving decimals for needed conversions, and verify with a DA equation. Evaluate answers: Is the equation balanced? Does the estimate support the answer? It would be helpful to write out the four steps of the DA equation before proceeding to problem 2.*

➤ Remember that the unit concentration supplied (on the label) and the dose ordered by the prescriber must be part of every medication dose calculation.

1   Ordered: 0.5 g tab PO daily. Label: dose concentration 250 mg per tab.

 a. Metric conversion factor needed: 1000 mg = 1 g

 b. Estimated dose: 0.5 g = 500 mg; 500 mg = 2 × 250 mg, or 2 tab

 c. Amount of tablets to administer:
    DA equation:

$$\frac{tab}{dose} = \frac{1\ tab}{\underset{1}{\cancel{250\ mg}}} \times \frac{\overset{4}{\cancel{1000\ mg}}}{1\ \cancel{g}} \times \frac{0.5\ \cancel{g}}{dose} = \frac{2\ tab}{dose}$$

 d. Evaluation: The equation is balanced. The estimate supports the answer.

2   Ordered: 0.25 g tab PO daily. Label: dose concentration 125 mg per tab scored.

 a. Metric conversion factor needed: _____

 b. Estimated dose: _____

 c. Amount of tablets to administer:
    DA equation:

 d. Evaluation: _____

3 Ordered: 0.1 g tab PO daily. Label: dose concentration 0.05 g per tab.

    a. Metric conversion factor needed: _____

    b. Estimated dose: _____

    c. Amount of tablets to administer:
       DA equation:

    d. Evaluation: _____

4 Ordered: 75 mcg tab PO daily. Label: dose concentration 50 mcg per tab scored.

    a. Metric conversion factor needed: _____

    b. Estimated dose: _____

    c. Amount of tablets to administer:
       DA equation:

    d. Evaluation: _____

5 Ordered: 20 mEq tab PO bid. Label: dose concentration 10 mEq per tab.

    a. Metric conversion factor needed: _____

    b. Estimated dose: _____

    c. Amount of tablets to administer:
       DA equation:

    d. Evaluation: _____

6 Ordered: 0.2 g cap PO at bedtime. Label: dose concentration 100 mg per cap.

    a. Metric conversion factor needed: _____

    b. Estimated dose: _____

    c. Amount of capsules to administer:
       DA equation:

    d. Evaluation: _____

7 Ordered: 250 mg cap PO at bedtime. Label: dose concentration 0.25 g per cap.

   a. Metric conversion factor needed: _____

   b. Estimated dose: _____

   c. Amount of capsules to administer:
      DA equation:

   d. Evaluation: _____

8 Ordered: 0.25 g cap PO tid. Label: dose concentration 125 mg per cap.

   a. Metric conversion factor needed: _____

   b. Estimated dose: _____

   c. Amount of capsules to administer:
      DA equation:

   d. Evaluation: _____

9 Ordered: 0.175 mg tab PO daily. Label: dose concentration 350 mcg per tab scored.

   a. Metric conversion factor needed: _____

   b. Estimated dose: _____

   c. Amount of tablets to administer:
      DA equation:

   d. Evaluation: _____

10 Ordered: 0.1 mg tab PO daily. Label: dose concentration 50 mcg per tab.

   a. Metric conversion factor needed: _____

   b. Estimated dose: _____

   c. Amount of tablets to administer:
      DA equation:

   d. Evaluation: _____

1 What are the two pieces of information obtained from the order and label that must be entered in every dose calculation?

_____

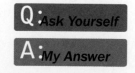

Q: Ask Yourself

A: My Answer

Converting Grams to Micrograms and Micrograms to Grams by Moving Decimal Places

When a problem calls for converting micrograms to grams or grams to micrograms, beginners enter *two* conversion factors in a DA equation: micrograms to milligrams and milligrams to grams, or grams to milligrams and milligrams to micrograms.

Microgram-milligram conversions are frequently encountered in dose calculations. Microgram-gram conversions are occasionally needed in calculations of intravenous doses. Medication errors can occur when the prescriber writes an order in micrograms and the nurse mistakes it for milligrams or vice versa.

Microgram-gram conversions can be reduced to one step if desired by using the conversion factor 1,000,000 mcg = 1 g, since *micro-* means one millionth of the base unit.

EXAMPLES

Conversion factor: 1,000,000 mcg = 1 g.

➤ To convert grams to micrograms, multiply by 1,000,000.
➤ To convert micrograms to grams, divide by 1,000,000.

Ordered		Equivalent	Decimal Movement
0.5 g	=	500,000 mcg	decimal moved six places to the right
250,000 mcg	=	0.250000 g	implied decimal moved six places to the left
0.004 g	=	4000 mcg	decimal moved six places to the right

TEST TIP: If you are comfortable with milligram conversions (milligrams to micrograms and milligrams to grams), use a stepped approach for microgram-gram conversions. First, change the ordered amount to milligrams and then to micrograms.

➤ Converting micrograms to grams and grams to micrograms involves two steps—1000 mcg = 1 mg, and 1000 mg = 1 g—for a total of 6 decimal place movements. It is expedient to study the relationships among the mcg/mg/g conversions at one time.

RAPID PRACTICE 5-4

Moving Decimal Places for Microgram-Gram Conversions

Estimated completion time: 5-10 minutes   Answers on page 501

Directions: *Convert the units ordered to milligrams and then micrograms (or grams).*

Ordered	Milligrams	Micrograms or Grams
1 0.3 g	300 mg	300,000 mcg
2 0.1 g	_____	_____ mcg
3 80,000 mcg	_____	_____ g
4 25,000 mcg	_____	_____ g
5 300,000 mcg	_____	_____ g

Decimal Conversions Using One or Two Conversion Factors

Estimated completion time: 10-15 minutes   Answers on page **502**

Directions: *Make the units equivalent.*

Needed Conversion	Number of Decimal Places to Be Moved	Answer
1 0.3 g = ? mg	_____	_____
2 200 mcg = ? mg	_____	_____
3 0.5 mg = ? mcg	_____	_____
4 15,000 mcg = ? g	_____	_____
5 0.004 g = ? mcg	_____	_____
6 2200 mg = ? g	_____	_____
7 350 mcg = ? mg	_____	_____
8 50,000 mcg = ? g	_____	_____
9 0.05 g = ? mg	_____	_____
10 500 mg = ? g	_____	_____

Metric Oral Medication Calculation Practice

Estimated completion time: 30 minutes   Answers on page **502**

Directions: *Study the medication order and the unit dose supplied. Estimate the answer and verify it with a DA equation. Evaluate the answer. Is the equation balanced? Does the estimate support the answer?*

➤ The desired answer unit is usually found in the available unit dose concentration. How is the ordered drug supplied: in tablets, capsules, or milliliters? That unit will be the desired answer unit for these kinds of problems.

1 Ordered: codeine sulfate 60 mg stat for a patient in pain.

   a. Estimated dose: _____
   b. Actual dose: _____
       DA equation:

   c. Evaluation:_____

2   Ordered: Ativan 1 mg PO prn at bedtime for a patient with anxiety.

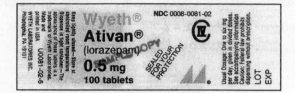

a. Estimated dose: _____
b. Actual dose: _____
   DA equation:

c. Evaluation: _____

3   Ordered: Biaxin 0.25 g PO daily for a patient with an infection.

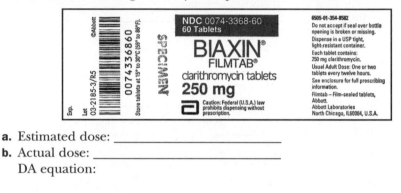

a. Estimated dose: _____
b. Actual dose: _____
   DA equation:

c. Evaluation: _____

4   Ordered: Lopressor 0.1 g PO daily at bedtime for a patient with hypertension (ATN).

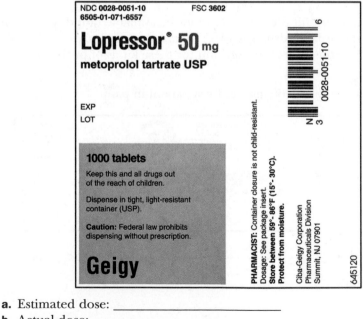

a. Estimated dose: _____
b. Actual dose: _____
   DA equation:

c. Evaluation: _____

➤ To prevent medication errors, always tell the patient and or family the name and dose of the medication being given and recheck when there's a question. Remember that generics are often substituted for brand names.

5   Ordered: clorazepate 15 mg tid PO for a patient with chronic anxiety.

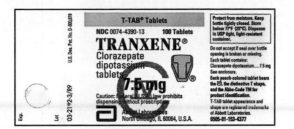

a. Estimated dose: _____

b. Actual dose: _____
  DA equation:

c. Evaluation: _____

Metric Oral Medication Calculation Practice

RAPID PRACTICE 5-7

Estimated completion time: 20 minutes   Answers on page 503

Directions: *Estimate answer and verify with DA equation. Evaluate the answer. Supply needed conversion factors.*

1   Ordered: alprazolam 0.5 mg PO q12h for a patient with anxiety.

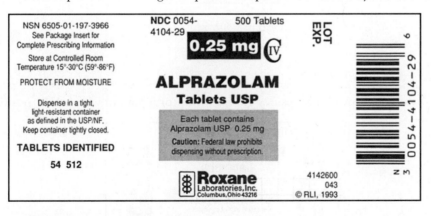

a. Estimated dose: _____
  DA equation:

b. Evaluation: _____

2 Ordered: sulfisoxazole 1000 mg PO tid for a patient with a recurrent urinary tract infection.

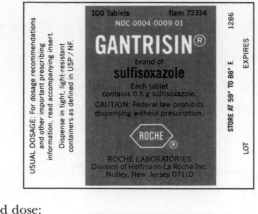

a. Estimated dose: _____
DA equation:

b. Evaluation: _____

3 Ordered: vasotec 5 mg daily at bedtime for a patient with hypertension.

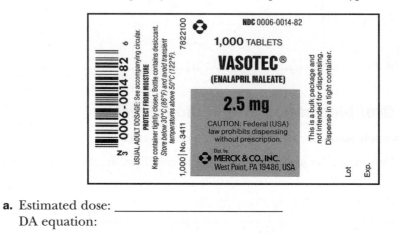

a. Estimated dose: _____
DA equation:

b. Evaluation: _____

4 Ordered: zidovudine capsules 0.3 g PO bid for a patient who is HIV positive.

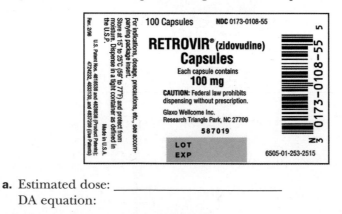

a. Estimated dose: _____
DA equation:

b. Evaluation:_____

5   Ordered: diltiazem HCl 0.12 g PO daily for a patient with hypertension (HTN).

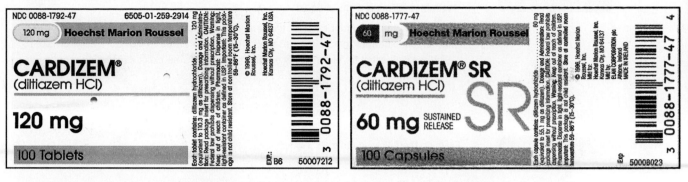

a. Which medication would you select?

b. Estimated dose: _____
    DA equation:

c. Evaluation:_____

Analyzing Liquid Dose Orders

Liquids may be supplied in a variety of containers. As with all dose calculations, the ordered dose and the drug concentration noted on the label must be included in the calculation. Liquid medications *ordered* and *supplied* in milligrams may require a calculation if the dose is supplied in more than 1 mL of solution. The estimate of the answer can be made right away if the metric units are matched. Compare the result with your estimate.

Estimating liquid doses

Ordered: 350 mg PO daily.

Available: dose concentration supplied: 250 mg per 5 mL.

The dose ordered and the drug supplied are in the same terms (milligrams). It is easy to see that the dose *ordered* (350 mg) will be *more than one* but *less than two* times the unit dose concentration supplied (250 mg in 5 mL, less than 2 × 5 mL).

EXAMPLES

Misinterpretation

Loss of focus may cause the nurse to reverse the order with the concentration supplied.

➤ Avoid distractions. Focus on the order in relation to the strength on hand.

Rounding numbers to simplify estimated liquid dose

➤ Rounding up helps the estimation in some instances.

EXAMPLES

Ordered: 300 mg.

Available: 75 mg in 1 mL of liquid

It is obvious that the order calls for *much more* than the unit dose per milliliter supplied. The nurse might approximate the dose by rounding the 75 up to 100 for easier division, giving a rough estimate of around 3 or more unit doses. The exact calculation requires a DA equation.

EXAMPLES

Examine the following order:

Ordered: 200 mg liquid.

Available: 80 mg per 5 mL concentration.

The terms are the same: milligrams. It is obvious that the order for 200 mg exceeds two times the dose (80 mg) per volume on hand. Thus, *the estimate is that more than 10 mL will be given.* Follow the estimate with an exact calculation in a DA equation. Compare the result with the estimate.

➤ Your calculation rounding is based on the measurements of the equipment you are using.

Metric Conversions and Estimating Answers for Liquid Medications

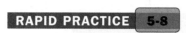

Estimated completion time: 10 minutes   **Answers on page 503**

Directions: *Examine the order and the label concentration. Follow the example in problem 1 to estimate the dose to be administered to the nearest milliliter or number of tablets.*

	Dose Ordered	Concentration Available	Conversion	Give Same, More, or Less of Available Dose per Volume	Estimated Amount
1	0.25 g	250 mg per mL	0.25 g = 250 mg	Same	1 mL
2	5000 mcg	2.5 mg per mL			
3	0.1 g	300 mg per mL			
4	750 mg	0.5 g per mL			
5	200 mg	0.1 g per mL			

CLINICAL RELEVANCE

Liquid unit dose concentrations are often written with a slash (e.g., 100 mg/5 mL). The slash mark (/) appears in printed drug literature for drug concentrations. It should *not be handwritten* in a patient's medical record. The slash can be misinterpreted as the number 1 if it occurs next to a number. For example, 100 mg/5 mL could be read as 100 mg per 15 mL instead of 5 mL. Write *per* instead of using the slash: 100 mg *per* 5 mL. The slash is clearly seen in printed materials.

➤ With oral liquid metric measurements, the final question is usually: How many milliliters should be given?

Setting Up DA-Style Equations for Liquid Dose Calculations

Review: The process required is to multiply a given quantity by one or more conversion factors to solve an equation. The process is the same for a liquid as for a solid.

- The given quantity in medication calculations is the *prescribed order.*
- The first entry in the equation is the *dose concentration on the label with the desired answer in the numerator.*

When ordered dose and available unit concentration match

EXAMPLES

Ordered: Valium 10 mg at bedtime for a patient with anxiety.

Available: Unit dose concentration (on label): Valium 20 mg per 5 mL.

How many milliliters (mL) (per dose implied) will you give?

Step 1	:	Step 2	×	Step 3		=	Answer
Desired Answer Units	:	Starting Factor	×	Given Quantity and and Conversion Factor(s)		=	Estimate, Multiply, Evaluate

$$\frac{mL}{dose} : \frac{5\ mL}{\overset{}{\underset{2}{20\ mg}}} \times \frac{\overset{1}{\cancel{10\ mg}}}{dose} = \frac{5}{2} = 2.5\ mL\ \text{per dose}$$

Liquids are often administered in mL	Label information	Per dose is entered in a denominator to <u>match</u> the desired answer

The final equation will be written like this:

$$\frac{mL}{dose} : \frac{5\ mL}{\overset{}{\underset{2}{20\ mg}}} \times \frac{\overset{1}{\cancel{10\ mg}}}{dose} = \frac{5}{2} = 2.5\ mL\ \text{of Valium per dose}$$

Analysis: This simple equation contains the ordered dose and the unit dose information from the medication label (5 mL per 20 mg or 20 mg per 5 mL). The unit dose information is selected for the Starting Factor and oriented to match up the desired answer units (mL) in the numerator. Per dose is related to the order as well as the answer. No other conversion factors are needed because the order and the label are both mg units. The nurse needs to calculate the individual dose to be given.

Evaluation: Only mL per dose remain in the answer. The estimate to give ½ of the available 5 mL unit dose supports the answer. (Math check: 50/20 = 2.5) The equation is balanced.

FAQ | *What is the most common error seen with liquid dose calculations?*

ANSWER | Sometimes the amount of drug is confused with the amount of solution. For example, *10 mg per 5 mL* means there are 10 mg of drug in *each 5 mL* of solution. The nurse needs to stay focused when doing the math.

When the ordered units do not match the available units

Metric equivalent conversion factor(s) are necessary when the ordered units do not match the available dose concentration. If another conversion is necessary, make room for it before entering the ordered dose.

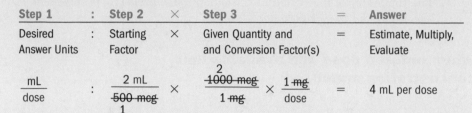

EXAMPLES

Ordered: 1 mg of a medicine.

Available: Dose concentration 500 mcg per 2 mL.

Conversion factor: 1000 mcg = 1 mg

How many milliliters will you give (per dose)?

Step 1	:	Step 2	×	Step 3	=	Answer
Desired Answer Units	:	Starting Factor	×	Given Quantity and and Conversion Factor(s)	=	Estimate, Multiply, Evaluate

$$\frac{mL}{dose} : \frac{2\ mL}{\underset{1}{\cancel{500\ mcg}}} \times \frac{\overset{2}{\cancel{1000\ mcg}}}{1\ \cancel{mg}} \times \frac{1\ \cancel{mg}}{dose} = 4\ mL\ per\ dose$$

The final equation will be written like this:

$$\frac{mL}{dose} : \frac{2\ mL}{\cancel{500\ mcg}} \times \frac{\overset{2}{\cancel{1000\ mcg}}}{1\ \cancel{mg}} \times \frac{1\ \cancel{mg}}{dose} = 4\ mL\ per\ dose\ of\ the\ medicine$$

Analysis: The available dose concentration stated on the label has a numerator and a denominator. This is a conversion factor that can be inverted without changing the value. For every 2 mL there are 500 mcg and in every 500 mcg there are 2 mL. Once again, the selected Starting Factor matches up to the desired answer permitting sequential cancellation.

Evaluation: The ordered information, the unit dose information on the label, and a conversion factor were entered in the correct orientation. An estimate that the answer would be about double the unit dose of 2 mL was made after all the data were entered. The estimate supported the answer (Math check: 2000 ÷ 500 = 4) The equation is balanced.

➤ TIP: The math is very simple if the units and numbers are cancelled.

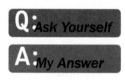

Q: *Ask Yourself*

A: *My Answer*

1 As you look at the previous example, which *three* key pieces of data are entered in the equation?

_____

2 If the units supplied and the units ordered were in the same measurement terms, milligrams, which entry in step 3 could be eliminated?

_____

Usual Unit Doses

➤ Most solid doses ordered are ½ to 2 times the supplied unit dose, such as ½ to 2 tablets or 1 to 2 capsules.
➤ With liquids, check current drug references for the usual dose; the amount can vary.

CLINICAL RELEVANCE

Sometimes a very frail person—a baby or an adult with a very low weight, or a person with a very serious illness—will receive a fractional dose (a very small amount of the unit dose), or because an illness is so aggressive or the person is larger than average, an unusually large dose will be ordered.

➤ Hold the medication, recheck the order, then a current drug reference and promptly clarify unusual doses with the prescriber if there is a question.

FAQ | *Why are DA equations required when the answer can be calculated more simply?*

ANSWER | Safe dose calculations require that the nurse has a solid back-up method for verification and for more complex problems. With repetition and practice, the nurse will find it easy to quickly and independently confirm calculations. It is unsafe to rely on peers who may make a calculation error.

➤ The nurse who administers the medication is legally responsible for that medication even if the order was incorrect.

Calculating Oral Liquid Doses Using DA

RAPID PRACTICE | **5-9**

Estimated completion time: 20-30 minutes   Answers on page 503

Directions: *Estimate, calculate, and evaluate the following ordered doses using DA.*

1   Ordered: cefixime oral susp. 0.2 g q 12 h for a patient with otitis media.

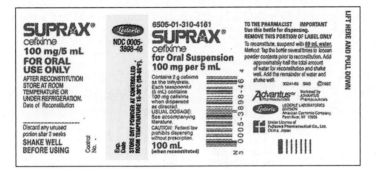

   a. Estimated dose: _____
      DA equation:

   b. Evaluation: _____

2   Ordered: prochlorperazine syrup 8 mg PO stat for a patient with preoperative anxiety.

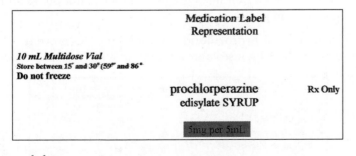

   a. Estimated dose: _____
      DA equation:

   b. Evaluation: _____

3 Ordered: Benadryl Elixir 15 mg PO at bedtime for a patient with skin allergies.

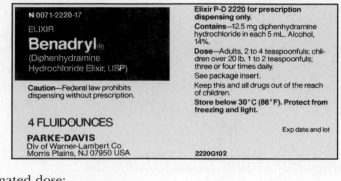

a. Estimated dose: _____

DA equation:

b. Evaluation: _____

4 Ordered: digoxin elixir pediatric 25 mcg PO daily in AM for a patient with an arrhythmia.

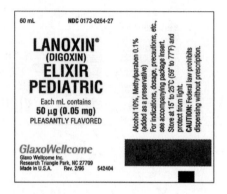

a. Estimated dose: _____

DA equation:

b. Evaluation: _____

➤ Note that the label has μg for micrograms. Write mcg, not μg. Refer to the TJC recommendations on p. 101.

5 Ordered: ondansetron hydrochloride oral sol 6 mg PO prevent chemotherapy-induced nausea and vomiting in a patient with cancer.

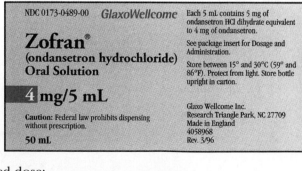

a. Estimated dose: _____

DA equation:

b. Evaluation: _____

Equipment for Administering Oral Liquid Doses

Depending on the medication, a 30-mL calibrated medicine cup, a special medicine teaspoon (5 mL), a calibrated dropper, a calibrated tablespoon, an oral syringe, or a needleless syringe may be selected if the agency does not have oral syringes.

Selecting the implement for oral liquid medications

The implement used to deliver an oral liquid unit dose is selected according to:

1 The amount of liquid to be administered
2 The ability of the patient to drink from a nipple or cup or to swallow from a medication spoon or dropper

Choosing the appropriate implement is not always age-related. Often, the medication is packaged with the equipment to be used, such as a medicine cup, a calibrated dropper, a teaspoon, or an oral syringe.

Many oral liquid medications are delivered in units of 5 mL (1 medication teaspoon) or 15 mL (1 medication tablespoon; Figure 5-1). Medication cups may be used for 5 to 30 mL (1 oz).

Sterile oral liquid medications may be prepared for infants, babies, immunosuppressed patients, and other at-risk populations. The nurse should check agency policies on the use of sterile oral liquid medications.

➤ Nurses do not use household implements because they vary greatly in capacity. Patients must be instructed to use calibrated measuring devices if they will be discharged on liquid oral medications.

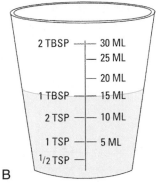

FIGURE 5-1 Medication cups. **A,** Filled to 5 mL. **B,** Filled to 15 mL.

Measuring Liquids

Measuring oral milliliter doses that call for more or less than the calibrated lines on the cup

Measuring oral doses may require the use of a syringe for more precise dosing if the dose is not a multiple of 5 mL. The metric measurements on the medication cups are calibrated in multiples of 5 mL (see Figure 5-1).

Reading Syringe Calibrations on the 3-mL and 5-mL Syringe

➤ The exact amount ordered to the nearest tenth of a mL should be poured. The nurse selects the syringe (Figure 5-2):

Follow these steps to read syringe calibrations on these two syringes:

• Identify the 1-mL marking if present.
• Count the number of lines within 1 mL (10 lines in 1 mL on the 3-mL syringe and 5 lines in 1 mL on the 5-mL syringe). Study Figure 5-2.
• The amount is read at the ring closest to the opening in the syringe (Figure 5-3).
• Locate the amount desired.

FAQ | *May the whole dose be prepared in a syringe and inserted in the cup?*

ANSWER | Yes, the dose needs to be drawn to the nearest tenth of a milliliter. Larger syringes do not have 0.1-mL calibrations. Select the syringe that will provide the nearest measurable dose.

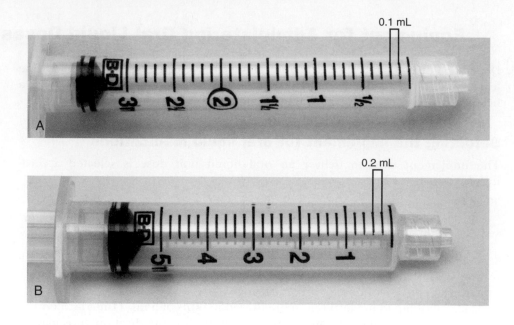

0.1 mL

0.2 mL

FIGURE 5-2 **A,** 3-mL syringe calibrated in 0.1-mL increments. **B,** 5-mL syringe calibrated in 0.2-mL increments.

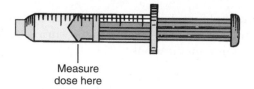

Measure
dose here

FIGURE 5-3 Reading measured amount of medication in a syringe. (From Perry AG, Potter PA: *Clinical nursing skills and techniques,* ed. 7, St. Louis, 2010, Mosby.)

EXAMPLES

Amount to give: Prepare 17.5 mL.

Procedure: Pour to 15 mL and add 2.5 mL with a syringe (Figure 5-4).

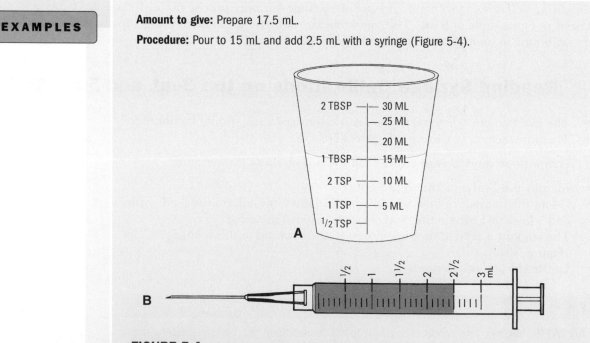

FIGURE 5-4 Total dose will be 17.5 mL: **(A)** 15 mL prepared in medicine cup and **(B)** 2.5 mL precise remainder added with syringe.

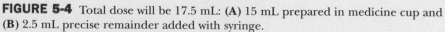

Amount to give: 12.4 mL.

Procedure: Pour to 10-mL calibration and add 2.4 mL with a 3-mL syringe.

Amount to give: 19 mL.

Procedure: Pour to 15-mL calibration and add 4 mL with a 5-mL syringe.

Review the steps:

➤ Pour the nearest measurable dose in a 30-mL medicine cup; when the dose is *not* a multiple of 5, pour the liquid to the *nearest* 5-mL calibration that is *less* than the dose.

➤ *Add* the precise additional amount needed to the *nearest tenth* of a milliliter with a syringe. The top center of the fluid is read at eye level (Figure 5-5).

EXAMPLES

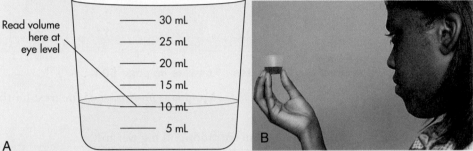

FIGURE 5-5 A, Pour the desired volume of liquid so that base of meniscus is level with line on scale. **B,** Hold cup at eye level to confirm volume poured.

➤ Avoid drawing excess amounts.

CLINICAL RELEVANCE

Measuring Liquid Doses with 30-mL Medicine Cup and Syringe

RAPID PRACTICE 5-10

Estimated completion time: 10 minutes   **Answers on page 504**

Directions: *Given the amount to prepare, state the nearest* measurable *amount to place in the 30-mL medicine cup and the amount to place in the syringe, and state whether a 3-mL or a 5-mL syringe is needed.*

Amount to Prepare	Amount to Place in Cup	Amount to Place in Syringe	Syringe Size (3-mL or 5-mL)
1 6.5 mL	_____	_____	_____
2 14 mL	_____	_____	_____
3 9 mL	_____	_____	_____
4 17 mL	_____	_____	_____
5 27.4 mL	_____	_____	_____

RAPID PRACTICE 5-11

Liquid Doses

Estimated completion time: 20-30 minutes   Answers on page 504

Directions: *Estimate, calculate, and evaluate the liquid dose problems to the* nearest tenth *of a milliliter.*

> ### ✳ Communication
>
> Nurse: "I have your liquid antibiotic erythromycin, Mrs. R."
>
> Patient: "Would you please get me some grapefruit or orange juice to kill the taste?"
>
> Nurse (returns with orange juice or some other alternative): "Would either of these work for you? As long as you're taking this medication, please don't take any grapefruit juice. It can cause very serious problems such as kidney damage. Orange juice is fine though. Do you have any questions?"

1 Ordered: 75 mg. Supplied dose concentration: 50 mg per mL.

   a. Estimated dose: _____
       DA equation:

   b. Evaluation: _____

2 Ordered: 20 mg. Supplied dose concentration: 5 mg per 5 mL.

   a. Estimated dose: _____
       DA equation:

   b. Evaluation: _____

3 Ordered: 35 mg. Supplied dose concentration: 15 mg per 2 mL.

   a. Estimated dose: _____
       DA equation:

   b. Evaluation: _____

4 Ordered: 125 mg. Supplied dose concentration: 75 mg per 8 mL.

   a. Estimated dose: _____
       DA equation:

   b. Evaluation: _____

5 Ordered: 45 mg. Supplied dose concentration: 25 mg per 10 mL.

   a. Estimated dose: _____
       DA equation:

   b. Evaluation: _____

Calculating and Measuring Liquid Dose Orders

Estimated completion time: 30 minutes Answers on page 505

Directions: *Identify and enter all the required elements in the DA equation. Estimate the answer, solve to the nearest tenth of a milliliter, and evaluate the equation. Shade in the medicine cup to the nearest 5 mL, and draw a vertical line through the calibrated line of the syringe for the remainder of the dose.*

1   Ordered: phenobarbital elixir* 25 mg PO at bedtime stat for sedation for an adolescent.

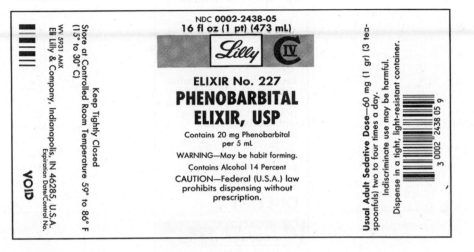

*High alert medication if given to children.

a. Estimated dose: _____
   DA equation:

b. Evaluation: _____

Shade in the dose in mL for the medicine cup and draw a vertical line through the calibrated line of the syringe.

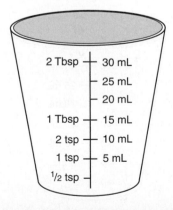

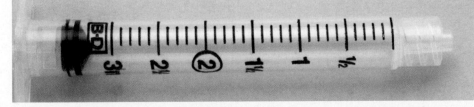

2 Ordered: potassium chloride 25 mEq PO daily 20% sugar-free solution.

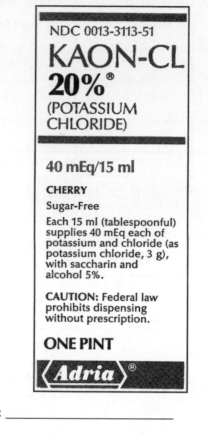

NDC 0013-3113-51

KAON-CL
20%®
(POTASSIUM CHLORIDE)

40 mEq/15 ml

CHERRY

Sugar-Free

Each 15 ml (tablespoonful) supplies 40 mEq each of potassium and chloride (as potassium chloride, 3 g), with saccharin and alcohol 5%.

CAUTION: Federal law prohibits dispensing without prescription.

ONE PINT

⟨*Adria*⟩®

a. Estimated dose: _____

DA equation:

b. Evaluation: _____

Shade in the dose in mL for the medicine cup and draw a vertical line through the calibrated line of the syringe.

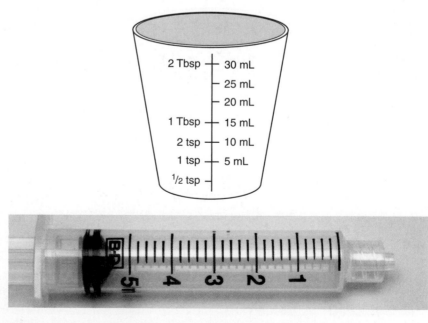

3 Ordered: Aprazolam sol 0.75 mg tid PO for a patient with an anxiety disorder.

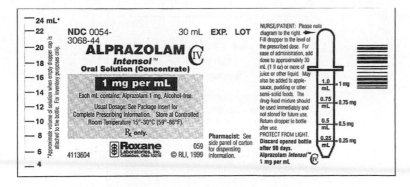

a. Estimated dose in mL: _____

b. Enclosed dropper dose in mL: _____

c. Evaluation: (Does your estimate agree with the dropper?) _____

d. Draw an arrow pointing to the dose on the dropper.

➤ Teach the patient to use the enclosed dropper when you give the medicine. Assess patient vision.

4 Ordered: Zithromax oral susp 0.5 g once daily for a patient with an infection.

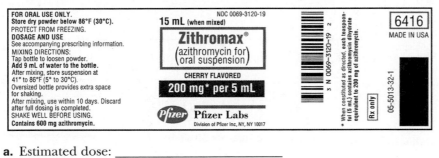

a. Estimated dose: _____

   DA equation:

b. Evaluation: _____

Shade in the dose in mL for the medicine cup and draw a vertical line through the calibrated line of the syringe.

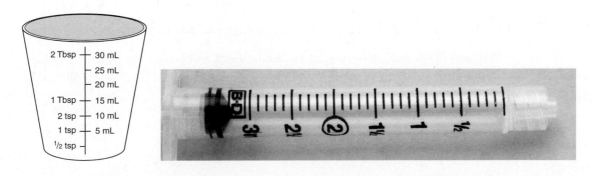

5 Ordered: lithium citrate 0.6 g PO tid for a patient with bipolar illness.

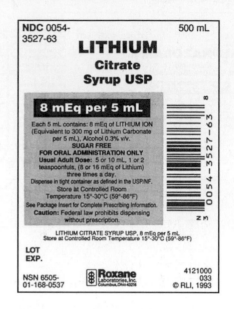

a. Estimated dose: _____

  DA equation:

b. Evaluation: _____

Shade in the dose in mL for the medicine cup.

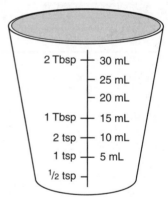

Safe Dose Ranges

Verifying SDRs (safe dose ranges) for medications and estimating doses for all medications are two techniques that protect patients and nurses from medication dose calculation errors.

Calculating safe dose ranges (SDRs)

Medications are approved by the FDA with guidelines for the safe amount to administer to the target audience, for example, "For adult use, 20 mg per day" or "Safe dose range 10-20 mg per day." The safe dose range may be even more specific for powerful drugs, for drugs that are supplied in various dose strengths or for intravenous routes, and for at-risk populations, such as infants, children, and frail adults (e.g., 1-2 mg per kg body weight per day).

The nurse must compare the prescribed order with the SDR in current pharmacologic references or drug package inserts to be sure that the order is within the SDR for a given dose and target population.

The SDR guidelines are usually for a 24-hour day. If the total dose cannot safely be administered on a once-a-day basis, the recommendation will include the *frequency schedule:* the number of times at which the total daily dose should be *divided* into individual doses.

The arithmetic to calculate the SDR is very simple:

- Calculate the low safe dose.
- Calculate the high safe dose.
- Evaluate the order in relation to the SDR and frequency schedule.
- Decision: *Hold* the medication and contact the prescriber because the order is not within the safe dose range or frequency, or *give* the medication because the order is within the safe dose range and frequency.

Three kinds of SDRs are commonly seen:

1 Simple range
2 Divided doses
3 Simple or divided based on weight

SDR with Simple Ranges

> Ordered: Drug A 10 mg tid. SDR: 10-30 mg per day.
>
> Order: 10 mg × 3 doses = 30 mg per day
>
> 10 mg is the *low safe dose* for 24 hours. 30 mg is the *maximum safe dose* for 24 hours.
>
> **Evaluation:** It can be seen at a glance that this order is within the SDR for the total daily dose.
>
> ➤ Take care to avoid confusing the SDR amount with the ordered amount. It is easier to avoid error if the SDR is placed above the order, as illustrated in the previous example.

EXAMPLES

SDR with Divided Doses

> Ordered: Drug B 10 mg tid. SDR: 30 mg per day in 2-3 divided doses.
>
> The phrase *divided doses* indicates that the entire daily dose cannot be given safely at one time. 30 mg/ day must be divided into two servings:
>
> $$\frac{30}{2} = 15 \text{ mg per dose}$$
>
> or into 3 servings: $\frac{30}{3} = 10$ mg per dose
>
> SDR: 30 mg per day in 2-3 divided doses.
>
> Order: 10 × 3 or 30 mg a day total in 3 divided doses.
>
> **Evaluation:** The order falls within SDR for both total daily dose and frequency.

EXAMPLES

Safe and Unsafe Orders

EXAMPLES

Safe Order	Unsafe Order
Ordered: Drug A 75 mg per day	Ordered: Drug B 200 mg per day
SDR: 50-100 mg per day	SDR: 50-100 mg per day
Order: 75 mg per day	Order: 200 mg per day
Evaluation: Safe to give.	**Evaluation:** Hold medication and contact prescriber promptly. Order exceeds maximum.

SDR with Range Based on Weight

EXAMPLES

Ordered: Drug A 150 mg four times daily.

Patient's weight: 88 lb.

SDR: 10-20 mg per kg per day in 3-4 divided doses.

Conversion factor: 1 kg = 2.2 lb

Step 1	:	Step 2	×	Step 3	=	Answer
Desired Answer Units	:	Starting Factor	×	Given Quantity and and Conversion Factor(s) (Quantity and Units)	=	Estimate, Multiply, Evaluate

The final equations will be written like this:

$$\frac{mg}{day} : \frac{10\ mg}{kg \times day} \times \frac{1\ \cancel{kg}}{\cancel{2.2\ lb}_1} \times \frac{\overset{40}{\cancel{88\ lb}}}{1} = 400\ mg\ per\ day\ low\ safe\ dose$$

$$\frac{mg}{day} : \frac{20\ mg}{kg \times day} \times \frac{1\ \cancel{kg}}{\cancel{2.2\ lb}_1} \times \frac{\overset{40}{\cancel{88\ lb}}}{1} = 800\ mg\ per\ day\ high\ safe\ dose$$

Analysis: For starting factor, we chose the SDR because it contains the desired answer and oriented it so that the desired answer units are in the numerator *to match the desired answer position.*

➤ Note **that a triple factor** mg per kg per day is placed **with the first unit mg in the** numerator and kg × day **in the** denominator. Remember this setup for more complex equations.

A number 1 in the denominator of 88 lb helps maintain correct alignment for numerators and denominators to avoid errors during multiplication. It does not change the answer.

➤ Before multiplication, recheck the setup: After all unwanted units were cancelled, are the only units remaining the same as those identified initially for the desired answer?

Evaluation: The order for 150 mg four times a day for a total of 600 mg is within the safe dose range and matches the frequency.

➤ Frequency is as important as dose. If given less often than recommended, the drug will not be therapeutic. If given too frequently, too much drug may be given, which can cause serious damage. The equation answers give only the desired answer units (mg per day). My estimate is that the kg will be about ½ the pound wt, supports the answer. (Math check: 10 × 40 = 400 and 20 × 40 = 800). The equation is balanced. The order is safe to give.

FAQ | *How do I know when to contact the prescriber?*

ANSWER | The prescriber must be contacted

- if the order is incomplete or contains TJC "Do Not Use" abbreviations (p. 101).
- if the total daily dose ordered is below or above SDR
- if the frequency schedule does not match the recommended schedule
- when an allergy to the drug or interaction with another drug might occur

Clarify with the prescriber promptly and document the clarification.

Safe Dose Range and Milligrams per Kilogram of Body Weight Calculator Practice

RAPID PRACTICE 5-13

Estimated completion time: 20 minutes   Answers on page 506

Directions: *Fill in the estimated weight, actual weight, and SDR in the spaces provided. Follow the example given for problem 1. Move decimal places to change the metric units to milligrams if necessary. Use a calculator to convert pounds to kilograms and calculate the SDR.*

➤ *Estimation helps prevent major math errors. It must be followed with exact math calculation. Enter your calculations twice.*

SDR	Patient's Weight (lb)	Estimated Weight (kg) to the Nearest Whole Number	Actual Weight (kg) to the Nearest Tenth	Total SDR to Nearest Tenth
1 10-20 mg per kg per day	66	33 (66 ÷ 2)	30 (66 ÷ 2.2)	10 × 30 = 300 mg per day 20 × 30 = 600 mg per day SDR = 300-600 mg per day
2 0.2-0.5 g per kg per day	44	_____	_____	_____
3 0.25-1.5 mg per kg per day	150	_____	_____	_____
4 2-5 mcg per kg per day	180	_____	_____	_____
5 10-20 mg per kg per day in 3 divided doses	200	_____	_____	_____

CLINICAL RELEVANCE

The SDR is particularly needed for unfamiliar medications and medications that represent a fraction of the unit dose or more than two times the unit dose. SDR checks are also needed for frail patients, immunocompromised patients, patients in the intensive care unit, and pediatric populations.

> **FAQ** | *What is a common math error with kg wt-based dosing?*
>
> **ANSWER** | Multiplying the pounds by 2.2 instead of dividing pounds by 2.2 is a common mistake. This affects the answer by over 4 times error.

RAPID PRACTICE **5-14**

Evaluation of Medication Orders According to SDR

Estimated completion time: 25 minutes   Answers on page 507

Directions: *Examine the example given for problem 1. Compare the frequency and total daily dose ordered with the SDR guidelines for problems 2-5. Evaluate the findings and make a decision to hold the medication, clarify the order promptly with the prescriber and document the clarification, or give the medication because the order is a safe dose. Use a calculator to calculate the SDR. Enter data twice.*

1 **Ordered:** Drug Y, 0.5 g tid PO.

   SDR: 25-50 mg per kg per day in 3 divided doses.

   a. Patient's weight: 100 lb. Estimated kilograms: 50 (nearest whole number). Actual kilograms: 45.5 (nearest tenth).
   b. SDR low and high dose based on actual kilogram weight.

   25 mg × 45.5 kg = 1137.5 mg per day = low safe dose

   50 mg × 45.5 kg = 2 × 1137.5, or 2275 mg per day = high (maximum) safe dose

   Conversion of order using decimal movement: 0.5 g = 500 mg tid = 1500 mg ordered per day

   SDR: 1137.5-2275 mg per day divided in 3 doses.

   c. Daily dose ordered: 1500 mg
   d. Evaluation: Within SDR and recommended frequency (circle one)? *Yes* or *No*.
   e. Decision: Order is within SDR and safe to give.

2 **Ordered:** Drug Y, 50 mg q4h.

   SDR: 1-2 mg per kg per day in 4-6 divided doses.

   a. Patient's weight: 160 lb. Estimated weight in kilograms: _____. Actual weight in kilograms: _____.
   b. SDR low and high dose based on actual kilogram weight:

   _____
   c. Daily dose ordered: _____
   d. Evaluation: Within SDR and recommended frequency (circle one)? *Yes* or *No*.
   e. Decision: _____

3 **Ordered:** Drug Y, 50 mg q6h.

   SDR: 2-4 mg per kg per day in 4 divided doses.

   a. Patient's weight: 120 lb. Estimated weight in kilograms: _____. Actual weight in kilograms: _____.
   b. SDR low and high dose based on actual kilogram weight:

   _____
   c. Daily dose ordered: _____
   d. Evaluation: Within SDR and recommended frequency (circle one)? *Yes* or *No*.
   e. Decision: _____

4 **Ordered:** Drug Y, 0.25 g tid.

SDR: 10-20 mg per kg per day in 2-3 divided doses.

   a. Patient's weight: 100 lb. Estimated weight in kilograms: _____. Actual weight in kilograms: _____.

   b. SDR low and high dose based on actual kilogram weight: _____

   c. Daily dose ordered: _____

   d. Evaluation: Within SDR and recommended frequency (circle one)? *Yes* or *No*.

   e. Decision: _____

5 **Ordered:** Drug Y, 25 mg bid.

SDR: 5-10 mg per kg per day in 2-3 divided doses.

   a. Patient's weight: 60 lb. Estimated weight in kilograms: _____. Actual weight in kilograms: _____.

   b. SDR low and high dose based on actual kilogram weight:

   _____

   c. Daily dose ordered: _____

   d. Evaluation: Within SDR and recommended frequency (circle one)? *Yes* or *No*.

   e. Decision: _____

1 What are three instances in which the medication ordered needs to be clarified with the prescriber?

_____

2 Why is documentation of the clarification important for the patient and the nurse?

_____

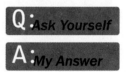

Q: Ask Yourself

A: My Answer

FAQ | *Are low or high doses outside of the SDR ever administered?*

ANSWER | ➤ Yes, but only the prescriber can make the decision. Beginning practitioners should hold the medication and clarify the order with the prescriber promptly. They should research the reason why the dose might be so low as to seem nontherapeutic or so high as to seem toxic. Always recheck the order and the label first. Document and report contacts with the prescriber and actions promptly.

Even if the medication order falls within safe dose range guidelines in the literature, the nursing assessments of the patient's record and of the patient may generate a decision to hold the medication pending clarification with the prescriber. Medication-related nursing assessments may disclose that one or more medications are unsafe for the patient at that point in time. For example, a change in the patient's mental status may render the patient unable to swallow food or fluids. This condition would necessitate a new order for a changed route of administration. Nausea and vomiting are also good reasons to withhold oral medications. If the medication is a critical one, such as a heart medication, the prescriber needs to be informed immediately.

CLINICAL RELEVANCE

➤ Interactions cited in the literature with one or more drugs already being administered would be another reason to hold the medication and clarify the order with the prescriber.

> **FAQ** | *How do I know whom to contact when there is a question about a medication order?*

ANSWER | The decision comes with experience. There are three good sources: the prescriber, the pharmacist, and a recent drug reference or drug information insert. The source to select depends upon the nature of the question. Here are some general guidelines:

➤ If the medication order is illegible, unclear, or incomplete, contact the prescriber.
➤ If the problem is with the amount of the *dose,* check a drug reference first and then the prescriber if necessary.
➤ If the medication *supplied is* in question, contact the pharmacist.
➤ Students should hold the medication, analyze the problem, use the references to determine the SDR and/or contact the pharmacist if appropriate, determine independently which action would be best, and promptly contact the instructor to confer regarding the decision, particularly if the prescriber is to be contacted.

RAPID PRACTICE 5-15   *Calculating Safe Doses with DA Verification*

Estimated completion time: 25 minutes   Answers on page **507**

Directions: *Examine and analyze the example in problem 1. Then complete problems 2-5, working out each step of the problem in order. If the decision is to hold the medication, stop calculations.*

1   Ordered: digoxin (Lanoxin) pediatric elixir 0.1 mg PO daily for an adult patient with heart failure.

  SDR for adult maintenance: 50 mcg-300 mcg per day.

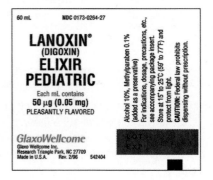

➤ Note that the label uses *μg* for *mcg.* Write mcg.*

a. Unit dose available: 50 mcg per mL, or 0.05 mg per mL
b. Order within SDR (circle one)? *Yes* or *No.* SDR is 50-300 mcg per day and the order (0.1 mg) is 100 mcg.
c. Estimated dose if safe to give: More than 1 mL would be given, 2 times the unit dose.
d. Actual dose to be given: 2 mL
  DA equation:

$$\frac{mL}{dose} : \frac{1\ mL}{0.05\ \text{mg}} \times \frac{0.1\ \text{mg}}{dose} = 2\ mL \text{ per dose (answer)}$$

e. Evaluation: The estimate supports the answer. The equation is balanced.

  Note: No math for conversions are necessary because the conversion is given on the label.

---

*μg can be misread as mg.

2 **Ordered:** lithium citrate 0.6 g bid PO daily for a patient with a bipolar disorder. Available: lithium citrate 300 mg per 5 mL.

SDR: 900-1200 mg daily in 2-3 divided doses.

NDC 0054-
3527-63   500 mL

LITHIUM
Citrate
Syrup USP

8 mEq per 5 mL

Each 5 mL contains: 8 mEq of LITHIUM ION
(Equivalent to 300 mg of Lithium Carbonate
per 5 mL), Alcohol 0.3% v/v.
SUGAR FREE
FOR ORAL ADMINISTRATION ONLY
Usual Adult Dose: 5 or 10 mL, 1 or 2
teaspoonfuls, (8 or 16 mEq of Lithium)
three times a day.
Dispense in tight container as defined in the USP/NF.
Store at Controlled Room
Temperature 15°-30°C (59°-86°F)
See Package Insert for Complete Prescribing Information.
Caution: Federal law prohibits dispensing
without prescription.

LITHIUM CITRATE SYRUP USP, 8 mEq per 5 mL
Store at Controlled Room Temperature 15°-30°C (59°-86°F)

LOT
EXP.

NSN 6505-
01-168-0537   Roxane
                     Laboratories, Inc.
                     Columbus, Ohio 43216

4121000
033
© RLI, 1993

a. Unit dose available in mg per mL: _____

b. Order with SDR (circle one)? *Yes* or *No.*

c. Estimated dose if safe to give: _____

d. Actual dose: _____

DA equation:

e. Evaluation: _____

Shade in the dose in mL for the medicine cup and draw a vertical line through the calibrated line of the syringe as applicable.

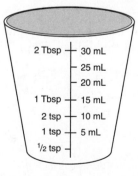

2 Tbsp — 30 mL
— 25 mL
— 20 mL
1 Tbsp — 15 mL
2 tsp — 10 mL
1 tsp — 5 mL
½ tsp —

➤ Remember that the estimate usually cannot be made until the measurement units are *the same.*

3 **Ordered:** loperamide hydrochloride sol. 2 mg PO after each loose stool up to 6 times daily. The patient has already received a 4-mg initial dose.

SDR: 4 mg initially, then 2 mg after each loose stool, not to exceed 16 mg per day.

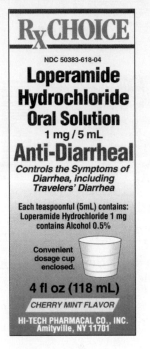

a. Unit dose available in mg per mL: _____

b. Order with SDR (circle one)? *Yes* or *No*.

c. Estimated dose if safe to give: _____

d. Actual dose: _____
DA equation:

e. Evaluation: _____

Shade in the dose in mL for the medicine cup and draw a vertical line through the calibrated line of the syringe as applicable.

4   Ordered: Kaon-Cl liquid 45 mEq PO stat for a patient with hypokalemia.
SDR for adult for potassium depletion: 40 mEq - 100 mEq per day PO.

NDC 0013-3113-51

KAON-CL
20%®
(POTASSIUM
CHLORIDE)

40 mEq/15 ml

CHERRY

Sugar-Free

Each 15 ml (tablespoonful)
supplies 40 mEq each of
potassium and chloride (as
potassium chloride, 3 g),
with saccharin and
alcohol 5%.

CAUTION: Federal law
prohibits dispensing
without prescription.

ONE PINT

⟨*Adria*⟩®

a. Unit dose available in mEq per mL: _____
b. Order with SDR (circle one)? *Yes* or *No.*

c. Estimated dose if safe to give: _____
d. Actual dose: _____
  DA equation:

e. Evaluation: _____

Shade in the dose in mL for the medicine cup and draw a vertical line
through the calibrated line of the syringe to the nearest measurable dose.

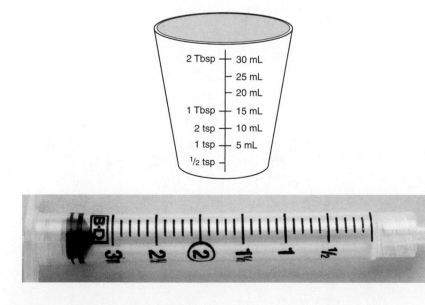

Check carefully for dilution directions.

5 **Ordered:** dyphylline elixir 120 mg PO for a child with asthma.

SDR for sedation of a child: 3-6 mg per kg per day in 3 divided doses.

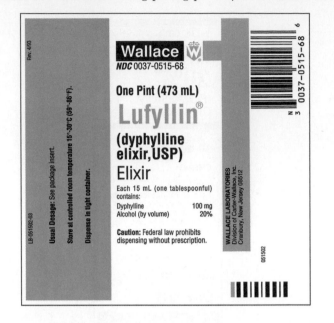

Child's weight: 44 lb. Estimated weight in kilograms (nearest whole number): _____. Actual weight in kilograms (nearest tenth): _____.

a. Unit dose available in mg per mL: _____
b. Order with SDR (circle one)? *Yes* or *No*.

c. Estimated dose if safe to give: _____
d. Actual dose: _____
DA equation:

e. Evaluation: _____

Shade in the dose in mL for the medicine cup and draw a vertical line through the calibrated line of the syringe as applicable.

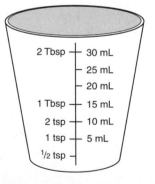

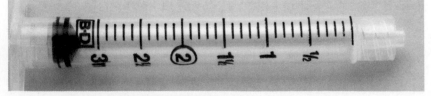

CHAPTER 5 MULTIPLE-CHOICE REVIEW

Estimated completion time: 10 minutes   Answers on page 509

Directions: *Select the best answer.*

1 One of the most important safety nets a nurse can use for catching major calculation errors is
   1. Performing metric conversions
   2. Estimating answers
   3. Using a calculator
   4. Carrying a math text to clinical

2 Which of the following pairs of units will need to have the decimal moved 6 places?
   1. Grams to micrograms
   2. Grams to milligrams
   3. Micrograms to milligrams
   4. Milliequivalents to milliliters

3 Which is the correct conversion for 50 mg to grams?
   1. 0.005 g
   2. 0.05 g
   3. 0.5 g
   4. 500 g

4 Which is the correct conversion for 25,000 mcg to grams?
   1. 250 g
   2. 25 g
   3. 0.25 g
   4. 0.025 g

5 The recommended way to write large numbers in the metric system for ease of reading, as in one hundred thousand micrograms, is
   1. With commas: 100,000
   2. With decimal points: 100.000
   3. With spaces: 100 000
   4. Without spaces or inserts: 100000

6 If 25 mg per kg per day is ordered in 2 divided doses and kg = 10, what will each dose be?
   1. 50 mg
   2. 100 mg
   3. 125 mg
   4. 250 mg

7 The SDR for 10-30 mg per kg per day for a patient weighing 44 lb is
   1. 300 mg per day
   2. 440 mg-1320 mg/ day
   3. 200-600 mg per kg per day
   4. 200-600 mg per day

8 Milligram-gram conversions require movement of how many decimal places?
   1. 3 places
   2. 5 places
   3. 6 places
   4. 1 million places

9 Select the appropriate measuring device and volumes when preparing an oral medication of 24 mL to be administered in a 30-mL calibrated medicine cup.
   1. Pour to 25 mL in the measuring cup and remove 1 mL.
   2. Pour to 20 mL in the measuring cup and administer 4 mL with a 3-mL syringe.
   3. Pour to approximately 24 mL, just short of the 25-mL line.
   4. Pour to 20 mL in the cup and add 4 mL with a 5-mL syringe.

10 Which of the following conversions is correct?
   1. 0.5 g = 50 mg
   2. 10,000 mcg = 20 mg
   3. 0.25 g = 250 mg
   4. 120 mg = 1.2 g

CHAPTER 5 FINAL PRACTICE

Estimated completion time: 40-50 minutes   Answers on page 509

Directions: *Evaluate the order and SDR. If safe to give, estimate and approximate dose.*
Verify the estimate with a DA style equation. Evaluate the answer. Use a calculator to
determine kg weights and SDR. Write the answers in the space provided.

1 Ordered: aspirin 0.65 g PO q4h prn for a 22-year-old patient with a painful
   sprained ankle.

   SDR (adult): (Consult label.)

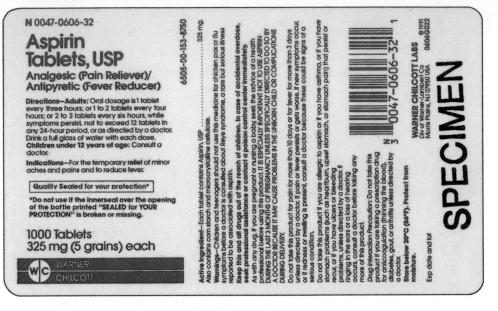

   a. SDR comparison with order: _____

   b. Decision: _____

   c. Estimate of number of tablets to be given: _____ More or less than unit
      dose? _____

   d. Actual number of tablets to be given: _____
      DA equation:

   e. Evaluation: _____

2 Ordered: acetaminophen liquid 0.65 g PO q6h for a patient with a fever.

   SDR (adult): 325-650 mg q4-6h up to 4 g per day.

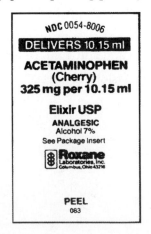

a. SDR comparison with order: _____

b. Decision: _____

c. Estimated dose: _____

d. Amount to give: _____

e. Evaluation: _____

Shade in the dose in mL for the medicine cup and draw a vertical line through the calibrated line of the syringe as applicable.

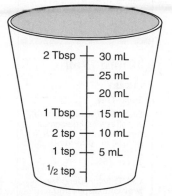

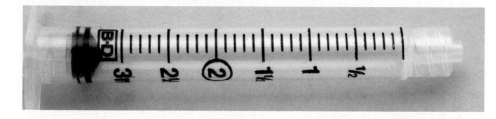

3 Ordered: raloxifene HCl 0.06 g bid PO daily for an adult patient with osteoporosis.

SDR (adult): 60 mg once a day.

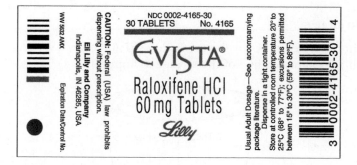

a. SDR comparison with order: _____

b. Decision: _____

c. Estimate: _____

d. Amount to give: _____
DA equation:

e. Evaluation: _____

4 Ordered: potassium chloride elixir 30 mEq PO daily for a patient on diuretics.
SDR: 20-40 mEq per day.

> NDC 0013-3113-51
>
> # KAON-CL
> ## 20%®
> (POTASSIUM CHLORIDE)
>
> **40 mEq/15 ml**
>
> **CHERRY**
>
> Sugar-Free
>
> Each 15 ml (tablespoonful) supplies 40 mEq each of potassium and chloride (as potassium chloride, 3 g), with saccharin and alcohol 5%.
>
> **CAUTION:** Federal law prohibits dispensing without prescription.
>
> **ONE PINT**
>
> 〈Adria〉®

a. SDR comparison with order: _____

b. Decision: _____

c. Estimate: _____

d. Amount to give: _____
   DA equation:

e. Evaluation: _____

Shade in the dose in mL for the medicine cup and draw a vertical line through the calibrated line of the syringe as applicable.

2 Tbsp ── 30 mL
       ── 25 mL
       ── 20 mL
1 Tbsp ── 15 mL
2 tsp ── 10 mL
1 tsp ── 5 mL
½ tsp ──

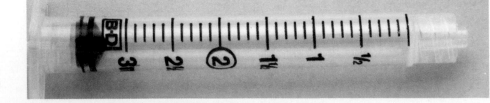

5 Ordered: valproic acid syrup 300 mg bid PO starting dose for a patient with a seizure disorder. Patient weight: 50 kg.

SDR: 10-15 mg per kg per day.

Directions: Immediately before use, dilute the medication with distilled water, acidified tap water, or juice.

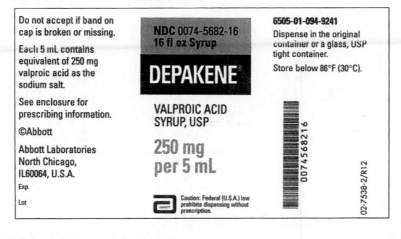

Do not accept if band on cap is broken or missing.

Each 5 mL contains equivalent of 250 mg valproic acid as the sodium salt.

See enclosure for prescribing information.

©Abbott

Abbott Laboratories
North Chicago,
IL60064, U.S.A.

Exp.

Lot

NDC 0074-5682-16
16 fl oz Syrup

DEPAKENE

VALPROIC ACID
SYRUP, USP

**250 mg
per 5 mL**

Caution: Federal (U.S.A.) law prohibits dispensing without prescription.

6505-01-094-9241

Dispense in the original container or a glass, USP tight container.

Store below 86°F (30°C).

a. SDR comparison with order: _____

b. Decision: _____

c. Estimate: _____

d. Amount to prepare before dilution: _____
DA equation:

e. Evaluation: _____

Shade in the dose in mL for the medicine cup and draw a vertical line through the calibrated line of the syringe as applicable.

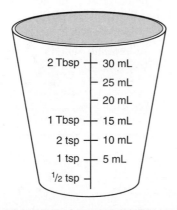

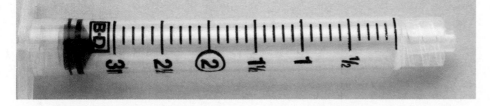

6 Ordered: phenobarbital tablets* 0.09 g bid PO for a patient with seizures.

SDR: 100-300 mg per day in divided doses or at bedtime.

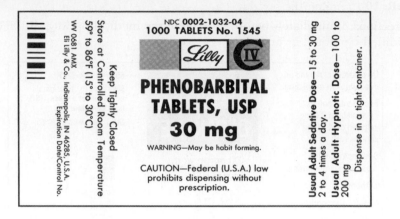

*High alert if given to a pediatric patient.

    a. SDR comparison with order: _____

    b. Decision: _____

    c. Estimate: _____

    d. Amount to give: _____

    DA equation:

    e. Evaluation: _____

7 Ordered: carbamazepine 0.2 g bid PO for a patient with *initial* treatment for seizures.

SDR: 200 mg bid to start; may be increased by 200 mg per day in divided doses.

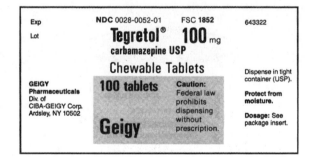

    a. SDR comparison with order: _____

    b. Decision: _____

    c. Estimate: _____

    d. Amount to give: _____

    DA equation:

    e. Evaluation: _____

8 Ordered: Synthroid 0.1 mg PO daily for a patient with hypothyroidism.

Maintenance: 75-125 mcg per day.

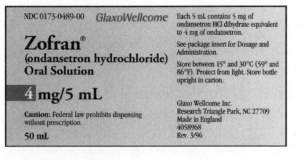

a. SDR comparison with order: _____

b. Decision: _____

c. Estimate: _____

d. Amount to give: _____

   DA equation:

e. Evaluation: _____

9 Ordered: ondansetron hydrochloride 14 mg 1 hr preoperatively PO stat for a patient to prevent postoperative nausea and vomiting.

SDR: 8-16 mg per dose 1 hr pre op.

a. SDR comparison with order: _____

b. Decision: _____

c. Estimate: _____

d. Amount to give: _____

   DA equation:

e. Evaluation: _____

Shade in the dose in mL for the medicine cup and draw a vertical line through the calibrated line of the syringe to the nearest measurable dose.

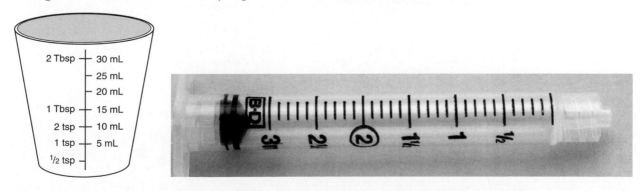

10 Ordered: penicillin V potassium tabs* 0.25 g PO q8h × 10 days for a patient with streptococcal infection.

SDR: 125-250 mg q6-8h × 10 days.

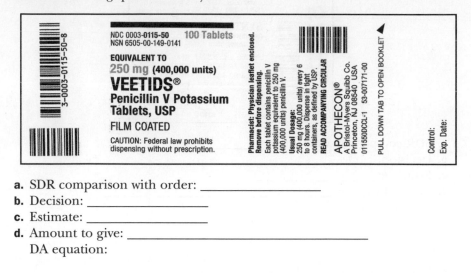

a. SDR comparison with order: _____

b. Decision: _____

c. Estimate: _____

d. Amount to give: _____
DA equation:

e. Evaluation: _____

_____

*Be sure to reassess for allergies to antibiotics and to the specific drug, Penicillin, in this case. If there is a problem, hold the drug and contact the prescriber.

Suggestions for Further Reading

Clayton BD, Stock YN, Cooper S: *Basic pharmacology for nurses,* ed. 15, St. Louis, 2010, Mosby.

PDR nurse's handbook, Montvale, NJ, 2009, Medical Economics Co.

Skidmore-Roth L: *Mosby's drug guide for nurses,* ed. 6, St. Louis, 2007, Mosby.

www.ampainsoc.org/advocacy/pdf/range.pdf
www.drhull.com/EncyMaster/M/measurement.html

 Additional practice problems can be found in the Calculating by Dimensional Analysis and Basic Calculations sections of the Student Companion on Evolve.

Chapter 6 covers syringe measurements in preparation for measuring injectable medication doses.

PART III

Reconstituted Medications

300 mg

20 ML

0.9%

1000 g = 1 kg

Syringe Measurements

- State the total volume capacity for various syringes.
- Differentiate the calibrations (quantity values) for various syringe sizes per milliliter.
- State the lowest and nearest measurable dose for syringes.
- Select the appropriate syringe size for stated volumes.
- Draw a vertical line through an accurate dose on a syringe.
- Select the appropriate syringe for selected purposes.
- Identify safety principles related to syringes and needles.
- Define needle gauge and three criteria for needle selection.

Essential Prior Knowledge

- Mastery of Chapters 1-5

Essential Equipment

- Basic syringe measurements can be learned from the chapter practice. Learning will be expedited if actual syringes are on hand.

Estimated Time To Complete Chapter

- 30 minutes to 1 hour

Introduction

Liquid doses in mL for oral medications have been covered in Chapter 4 as well as an introduction to measuring syringe volumes with the 3-mL and the 5-mL syringe. Sufficient drawings and practice will be offered in this chapter so that syringe volume measurements for any syringes can be identified for providing the nearest measurable dose.

Examining and handling a variety of syringes and needles in the laboratory will be necessary to obtain a more comprehensive view and competence in the use of the equipment.

ESSENTIAL *Vocabulary*

Hypodermic	General term used to describe injectables under the skin.
Insulin Syringe	Small syringe, with a 0.3- to 1-mL capacity, calibrated for specific insulin mixtures in standardized units.

Intradermal (ID)	Shallow injection to be given just under the skin between the dermis and the epidermis. Used mainly for skin tests. Not used to deliver medications. *0.1 mL* is the usual volume for skin test injections. A 1-mL syringe is used.
Intramuscular (IM)	Into the muscle. The muscle is able to accept more irritating substances than other injectable routes.
Intravenous (IV)	Into the vein. These injections provide *instant* drug access to the circulation.
Needle Gauge	Diameter (thickness) of the needle shaft. The lower the gauge number, the larger the diameter of the needle. An 18-gauge needle is much larger than a 27-gauge needle.
Parenteral Medications	Injectable medications. Excludes oral, nasogastric, gastric, topical, and intestinal routes.
Prefilled Syringe	Syringe prefilled by manufacturer or pharmacy with specific frequently ordered doses of medication. This method is thought to reduce dose measurement errors.
Safety Syringe	Syringe designed with a variety of locking sheath covers to protect needle sterility and prevent accidental injury during and after disposal.
Subcutaneous	Under the skin into the fatty layer. Used for less irritating substances than are intramuscular injections. Insulin and heparin are given subcutaneously.
Syringe Holder	Specially designed device to be used only with an inserted prefilled medication cartridge.
Tuberculin Syringe	Small-volume syringe, with a 1-mL capacity, used for intradermal skin tests and small-volume injections in frail at-risk populations.
Viscosity	Ability to flow; thickness of a solution. A solution that is viscous may have directions for dilution. Blood is viscous, as are some reconstituted medications. Viscous solutions require larger-gauge needles. Refer to needle gauge above.

Vocabulary Review

Estimated completion time: 5-10 minutes   Answers on page 512

Directions: *Review the vocabulary list and fill in the definitions with one- or two-word phrases.*

1   The marked lines on a syringe that indicate the capacity are called _____.

2   The route that is used for skin tests is called _____, and the syringe used for that route has a _____-mL capacity.

3   Injectable medications are given through various routes called _____, as opposed to the oral route.

4   The size of a needle diameter is called _____.

5   Do needles that have a larger gauge number have a larger or smaller diameter?
_____

Syringe Sizes

20-mL, 10-mL, 5-mL, 3-mL, and 1-mL syringes

Syringes are available in many sizes, ranging from *0.3-mL* insulin syringe to *60-mL* or greater capacity. The decision to use a specific syringe is based on the volume of medication to be administered and the route of administration.

The 3-mL and 5-mL syringes were introduced in Chapter 5 for oral liquid medications.

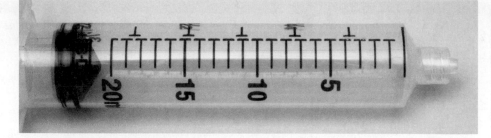

FIGURE 6-1 20-mL syringe with 1-mL calibrations.

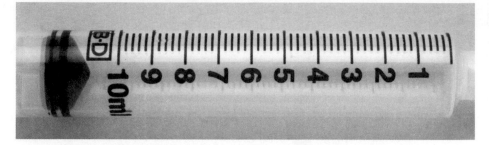

FIGURE 6-2 10-mL syringe with 0.2-mL calibrations.

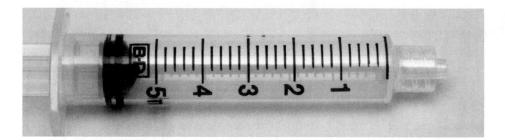

FIGURE 6-3 5-mL syringe with 0.2-mL calibrations.

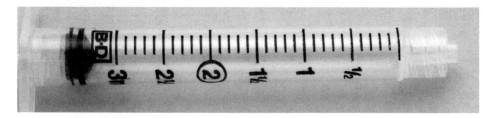

FIGURE 6-4 3-mL syringe with 0.1-mL calibrations.

Intravenous medications should be given with large volume syringes to avoid excessive pressure in the line (Figures 6-1 and 6-2).

Intramuscular injections may be given with a 5-mL syringe. It is used for doses of 5 mL or less (Figure 6-3)

Many subcutaneous and intramuscular injections are given with a 3-mL syringe, used for doses of 3 mL or less (Figure 6-4).

A 1-mL syringe is used for skin tests and some vaccines and may be used for infants' injections and for very small doses. It is selected for doses of 1 mL or less (Figure 6-5).

Be sure you can identify the lowest measurable dose on each of the following syringes.

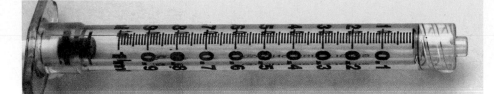

FIGURE 6-5 1-mL tuberculin syringe with 0.01-mL calibrations.

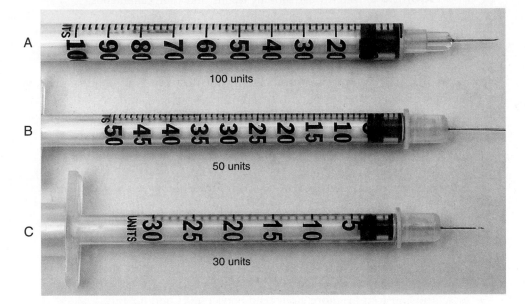

FIGURE 6-6 Insulin syringes. **A,** 100 units (1 mL). **B,** 50 units (0.5 mL). **C,** 30 units (0.3 mL).

FIGURE 6-7 A, 1-mL tuberculin syringe. **B,** 100-Unit 1-mL insulin syringe. (From Potter PA, Perry AG: *Fundamentals of nursing*, ed. 7, St. Louis, 2009, Mosby.)

Insulin syringes

Insulin syringes are sized in 100 units, 50 units, and 30 units (Figure 6-6).

A 100-unit insulin syringe is selected for insulin doses up to 100 units.

A 50-unit insulin syringe is selected for better visualization of insulin doses up to 50 units. A 30-unit insulin syringe is selected for better visualization of insulin doses up to 30 units.

➤ Do not use insulin syringes for anything but insulin. Insulin doses are ordered in units. Avoid confusing insulin syringes with tuberculin syringes.

➤ All used needles as well as their attached used syringes must be placed in hazardous waste sharps containers immediately after use. They may not be thrown in trash baskets.

➤ Do not confuse 1-mL syringes or tuberculin syringes marked in milliliters (or cubic centimeters) with 1-mL *insulin* syringes, which are marked with the word *insulin* and calibrated in *units* (Figure 6-7).

➤ Do not substitute a tuberculin syringe for insulin.

Parts of the Syringe

Figure 6-8 shows the parts of a syringe. Syringes are supplied without needles or with attached needles. Supervised clinical practice is required in order to learn safe handling of syringes and needles.

The 3-mL syringe is the most commonly used syringe for subcutaneous and intramuscular injections. The arrows illustrate the location of the 1- and 0.5-mL markings (Figure 6-9). The lowest measurable dose is 0.1 mL.

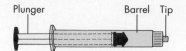

FIGURE 6-8 Parts of a syringe. (From Potter PA, Perry AG: *Fundamentals of nursing,* ed. 7, St. Louis, 2009, Mosby.)

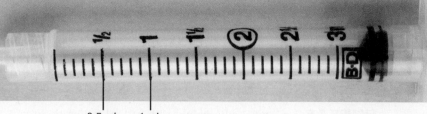

FIGURE 6-9 3-mL-syringe showing 0.5-mL and 1-mL calibrations.

Total Capacity and Lowest Measurable Dose

Finding the total capacity and the lowest measurable dose involves the same process for all syringes. Syringe size selection is based on the medication dose ordered, the total volume of the syringe, and nearest: *measurable* dose on the syringe. Examine the empty 3-mL syringe shown in Figure 6-9 for a review:

- The total capacity is 3 mL.
- The lowest measurable dose is 0.1 mL.
- Medications for this syringe can be given to the *nearest tenth of a milliliter* (e.g., 2.2 mL, 2.3 mL, etc.) because that is the *lowest measurable dose.*
- The calibrations are slightly more prominent for the *whole*-milliliter marks.
- It is sometimes easier to count the lines to a whole number, if present, such as 0 to 1 mL, or between whole numbers, such as 1 and 2 mL. Keep in mind that smaller syringes may not have whole numbers. Examine the 1-mL syringe illustrated in Figure 6-5. It has 100 calibrations between 0 and 1 mL. In this case, the line count is more easily read between 0.1 and 0.2 mL.

EXAMPLES

$$\frac{1 \text{ mL}}{100 \text{ calibrations}} = 0.01 \text{ mL lowest measurable dose}$$

$$\frac{1 \text{ mL}}{10 \text{ calibrations}} = 0.1 \text{ mL lowest measurable dose}$$

$$\frac{1 \text{ mL}}{5 \text{ calibrations}} = 0.2 \text{ mL lowest measurable dose}$$

FAQ | *Why do I need to look at the total volume and the 1-mL markings?*

ANSWER | To avoid medication dose errors, you need to know the precise measurements. After the dose is calculated, select a syringe that will contain the total number of milliliters that you need to give. You would not select a 3-mL syringe if you had to give 4.5 mL. The patient would not appreciate two injections instead of one. The best way to avoid making a syringe measurement error is to locate the 1-, 0.5-, or other major mL mark if available and then to observe the value of each calibration. Larger syringes will not have all the smaller calibrations. Misreading *1.5 mL* for *0.5 mL* is a major error. Nevertheless, it has occurred.

Where to Measure the Dose on Syringes

The dose in syringes is measured at the upper flat ring of the plunger, the ring closest to the needle end. For practice measurements, the plunger will not be shown (Figure 6-10).

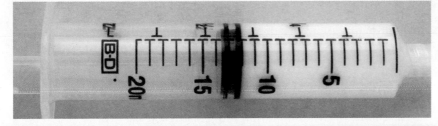

FIGURE 6-10 20-mL syringe illustrating a 12-mL measurement reading at the upper ring of the plunger. (From Macklin D, Chernecky C, Infortuna H: *Math for clinical practice,* ed. 2, St. Louis, 2011, Mosby.)

Measuring Syringe Capacities

RAPID PRACTICE   6-2

Estimated completion time: 10-15 minutes   Answers on page 513

Directions: *Examine the numbers and calibrations on the syringe, and provide the answer in the space provided.*

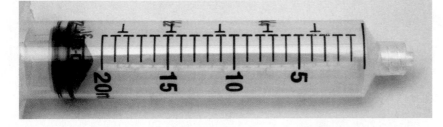

1 What is the total capacity of this syringe in milliliters? _____

2 How many calibrations are there between 0 and 5 mL? _____

3 What is the smallest measurable dose (the first space up to the first line) on the syringe? _____

4 Draw a vertical line through the syringe below at 1 mL.

5 Draw a second vertical line through the syringe below at 14 mL.

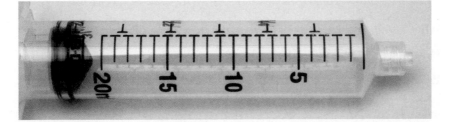

Problems 6-10 pertain to the syringe below.

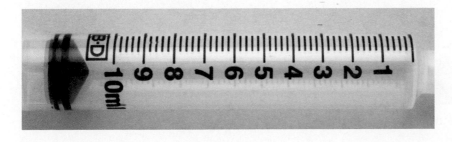

6 What is the total capacity of the syringe in milliliters? _____

7 How many calibrations are there between 0 and 1 mL? _____

8 What is the smallest measurable dose on the syringe? _____

9 Draw a vertical line through the syringe at 5.6 mL.

10 Draw a second vertical line through the syringe at 8.8 mL.

Q: Ask Yourself

A: My Answer

1 How do the lowest measurable doses on the 10- and 20-mL syringe shown in the text differ from the lowest measurable doses on the 3- and 5-mL syringe?

_____

RAPID PRACTICE 6-3

Measuring Syringe Capacities

Estimated completion time: 10 minutes   Answers on page 513

Directions: *Problems 1-5 pertain to the syringe below. Examine the numbers and calibrations on the syringe and provide the answers in the space provided.*

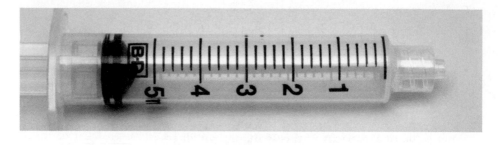

1 What is the total capacity of the syringe above in milliliters? _____

2 How many calibrations are there between 0 and 1 mL? _____

3 What is the smallest measurable dose on the syringe? _____

4 Draw a vertical line through the syringe above at 0.6 mL. (Note: There are also 5-mL syringes that have 10 calibrations per milliliter.)

5 Draw a second vertical line through the syringe above at 3.4 mL.

6 What is the total capacity of the syringe below in milliliters? _____

7 How many calibrations are there between 0 and 0.1 mL? _____

8 What is the smallest measurable dose on the syringe? _____

9 Draw a vertical line through the syringe below at 0.05 mL.

10 Draw a second vertical line through the syringe below at 0.1 mL.

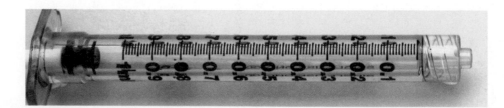

➤ Pay special attention to the decimal place in the doses for the 1-mL syringe.

1 What are the two most commonly used sizes of syringes?

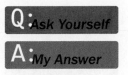

Q:*Ask Yourself*

A:*My Answer*

RAPID PRACTICE   6-4

Measuring Syringe Capacities

Estimated completion time: 5 minutes   **Answers on page 514**

Directions: *Examine the numbers and calibrations on the syringe and provide the answers in the space provided or by putting a line on the syringe drawing.*

1 What is the total capacity of the syringe below in milliliters? _____

2 What is the smallest measurable dose on this syringe? _____

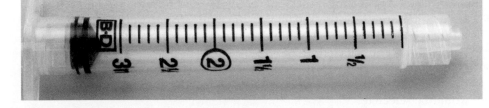

3 Draw a vertical line through the syringe below at 2.7 mL.

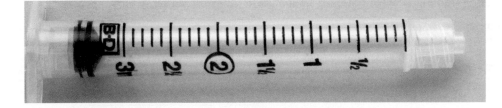

4 Draw a vertical line through the syringe below at 1.6 mL.

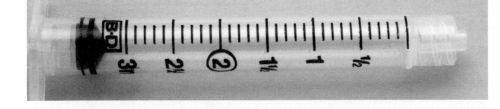

5 Draw a vertical line through the syringe below at 0.9 mL.

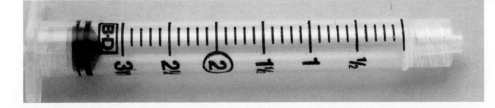

The 3- and 5-mL syringes are the most commonly used. However, nurses must know how to distinguish the differences in calibrations in the other sizes to avoid a dose measurement error.

Q: Ask Yourself

A: My Answer

1 What is the difference in the lowest measurable dose between the 3-mL and the 5-mL syringe shown in this text?

_____

2 Of the 3- and the 5-mL syringe shown in this text, which one can accommodate a 2.7-mL ordered dose?

_____

Examining the Calculated Doses for Correct Syringe Selection

- If the amount ordered is a whole number (e.g., 3 mL) or in tenths of a milliliter (e.g., 2.8 or 0.8 mL), the 3-mL syringe would be appropriate.
- If the amount to be given is 0.08 mL, the 3-mL syringe would not be used because it is not calibrated in hundredths of a milliliter. A 1-mL (tuberculin) syringe would be selected.
- If the amount to be given is 3.6 mL, the 3-mL syringe would not be used because the patient would have to receive two injections. A 5-mL syringe would be selected.

RAPID PRACTICE **6-5**

Identifying the Syringe for the Dose Ordered

Estimated completion time: 10-15 minutes   **Answers on page 514**

Directions: _State the preferred syringe size in mL that provides the nearest measurable dose for the dose ordered. Note that a TB syringe is a 1-mL syringe._

Ordered Dose Volume	Syringe Size
1 2.8 mL	_____
2 3.2 mL	_____
3 6.4 mL	_____
4 0.08 mL	_____
5 1.7 mL	_____
6 9.6 mL	_____
7 12.6 mL	_____
8 0.6 mL	_____
9 1.5 mL	_____
10 0.1 mL	_____

Syringe Selections and Disposal

Estimated completion time: 5 minutes   Answers on page 515

Directions: *Refer to the preceding text and syringe photographs that follow to answer the following questions.*

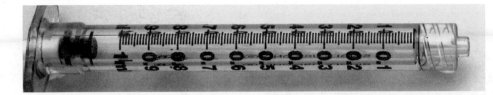

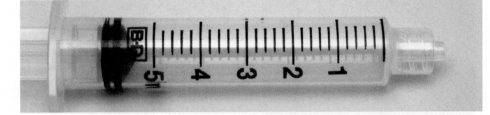

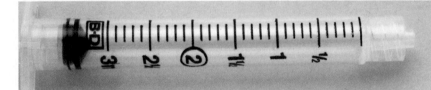

1   What is the main criterion for selection of syringe size? _____

2   Can used syringes without needles be placed in ordinary trash containers? _____

3   If a nurse prepares 0.06 mL of a medication, which size syringe should the nurse select? _____

4   If a nurse calculates a dose of 2.9 mL of a medication, which size syringe should the nurse select? _____ How much medication will be drawn up in the syringe for the nearest measurable dose? _____

5   If a nurse calculates a dose of 3.19 mL of a medication, which size syringe should the nurse select? _____ What will be the nearest measurable dose on the syringe? _____

Oral Syringes

Oral syringes have milliliter marks on one side, and some have household *teaspoon* mark on the other (Figure 6-11). Their tips may be off center. Some of them are capped (Figure 6-12).

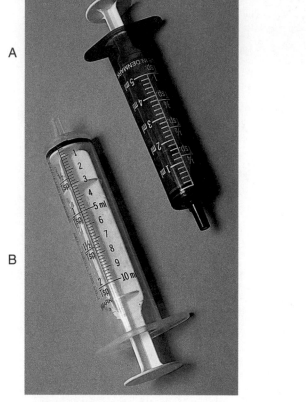

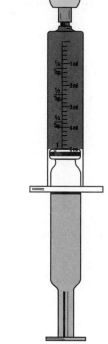

FIGURE 6-11 Oral syringes. **A,** 5-mL. **B,** 10-mL. (From Clayton BD, Stock YN, Cooper S: *Basic pharmacology for nurses,* ed. 15, St. Louis, 2010, Mosby.)

FIGURE 6-12 Prefilled, capped oral syringe. (From Brown M, Mulholland J: *Drug calculations: process and problems for clinical practice,* ed. 8, St. Louis, 2008, Mosby.)

Oral Syringes Versus Injectable Syringes

Empty and prefilled oral syringes are not always available in all clinical facilities. Nurses may measure and administer oral medications with a regular syringe with the needle removed. They may also transfer the medication to a medicine cup or a nipple.

> **CLINICAL RELEVANCE**
>
> ➤ Oral syringes are not to be used for injections. Do not confuse oral syringes with parenteral syringes. Oral syringes have milliliter calibrations and may have teaspoon or tablespoon marks as well. Their tips do not fit needles. They are *not sterile.* Errors have been caused by jamming needles onto oral syringes. The needles do not fit properly and can fall off during "injection."

Prefilled Injectable Syringes

Prefilled injectable syringes contain a single-dose of medication. They have a needle attached and are disposable (Figure 6-13). If the order calls for less than the supplied amount, the nurse adjusts the dose by discarding unneeded amounts before administration.

➤ Doses for prefilled syringes must be calculated before administration. There *may* be extra medication and air in the syringe that need to be expelled before administration. Check the package and/or label directions.
➤ Check agency protocols for discard of controlled substances.
➤ Many prefilled syringe medications look similar. The nurse must check all the information on the syringe to avoid giving the wrong medicine or dose.

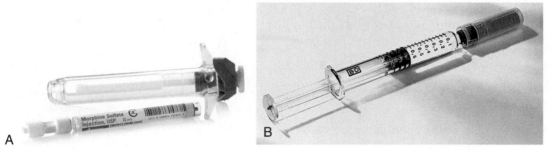

FIGURE 6-13 A, Carbujet syringe holder and needleless prefilled sterile cartridge. **B,** BD Hypak prefilled syringe. (**A,** From Hospira, Inc., Lake Forest, IL. **B,** From Becton, Dickinson, and Company, Franklin Lakes, NJ.)

Prefilled Medication Cartridges for Injection

Injectables may be supplied in a cartridge with an attached needle. The cartridge containing the medicine is to be locked in the plastic holder for injection of the medication.

Dexterity with this equipment requires *intermittent* practice sessions for insertion, locking, unlocking, and needle safety techniques (Figure 6-14). The cartridges usually have 0.1 or 0.2 mL extra medication in case of loss. The label and calibrations must be read and compared with the order *before* the cartridge is inserted. The cartridge can be rotated so that the calibrations are in view for adjusting the dose.

➤ Be especially careful to examine prefilled syringe labels and cartridge calibrations before administering them. Rotate the cartridge after placement in the holder so that the amounts and calibrations can be clearly seen.

There have been ADE because a prefilled syringe cartridge containing potassium was given intravenously instead of a normal saline cartridge. The cartridges "looked similar" but obviously the nurse did not examine and read the labels. Arrhythmias and cardiac arrest are some of the ADE connected with concentrated and/or high potassium levels.

CLINICAL RELEVANCE

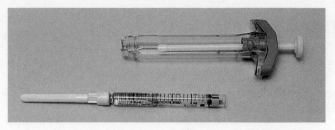

FIGURE 6-14 Carpuject syringe and prefilled sterile cartridge with needle. (From Potter PA, Perry AG: *Fundamentals of nursing,* ed. 6, St. Louis, 2005, Mosby.)

Needle Sizes

Needle size refers to length and gauge. There are many options available (Figure 6-15). Supervised laboratory and clinical experience is needed to master needle size selection, dexterity, and safe handling.

Needle lengths are as follows:

- Intramuscular: 1 to 2 inches
- Subcutaneous: $\frac{3}{8}$ to $\frac{5}{8}$ inch
- Intradermal: $\frac{3}{8}$ to $\frac{1}{2}$ inch

Basics of needle selection

Needle selection, length, and gauge depend on three criteria:

1 Purpose and route of the injection
2 Size and skin integrity of the patient
3 Viscosity of the solution

Intramuscular injections require longer needles than do intradermal and subcutaneous injections. Irritating substances are not injected into *subcutaneous* tissue because they are not absorbed as quickly into the circulation. The muscle would be a better alternative for such a substance because it has a better blood supply. Larger adults require a longer needle than a frail adult or a child. The shortest needles are reserved for intradermal use. See Table 6-1 for usual needle sizes and their purposes. In addition to altering needle size, the angle of injection is altered for different-sized patients. This is learned in supervised clinical practice.

> ✳ **Mnemonic**
>
> LL: **L**ower gauge number, **L**arger needle.

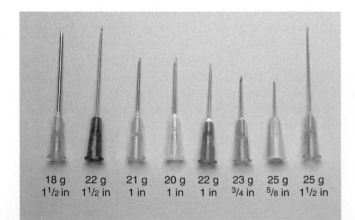

| 18 g | 22 g | 21 g | 20 g | 22 g | 23 g | 25 g | 25 g |
| 1½ in | 1½ in | 1 in | 1 in | 1 in | ¾ in | ⅝ in | 1½ in |

FIGURE 6-15 Needles of various gauges and lengths. (From Lilley LL, Collins SR, Harrington S, Snyder JS: *Pharmacology and the nursing process,* ed. 6, St. Louis, 2011, Mosby.)

TABLE 6-1	Usual Needle Sizes and Purposes	
Usual Needle Size*	**Purpose**	
27-30 gauge	Intradermal skin tests, subcutaneous insulin administration	
25-27 gauge	Subcutaneous injections, heparin administration	
22 gauge	Spinal canal insertion	
20-23 gauge	Intramuscular injections	
16-20 gauge	Intravenous injections	
18 gauge	Preferred for blood administration because blood is viscous	

*Check your agency supply and protocols. There are other sizes available.

1 If you were going to have an intramuscular injection, which gauge would you prefer for the injection, provided your body size was appropriate for any of them: 20, 21, 22, or 23?

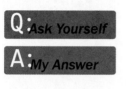

_____

2 If a solution is viscous, might you need a lower or higher gauge needle?

_____

The tips of glass ampules are broken off by the nurse to gain access to the contents.

➤ Special filter needles *must* be used when withdrawing medications from glass ampules so that small particles of glass cannot enter the syringe (Figure 6-16).

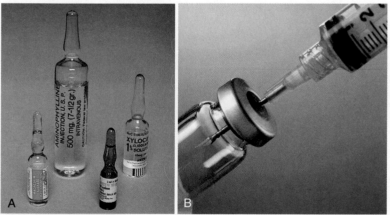

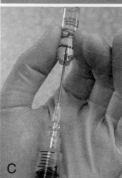

FIGURE 6-16 A, Ampules containing medications come in various sizes. The ampules must be broken carefully to withdraw the medication. **B,** BD Filter Nokor™ needle. Some agencies require that filter needles be used for vials as well as ampules. **C,** Using a filter needle to withdraw medication from an ampule. (**A,** From Perry AG, Potter PA: *Clinical nursing skills and techniques,* ed. 7, St. Louis, 2010, Mosby. **B,** From Becton, Dickinson, and Company, Franklin Lakes, NJ. **C,** From Lilley L, Collins SR, Harrington S, Snyder JS: *Pharmacology and the nursing process,* ed. 6, St. Louis, 2011, Mosby. From Rick Brady, Riva, MD.)

➤ Discard the filter needle and replace it with an appropriately sized needle for injection of the medication into the patient.
➤ Do not use a filter needle for injection into a patient.

Q: *Ask Yourself*

1 Why must the filter needles be replaced before injection?

A: *My Answer*

_____

Safety Syringes

CLINICAL RELEVANCE

➤ The greatest risks for needle-stick injury are during the handling and disposal of used needles *after* injection. Risks of needle-stick injury include transmission of blood-borne pathogens such as hepatitis B and C and AIDS.

There is a trend to provide prepared medicines and needles with safety features to prevent needle-stick injuries. Many syringes are supplied with a variety of sheaths and sliding or retracting devices to cover the needle as soon as it is withdrawn from the patient to prevent needle-stick injuries (Figures 6-17 and 6-18).

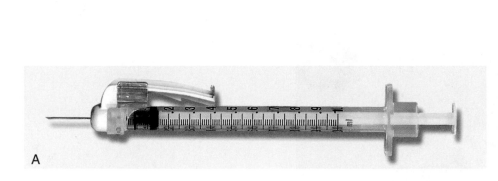
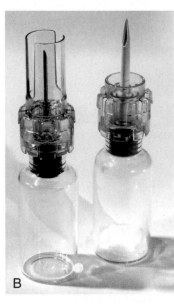

FIGURE 6-17 **A,** BD Safety Glide™ single-handed syringe device with needle cover. **B,** BD Monovial™. (From Becton, Dickinson, and Company, Franklin Lakes, NJ.)

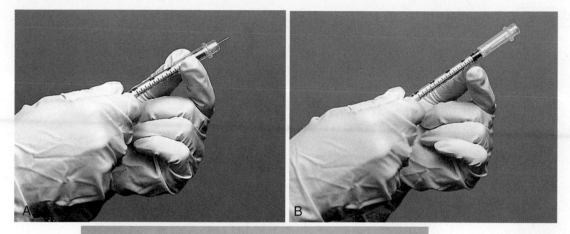

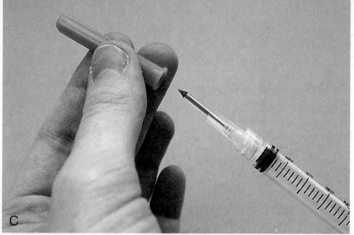

FIGURE 6-18 Needle with plastic guard to prevent needle-sticks. **A,** Position of guard before injection. **B,** After injection, the guard locks in place, covering the needle. **C,** Syringe with needleless vial access adapter. (**A** and **B,** From Potter PA, Perry AG: *Fundamentals of nursing,* ed. 6, St. Louis, 2005, Mosby. **C,** From Perry AG, Potter PA: *Clinical nursing skills and techniques,* ed. 7, St. Louis, 2010, Mosby.)

Do not recap used needles.

Beware of needles projecting from overfilled containers.

Beware of human traffic when crossing a room or exiting a curtained area with an exposed contaminated needle. The needle needs to be pointed away from the carrier and toward the floor (not angled toward the ceiling).

Sharps containers need to be replaced when they are $\frac{2}{3}$ full.

Do not attempt to push a syringe into a filled sharps container. Your hand may be stuck by an upright needle in the container.

Be very careful if a bedside treatment that included an injection (e.g., a spinal tap) has been performed. A used needle inadvertently dropped in the bedding poses a needle-stick risk.

➤ During orientation to any new clinical agency, nurses need to familiarize themselves with the types and uses of syringes and needles, the needleless equipment available, and the location of sharps disposal containers. Agency policies pertaining to handling of the equipment must also be checked.

CLINICAL RELEVANCE

Safety Issues and Disposal of Sharps

Used syringes and needles must be disposed *of immediately* in special hazardous waste containers (Figure 6-19). Check your agency policies for needle and syringe disposal. The trend is to use needleless equipment and safety syringes.

RAPID PRACTICE **6-7**   *Reading Syringe Volumes*

Estimated completion time: 10 minutes   **Answers on page 515**

Directions: *Examine the calibrations of the syringes pictured to answer the questions. Follow these three steps to rapidly interpret syringe calibrations:*

- Identify the total capacity.

- Note the volume and number of calibrations between two adjacent dark lines.

- Calculate the smallest measurable dose (specific volume ÷ number of calibrations).

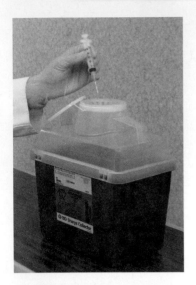

FIGURE 6-19 Never recap a used needle! Always dispose of uncapped needles in the appropriate sharps container. (In Lilley LL, Collins SR, Harrington S, Snyder JS: *Pharmacology and the nursing process,* ed. 6, St. Louis, 2011, Mosby.)

1

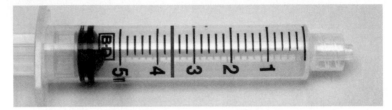

a. Total volume of this syringe: _____

b. Number of calibrations between 0 and 1 mL: _____

c. Value of each calibration (smallest measurable dose): _____

d. What is the amount marked on the syringe? _____

2

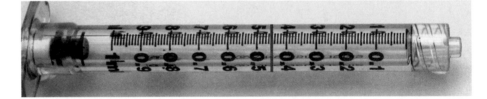

a. Total volume of this syringe: _____

b. Number of calibrations between 0 and 0.1 mL: _____

c. The value of each calibration (smallest measurable dose): _____

d. What is the amount marked on the syringe? _____

3

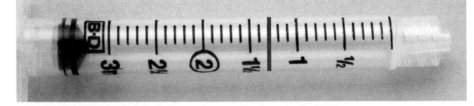

a. Total volume of this syringe: _____

b. Number of calibrations between 0 and 1 mL: _____

c. The value of each calibration (smallest measurable dose): _____

d. What is the amount marked on the syringe? _____

4

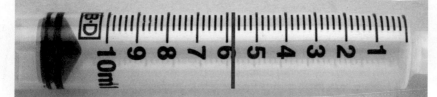

   a. Total volume of this syringe: _____

   b. Number of calibrations between 0 and 1 mL: _____

   c. The value of each calibration (smallest measurable dose): _____

   d. What is the amount marked on the syringe? _____

5

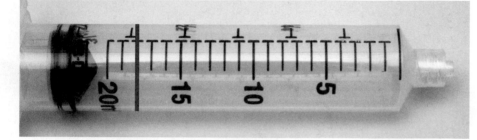

   a. Total volume of this syringe. _____

   b. Number of calibrations between 0 and 1 mL. _____

   c. The value of each calibration (smallest measurable dose) _____

   d. What is the amount marked on the syringe? _____

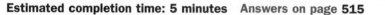

Measuring Syringe Volumes in 5-, 10-, and 20-mL Syringes   **RAPID PRACTICE** 6-8

Estimated completion time: 5 minutes   **Answers on page 515**

Directions: *Draw a vertical line through the calibrated line for the requested volume on each syringe.*

1   3.8 mL

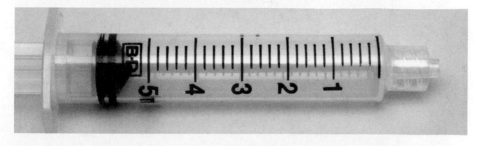

2   4.2 mL

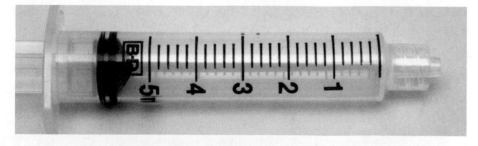

3   8.2 mL

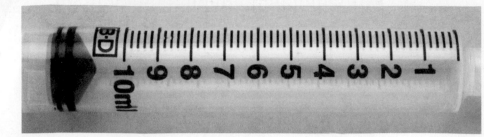

4   14 mL

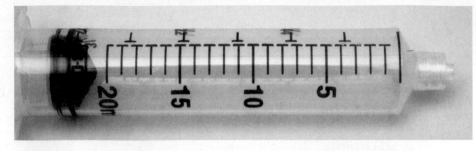

5   7.2 mL

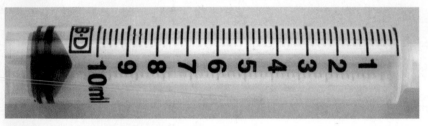

1-mL Syringe Measurements

Estimated completion time: 5-10 minutes   **Answers on page 516**

Directions: *Draw a vertical line through the calibrated line of each syringe for the dose to be given. The top ring of the plunger,* closest to the needle, *must rest on that calibrated line of the dose in milliliters when the medication is drawn into the syringe.*

1   0.24-mL

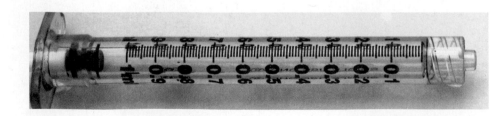

2   0.86-mL

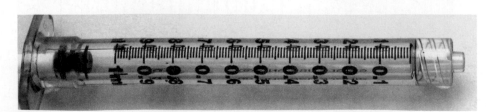

CHAPTER 6

3   0.55-mL

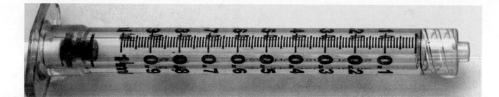

4   0.3-mL

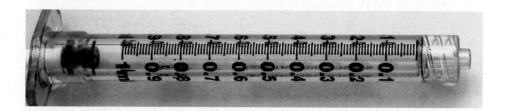

5   Draw an arrow pointing to 0.1 mL, the volume used for most skin tests (such as that for tuberculosis).

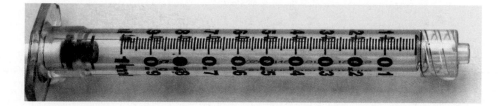

3-mL Syringe Measurements

RAPID PRACTICE 6-10

Estimated completion time: 5-10 minutes   Answers on page **517**

Directions: *Draw a vertical line through the calibrated line of each syringe for the dose requested.*

1   1.4-mL

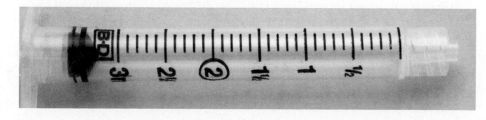

2   1.8-mL

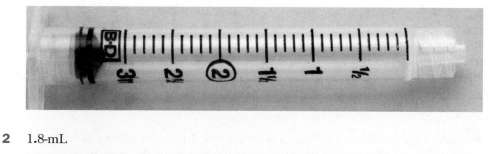

3   0.6-mL

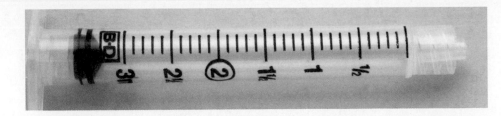

4   2.8-mL

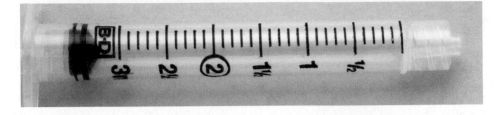

5   0.7-mL

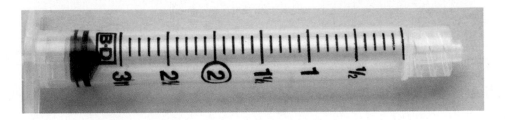

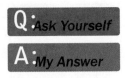

1   When you read and check volumes on a syringe, why is it advisable to have the calibrations at eye level and eyeglasses on hand?

_____

Recommended Fluid Volume for Selected Sites

An excess of injected fluid volume into tissue is not absorbed within a reasonable amount of time, and it causes discomfort for the patient. The recommended fluid volumes for selected sites are as follows:

- 0.1 mL for intradermal skin tests
- 0.5-1 mL for subcutaneous injections at a single site
- Up to 3 mL for intramuscular injections at a single site
- 1-60 mL for intravenous injections

➤ Assuming the correct syringe is selected, the nurse rounds the number of milliliters of medication to the *nearest measurable dose* on the syringe. If the syringe is calibrated in *tenths* of a milliliter, the medication is prepared to the *nearest tenth*. If the syringe is calibrated in *hundredths* of a milliliter, the medication prepared to the *nearest hundredth*.

➤ Do *not* round up to whole numbers, such as from 0.8 to 1 mL or from 0.5 to 1 mL on a syringe. For a review of rounding instructions, see p. 20.

CHAPTER 6 MULTIPLE-CHOICE REVIEW

Estimated completion time: 10-15 minutes   **Answers on page 517**

Directions: *If necessary, review the syringe measurements presented in this chapter. Then circle the number of the correct response, as shown in problem 1.*

1 A 1-mL syringe is calibrated in which of the following increments?
  1. Hundredths of a milliliter   **3.** 0.2 mL
  2. Tenths of a milliliter   **4.** 1 mL

2 A 3-mL syringe is calibrated in which of the following increments?
  1. Hundredths of a milliliter   **3.** 0.2 mL
  2. Tenths of a milliliter   **4.** 1 mL

3 The most commonly used size of syringe for adult intramuscular injections is
  1. 1 mL   **3.** 5 mL
  2. 3 mL   **4.** 10 mL

4 The *syringe* size and amount used for skin tests is
  1. 1-mL size, 0.1-mL amount   **3.** 5-mL size, 0.2-mL amount
  2. 3-mL, size, 1-mL amount   **4.** 10-mL size, 1-mL amount

5 Which of the following is the major criterion in *syringe* selection?
  1. Volume of medication to be given
  2. Route of administration specified by prescriber
  3. Trade and generic names of the drug
  4. Size of the patient in lb or kg

6 When do most needlestick injuries occur?
  1. During medication preparation   **3.** After medication administration
  2. During medication administration   **4.** When the patient self-administers

7 Which of the following are the main criteria for selection of needle size?
  1. Medication viscosity, medication route, size of patient, and skin condition of patient
  2. Volume of fluid to be administered and number of milligrams of medication to be administered
  3. Frequency of medication administration
  4. Gauge and length of needle

8 Which of the following statements pertaining to needle gauge is true?
  1. The highest-gauge needles have the smallest diameters.
  2. An 18-gauge needle is narrower than a 23-gauge needle.
  3. The needles with the smallest gauges are used for intradermal skin tests.
  4. The needles with the largest gauges are used for intramuscular tests.

9 If the dose ordered is 2.54 mL, to be administered with a 3-mL syringe, how many milliliters should the nurse administer?
  1. 2.5 mL   **3.** 2.6 mL
  2. 2.54 mL   **4.** 3 mL

10 If the dose ordered is 0.88 mL, to be administered with a 1-mL syringe, how many milliliters should the nurse administer?
  1. 0.8 mL   **3.** 0.88 mL
  2. 0.85 mL   **4.** 0.9 mL

CHAPTER 6 FINAL PRACTICE

Estimated completion time: 1 hour   **Answers on page 517**

Directions: *Estimate and calculate the dose using mental arithmetic and DA verification when requested. Evaluate the answer. Does the estimate support the answer? Draw a vertical line through the calibrated line of each syringe to indicate the dose to be given.*

1 Ordered: 200 mg of Drug Y. Available: 100 mg per mL.

   a. Estimated dose: Will you need to give *more or less* than the unit mL dose available? (Circle one.)

   b. How many mL will you give? (Use mental arithmetic.) _____

   c. Evaluation: _____

Draw a vertical line through the nearest measurable amount on the 3-mL syringe shown.

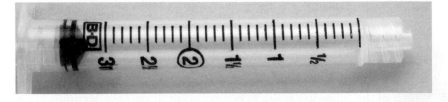

2 Ordered: 15 mg of Drug Y. Available: 30 mg per mL.

   a. Estimated dose: Will you need to give *more or less* than the unit mL dose available? (Circle one.)

   b. How many mL will you give? (Use mental arithmetic.) _____

   c. Evaluation: _____

Draw a vertical line through the nearest measurable amount on the 3-mL syringe shown.

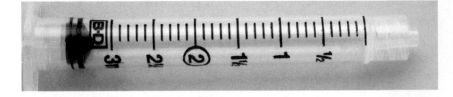

3 Ordered: 320 mg of Drug Y. Available: 50 mg per mL.

   a. Estimated dose: Will you need to give *more or less* than the unit mL dose available? (Circle one.)

   b. How many mL will you give?

   DA equation:

   c. Evaluation: _____

Draw a vertical line through the nearest measurable amount on the 10-mL syringe shown.

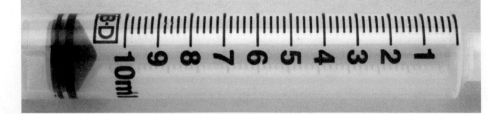

4 Ordered: 80 mg of Drug Y. Available: 75 mg per mL.

    a. Estimated dose: Will you need to give *more or less* than the unit mL dose available? (Circle one.)

    b. How many mL will you give?

    DA equation:

    c. Evaluation: _____

Draw a vertical line through the nearest measurable amount on the 3-mL syringe shown.

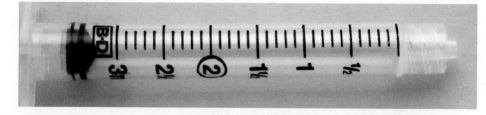

5 Ordered: 50 mg of Drug Y. Available: 10 mg per mL.

    a. Estimated dose: Will you need to give *more or less* than the unit mL dose available? (Circle one.)

    b. How many mL will you give? (Use mental arithmetic.) _____

    c. Evaluation: _____

Draw a vertical line through the nearest measurable amount on the 5-mL syringe shown.

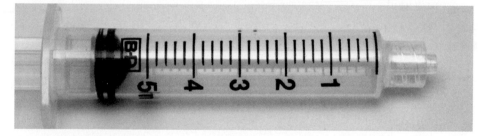

6 Ordered: 40 mg of Drug Y. Available 50 mg per mL.

    a. Examine the ordered dose and the dose available. Estimate your dose calculation. Will you need to give *more or less* than the unit mL dose available? (Circle one.)

    b. How many mL will you give?

    DA equation:

    c. Evaluation: _____

Draw a vertical line through the nearest measurable amount on the 3-mL syringe shown.

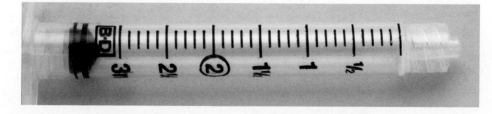

7 Ordered: 120 mg of Drug Y. Available: 10 mg per mL.

    a. Examine the ordered dose and the dose available. Estimate your dose calculation. Will you need to give *more or less* than the unit mL dose available? (Circle one.)

    b. How many mL will you give?

    DA equation:

    c. Evaluation: _____

Draw a vertical line through the nearest measurable amount on the 20-mL syringe shown.

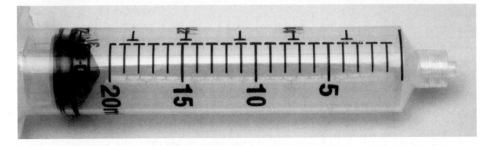

8 Ordered: 15 mg of Drug Y. Available: 100 mg per mL.

    a. Examine the ordered dose and the dose available. Estimate your dose calculation. Will you need to give *more or less* than the unit mL dose available? (Circle one.)

    b. How many mL will you give for the nearest measurable dose on the syringe provided?

    DA equation:

    c. Evaluation: _____

Draw an arrow pointing to the nearest measurable amount on the 1-mL syringe provided.

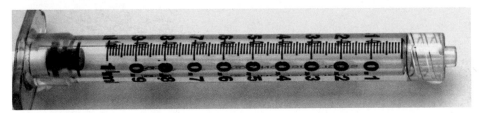

9 a. What is the most important criterion for syringe selection in relation to the ordered dose? _____

    b. Should you select the syringe *before* or *after* calculating the dose volume in mL? _____

10 a. List two special precautions that must be taken when disposing of used and/or contaminated needles? _____

    _____

    b. Name two diseases mentioned in the chapter that can be acquired through needle-stick injuries. _____

Suggestions for Further Reading

Perry AG, Potter PA: *Clinical nursing skills and techniques,* ed. 7, St. Louis, 2010,
    Mosby.

www.bd.com
www.cdc.gov/niosh/docs/2000-108
www.fda.gov/cder/drug/MedErrors
www.ismp.org
www.usp.org/hqi/patientSafety/standards.html

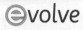 Additional information can be found in the Safety in Medication Adminis-
tration section of the Student Companion on Evolve.

Chapter 7 covers the calculations for reconstitution of powder and liquid medications. Syringes are often used to reconstitute medications. DA equations will be
needed to calculate a variety of doses.

Reconstitution of Powders and Liquids

OBJECTIVES

- Distinguish routes of drugs for reconstitution.
- Interpret directions for dilution of reconstituted medications.
- Select the appropriate concentration to prepare for the ordered dose.
- Calculate doses for reconstituted medications using DA equations.
- Measure the appropriate dose using a medicine cup and a syringe.
- Identify appropriate notation on reconstituted multidose medication labels.
- Interpret directions for safe storage of reconstituted medications.
- Calculate ratio dilutions for partial-strength solutions.

Essential Prior Knowledge

- Mastery of Chapters 1-6

Essential Equipment

- The mathematics can be mastered without equipment, but eventually supervised clinical laboratory experience with vials, syringes, and powders will be necessary.

Estimated Time To Complete Chapter

- 1-2 hours

Introduction

Campers who have reconstituted dried food and care-givers who have mixed powdered baby formula with water to prepare a bottle have applied the technique of reconstitution of dry products. Some medications are supplied in the form of powders or crystals to which a liquid must be added for reconstitution shortly before use.

The medications are supplied in dry form because the product can be stored for a long time in dry form but becomes unstable and deteriorates in solution within a relatively short time. Such solutions are said to have a "short shelf life." The equipment used to reconstitute medications must be calibrated for the medicines being dispensed. The capacity of syringes, medicine droppers, and "medication teaspoons" is precise, while that of household equipment varies greatly from spoon to spoon and cup to cup.

ESSENTIAL *Vocabulary*

Diluent	Fluid that makes a mixture less concentrated or viscous. The fluid dilutes the mixture. It is also used to convert a dry form of a substance to a liquid form. For example, water is used to liquefy a dry form of baby formula. When reconstituting medications, read the directions to find out which diluent needs to be used. Water or normal saline (NS) solution is often used to dilute medicines and to liquefy dry, powdered forms of medicines.
Dilution	Extent to which the concentration of a mixture is reduced.
Dilution Ratio	Special ratio indicating the number of parts of an active ingredient to the number of parts of inactive ingredients in a solution. For example, a 1:4 dilution ratio means that, out of 5 total parts, 1 part is active and 4 parts are inactive. Adding 4 parts water to 1 part powdered milk would provide a dilution ratio of 1:4.
Displacement	Volume occupied by a powder when a diluent is added during reconstitution.
Reconstitution	Process of combining the dry form of a mixture with a fluid to achieve a usable state. Process of diluting a liquid concentrate to achieve a usable state.
Solution Concentration (Strength)	Amount of drug in a quantity of solution expressed as a ratio (e.g., 100 mg per 100 mL, or 1:1) or as a fraction or a percentage (e.g., $\frac{1}{2}$ strength, or 50% solution).
Suspension	Liquid in which fine particles are dispersed throughout a fluid, where they are supported by the buoyancy of shaking or stirring. If a suspension is left standing, the solid particles settle. Antibiotics are often supplied as oral suspensions.
SW	Sterile water.
Bacteriostatic SW	Sterile water with an antimicrobial agent, such as benzyl alcohol.
	➤ Sterile water and bacteriostatic sterile water cannot be used interchangeably with each other or with tap water. The product label specifies the diluent.
Unit	Standardized laboratory measure of the therapeutic strength, as opposed to the weight or volume, of a drug. Often used as a standard of measure for medications that are derived from plants and animals and that have components with variable strengths. Substances, such as hormones and penicillin, that are partially derived from animal and plant sources are easily broken down to an unstable state of diminished effectiveness. The term *units* is also used to describe metric units of measurement.
Unstable	Easily broken down to a state of diminished effectiveness. Breakdown can occur rapidly with reconstituted solutions. Foods, solutions, and certain medications that are unstable, such as reconstituted medications, have a short shelf life. They must be discarded if they are not used in a timely fashion. Refrigeration may extend shelf life. Consult the label.

Vocabulary Review

RAPID PRACTICE   7-1

Estimated completion time: 5 minutes   Answers on page 520

Directions: *Circle the correct definition for the following.*

1   The amount of drug in a quantity of solution expressed as a ratio is called

    1. An emulsion   **3.** A suspension

    2. The concentration   **4.** A diluent

2   The solution used to reconstitute powders and crystals from a dry form of medicine to a liquid form is called

    1. An emulsion   **3.** A suspension

    2. An elixir   **4.** A diluent

3 Solutions that deteriorate rapidly in liquid form are considered to have a short shelf life and are described as:

    1. Crystals   **3.** Bacteriostatic

    2. Unstable   **4.** Diluents

4 The process of combining a liquid with a solid form of medication so that the medication can be used is called

    1. Reconstitution   **3.** Calibration

    2. Dilution   **4.** Concentration

5 Accurate measurement of liquid medications requires which type of equipment?

    1. Household teaspoons and tablespoons

    2. Equipment with metric calibrations

    3. Household droppers and cups

    4. A syringe and needle

Reconstituted Medications

Some medicines are very unstable in liquid form. Therefore, they are supplied in a dry form to which an inactive diluent is added just before use. The information about the specific type and amount of diluent to be added to achieve specific concentrations is provided on the label. The nurse selects the amount of diluent that will provide the concentration closest to the dose ordered.

Interpreting orders and reading labels for reconstituted medications

Examine the following order: Augmentin suspension 125 mg tid PO × 5 days. The order includes the form, oral *suspension,* but does *not* mention that the drug requires reconstitution or describe how to prepare it. The nurse must read the medication label and insert to determine how to prepare the medication.

➤ Pharmacists usually reconstitute large volume oral suspensions and relabel with the quantity per dose to be given.

Reading Labels Directions on the label state the precise amount and type of liquid diluent to add in order to achieve specific dilutions or concentrations of the drug per milliliter. The directions always state conditions and time limits for storage after reconstitution to liquid form. Some products must be discarded immediately, while others may be refrigerated for several hours or days so that they can be used for additional doses.

There is a lot of information on the label, but most of it is self-explanatory once you have read one or two types of labels. Examine the directions on the following label for an oral suspension to be reconstituted:

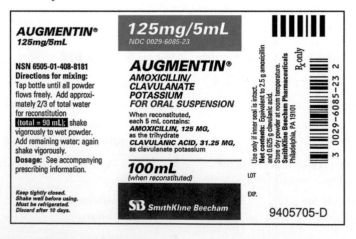

➤ The route is oral. This is important to note because there are injectable antibiotics and other drugs with similar names made specifically for intramuscular or intravenous routes.

➤ The type of *diluent* is water. Most oral suspension diluents use tap water unless otherwise specified. Pediatric patients and immunocompromised patients may need SW.

➤ The total *amount of diluent* to be added is 90 mL, added in two parts: 60 mL for the first mix and 30 mL for the second.

➤ After reconstitution, the unit drug *concentration* (unit dose concentration) will be 125 mg per 5 mL water. The total amount of medication will be 100 mL, although only 90 mL of water was added. This discrepancy is due to displacement of liquid by the powder. Both ingredients occupy space. Discard after 10 days.

➤ Reconstitution of an injectable is illustrated on p. 217.

It is critical to communicate the date and time of preparation and the specific concentration of reconstituted solutions to nursing staff on subsequent shifts with a *clearly marked added label.*

CLINICAL RELEVANCE

Marking the label for reconstituted medications

The label is marked by the nurse only under the following conditions:

1 The drug label states that the medication may be used more than once after reconstitution.

2 The patient is eligible to receive another dose before the drug must be discarded.

➤ The label for reconstituted medications must contain the patient's name, the date and time of preparation, the diluent type and amount added, the concentration per milliliter after dilution, and the nurse's initials or name, according to agency policy. Discard date and time are added according to agency policy. Refer to the Augmentin label on p. 206 and the reconstituted label below.

RECONSTITUTED AUGMENTIN ORAL SUSPENSION BOTTLE
Patient: John B. Doe
01/05/11 1800: 90 mL SW added; 125 mg per 5 mL, JM, RN
Discard date and time*:

_____

*Check institutional policies for specific agency requirements, especially discard date requirements. Some agencies require that the nurse add the discard date and *time* for the prepared reconstituted drug to the label. Other agencies prefer that the expiration or discard date and time be redetermined from the reconstitution date and label directions by *each* nurse administering the medication.

EXAMPLES

➤ Reconstituted medications for multidose use are the one exception to the rule, "Never give a medication prepared by someone else."

➤ The exception may be made only if the label is clearly marked with all the required data.

➤ Reconstituted medications with labels that are not annotated with all the required data must be discarded to avoid giving an ineffective drug or a spoiled liquid.

CLINICAL RELEVANCE

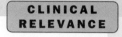

Expired Reconstituted Drugs

Single-dose preparations cannot be stored. The remainder must be discarded. Only multidose preparations may be stored and reused according to label directions and hospital policy.

CLINICAL RELEVANCE	Because of the cost and short shelf life of reconstituted medications, it is appropriate that the nurse review the patient's records and recent orders to be sure that the medication order has not expired before preparing the medication.

RAPID PRACTICE **7-2**

Interpreting Labels for Reconstituted Medications

Estimated completion time: 25 minutes   **Answers on page 520**

Directions: *Read the labels for the medications and supply the required information. Use brief phrases.*

1

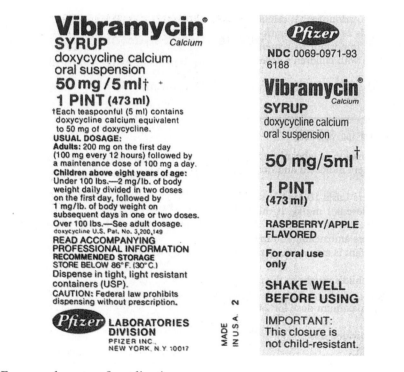

a. Form and route of medication: _____

b. Generic name: _____

c. Unit dose concentration after reconstitution (mg per mL)*: _____

d. Unit dose or multidose container: _____

e. Total volume in container after reconstitution: _____

f. Storage directions: _____

---

*milligram(s) per milliliter(s). The unit dose (drug) concentration is a multiple of the usual doses ordered. Note that mL is both the singular and plural abbreviation. Do not write mLs.

2

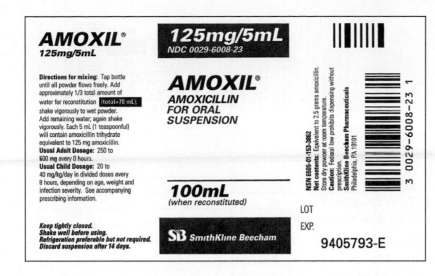

a. Form and route of medication: _____

b. Type of diluent to be used: _____

c. Total amount of diluent to add to bottle: _____

d. Mixing directions: _____

e. Unit dose concentration after reconstitution: _____

f. Usual adult dose: _____

g. Usual child dose: _____

h. Unit dose or multidose container: _____

i. Expiration, or discard time, after reconstitution: _____

➤ If a slash (/) is used on a drug label or in a drug order, be careful to avoid reading it as the number 1. For example, 5 mg/5 mL may be misread as 5 mg per 15 mL.

3

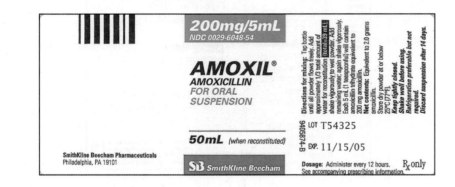

a. Form and route of medication: _____

b. Type and amount of diluent to be used: _____

c. Total volume in container after reconstitution: _____

d. Unit dose concentration after reconstitution: _____

e. Storage directions: _____

f. Mixing directions after reconstitution: _____

g. Discard directions: _____

Note that the labels in problems 2 and 3 are for the same medication but contain different unit dose concentrations per 5 mL (1 medication teaspoon). Remember to use special calibrated medication teaspoons and/or droppers if those implements are needed. Use a syringe without a needle for measurement of oral suspensions if the implements are not provided.

4

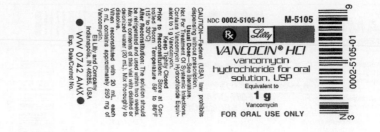

a. Trade name: _____

b. Generic name: _____

c. Route: _____

d. Total amount in vial: _____

e. Unit dose concentration after reconstitution: _____

5   Ordered: Nystatin oral suspension 400,000 units swish and swallow four times daily while awake for an adult with an oral candidiasis (yeast) infection secondary to antibiotic administration.*

Directions: Administer ½ of dose each side of the mouth and have patient swish thoroughly and swallow.

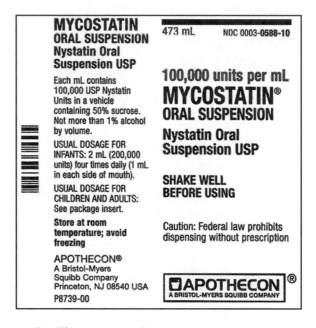

a. How many mL will you prepare? _____

b. How many mL will you administer each side of the mouth? _____

c. Where should the product be stored? _____

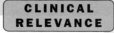
CLINICAL RELEVANCE

The medications in problems 1 and 5 have already been reconstituted by the pharmacy prior to dispensing. This can reduce errors. Directions for storage and discard need to be emphasized when teaching patients.

*Problem 5 is an example of a prepared suspension that does not need further dilution.

Reconstituting, Calculating, and Measuring Oral Doses

Estimated completion time: 30 minutes   Answers on page 521

Directions: *Read the order and the label, then estimate and calculate the dose using a DA equation. Shade in the medicine cup to the nearest multiple of 5 mL. Indicate the balance of the dose that will be added with the syringe, as shown in problem 1.*

1   Ordered cephalexin oral suspension 0.3g PO q6h for a patient with a respiratory tract infection

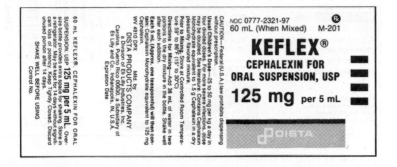

a. Total amount and type of diluent to be added: _____36 mL_____ (*all at once* or *divided*?)

b. Estimate: *more than* or *less than* the dose per 5 mL after reconstitution (circle one)

c. How many mL will you prepare (per dose)? _____12 mL_____ to the nearest tenth of a mL?

DA equation:

$$\frac{mL}{dose} : \frac{5\ mL}{\overset{}{\underset{1}{125\ mg}}} \times \frac{\overset{8}{\cancel{1000\ mg}}}{1\ g} \times \frac{0.3\ g}{dose} = \frac{12\ mL}{dose}$$

d. Evaluation: _The answer supports the estimate. The equation is balanced._

Shade in the nearest measurable dose in mL on the medicine cup and draw a vertical line through the calibrated line of the syringe for the remaining mL as applicable.*

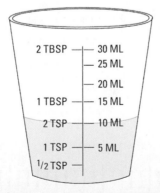

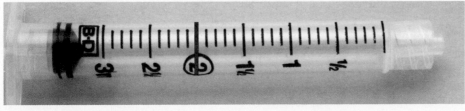

---

*Throughout, shade in the medicine cup in multiples of 5 mL as applicable; measure the balance of the dose in the syringe.

2 Ordered: Augmentin oral susp 0.25 g q8h PO for a patient with otitis media.

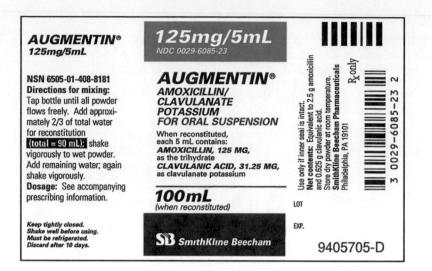

a. Amount and type of diluent to be added: _____

b. Estimate: *more than* or *less than* unit dose after reconstitution? (Circle one.)

c. How many milliliters will you prepare? _____

DA equation:

d. Evaluation: _____

Shade in the dose in mL on the medicine cup and draw a vertical line through the calibrated line of the syringe as applicable.

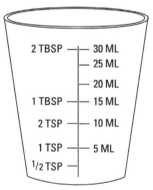

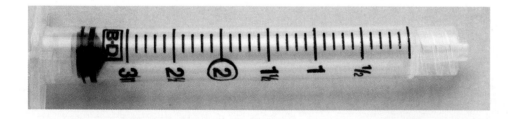

3 Ordered: amoxicillin oral susp 0.2 g PO q8h for a patient with an infection.

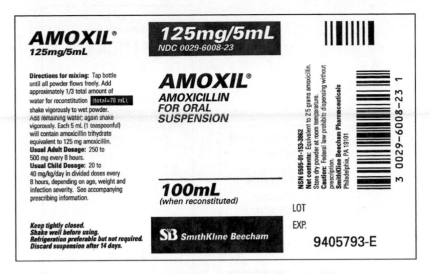

a. Estimate: *more than* or *less than* unit dose after reconstitution? (Circle one.)

b. How many milliliters will you prepare? _____

DA equation:

c. Evaluation: _____

Shade in the dose in mL on the medicine cup and draw a vertical line through the calibrated line of the syringe as applicable.

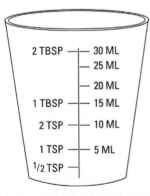

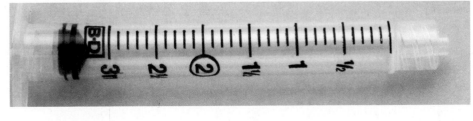

4 Ordered: fluconazole oral susp 0.03 g PO daily for a patient with oral candidiasis.

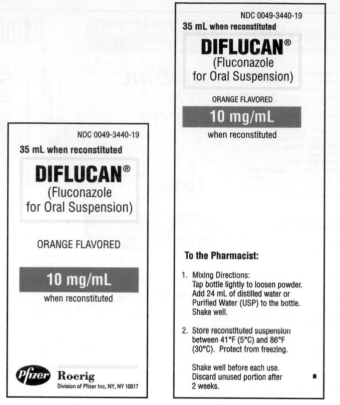

a. Amount and type of diluent to be added: _____

b. Estimate: *more than* or *less than* unit dose after reconstitution? (Circle one.)

c. How many milliliters will you prepare? _____

DA equation:

d. Evaluation: _____

Draw a vertical line through the calibrated line of the syringe as applicable.

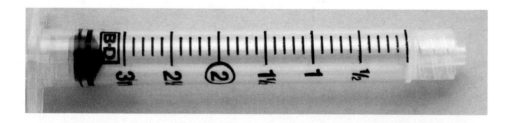

5   Ordered: Amoxicillin susp 0.25g PO TID for a adult patient with an infection.

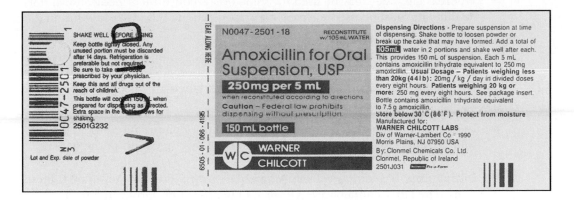

a. Amount and type of diluent to be added: _____

b. Estimate: *more than* or *less than* dose after reconstitution? (Circle one.)

c. How many milliliters will you prepare to the nearest tenth of a mL? _____

   DA equation:

d. Evaluation: _____

Shade in the dose in mL on the medicine cup and draw a vertical line through the calibrated line of the syringe as applicable.

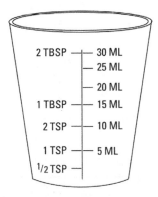

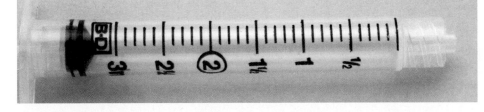

Reconstituted Parenteral Drugs

➤ Parenteral medications must be sterile and have a much shorter shelf life than do drugs administered by other routes.

Diluents

➤ Whereas tap water may be used for some oral reconstituted medications, sterile diluents must be used for parenteral medications. Always read dilution directions.

Although sterile water *for injection* and sterile NS solution are the most commonly used diluents, occasionally, custom diluents or dextrose solutions are required. Some labels permit either SW *or* NS. Other labels are specifically limited to one choice of diluent because of incompatibility.

➤ Incompatibility can result in crystallization and/or clumping of the drug in solution and can cause a problem in the tissue or circulation of the patient.

➤ Distinguish *SW for injection* from *bacteriostatic water for injection* on diluent directions. The latter contains a *preservative*. One cannot be substituted for the other. The label must be read and followed exactly. Some references use the abbreviation *SW* for *sterile water for injection* and *NS* for *sterile normal saline solution for injection*. Bacteriostatic water is spelled out in the dilution directions on the label.

Selecting the Appropriate Unit Dose Concentration Based on Dilution Directions When More Than One Dilution Is Offered

If a 1:100 concentration of sugar water was needed for your hummingbird feeder and you had on hand a 1:30 solution, a 1:50 solution, and a 1:100 solution, you would select the more dilute 1:100 concentration for the feeder. Giving the more concentrated solutions would overdose the hummingbirds with sugar. Similarly, with medications the nurse prepares the strength that provides the dose needed and the most convenient volume for the route ordered.

In selecting the appropriate amount of diluent, the nurse considers the relevant factors in the following sequence when reading the label:

- Route ordered
- Dose ordered and amount needed
- Drug concentrations and volumes available that are close in amount to the ordered dose for that route

Based on the ordered amount, the nurse examines the label to make critical decisions. For example, consider an order of Drug A 200 mg IM. The label dilution directions state:

For IM injection:
Add 1.8 mL SW for injection to obtain 200 mg per mL.
Add 3.6 mL SW for injection to obtain 100 mg per mL.
Add 5.2 mL SW for injection to obtain 75 mg per mL.
For IV injection:
Add 8.4 mL SW for injection to obtain 50 mg per mL.

According to the label, three concentrations are safe to inject into the muscle. The nurse chooses a concentration based on the order. In this example, the first intramuscular option allows the patient to receive a smaller injected *volume*.

Q: Ask Yourself

A: My Answer

1 Which is the more concentrated solution after reconstitution according to the reconstitution directions cited above for Drug A above?

_____

2 Can I use SW, NS, and bacteriostatic water interchangeably to dilute medicines?

_____

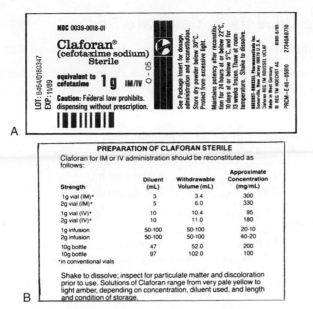

A

B

PREPARATION OF CLAFORAN STERILE

Claforan for IM or IV administration should be reconstituted as follows:

Strength	Diluent (mL)	Withdrawable Volume (mL)	Approximate Concentration (mg/mL)
1g vial (IM)*	3	3.4	300
2g vial (IM)*	5	6.0	330
1g vial (IV)*	10	10.4	95
2g vial (IV)*	10	11.0	180
1g infusion	50-100	50-100	20-10
2g infusion	50-100	50-100	40-20
10g bottle	47	52.0	200
10g bottle	97	102.0	100

*in conventional vials

Shake to dissolve; inspect for particulate matter and discoloration prior to use. Solutions of Claforan range from very pale yellow to light amber, depending on concentration, diluent used, and length and condition of storage.

This label is included to illustrate medications that need to be reconstituted for routes other than oral and that offer *multiple options for dilution.* If the label permits several choices of dilution in order to obtain different unit dose strengths, the nurse must take special care to focus on the appropriate dilution. Several choices of dilution are more likely to be found with reconstituted parenteral drugs.

1   What are the amounts of diluent recommended for the 1 g reconstituted intramuscular preparation and for the 1 g intravenous preparation?

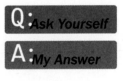

_____

2   What will be the concentration of the 1 g reconstituted intramuscular preparation and the 1 g intravenous infusion preparation?

_____

➤   If you require reading glasses, keep them handy for reading the reconstitution directions.

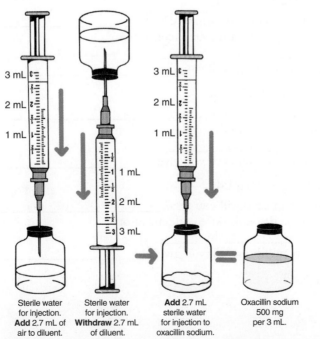

Diluting oxacillin sodium in sterile water for injection. (From Brown M, Mulholland J: *Drug calculations: process and problems for clinical practice,* ed. 8, St. Louis, 2008, Mosby.)

Selecting Diluents to Calculate Doses

Estimated completion time: 20-30 minutes   Answers on page 523

Directions: *Examine the following reconstitution directions and the example in problem 1. Select the appropriate dilution for problems 2-5 using the reconstitution directions provided. Evaluate your equations for problems 4-5.*

Reconstitution directions for Drug Y for IM administration:

Diluent SW	Total Volume	Solution Concentration
1 mL	1.4 mL	480 mg per mL
2 mL	3 mL	250 mg per mL
4 mL	5.8 mL	100 mg per mL
For IV administration:		
12 mL	15.8 mL	50 mg per mL

➤ The more diluent added, the weaker the concentration of the solution.

CLINICAL RELEVANCE

➤ Keep in mind that the average-sized adult should receive no more than 3 mL in one intra-muscular site and that the nurse should select a dilution that permits at least 0.5 mL of in-tramuscular injection.

Select the dilution from the list above that is closest to the unit dose you need and that meets the foregoing criteria. Calculate doses to the *nearest tenth of a milliliter.* Examine the routes first. Then compare the order to the concentrations to find a reasonable low-volume dose. Verify the answer with a DA equation where requested.

1   Ordered: Drug Y, 50 mg IM.

   a. How much diluent will you add? <u>4 mL</u>

   b. What will be the unit dose concentration? <u>100 mg per mL</u>

   c. How many milliliters will you give? <u>0.5 mL</u>

2   Ordered: Drug Y, 0.1 g IM.

   a. How much diluent will you add? _____

   b. What will be the unit dose concentration?

   _____

   c. How many milliliters will you give? _____

3   Ordered: Drug Y, 0.25 g IM.

   a. How much diluent will you add? _____

   b. What will be the unit dose concentration?

   _____

   c. How many milliliters will you give? _____

4   Ordered: Drug Y, 0.3 g IM.

   a. How much diluent will you add? _____

   b. What will be the unit dose concentration?

   _____

   c. How many milliliters will you give? _____

   DA equation:

   d. Evaluation: _____

5 Ordered: Drug Y, 0.5 g IV.
   a. How much diluent will you add? _____
   b. What will be the unit dose concentration?
   _____
   c. How many milliliters will you give? _____

   DA equation:

   d. Evaluation: _____

1 If you were to receive 150 mg of an intramuscular injection and the directions for reconstitution of the medicine specified (a) add 20 mL to obtain 50 mg per mL or (b) add 10 mL to obtain 100 mg per mL, which concentration would you select for reconstitution?

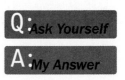

Reconstituted Drug Prefilled Containers

Some parenteral medications for reconstitution are supplied with diluents that are in prefilled syringe cartridges, ampules, or vials. Others are attached to the vial (Figure 7-1) and can be mixed by depressing the stopper without opening the vials. There is less chance for contamination of the contents when the ingredients are not exposed to air.

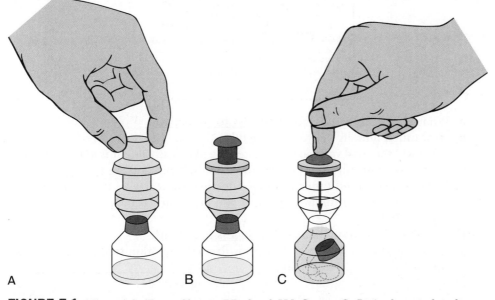

A   B   C

FIGURE 7-1 Mix-o-vial. (From Clayton BD, Stock YN, Cooper S: *Basic pharmacology for nurses,* ed. 15, St. Louis, 2010, Mosby.)

Interpreting Directions and Calculating Reconstituted Injectables

Estimated completion time: 30 minutes   Answers on page 523

Directions: *Examine the worked-out problem 1. Read the labels to answer the questions for problems 2-5. Calculate doses to the nearest measurable dose on the syringe provided.*

1   Ordered: ceftazidime 0.5 g IM, an antibiotic, for a patient with *Klebsiella* pneumonia.

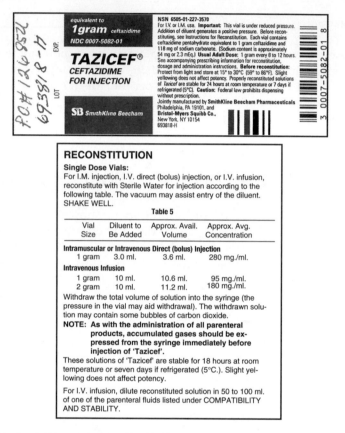

a. What kind of diluent is specified? <u>SW for injection</u>

b. How much diluent will you add? <u>3 mL</u>

c. What will the total volume in milliliters be after the diluent is added? <u>3.6 mL</u>

d. Unit dose concentration IM per mL after dilution: <u>280 mg per mL</u>

e. Is the dose ordered (after you move decimal places) (more than) or *less than* the unit dose after dilution? <u>0.5 g = 500 mg, which is more than the unit dose of 280 mg</u>

f. Estimated dose in milliliters: <u>A little less than 2 mL</u>

g. Actual dose in milliliters calculated with a DA equation to the nearest measurable dose on a 3-mL syringe: _____

$$\frac{mL}{dose} : \frac{mL}{\underset{14}{\cancel{280\ mg}}} \times \frac{\overset{25}{\cancel{500\ mg}}}{dose} = \frac{25}{14} = 1.78,\ \text{rounded to 1.8 mL per dose for the 3-mL syringe}$$

e. Draw a vertical line through the calibrated line of the nearest measurable dose on the syringe.

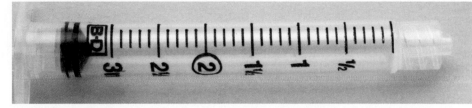

5 Ordered: penicillin G potassium 400,000 units IM q 8 h for 10 days for a patient with a streptococcal infection.

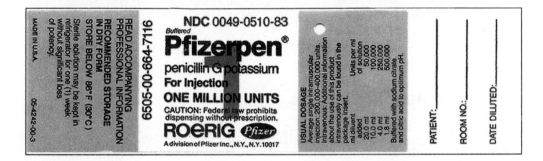

a. Which volume of diluent will you select for this dose to give a minimum of 1 mL? _____

b. Will you give more or less than the units per mL for this dilution? _____

c. How many mL will you administer per dose?

DA equation:

d. Evaluation: _____

e. If satisfactory, draw a vertical line through the calibrated line of the nearest measurable dose on the syringe.

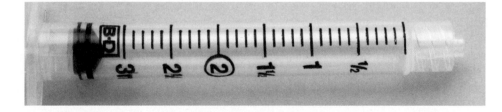

Many of the medications for reconstitution are antibiotics. They may be supplied in several forms and a variety of concentrations for oral, topical, intramuscular, or intravenous routes. Some have similar-sounding generic and trade names. Take care when comparing the order to the label.

➤ Each antibiotic is targeted for specific kinds of infections.

CLINICAL RELEVANCE

Generic Name	Trade Name
cefaclor	Ceclor
cefprozil	Cefzil
cefuroxime	Ceftin
cephalexin	Keflex
cephazolin	Kefzol
ciprofloxacin	Cipro
	Cipro XR

CLINICAL RELEVANCE

Some patients are allergic to certain antibiotics and need a reminder. Assess lung sounds for wheezes and the skin for rashes, and ask the patient if there have been any bowel changes (e.g., diarrhea). These are the most common symptoms of allergic reactions. A skin rash may precede more serious symptoms.

Liquid Concentrates: Diluting Liquids

The pharmacy usually dilutes medication solutions to the ordered strength. Occasionally, the nurse will need to dilute a medication, nutritional beverage supplement, or irrigation solution based on a dilution ratio or percent concentration. Dilution is done to protect the patient from side effects of an overly strong concentration.

➤ Always look for dilution instructions when you see the word *concentrate* on a medication label. Failure to do so could result in serious injury to the patient.

Liquids administered through feeding tubes full strength may cause gastrointestinal distress. Solutions for irrigation treatments may need to be diluted to avoid tissue injury.

Orders may be written in one of three ways to indicate the strength or concentration of a solution:

Order	Meaning
Percentage	*Percent* means "per 100." For example, *50% strength* denotes a solution that contains 50% active ingredient (the drug) plus 50% inactive ingredient (the diluent).
Fraction	For example, $\frac{1}{2}$ or "half strength" indicates that 1 part out of a total of 2 parts is the active ingredient and the other part is the inactive ingredient. The *denominator* of the fraction denotes the total number of parts.
Ratio	For example, 1:1 denotes 2 total parts: 1 part active ingredient *added to* 1 part inactive ingredient. The *left* number is the *active* ingredient, or the drug. The right number is the inactive ingredient, or the diluent.

Inactive Ingredients Used for Dilutions

Water or normal saline (NS) is often the *inactive* ingredient used for dilution. Check the order and label for the diluent. Sterile solutions may be indicated for wound irrigations, pediatric formulas, or immunocompromised patients. Normal saline solution is supplied as a sterile solution. Read the label and check agency protocols. Order the supplies from the pharmacy or central supply, according to agency guidelines.

Percent or fractional strengths are written more frequently for dilution than are ratios.

➤ The two sides of a ratio need to be added to obtain the total number of parts (e.g., 1:3 = 4 total parts).

➤ The nurse must be able to interpret any of the three ways the order may be written.

The order may read as follows:

"Ensure $\frac{1}{2}$ strength, for 3 days PO,"

"Irrigate abdominal wound bid with equal parts NS sol. and hydrogen peroxide (H_2O_2) and NS,"

"Baby formula 60 mL 1:3 sol q2h. If tolerated, increase to 1:2 sol tomorrow."

Converting Dilution Ratios to Fractions and Percentages

➤ To convert a ratio to a fraction, add the *total number of parts* to create a *denominator*. Place the number of active-ingredient parts in the numerator.
➤ To convert a fraction to a percentage, multiply the fraction by 100 and add a percent sign.
➤ To convert a percentage to a fraction, divide the percentage by 100, remove the percent sign, and reduce the fraction.

EXAMPLES

1 **Ordered:** 120 mL q2h Ensure 50%. Preparation: 60 mL Ensure plus 60 mL water to make a 1:1 ratio, $\frac{1}{2}$ strength, or 50% solution. 1:1 = 1 part active ingredient per, to, or plus 1 part inactive ingredient (ratio of Ensure to water). Total parts = 2 = $\frac{1}{2}$ strength = 50% solution ($\frac{1}{2} \times$ 100).

2 **Ordered:** Irrigation with peroxide solution: 1:4. 1:4 = 1 part active ingredient (peroxide) "per", "to", or "plus" 4 parts inactive ingredient (water). Total parts = 5, $\frac{1}{5}$, or 20% solution. Use 1 part active ingredient, and add 4 parts diluent.

➤ Note that the dilution ratio 1:4 does not convert to the fraction $\frac{1}{4}$.
➤ Think of the dilution ratio 1:4 as 1 part added to 4 parts (1 + 4 =5 total parts).
➤ Read the fraction as 1 part out of 5 total parts, or $\frac{1}{5}$.
➤ Read 20% strength as 20 parts per 100 parts, or $\frac{1}{5}$.

Recall from Chapter 1, Essential Math Review, that the denominator of a fraction indicates the *number of total parts* and that *percent* means "per 100." Read $\frac{1}{5}$-strength concentration as 20%.

Using a DA Equation to Calculate the Amount of Concentrate

Most dilution orders can be solved with mental arithmetic or simple arithmetic. The nurse needs to know the concentration and the total amount to be given in order to calculate the amount of active ingredients per the amount of inactive ingredients in milliliters.

➤ Simple DA-style equations are solved using fraction forms. Change the percentage in the order to a fraction.

EXAMPLES

Ordered: 120 mL of 25% formula per feeding tube q2h for 12 hours per day. 25% $= \dfrac{25}{100} = \dfrac{1}{4}$. The desired answer is the amount in milliliters of the *active ingredient*:

mL active ingredient:	Total mL	×	fraction	= answer
(formula)	120 mL	×	$\frac{1}{4}$	= 30 mL *active ingredient*

120 mL total −30 mL active ingredient = 90 mL *diluent* (water)

Evaluation: 30 is 25%, or $\frac{1}{4}$, of 120. 30 + 90 = 120 = 1:3 ratio. Both sides of the equation balance mathematically.

➤ When in doubt about dilutions, consult the agency pharmacist.

RAPID PRACTICE   7-6   *Interpreting Dilution Orders*

Estimated Completion Time: 25 minutes   Answers on page 524

Directions: *Fill in the dilution tables from left to right with the correct equivalent terms and solution amounts, as shown in the first row of the table that follows.*

	Fractional Strength	Ratio of Active to Inactive Ingredients	Percent	Order	Amount of Active Ingredient	Amount of Diluent (Inactive Ingredient)
1	$\frac{1}{4}$	1:3	25%	100 mL q1h	25 mL	75 mL
2			50%	60 mL tid		
3			75%	1000 mL q8h		
4			20%	240 mL four times daily		
5			10%	50 mL once a day		

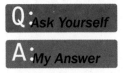

Q: Ask Yourself

A: My Answer

1   What is the difference between a dilution ratio and a fraction? How will I remember? Which one is easier (one less step) to convert to a percentage: the ratio or the fractional strength?

_____

CHAPTER 7 MULTIPLE-CHOICE REVIEW

Estimated completion time: 20-30 minutes   Answers on page 525

Directions: *Circle the correct answer for the following.*

1 Which of the following statements defines *displacement?*
  1. Liquid oral medications are prepared using clean technique and nonsterile equipment.
  2. The diluent for oral liquid medications is usually water.
  3. The volume after reconstitution exceeds the amount of liquid diluent added.
  4. Oral liquid medications are usually prepared to the nearest tenth of a milliliter for adults.

2 Which of the following statements can lead to medication calculation errors?
  1. Suspensions must be combined with a precise amount of diluent and thoroughly mixed.
  2. Elixirs are solutions that contain alcohol.
  3. Extracts are solutions that are concentrated.
  4. It is acceptable to use household teaspoons and tablespoons to measure liquids.

3 Most plastic medication cups have the following milliliter calibrations:
  1. Multiples of 5   **3.** Multiples of 15
  2. Multiples of 10   **4.** Multiples of 30

4 If a liquid oral medication order calls for 13 mL, how will the nurse prepare it?
  1. Pour at eye level to just below the 15 mL line
  2. Pour to 10 mL at eye level and add 3 mL with a needleless syringe.
  3. Pour to 15 mL, remove 2 mL, and return the 2 mL to the medication bottle.
  4. Draw 20 mL in a 20-mL syringe and discard 7 mL.

5 If a liquid oral medication order calls for 7.5 mL, how will the nurse prepare it?

  1. Pour at eye level to 5 mL and add 2.5 mL with a needleless syringe.
  2. Pour to 10 mL, remove 2.5 mL, and return the 2.5 mL to the medication bottle.
  3. Withdraw 7.5 mL in a 10-mL syringe and place it in the medication cup.
  4. Give $1\frac{1}{2}$ medication teaspoonful.

6 One way to detect major errors in the dose calculations is to:

  1. Estimate the answer.
  2. Pour oral medications to the nearest tenth of a milliliter.
  3. Move decimal places to obtain equivalent measurements.
  4. Rely on the calculations from another nurse.

7 Which conversion is most commonly used in medication problems?

  1. 2.2 lb = 1 kg   **3.** 1,000,000 mcg = 1 g
  2. 1000 mg = 1 g   **4.** 1000 mL = 1 L

8 The usual adult dose for oral liquid medications is measured to the:

  1. Nearest tenth of a milliliter   **3.** Nearest 0.5 mL
  2. Nearest hundredth of a milliliter   **4.** Nearest whole milliliter

9 If a drug label states 250 mg per 5 mL, which of the following statements would be correct?

  1. There are 5 mL of active drug concentrated in the solution.
  2. The medicine has a concentration of 250 mg of drug in each 5 mL of solution.
  3. There is 250 mg of diluent in each 5 mL of solution.
  4. A ratio of 125 mg per 5 mL of the same drug would be more concentrated.

10 An order calls for a wound irrigation with 120 mL of a mixture of hydrogen peroxide solution and sterile normal saline at a 1:1 ratio, followed by a normal saline rinse. How many mL of hydrogen peroxide will be used?

  1. 240   **2.** 120   **3.** 60   **4.** 30

CHAPTER 7 FINAL PRACTICE

Estimated completion time: 1 hour   Answers on page 525

Directions: *Examine the labels, change the units to equivalents by moving decimal places, estimate the answer, calculate the dose to the nearest tenth of a milliliter, and evaluate your answer. Then shade in the dose on the medicine cup and draw a vertical line through the calibrated line of each syringe for the dose to be given.*

  1 Ordered: amoxicillin clavulanate potassium oral susp 0.3 g q8h for a patient with a sinus infection.

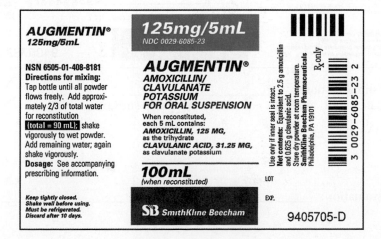

This drug is a combination drug.

a. Estimated dose: _____

b. Calculated dose with equation to the nearest tenth of a milliliter:

DA equation:

c. Evaluation: _____

Shade in the dose in mL on the medicine cup and draw a vertical line through the calibrated line of the syringe as applicable.

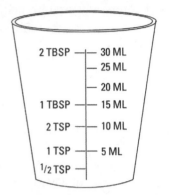

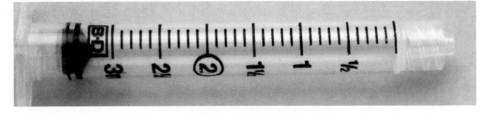

2 Order: amoxicillin 0.2 g PO q8h for a patient with cystitis.

AMOXIL®
250mg/5mL

Directions for mixing: Tap bottle until all powder flows freely. Add approximately 1/3 total amount of water for reconstitution (total=59 mL); shake vigorously to wet powder. Add remaining water; again shake vigorously. Each 5 mL (1 teaspoonful) will contain amoxicillin trihydrate equivalent to 250 mg amoxicillin.
Usual Adult Dosage: 250 to 500 mg every 8 hours.
Usual Child Dosage: 20 to 40 mg/kg/day in divided doses every 8 hours, depending on age, weight and infection severity. See accompanying prescribing information.

Keep tightly closed.
Shake well before using.
Refrigeration preferable but not required.
Discard suspension after 14 days.

250mg/5mL
NDC 0029-6009-21

AMOXIL®
AMOXICILLIN
FOR ORAL
SUSPENSION

80mL (when reconstituted)

SB SmithKline Beecham

NSN 6505-01-153-3442
Net contents: Equivalent to 4.0 grams amoxicillin.
Store dry powder at room temperature.
Caution: Federal law prohibits dispensing without prescription.
SmithKline Beecham
Pharmaceuticals
Philadelphia, PA 19101

3 0029-6009-21 4

LOT

EXP.

9405783-E

a. Estimated dose: _____

b. Calculated dose with equation to nearest tenth of a milliliter:

DA equation:

c. Evaluation: _____

Shade in the dose in mL on the medicine cup and draw a vertical line through the calibrated line of the syringe as applicable.

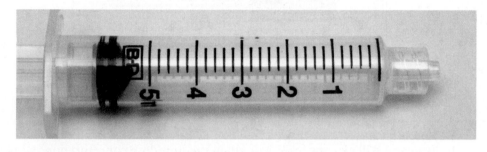

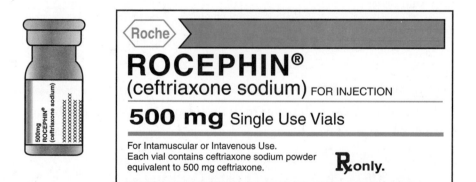

3 Ordered: Rocephin 0.45 g IM bid for a patient with a skin infection.

⟨Roche⟩

ROCEPHIN®
(ceftriaxone sodium) FOR INJECTION

500 mg Single Use Vials

For Intamuscular or Intavenous Use.
Each vial contains ceftriaxone sodium powder
equivalent to 500 mg ceftriaxone.

℞only.

Directions: For IM use, add SW for injection and withdraw entire contents (500 mg).

  A. *1.8 mL SW yields 250 mg per mL.*

  B. *1 mL SW yields 350 mg per mL.*

a. Which concentration will you select: A or B (to yield a minimum of 1 mL)?

_____

b. How much medication will you give?
Estimate: more or less than unit dose?

DA equation:

c. Evaluation: _____

Draw a line through the nearest measurable dose on the syringe provided.

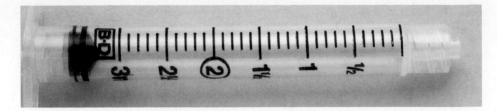

4 Ordered: ceftazidime 750 mg q 12 hr IM for a patient with a genitourinary infection.

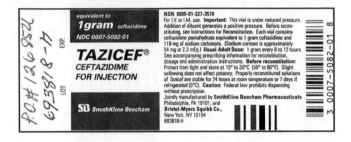

a. Unit dose concentration after dilution: __280 mg per mL__

b. Estimate: Will you give *more* or *less* than the unit dose concentration. (circle one)

c. Estimated round dose in milliliters: _____

d. Actual dose: _____

DA equation:

e. Evaluation: _____

f. If satisfactory to give, draw a vertical line through the calibrated line of the dose on this syringe.

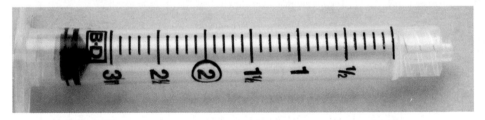

5 Ordered: clarithromycin oral susp 0.15 g for a patient with tonsilitis. Note the form of this oral solid drug before reconstitution.

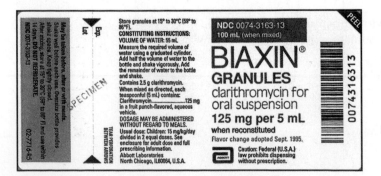

a. Estimated dose: _____

b. Calculated dose with equation to nearest tenth of a milliliter:

DA equation:

c. Evaluation: _____

Shade in the dose in mL on the medicine cup and draw a vertical line through the calibrated line of the syringe as applicable.

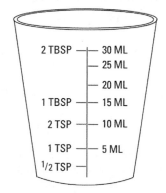

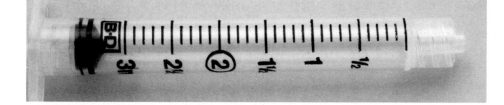

6 Ordered: Ensure food supplement 200 mL 25% strength q8h for 3 days.

   a. What will be the ratio of Ensure to the water diluent? _____

   b. How would the 25% concentration be expressed as a fraction? _____

   c. How many milliliters of Ensure will be used for the dose? _____

   d. How many milliliters of water will be added? _____

7 Ordered: Baby formula $\frac{1}{3}$ strength, 30 mL/hr to be diluted with SW.

   a. What is the equivalent percent concentration to the nearest whole number? _____

   b. What is the equivalent ratio of active to inactive ingredients? _____

   c. How much formula will the nurse pour per hr? _____

   d. How much diluent will the nurse add per hr? _____

8 The baby in problem 7 tolerated the $\frac{1}{3}$ strength formula without vomiting or diarrhea. The prescriber changed the order 48 hours later to, "Increase formula to 1:1 concentration qh."

   a. What is the equivalent percent concentration of this order? _____

   b. What is the equivalent fractional concentration of this order? _____

   c. How much formula will the nurse pour per hr? _____

   d. How much diluent will the nurse add per hr? _____

9 An NS solution has a concentration of sodium chloride (NaCl) 0.9%. NaCl is supplied in grams. The diluent is SW.

    a. Is the NS concentration more or less than a 1% solution? _____

    b. How many grams of solute (0.9 g solute NaCl concentrate) are contained in 100 mL of NS? _____

    c. How many grams of solute are contained in 1000 mL (1 L) of NS? _____

10 A wound irrigation order calls for 50 mL $\frac{1}{2}$ strength NS irrigations tid. The nurse needs to prepare the irrigation from full-strength NS by adding SW.

    a. What will be the ratio of NS solution to SW? _____

    b. How much NS solution will the nurse pour? _____

    c. How much SW will the nurse add? _____

Suggested References

www.emea.europe.eu/htms/vet/presub/q11.htm
www3.niaid.nih.gov/topics/allergicDiseases/default.htm
www.rxmed.com
www.uihealthcare.com/vh

 Additional practice problems can be found in the Basic Calculations section of the Student Companion on Evolve.

    Chapter 8 builds on early chapters to provide a variety of practice problems for subcutaneous and intramuscular dose calculations, with labels of commonly used medications. Injection sites are illustrated.

PART IV

Parenteral Medication Calculations

Injectable Medication Calculations

OBJECTIVES

- Calculate and measure intradermal, subcutaneous, and intramuscular doses.
- Calculate and combine doses for two medications to be mixed in one syringe to the nearest measurable dose.
- Identify safety hazards of injectable medications.

Essential Prior Knowledge

- Mastery of Chapters 1-7

Essential Equipment

- No special equipment is required. It would be helpful to have a 3-mL syringe on hand and some food coloring for practice injection mixes. If two separate colors are used for two simulated liquid medicines, it will be easy to see if any contamination takes place when drawing up the second "medication."

Estimated Time To Complete Chapter

- 1-2 hours

Introduction

This chapter offers a variety of practice problems involving subcutaneous and intramuscular dose calculations. Work out all the problems. This practice will improve your calculations in the clinical setting so that you can focus on injection technique. Selected injectable drugs are mixed in one syringe to spare the patient two injections. Technical competence in preparing parenteral medications requires supervised clinical practice.

ESSENTIAL *Vocabulary*

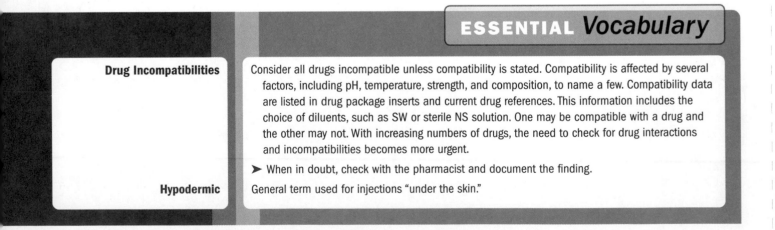

Drug Incompatibilities	Consider all drugs incompatible unless compatibility is stated. Compatibility is affected by several factors, including pH, temperature, strength, and composition, to name a few. Compatibility data are listed in drug package inserts and current drug references. This information includes the choice of diluents, such as SW or sterile NS solution. One may be compatible with a drug and the other may not. With increasing numbers of drugs, the need to check for drug interactions and incompatibilities becomes more urgent.
	➤ When in doubt, check with the pharmacist and document the finding.
Hypodermic	General term used for injections "under the skin."

Intradermal (ID) Injection	Injection into the dermal layer, just under the epidermis, as for many skin tests.
Intramuscular (IM) Injection	Injection into a muscle.
Parenteral	Medications given outside the gastrointestinal (GI) tract. Includes medications delivered via a needle.
Parenteral Mix	Two or more compatible liquid medications combined in one syringe for injection. Medication combinations may include a narcotic and an anticholinergic agent to reduce nausea or dry secretions. Mixes relieve the patient from having to receive two separate intramuscular injections.
Subcutaneous (Subcut) Injection	Injection into loose connective tissue, or fatty layer, underlying the dermis.

Vocabulary Review

RAPID PRACTICE 8-1

Estimated completion time: 5 minutes Answers on page 527

Directions: *Study the essential vocabulary and select the correct injection-related definition.*

1 An injection into the fatty layer beneath the dermis is called _____.

   1. Subcutaneous   **3.** Intravenous
   2. Intramuscular   **4.** Intradermal

2 Medications administered outside the GI tract, including those administered with a needle, are called _____.

   1. Subcutaneous   **3.** Intradermal
   2. Parenteral   **4.** Intramuscular

3 When two or more medications, such as a narcotic and an anticholinergic agent, are combined in a single syringe, they are referred to as _____.

   1. Intramuscular   **3.** Parenteral mix
   2. Therapeutic   **4.** Hypodermic

4 The route used to administer skin tests is called _____.

   1. Subcutaneous   **3.** Hypodermic
   2. Intramuscular   **4.** Intradermal

5 Medications that, when combined, cause an undesired change in the effect or composition of one or both of the individual medications are referred to as _____.

   1. Hypodermic   **3.** Incompatible
   2. Parenteral   **4.** Diluted

Intradermal Injections

Small-volume injections usually administered as skin tests are injected intradermally just under the epidermis at a very shallow angle. A small fluid-filled wheal or bleb like a mosquito bite forms. The area is examined daily for a few days to see if there is an antibody reaction to the antigen injected. The observations are measured and documented.

Medications are not delivered via the ID route because this route offers poor absorption capability.

0.1 mL is the usual dose for a skin test administered with a 1-mL syringe and a 26- to 29-gauge needle (Figure 8-1).

Many patients are afraid of "needles." When giving vaccines and administering skin tests, the nurse can reassure patients about ID injections by showing them how little medicine will be given and how small and fine the needle is, if the patient is willing to take a look. Do not give false reassurances, such as, "Oh, you won't feel a thing." Prepare the patient for some discomfort even though there usually is minimal pain with these types of injections: "Mrs. Brown, most people dislike injections. This is just a drop or two of medicine. This will just feel like a little mosquito bite."

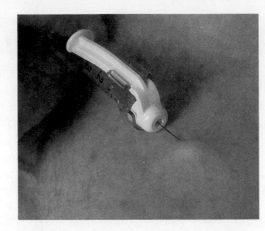

FIGURE 8-1 During intradermal injection, note formation of small bleb on the skin's surface. (From Perry AG, Potter PA: *Clinical nursing skills and techniques,* ed. 7, St. Louis, 2010, Mosby.)

Subcutaneous Injections

Nonirritating substances up to 1 mL may be injected into subcutaneous fatty tissue sites, usually with a 25- to 29-gauge needle. Insulin and anticoagulants, such as heparin and Fragmin, are medications that are delivered through the subcutaneous route. The fluid volume needle gauge, needle length (average ½ inch), and angle of injection depend on the patient's size, skin thickness, and condition.

The most common sites for subcutaneous injection are the subcutaneous fatty areas of the upper posterior arm, the abdomen, and the anterior thigh (Figure 8-2).

➤ A 2-inch zone around the umbilicus is to be avoided. As with all injections, the sites must be rotated systematically to avoid tissue injury.
➤ It is best to write out *subcutaneous* or *subcut* on medical records to avoid misinterpretation. *Subq* and *subc* can be misinterpreted. Printed materials do use abbreviations such as *subc* or *subQ* but are less likely to be misinterpreted than is handwriting.

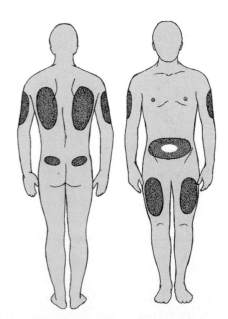

FIGURE 8-2 Sites recommended for subcutaneous injections. (Modified from Perry AG, Potter PA: *Clinical nursing skills and techniques,* ed. 7, St. Louis, 2010, Mosby.)

Intramuscular Injections

Intramuscular injection sites are selected to deliver medications for faster absorption and tolerate more concentrated substances than do subcutaneous sites. Solutions up to 3 mL may be injected with a 20- to 23-gauge needle into a single muscle site, depending on the patient's skin integrity and muscle size. The volume of fluid and the length, gauge, and angle of needle are scaled down for smaller adults, children, and infants.

The most common sites for intramuscular injection are the deltoid, the ventrogluteal muscle, and the vastus lateralis (Figure 8-3).

➤ Check workplace policies and procedures for acceptable injection sites. Assess integrity of skin sites prior to injection.

Administering Injections

Mastery of the technique of delivering injections to the correct layer of tissue requires supervised laboratory and clinical practice with anatomical models and a variety of different-sized patients.

Medications for subcutaneous and intramuscular injections are administered with a variety of equipment, including vials, ampules, prefilled syringes, and syringe cartridges, as illustrated below. Ampules are single-dose glass containers containing liquid medications and solutions. Vials are supplied as single-

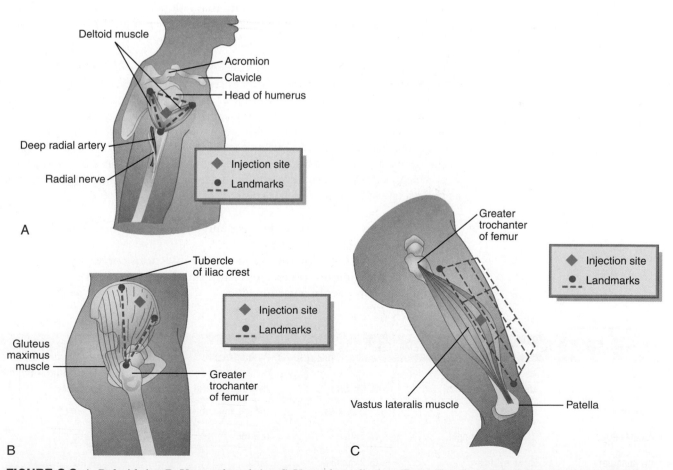

FIGURE 8-3 A, Deltoid site. **B,** Ventrogluteal site. **C,** Vastus lateralis site. (From Kee JL, Marshall SM: *Clinical calculations: with applications to general and specialty areas,* ed. 6, St. Louis, 2009, Saunders.)

Ampules   Vials

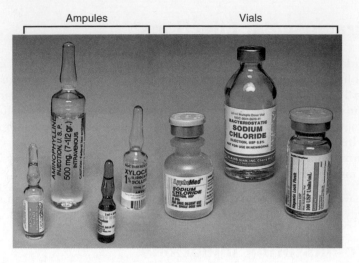

FIGURE 8-4 Assorted ampules and vials. (Modified from Perry AG, Potter PA: *Clinical nursing skills and techniques,* ed. 7, St. Louis, 2010, Mosby.)

dose or multidose glass containers and may contain liquid or dry medication forms (Figure 8-4).

➤ Remember that a filter needle must be used to withdraw medicines from glass ampules.

Prefilled syringes reduce the chance of contamination during preparation of the medication.

➤ However, they do not entirely eliminate that risk because dose adjustments may be required with prefilled syringes. They may contain 0.1 to 0.2 mL of extra medication in case of loss during preparation.

FAQ | What is the quickest way to learn selection of syringe and needle sizes?

ANSWER | There is no substitute for supervised and, later, independent experience, but learning can be greatly expedited. Assuming that you have learned to identify syringe capacities and calibration amounts (covered in Chapter 6), focus on a commonly used syringe size for each route and an approximate needle size and usual amount. Try to learn syringe and needle size selection in sequential order from the intradermal to intramuscular or vice versa (Table 8-1). Then, in the clinical setting, modifications and the selection of needles and the appropriate angle of injection for specific-sized patients can be added to the body of knowledge.

➤ There are many variations on the sizes and amounts shown in Table 8-1. These figures are just averages.
➤ Note that the 3-mL syringe for intramuscular injections corresponds to the maximum 3-mL amount preferred for intramuscular injections in one site.
➤ Remember: Never recap a used needle.

TABLE 8-1	Usual Syringe Size, Needle Size, and Doses			
Route	Usual Syringe Size	Needle Size	Average/Usual Amount	Maximum Amount per Site
Intradermal*	1-mL syringe	$\frac{1}{2}$ inch or less	0.1-mL injection	0.5 mL*
Subcutaneous	1- to 3-mL syringe	$\frac{1}{2}$ to 1 inch	0.5 mL	1 mL
Intramuscular	3-mL syringe	1 to 2 inches	2 mL	3 mL

*The intradermal route is not used for medication administration. Skin test amounts are usually 0.1 mL.

Parenteral Dose Calculations

Estimated completion time: 20-30 minutes   Answers on page 527

Directions: *Estimate the dose, verify it with a DA-style equation to the nearest tenth of a mL, and evaluate. Draw a vertical line through the calibrated line of each syringe for the dose to be given.*

1 Ordered: nafcillin 0.45 g IM q4h, an antibiotic, for a patient with infection.

NDC 0015-7226-20
EQUIVALENT TO
2 gram NAFCILLIN
**NAFCILLIN SODIUM
FOR INJECTION, USP**
Buffered-For IM or IV Use
CAUTION: Federal law prohibits
dispensing without prescription.
APOTHECON®

When reconstituted with 6.6 mL diluent, (SEE INSERT-INTRAMUSCULAR ROUTE), each vial contains 8 mL solution. Each mL of solution contains nafcillin sodium, as the monohydrate, equivalent to 250 mg nafcillin, buffered with 10 mg sodium citrate. Read accompanying circular for complete stability data.
Usual Dosage: Adults—500 mg every 4 to 6 hours. Read accompanying circular for directions for IM or IV use.
APOTHECON®
A Bristol-Myers Squibb Company
Princeton, NJ 08540 USA

72262DRL-2

a. Drug concentration after reconstitution:

_____

b. Estimated dose: _____

c. How many mL will you prepare for the syringe provided below?

DA equation:

d. Evaluation: _____

Draw a vertical line through the nearest measurable amount on the syringe provided.

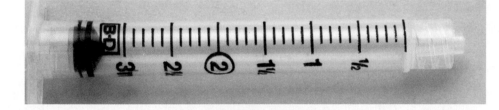

2 Ordered: diazepam 6 mg stat for a patient with anxiety.

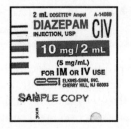

2 mL DOSETTE® Ampul   A-14088
DIAZEPAM CIV
INJECTION, USP
10 mg / 2 mL
(5 mg/mL)
FOR **IM** OR **IV** USE
ESI ELKINS-SINN, INC.
CHERRY HILL, NJ 08003
SAMPLE COPY

a. Drug concentration: _____

b. Estimated dose: _____

c. How many mL will you prepare?

DA equation:

d. Evaluation: _____

Draw a vertical line through the nearest measurable amount on the syringe provided.

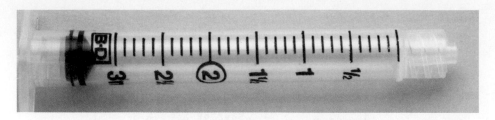

3 Ordered: morphine sulfate 9 mg IM stat, an opioid narcotic, for a patient in pain.

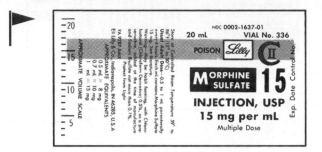

   a. Drug concentration: _____

   b. Estimated dose: _____

   c. How many mL will you prepare?

➤ Write out morphine sulfate. Do not abbreviate.

   DA equation:

   d. Evaluation: _____

Draw a vertical line through the nearest measurable dose on the syringe provided.

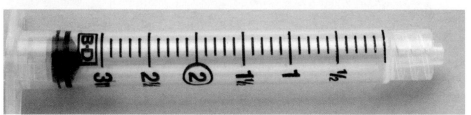

➤ Note the *C II* on the morphine label. Recall that it means that the drug is a federally controlled substance, Schedule II, a category of drugs with strong potential for abuse as well as useful medical purposes. Morphine is an opium-derived narcotic. There are strict record-keeping requirements for controlled drugs as well as limitations on the number of doses that can be prescribed before a renewal is required.

CLINICAL RELEVANCE

➤ Assess the patient for respiratory depression before giving an opioid and thereafter until the drug effect has diminished. There are several visual analog scales (VAS) available for assessing current pain levels. The patient identifies the current level on a "no pain" to "worst pain" or "severest pain" subjective rating. Find out which scale your agency prefers. This practice may reduce the risk of overmedication.

4 Ordered: lorazepam 2 mg IM stat, a sedative and anti-anxiety agent, for an agitated elderly patient.

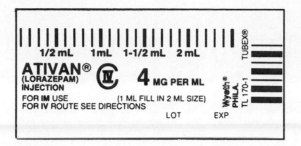

a. Drug concentration: _____

b. Estimated dose: _____

c. How many mL will you prepare?

   DA equation:

d. Evaluation: _____

Draw a vertical line through the nearest measurable dose on the syringe provided.

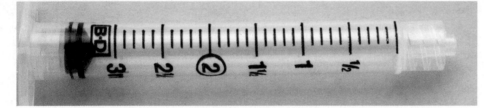

Note that Ativan (lorazepam) is labeled *C IV* (i.e., controlled substance Schedule IV). Drugs in this category have *less* potential for abuse or addiction than do Schedule I, II, or III drugs. Schedule IV drugs include phenobarbital and certain other anti-anxiety agents.

5 Ordered: digoxin 0.125 mg IM daily, for a patient with heart failure.

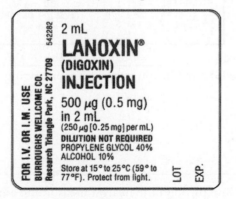

a. Drug concentration: _____

b. Estimated dose: _____

c. How many mL will you prepare?

   DA equation:

d. Evaluation: _____

Draw a vertical line through the nearest measurable dose on the syringe provided.

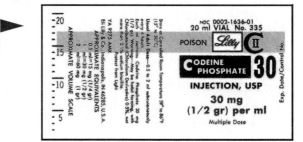

➤ Focus intently on decimals when they appear in medication orders or drug labels. Review decimal calculations in Chapter 1 as needed to ensure that you are comfortable with decimal addition, division, and multiplication. Dose calculation errors are large if a decimal point is misplaced. Write neatly and make decimal points prominent.

Q: *Ask Yourself*

A: *My Answer*

1 How many times does 0.05 go into 0.1? How many times does 0.25 go into 0.5? How many times does 0.5 go into 1? How many times does 0.025 go into 0.05?

_____

RAPID PRACTICE **8-3**

More Parenteral Dose Calculation Practice

Estimated completion time: 20-30 minutes   **Answers on page 529**

Directions: *Examine the order and calculate the dose. Recalculate if the estimate does not support the answer.*

1 Ordered: codeine 0.02 g IM q3-4h prn for pain, a narcotic analgesic, for a patient in pain.

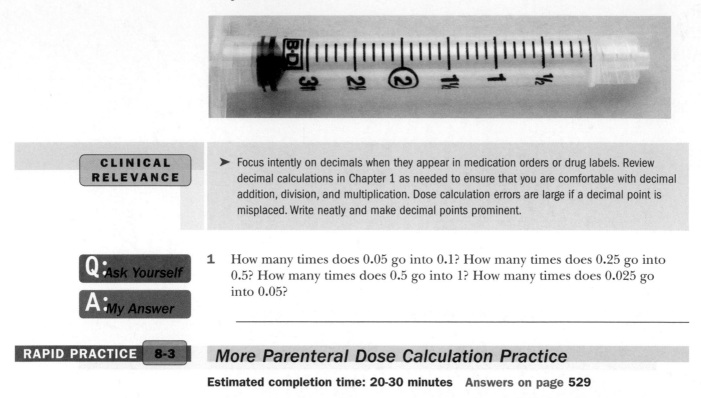

a. Estimated dose: _____

b. How many milliliters will you prepare for this syringe to the nearest tenth of a mL?

DA equation:

c. Evaluation: _____

Draw a vertical line through the nearest measurable amount on the syringe provided.

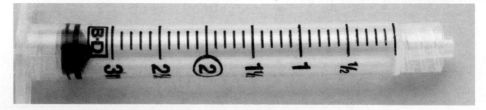

2 Ordered: furosemide 38 mg IM, a diuretic, for a patient with edema.

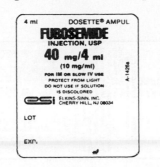

a. Estimated dose: _____

b. How many milliliters will you prepare for this syringe?

DA equation:

c. Evaluation: _____

Draw a vertical line through the nearest measurable amount on the syringe provided.

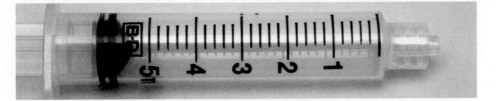

d. What is the smallest measurable dose in a 5-mL syringe?

3 Ordered: Solu-Cortef 0.3 g IM, an anti-inflammatory steroid, for a patient with severe inflammatory response.

Single-Dose Vial For IV or IM use	2 mL Act-O-Vial®	NDC 0009-0909-08
Contains Benzyl Alcohol as a Preservative	**Solu-Cortef**® Sterile Powder	
See package insert for complete product information.	hydrocortisone sodium succinate	
Per 2 mL (when mixed): * hydrocortisone sodium succinate equiv. to hydrocortisone, 250 mg. Protect solution from light. Discard after 3 days.	for injection, USP	
814 070 205 Reconstituted	**250 mg***	
The Upjohn Company Kalamazoo, MI 49001, USA		

a. Estimated dose: _____

b. How many milliliters will you prepare for this syringe?

DA equation:

c. Evaluation: _____

Draw a vertical line through the nearest measurable amount on the syringe provided.

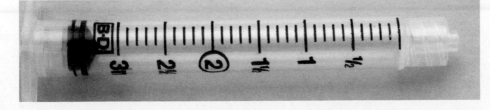

4   Ordered: atropine 0.3 mg IM on call to OR, an anticholinergic for a preoperative patient.

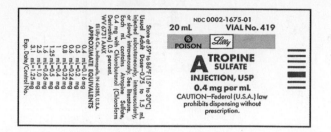

a. Estimated dose: _____

b. How many milliliters will you prepare for the 1-mL syringe?

DA equation:

c. Evaluation: _____

Draw a red arrow pointing to the nearest measurable amount on the syringe provided.

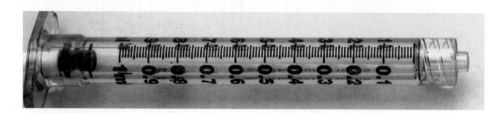

5   Ordered: tuberculin skin test ID for an adult patient. The volume for this skin test is 0.1 mL.

Draw an arrow pointing to the nearest measurable dose on the tuberculin syringe provided.

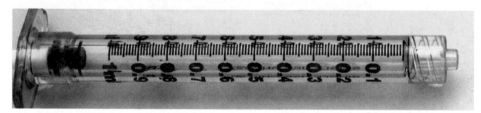

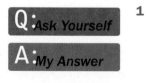

1   Why is it important to make a habit of evaluating the equations and comparing the answers to the estimates? What are the risks if this step is skipped?

_____

Parenteral Mixes

When two medications are administered together in one syringe, the order is bracketed:

        morphine 5 mg IM   } on call to OR
        atropine 0.2 mg IM

| TABLE 8-2 | Drug Compatibility Chart (Excerpt) |

	Atropine	Buprenorphine	Butorphanol	Chlorpromazine	Codeine	Diazepam	Dimenhydrinate	Diphenhydramine	Droperidol	Fentanyl	Glycopyrrolate	Heparin	Hydroxyzine	Meperidine	Metoclopramide	Midazolam	Morphine
Atropine			C	C		I	C	C	C	C	C		C	C	C	C	C
Buprenorphine																	
Butorphanol	C			C		I	I	C	C	C			C	C	C	C	C
Chlorpromazine	C		C			I	I	C	C	C	C	C	C	C	C	C	C

C, Compatible; I, incompatible
Excerpt from Skidmore-Roth L: *Mosby's drug guide for nurses,* ed. 9, St. Louis, 2011, Mosby.

Compatibility between medications to be mixed must be checked in a current drug reference. Many drug references have compatibility charts. Note the example shown in Table 8-2.

➤ When in doubt about drug compatibility, call the pharmacy. Consider all drugs incompatible unless otherwise documented.

Example of parenteral mix order

Ordered:

hydromorphone 2 mg ⎱ IM q4h prn pain
hydroxyzine 25 mg ⎰

Sometimes the order states "mix" after the route.

There is an automatic expiration date on narcotics and medications that have the potential for dependence or abuse or that are ineffective if given beyond a specified period. Check agency policy. It is usually 48-72 hours for controlled substances. In order to continue the medications, the order must be renewed in a timely manner so that the medication schedule proceeds without interruption.

CLINICAL RELEVANCE

➤ The nurse cannot legally continue to administer any drug after the expiration date, be it automatic or written out. The prescriber must be contacted promptly if the medication is still perceived to be needed. By giving an expired drug, the nurse becomes a prescriber without the license to prescribe, an illegal practice. When medications expire, the medication must be renewed by the prescriber.

The use of parenteral mixes spares the patient the discomfort of two separate injections. The mixes usually consist of a narcotic and an anticholinergic or antihistamine type of medication that extends the action of the narcotic and decreases nausea, a common side effect of narcotics, or dries respiratory secretions for patients who are to receive general anesthesia.

Mixing two medications in one syringe

Mixtures may be combinations of vial, ampule, prefilled syringe, and/or prefilled cartridge medications. This technique requires supervised clinical practice (Figure 8-5).

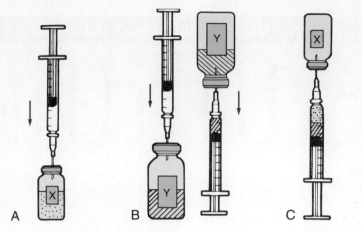

FIGURE 8-5 Mixing medications from a vial. **A,** Injecting air into first vial. **B,** Injecting air into the second vial and withdrawing dose. **C,** Withdrawing medication from first vial.

Containers:	First Vial	Second Vial	First Vial
Steps:	Air in	Air in & Medicine Out	Medicine Out

Medications are now mixed. (Modified from Perry AG, Potter PA: *Clinical nursing skills and techniques,* ed. 7, St. Louis, 2010, Mosby.)

Calculating the dose for a parenteral mix

Calculate each dose separately to the nearest tenth of a milliliter. Add them together. Round the dose to the nearest tenth of a milliliter, for example,

morphine sulfate   0.4 mL
atropine sulfate <u>+0.2 mL</u>
             0.6 mL total volume for syringe

RAPID PRACTICE 8-4   *Calculating Parenteral Mix Doses*

Estimated completion time: 10-15 minutes   Answers on page 530

Directions: *Examine the order and the labels. Estimate the ordered doses. Calculate the two individual doses to the nearest tenth of a milliliter using DA-style equations. Evaluate the equation. Is the equation balanced? Does the estimate support the answer? Draw a vertical line through the* total *desired amount to the nearest measurable dose on the available 3-mL syringe. Follow the example given in problem 1. The order of the questions for each problem suggests the order to follow to solve these problems.*

1   Ordered: meperidine hydrochloride 75 mg   IM q4–6h prn pain for a
               hydroxyzine hydrochloride 25 mg   patient allergic to morphine
                                             and codeine

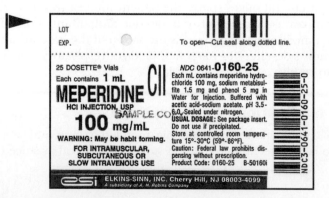

LOT
EXP.

To open—Cut seal along dotted line.

25 DOSETTE® Vials
Each contains **1 mL**

MEPERIDINE CII
HCl INJECTION, USP
SAMPLE CO
100 mg/mL
WARNING: May be habit forming.
FOR INTRAMUSCULAR,
SUBCUTANEOUS OR
SLOW INTRAVENOUS USE

NDC 0641-**0160-25**
Each mL contains meperidine hydro-
chloride 100 mg, sodium metabisul-
fite 1.5 mg and phenol 5 mg in
Water for Injection. Buffered with
acetic acid-sodium acetate. pH 3.5-
6.0. Sealed under nitrogen.
USUAL DOSAGE: See package insert.
Do not use if precipitated.
Store at controlled room tempera-
ture 15°-30°C (59°-86°F).
Caution: Federal law prohibits dis-
pensing without prescription.
Product Code: 0160-25 B-50160i

ELKINS-SINN, INC. Cherry Hill, NJ 08003-4099
A subsidiary of A. H. Robins Company

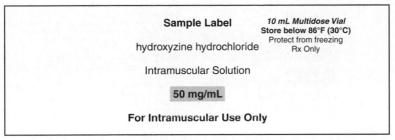

<table>
<tr><td>**Sample Label**

hydroxyzine hydrochloride

Intramuscular Solution

50 mg/mL

For Intramuscular Use Only</td><td>**10 mL Multidose Vial**
Store below 86°F (30°C)
Protect from freezing
Rx Only</td></tr>
</table>

Meperidine

a. Estimate: Does the order call for *more* or *less* than the unit dose available? Less. Estimated dose: about $\frac{3}{4}$ mL.

b. How many mL will you prepare?

DA equation:

$$\frac{mL}{dose} = \frac{1\ mL}{\underset{4}{\cancel{100\ mg}}} \times \frac{\overset{3}{\cancel{75\ mg}}}{dose} = 0.75\ mL,\ rounded\ to\ \frac{0.8\ mL\ meperidine}{dose}$$

c. Evaluation: Is the equation balanced? <u>Yes.</u> Does the estimate support the answer? <u>Yes.</u>

Hydroxyzine

d. Estimate: Does the order call for *more* or *less* than the dose available? Less. Estimated dose: about $\frac{1}{2}$ of 1 mL.

e. How many mL will you prepare?
DA equation:

$$\frac{mL}{dose} = \frac{1\ mL}{\underset{2}{\cancel{50\ mg}}} \times \frac{\overset{1}{\cancel{25\ mg}}}{dose} = \frac{0.5\ mL\ hydroxyzine}{dose}$$

f. Evaluation: Is the equation balanced? <u>Yes.</u> Does the estimate support the answer? <u>Yes.</u>

Total Dose

g. *Total combined volume* in milliliters *to nearest tenth:* <u>0.8 + 0.5 mL = 1.3 mL</u>

Draw a vertical line through *the nearest measurable amount* for the total dose on the syringe.

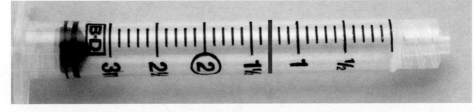

The only difference between this calculation and other calculations of liquid doses learned earlier is the addition of the two doses together.

2 Ordered: hydromorphone HCL 1.5 mg $\Big\}$ IM at 0800
         atropine 0.4 mg

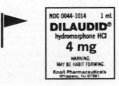

NDC 0044-1014   1 mL
DILAUDID®
hydromorphone HCl
4 mg
WARNING:
MAY BE HABIT FORMING.
Knoll Pharmaceuticals
Whippany, NJ 07981

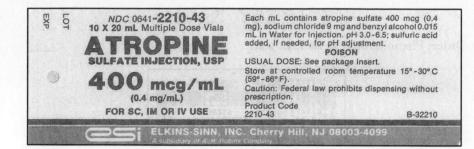

Dilaudid

a. Estimated dose: _____

b. How many mL will you prepare?

DA equation:

c. Evaluation: Is the equation balanced? Does the estimate support the answer? _____

Atropine

d. Estimated dose: _____

e. How many mL will you prepare?

DA equation:

f. Evaluation: Is the equation balanced? Does the estimate support the answer? _____

Total Dose

g. Total combined volume: _____

Draw a vertical line through the nearest measurable amount for the total dose on the syringe provided.

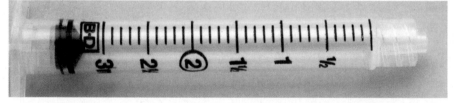

➤ Do not confuse morphine and hydromorphone (Dilaudid). Hydromorphone is considerably more powerful than morphine.

3 Ordered: morphine sulfate 8 mg ⎫ IM stat.
　　　　 atropine 0.6 mg ⎭

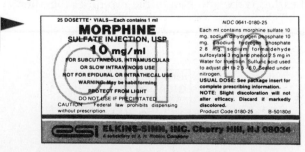

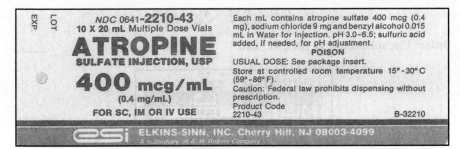

Morphine

a. Estimated dose: _____

b. How many mL will you prepare?

DA equation:

c. Evaluation: Is the equation balanced? Does the estimate support the answer? _____

Atropine

d. Estimated dose: _____

e. How many mL will you prepare?

DA equation:

f. Evaluation: Is the equation balanced? Does the estimate support the answer? _____

Total Dose

g. Total combined volume: _____

Draw a vertical line through the nearest measurable amount for the total dose on the syringe provided.

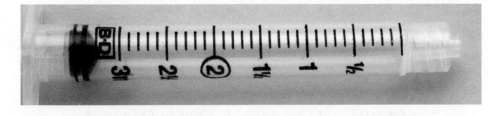

4   Ordered: hydromorphone HCl 3 mg ⎱ IM stat
          Promethazine 10 mg   ⎰

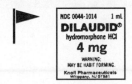

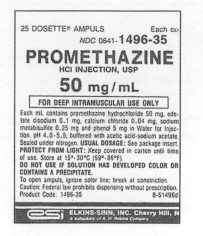

Dilaudid

a. Estimated dose: _____

b. How many mL will be prepared?

    DA equation:

c. Evaluation: Is the equation balanced? Does the estimate support the
answer? _____

Promethazine

d. Estimated dose: _____

e. How many mL will you prepare?

    DA equation:

f. Evaluation: Is the equation balanced? Does the estimate support the
answer? _____

Total Dose

g. Total combined volume: _____

Draw a vertical line through the nearest measurable amount for the total dose
on the syringe provided.

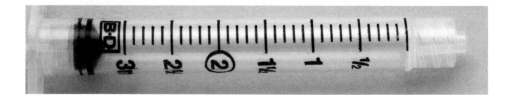

5 Ordered: morphine 12 mg ⎫ IM q6h prn pain
　　　　　atropine 0.3 mg ⎭

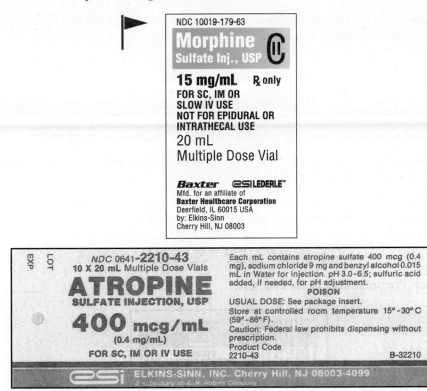

Morphine Sulfate

a. Estimated dose: _____

b. How many mL will you prepare?

　　DA equation:

c. Evaluation: Is the equation balanced? Does the estimate support the answer? _____

Atropine

d. Estimated dose: _____

e. How many mL will you prepare?

　　DA equation:

f. Evaluation: Is the equation balanced? Does the estimate support the answer? _____

Total Dose

g. Total dose in milliliters to nearest tenth: _____

Draw a vertical line through the nearest measurable amount for the total dose on the syringe provided.

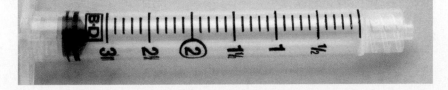

☐ Medicines Supplied in Units

Medicines that are supplied in units and also may be administered via the subcutaneous route are covered in Chapters 11 and 12.

CHAPTER 8 MULTIPLE-CHOICE REVIEW

Estimated completion time: 30 minutes to 1 hour   Answers on page 532

Directions: *Place a circle around the letter of the correct answer. Select reconstituted drugs for an IM injection with a 3-mL syringe.*

1 Ordered: Stadol 1 mg   ⎱ IM stat for a patient with a severe
            Promethazine 10 mg ⎰ migraine headache

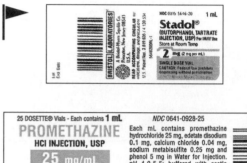

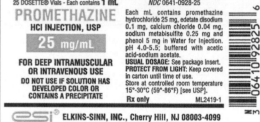

How many total milliliters will you administer?

1. 1.1   **3.** 1.3
2. 1.2   **4.** 1.4

2 Skin tests are administered via which route?

1. Subcutaneous   **3.** Intramuscular
2. Intradermal   **4.** Intravenous

3 The most commonly used syringe size for intramuscular injections is:

1. 1 mL   **3.** 3 mL
2. 2 mL   **4.** 5 mL

4 Parenteral mixes most often include which types of medications?

1. A narcotic and another medication, for example, to control nausea
2. Potassium and bacteriostatic sterile water for injection
3. Two different kinds of antibiotics
4. An intravenous medication and an intramuscular medication

5 The maximum amount of fluid that is recommended for one site for adult intramuscular injections is:

1. 1 mL   **3.** 3 mL
2. 2 mL   **4.** 5 mL

6 Ordered: morphine sulfate 6 mg. Available: morphine sulfate 10 mg/ mL. What is the estimated dose?

   1. 0.06 mL   **3.** 1.2 mL

   2. 0.6 mL   **4.** 6 mL

7 Examine the following dose concentrations. Which dilution would be most appropriate for a 10-mg IM dose? (Consider the volume to be administered.)

   1. Add 20 mL to make 1 mg per mL

   2. Add 10 mL to make 2 mg per mL

   3. Add 5 mL to make 5 mg per mL

   4. Add 1 mL to make 40 mg per mL

8 Examine the following dose concentrations. Which dilution would be appropriate for a 50-mg IM dose? (Consider the volume of the prepared dose.)

   1. Add 10 mL to make 5 mg per mL

   2. Add 8 mL to make 10 mg per mL

   3. Add 5.6 mL to make 12 mg per mL

   4. Add 3 mL to make 25 mg per mL

9 Identify the difference between SW and bacteriostatic water, if any.

   1. Bacteriostatic water contains a preservative and may be used as a diluent only if the medication label so states.

   2. Both solutions are sterile and may be used interchangeably.

   3. SW may be used in place of bacteriostatic water.

   4. Both are bacteriostatic.

10 What is the first step the nurse must take after reading an order for a parenteral mix?

   1. Estimate the doses.

   2. Prepare each medication separately, maintaining sterile technique.

   3. Evaluate the DA dose calculation against the estimated dose.

   4. Check current drug literature for drug compatibility.

CHAPTER 8 FINAL PRACTICE

Estimated completion time: 1 hour   Answers on page **532**

Directions: *Analyze the problems. Estimate and calculate the requested doses to the nearest tenth of a mL. Use a calculator for long division and multiplication. Evaluate your equations and answers on your own.*

1 Ordered: morphine 10 mg ⎫ IM for postoperative pain and nausea
             atropine 200 mcg ⎬

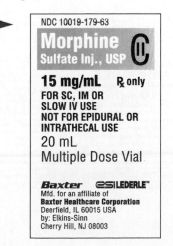

NDC 10019-179-63

Morphine
Sulfate Inj., USP Ⓒ Ⅱ

15 mg/mL   ℞ only
FOR SC, IM OR
SLOW IV USE
NOT FOR EPIDURAL OR
INTRATHECAL USE
20 mL
Multiple Dose Vial

Baxter ℮SⅠLEDERLE™
Mfd. for an affiliate of
Baxter Healthcare Corporation
Deerfield, IL 60015 USA
by: Elkins-Sinn
Cherry Hill, NJ 08003

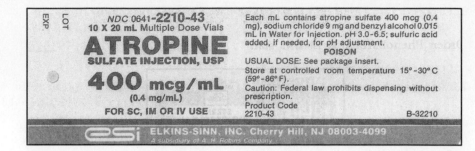

Morphine

a. Estimated dose: _____

b. How many mL will be prepared?

DA equation:

Evaluation: _____

Atropine

c. Estimated dose: _____

d. How many mL will be prepared?

DA equation:

Evaluation: _____

Total Combined Dose

e. Total dose in mL to nearest tenth: _____

Draw a vertical line through the nearest measurable amount on the syringe provided.

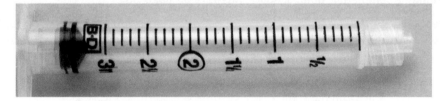

2 Ordered: morphine sulfate 7 mg } IM for postoperative discomfort
promethazine 20 mg

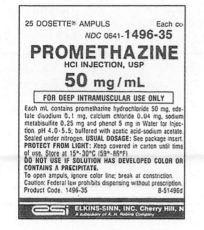

Morphine

a. Estimated dose: _____

b. How many mL will be prepared?

   DA equation:

Evaluation: _____

Promethazine

c. Estimated dose: _____

d. How many mL will be prepared?

   DA equation:

Evaluation: _____

Total Combined Dose

e. Total dose in mL to nearest tenth: _____

Draw a vertical line through the nearest measurable amount on the syringe provided.

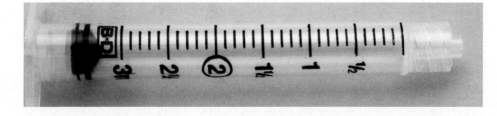

3 Ordered: morphine 12 mg ⎫ IM, a narcotic and an anticholinergic,
glycopyrrolate 0.3 mg ⎬ on call to OR

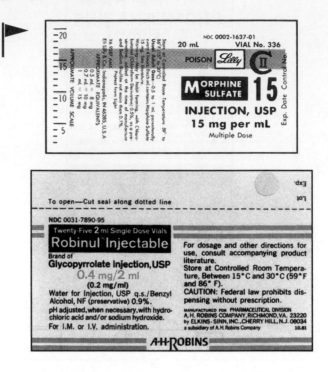

Morphine

a. Estimated dose: _____

b. How many mL will be prepared?

DA equation:

Evaluation: _____

Robinul

c. Estimated dose: _____

d. How many mL will be prepared?

DA equation:

Evaluation: _____

Total Combined Dose

e. Total dose in milliliters to nearest tenth: _____

Draw a vertical line through the nearest measurable amount on the syringe
provided.

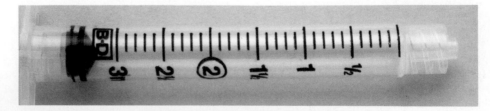

4 Ordered: codeine 10 mg IM stat, for a child with complaints of pain.

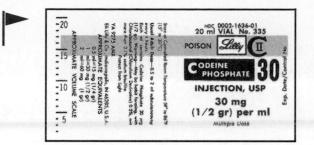

   a. Estimated dose: _____

   b. How many mL will be prepared?

     DA equation:

   Evaluation: _____

If estimated dose is confirmed, draw a vertical line through the nearest measurable amount on the syringe provided.

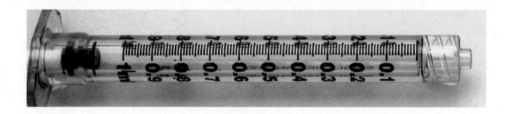

5 Ordered: nafcillin sodium 0.4 g IM, an antibiotic, for a patient with an infection.

   a. Total dose in vial in g and mg: _____

   b. Amount of diluent needed:

   _____

   c. Dose concentration after reconstitution: _____

   d. Estimated dose: _____

   e. How many mL will you prepare?

     DA equation:

   Evaluation: _____

Draw a vertical line through the nearest measurable amount on the syringe provided.

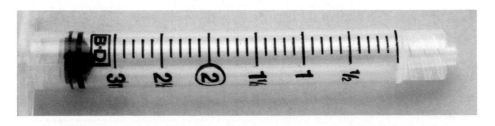

6 Ordered: ampicillin 0.2 g IM q6h, an antibiotic, for a patient with an infection.

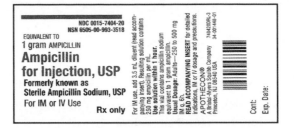

a. Total dose in vial in g and mg: _____

b. Amount of diluent needed:

_____

c. Dose concentration after reconstitution: _____

d. Estimated dose: _____

e. How many mL will you prepare?

DA equation:

Evaluation: _____

Draw a vertical line through the nearest measurable amount on the syringe provided.

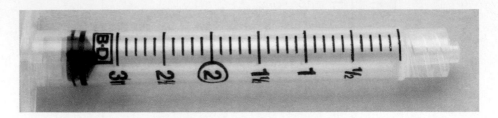

7 Ordered: phenobarbital sodium 0.1 g IM, a barbiturate, for a patient who needs sedation. Available: phenobarbital sodium 120 mg per mL.

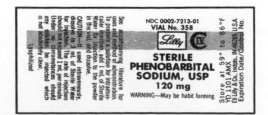

a. Total dose in vial: _____

b. Amount of diluent needed:

_____

c. Dose concentration after reconstitution: _____

d. Estimated dose: _____

e. How many mL will you prepare?

DA equation:

Evaluation: _____

Draw a vertical line through the nearest measurable amount on the syringe provided.

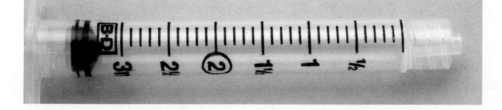

8 Ordered: penicillin G potassium IM 400,000 units q6h, an antibiotic, for a patient with infection. Directions: Add 4.6 mL SW to make 200,000 units per mL.

NDC 0002-1406-01
VIAL No. 526

℞ *Lilly*

PENICILLIN G POTASSIUM FOR INJECTION USP
(BUFFERED)

1,000,000 Units

CAUTION—Federal (U.S.A.) law prohibits dispensing without prescription.

Sterile solution may be kept in refrigerator for 7 days without significant loss of potency.

Add diluent	Conc. of Solution
9.6 ml	100,000 Units/ml
4.6 ml	200,000 Units/ml
1.6 ml	500,000 Units/ml

Usual Adult Dose—Intramuscularly, 400,000 units 4 times a day. Intravenously, 10,000,000 units a day.

See literature. Contains sodium citrate-citric acid buffer.

YA 3125 AMX
Eli Lilly & Co., Indianapolis, IN 46285, U.S.A.

Exp. Date/Control No.

a. Total number of units in vial: _____

b. Dose concentration after reconstitution: _____

c. Estimated dose: _____

d. How many mL will you prepare?

DA equation:

Evaluation: _____

Draw a vertical line through the nearest measurable amount on the syringe provided.

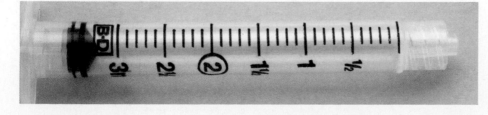

9 Ordered: streptomycin 0.3 g IM bid, an antibiotic, for a patient with an infection.

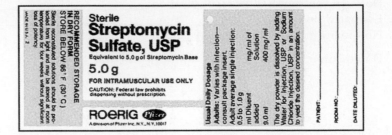

a. Total dose in vial: _____

b. Dose concentration after reconstitution: _____

c. Estimated dose: _____

d. How many mL will you prepare?

DA equation:

Evaluation: _____

Draw a vertical line through the nearest measurable amount on the syringe provided.

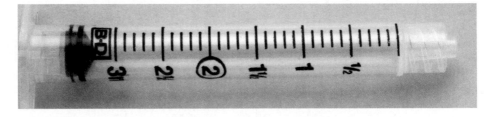

10 Ordered: atropine 0.2 mg IM stat, for a preoperative child.

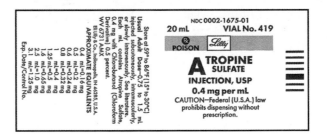

a. Dose concentration in micrograms and milligrams: _____

b. Estimated dose: _____

c. How many mL will you prepare?

DA equation:

Evaluation: _____

Draw an arrow pointing to the nearest measurable amount on the syringe provided.

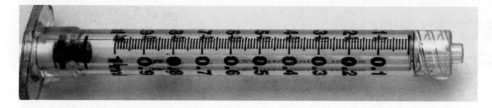

Suggestions for Further Reading

Clayton BD, Stock YN, Cooper S: *Basic pharmacology for nurses,* ed. 15, St. Louis, 2010, Mosby.

Lilley LL, Collins SR, Harrington S, Snyder JS: *Pharmacology and the nursing process,* ed. 6, St. Louis, 2011, Mosby.

Perry AG, Potter PA: *Clinical nursing skills and techniques,* ed. 7, St. Louis, 2010, Mosby.

http://opioids.com
www.ccforpatientsafety.org
http://professional.medtronic.com
www.nysna.org

evolve   Additional practice problems can be found in the Basic Calculations section of the Student Companion on Evolve.

Chapter 9 introduces basic intravenous flow rate calculations and the equipment used to deliver intravenous medications. These calculations are used daily in most clinical agencies. Much of the math needed to solve intravenous dose and rate problems has been covered in earlier chapters and can be applied to the intravenous route with some modifications.

Basic Intravenous Calculations

Introduction

Most patients receive at least one IV solution during hospitalization. Students often care for patients with IV lines before learning to prepare and give oral and injectable medications. Monitoring the site and flow rate is a basic skill. Reporting concerns to the primary nurse is appropriate to protect the patient from fluid drug overload or underdose as well as to protect the site from tissue damage due to a displaced venous access cannula or needle. Additional IV therapy skills and theory can take place later and will progress faster because of the experience gained with the orders, site, and flow rate.

Basic IV calculations require only the simplest arithmetic. Examining each piece of IV equipment encountered in the laboratory and clinical agency and noting the key features, functions, similarities, and differences will expedite understanding.

➤ Be aware that IV equipment changes with facility purchase agreements.

➤ Patients may have some ability to monitor their therapy with oral medications because they may have knowledge and experience with them at home. However, patients are totally dependent on the nurse for safe IV administration. Hazards from improper IV administration occur more rapidly than from other, slower routes of absorption and may not be reversible.

➤ This vocabulary is essential for interpreting IV solution orders. The calculations are dependent on the type of equipment used.

ESSENTIAL *Vocabulary*

Bolus	Fluids or concentrated medication solution given by IV route over a relatively brief period of time. Equipment used to deliver varies, depending on existing IV lines, volume, and time to be infused. Often given by injection into a peripheral venous access device (IV push).
Continuous IV Infusion	IV solution that flows continuously (until further notice) as the name implies (e.g., dextrose 5% in water at 75 mL per hr). Patients who are NPO and surgical patients are two of the many types of patients who receive continuous infusions.
Drop Factor (DF)	Number of drops per milliliter delivered through various sizes of IV tubing devices. The tubing diameter affects the size of the drop. The DF is used to calculate flow rates on gravity devices. DF is also known as tubing factor.
	The abbreviation *gtt(s)* is an outdated apothecary term for *drop(s)*. It may be seen on some prescriber's orders. It is recommended that the word *drops* be written out.
Electronic Infusion Devices (EIDs)	Variety of devices that deliver IV fluids and medications at a preselected rate.
Controllers (Nonvolumetric)	Flow rate controllers that are *gravity* dependent use drop sensors and pinching action to regulate rate. They are used for many IV solutions in large clinical agencies.
Pumps (Volumetric)	Cassette pumps are not gravity dependent. They deliver fluids under positive pressure and are used for powerful drugs, high-risk patients, and more accurate controlled flow rates.
Flow Rate	Rate at which fluid is delivered by IV infusion devices, most often ordered in whole milliliters per hour (mL/hr) (e.g., "Infuse [solution] at 100 mL/hr (100 mL per hr)." Write "per."
Gravity Infusion Device	IV delivery device with flow rate affected by the height of solution and the patient's position. The most elementary devices use a manually operated plastic slide or ball-roller clamp to control flow rate.
Infusion Line, Primary	Main IV line or lines connected to the patient. Also called primary tubing on the IV administration set label. A patient may have more than one primary line. The first one is usually "dedicated" to fluid delivery and maintenance. Additional primary and secondary lines are usually reserved for medications or medicated solutions that are incompatible with other fluids. Primary lines may be vented or nonvented.
Infusion Line, Secondary	Tubing that connects to ports on the primary line and permits a variety of additional medications and fluids to be added without disruption of the primary line. Use of a secondary infusion line spares the patient additional injections into the veins. Labels on the administration sets indicate "secondary."
	➤ Compatibility must be carefully checked before "mixing" additional substances into the primary line.
IV Injection Ports	Latex or rubber ports located on IV lines and solution containers to permit access for injection of additional fluids or medications. A port adapter may also be attached directly to a cannula that is in a vein (also known as an IV lock, med lock, heparin lock, or saline lock).
Intermittent Infusions	Usually small-volume (up to 250-mL) medicated IV solutions delivered at intervals. A variety of devices and methods are available, the most common being IV piggyback equipment, syringe pumps, and calibrated volume-control burette chambers.
IV Containers	Variously sized plastic bags are the most common. Glass bottles are used for medications that cause plastic to deteriorate.
IV Piggyback (IVPB)	Small-volume infusions, usually 50 or 100 mL, infused through a short secondary tubing line that is "piggybacked" to a port on a primary line. Intermittent medicated infusions are delivered over 20 to 60 minutes, as specified by the pharmacy or manufacturer in drug references.

IV Push	IV concentrated, medicated, intermittent bolus dose of 1-50 mL, usually administered by manual direct injection with a syringe, sometimes via an infusion pump.
	➤ It is occasionally written incorrectly as "IVP," which can be confused with the common abbreviation for the intravenous pyelogram (IVP) test. Also, do not confuse with IVPB (IV piggyback).
Macrodrip	Gravity IV infusion tubing set that has a wide diameter to deliver large drops (10-20 drops/mL drop factor) and faster flow rates.
Microdrip	Gravity IV infusion tubing set that has a narrow diameter to deliver small drops (60 drops/mL drop factor) and slower flow rates. Also known as pediatric tubing.
Osmolarity	Solute concentration in solution. The unit of measurement is the osmol. The milliosmol (mOs) is the unit of measurement in *plasma* and is used as a basis for comparison with the contents of IV solutions. *Isotonic* solutions, such as normal saline solution, 5% dextrose in water, and lactated Ringer's solution, approximate plasma osmolality. *Hyper*tonic solutions contain a higher number of milliosmols per liter and have higher tonicity. *Hypo*tonic solutions contain a lower number of milliosmols per liter and have lower tonicity.
Parenteral Fluids	Fluids administered outside of the digestive tract (e.g., IM, IV).
Patency	State of being open and unblocked, such as a "patent IV site" or "patent airway." Sites are checked for patency during every visit to the bedside to ensure that the ordered fluids and medications are flowing into the vein and not into tissue.
PCA Pump	Patient-controlled analgesia pump. An electronic IV device with a syringe or narcotic injector vial programmed to dispense prescribed amounts of analgesic narcotics and other medications at prescribed intermittent intervals with intermittent lockout intervals. Patients self-administer boluses of medication in solution to control pain by remote push-button control.
	Mnemonic: PC, Pain Control.
Port	Resealable *access* device that permits additional IV lines or medications to be added into or on primary (main) IV tubing without initiating another injection site or disrupting the main IV line. Ports may also be indwelling venous cannulas that can be capped and kept patent with a saline or heparin (lock) flush solution and accessed when needed. The latter type of port frees the patient of the need to have IV solutions and tubing connected continuously.
TKO **KVO**	"To keep open" or "Keep vein open," a flow rate order that may be given for gravity devices for the minimum rate that will keep the IV line patent and prevent coagulation. This order has mostly been replaced by the insertion of an indwelling IV access port. See "Port." Some institutions specify a TKO rate in their procedure manuals. The nurse needs to check the agency policy. EIDs can be programmed for specific minimum rates.
Tonicity	Solute concentration in a parenteral fluid to permit water transport across a semi-permeable cell membrane. Osmotic pressure can cause cells to shrink or swell.
Volume-Control Burette Device	Transparent, calibrated small-volume container, with a capacity of 100, 110, or 150 mL, that is manually connected to an IV line just below the main IV solution container. It is filled with only 1 or 2 hours' worth of IV fluid and/or smaller amounts of medicated solution at a time, depending on agency policy. As the name implies, it protects at-risk patients from fluid or medication overload by limiting the total amount of solution available in case of equipment or a rate failure incident.

RAPID PRACTICE | **9-1**

Vocabulary Review

Estimated completion time: 10-15 minutes   Answers on page 536

Directions: *Examine the IV-related vocabulary to expedite comprehension of the material in this chapter. Fill in* very brief *descriptions of the vocabulary terms supplied.*

1   What is the difference between a continuous IV solution order and an intermittent IV order? _____

2 What is the difference between a primary and a secondary infusion line?

_____

3 **a.** What is a DF, and which kind of IV equipment requires the DF to determine flow rate?

_____

    b. Which type of administration set delivers the smallest drops and is used for low flow rates?

_____

4 What is the difference between a nonvolumetric and a volumetric EID?

_____

5 Flow rates for IV solutions are usually ordered in which measurement terms?

_____

Overview of Intravenous Therapy

Oral medications and IV solutions that may be medicated are the two most common routes of medication administration. The nursing responsibilities related to the patient's safety during oral and IV medication therapy are paramount.

Purpose of intravenous solutions

Intravenous solutions are ordered to:

- Provide daily maintenance fluid and electrolyte therapy.
- Replace prior deficits.
- Administer medications and nutrients.

The fluids may contain dextrose solutions, electrolytes, medications, nutrients, or blood products as needed. They may be _isotonic, hypotonic,_ or _hypertonic,_ based on the prescriber's assessment of current laboratory test results and the patient's clinical needs.

Intravenous solutions are ordered to be either _continuous_ or _intermittent,_ depending on the patient's fluid and medication needs and fluid intake status. They are administered through peripheral or larger-diameter central veins. They are supplied in _nonvented plastic_ or _vented_ and nonvented glass containers.

Continuous IV lines are placed on _primary infusion administration lines. Intermittent_ infusions are administered in a variety of ways but are frequently connected (piggybacked) to a port on a primary line via a _secondary_ tubing set.

1 What are three purposes for ordering IV solutions? (Use one- or two-word answers.)

_____

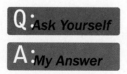

Q: _Ask Yourself_

A: _My Answer_

Maintenance intravenous flow rates

The average-sized adult patient who is to be NPO for a short period of time but is otherwise well hydrated, with good heart, lung, and renal function, may have a _maintenance isotonic_ continuous IV solution ordered at about _75-125 mL per hr._ When an order calls for much less or more than this flow rate, the nurse needs to research the need for the variation. It is easier to keep in mind an average of about 1 L q8h or 2-3 L q24h for the hypothetical hydrated adult who is NPO for a limited period of time. Often, the reason for variation is clear.

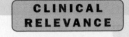

CLINICAL RELEVANCE

A dehydrated patient will receive a higher-than-average volume and flow rate, depending on clinical tolerance. A patient with compromised heart, lung, or renal function or a baby will receive a lower-than-average flow rate. The more the patient is able to drink, the less the need for a high flow rate or a continuous IV infusion. Even if the patient is able to take 2-3 L of fluid a day by mouth, an IV access line is frequently established and "capped" in order to provide prompt access for IV medications or fluids if needed.

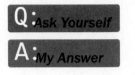

Q: Ask Yourself

A: My Answer

1   What are examples of the patient-related criteria that the prescriber uses to make an informed decision about the flow rate for an IV order? (Give a brief answer.)

_____

2   What are the main purposes of a primary line, a secondary line, and a port?

_____

_____

3   What is an average range of isotonic maintenance solution flow rates that might be ordered for a maintenance IV for an adult patient who is NPO and has good heart, lung, and renal function?

_____

RAPID PRACTICE   9-2

More Vocabulary Review

Estimated completion time: 10-15 minutes   **Answers on page 536**

Directions: *Select the IV-related term or phrase that best completes the sentence.*

1   The name for the main infusion administration set is _____.
   1. Intermittent   **3.** Primary
   2. Drop factor   **4.** Secondary

2   An IV solution that does not have a discontinue date or time is _____.
   1. 5% dextrose in water   **3.** Intermittent
   2. Continuous   **4.** PCA

3   The term for the *calibrated container* that can be used to deliver intermittent infusions is _____.
   1. Gravity infusion device   **3.** Electronic infusion device
   2. Volume-control burette device   **4.** IV piggyback

4   The term that describes undesired reactions that can result from a mixture of certain combinations of IV medications, diluents, and/or other solutions is _____.
   1. Incompatibility   **3.** Constant
   2. IV push   **4.** KVO

5   When a medication is manually injected directly into a venous access device by the nurse, the procedure is referred to as _____.
   1. IV piggyback   **3.** IV push
   2. TKO   **4.** PCA

Basic Intravenous Equipment

The essential elements of infusion equipment are

   • A prescribed unmedicated or medicated solution
   • A pole or stand to hold the solution and delivery devices

- A rate controller or cassette pump(s) as needed
- Infusion tubing of various sizes and types to connect the solution to the access device, needle, or needleless port
- Dressings and tape to protect and secure the injection site

---

Safety trends pertaining to IV equipment include increasing use of premixed medicated IV solutions supplied by the pharmacy or the manufacturer; needleless equipment; and sophisticated electronic devices that can handle up to four IV lines for one patient and have the capability of extensive programming of alarms, drug doses, and flow rates.

CLINICAL RELEVANCE

Types of Intravenous Solutions

There are many types of IV solutions. The contents depend on the purpose of the IV order, the condition of the patient as evidenced by laboratory test results, the hydration and fluid and electrolyte status of the patient, and compatible parenteral medications that need to be added to the solution.

The following are some of the most frequently ordered solutions to which medications can be added if necessary. Their names and abbreviations must be learned. Dextrose (D), normal saline (NS) solution, water (W), and lactated Ringer's (L/R) solution may contain varying percentages of dextrose or electrolytes. The nurse needs to focus on the percentage of contents ordered and match that with the label.

➤ A number indicates the % of grams of solute per 100 mL; for example, 5D = 5% dextrose or 5 grams of dextrose per 100 mL of solution.

Tonicity of Intravenous Solutions

➤ Examine and learn the names and contents of the isotonic solutions *first.* Then contrast the isotonic solution with the selected hypo- and hypertonic solutions.

Hypotonic	Isotonic (290 mOs)	Hypertonic
2.5% dextrose in water (2.5% DW)	5% dextrose in water (D5W or 5DW)	10% dextrose in water or (10DW)
0.45% NaCl (sodium chloride) solution (0.45NS, $\frac{1}{2}$ NS, or $\frac{1}{2}$-strength NS)	Normal saline (NS) solution (0.9% NaCl solution)	5DW in 0.45% NaCl solution or D5W in $\frac{1}{2}$ NS
	Lactated Ringer's solution (L/R, R/L, or LRS)	D5LR or D5RLS solution

Additives such as vitamins, minerals, potassium chloride (KCl), and many other medications may be ordered for inclusion in these solutions. Figure 9-1 shows labels of selected isotonic solutions.

1 Which type of solution most closely approximates the tonicity of plasma—hypotonic, isotonic, or hypertonic? Refer to "Osmolarity" in the Essential Vocabulary.

Q: *Ask Yourself*

A: *My Answer*

2 How does the percentage of solute in hypotonic and hypertonic solutions differ from that in isotonic solutions? (Give a brief answer and refer to Essential Vocabulary if necessary.)

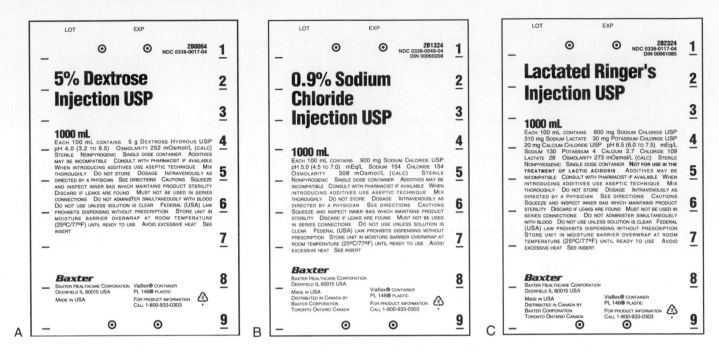

FIGURE 9-1 Labels of isotonic solutions. **A,** 5% dextrose. **B,** 0.9% sodium chloride. **C,** Lactated Ringer's solution.

FAQ | *Why is $\frac{1}{2}$ NS labeled 0.45% rather than 0.5% NaCl?*

ANSWER | Because it contains half the NaCl content of NS solution. NS solution contains 0.9%, not 1%, NaCl.

➤ All IV solutions and medications must be checked for compatibility using a current drug reference before being administered. When in doubt, the nurse should consult the pharmacy. In some large agencies, the pharmacy has an IV telephone "hotline."

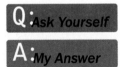

1 What are five types of equipment needed for all IV infusions?

_____

_____

Intravenous Solution Volume

Volumes of solution per IV container are usually 500 or 1000 mL but can vary from less than 50 to more than 1000 mL. Some medicated solutions are provided in 100- and 250-mL containers. Volumes of 500 and 1000 mL are among the most frequently encountered for maintenance and continuous solutions.

If the order calls for a liter, the nurse selects a 1000-mL container. Often, the order for a continuous IV infusion states only the name of the solution and the flow rate per hour. The nurse selects the volume for the infusion that will last a reasonable amount of time.

➤ A superscript *o* may be seen on orders to designate *hour* (e.g., q8°). Do not use this notation. The *o* may be mistaken for a zero.

Intravenous Solution Orders for Milliliters per Hour

➤ One calculation needed for *all* infusions so that flow rate can be monitored is a determination of the number of milliliters per hour (mL per hr).

The following are two typical orders for a *continuous* IV infusion:

Order	Meaning
1000 mL 5DW at 125 mL per hr	1 Liter of 5% dextrose in water to flow at a rate of 125 mL per hour until further notice
1 liter L/R solution q8h	1000 mL of lactated Ringer's solution every 8 hours

- Identify the ordered flow rate in mL per hr and any special instructions.
- Determine how long the IV solution will last.
  The calculations are usually very basic.
- If the prescriber orders D5W at 125 mL per hr, the nurse administers a *continuous* flow rate of *125 mL per hr* until the order is discontinued or changed. The equipment may vary and require further calculations, but the essential rate in mL per hr must be known.
- If the prescriber orders 1 L D5W q8h, the flow rate is derived with a simple calculation:

$$\frac{mL}{hr} : \frac{1000\ mL}{8\ hr} = 125\ mL\ per\ hr$$

- Milliliters and hours are both desired in the answer. This distinguishes hours from minutes or other time frames that may be ordered. The *initial* entry in the equation setup is the matched units in the numerator (milliliters). Hours (hr) must be entered in a denominator.
- Round flow rates to the nearest whole number.

1 What is the one calculation that is needed for all infusion rates?

_____

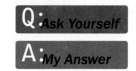

Q: *Ask Yourself*

A: *My Answer*

Determining Infusion Durations

- If the order states *1 L q8h*, it is obvious that the IV infusion will require replacement in 8 hours. If the order states only the mL per hour, a simple calculation is required.

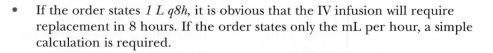

If the order states mL per hr such as *120 mL per hr*, and a liter (1000 mL) will be supplied:
1. Determine the hours of duration first (total mL ÷ mL per hr)
2. Convert any remainder of hours to minutes using a conversion factor: 60 minutes = 1 hr (60 × hr = minutes).

$$hr : \frac{1\ hr}{120\ mL} \times \frac{1000\ mL}{1} = 8.3\ hr$$

$$minutes : \frac{60\ minutes}{1\ hr} \times \frac{0.3\ hr}{1} = 18\ min$$

Total expected duration of 1000 mL flowing at 120 mL per hr = 8 hr and 18 min.

EXAMPLES

★ Communication

After the nurse identifies the patient, she or he briefly explains the purpose for administering the IV solution: "Mr. Smith, your doctor has ordered some fluids and (name) medications in your vein to help your (state the condition)." It is better to say "help" than "prevent." Accentuate the positive. "Have you had an IV before? How did it go?" or "How did you do with them?" "Do you have any allergies to these medications or any other medications? What kind of reaction did you have?" *Listen carefully* to the patient's responses to these questions.

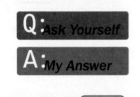

Q: Ask Yourself

A: My Answer

RAPID PRACTICE **9-3**

Calculating simple milliliter per hour (mL per hr) orders

Experienced nurses calculate simple orders, such as 1 L q8h, by converting 1 L to 1000 mL and performing simple division, 1000 mL ÷ 8 (total volume of the container divided by hours), yields a flow rate of 125 mL per hr.

➤ When the question is, How many mL per hr, think of *per* as a *division line:*
  total milliliters ÷ total hours = $\dfrac{\text{mL}}{\text{hr}}$.

➤ Always double check your answers.

Check agency policy pertaining to IV solution, tubing, and needle replacement. Some solutions need to be changed every 24 hours, others every 48 hours. TJC regulations present replacement guidelines. The contents of solution are factors in the policies. The product label may indicate an expiration date.

1 What are the abbreviations for three commonly ordered isotonic IV solutions?

_____

➤ With all patient communications, it pays to *stop*, *look*, and *listen* and respond accordingly.

If you are comfortable with multiplication and division skills, use a calculator for multiplication and long division.

Flow Rates and Infusion Times for Intravenous Solutions

Estimated completion time: 15-20 minutes   **Answers on page 536**

Directions: *Using the flow rate supplied, fill in the abbreviations for the* solution *ordered, the flow rate in mL/hr, the nearest whole number, and the infusion time in hours and minutes, if applicable. Use a calculator for long division and multiplication.*

Order	Abbreviation(s) for Solution	Flow Rate (mL per hr)	Infusion Time, Hours (and Minutes, If Applicable)
1 Infuse 500 mL normal saline over 6 h	_____	_____	_____
2 1000 mL 5% dextrose in water at 125 mL per hr	_____	_____	_____
3 1 L lactated Ringer's q10h	_____	_____	_____
4 250 mL half-strength normal saline q4h	_____	_____	_____
5 500 mL 5% dextrose in lactated Ringer's @40mL per hr	_____	_____	_____

FAQ | *How do I know which size, in milliliters, of IV bag to select?*

ANSWER | There are three criteria:
• Infusion time
• Flow rate ordered
• Solutions available or supplied

The commonly available solutions are packaged in amounts of 250, 500, and 1000 mL. Smaller amounts, including medicated solutions, are also supplied by the pharmacy. If the infusion is to last 8 hours and the flow rate is 100 mL per hr, 800 mL would be the minimum needed. The closest amount that can be selected would be a 1000 mL bag. If the solution is to infuse at 50 mL per hr continuously, most nurses will select a bag that contains at least enough to last for an 8- or 12-hour shift: 50 mL × 8 = 400 mL, or 50 mL × 12 = 600 mL. The nurse would probably select a 500 or 1000 mL bag even for the 50 mL per 8 hr order, assuming that the IV infusion would be reordered.

Intravenous Flow Rate Entries for Electronic Infusion Devices

When electronic controllers or pumps are used for IV infusion, the nurse must enter the ordered flow rate on the digital device. The LED screen displays the number of milliliters being infused per hour, the total number of milliliters that have been infused, and various other information, depending on the sophistication of the device (Figure 9-2).

For an order of 1000 mL q8h, the nurse would set up the equipment and enter a flow rate of 125 mL per hr.

➤ It is preferable to administer medicated solutions through EIDs. Critical care units do not usually use gravity infusions.

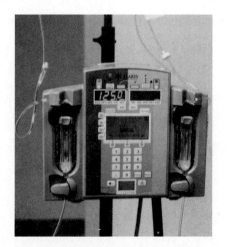

FIGURE 9-2 Dual-channel electronic infusion pump. (From Kee JL, Marshall SM: *Clinical calculations: with applications to general and specialty areas*, ed. 6, St. Louis, 2009, Saunders.)

Gravity Infusions

Some agencies use simple gravity devices with manual rate controllers for temporary emergency purposes, for administering unmedicated solutions or less powerful medicated solutions, and for maintenance unmedicated IV therapy (Figure 9-3).

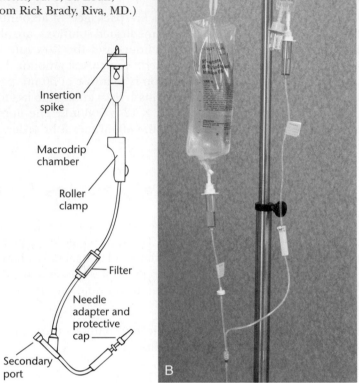

FIGURE 9-3 A, Gravity flow intravenous infusion equipment. (**A,** Modified from Clayton BD, Stock YN, Harroun RD: *Basic pharmacology for nurses,* ed. 15, St. Louis, 2010, Mosby. **B,** From Lilley LL, Harrington S, Snyder JS: *Pharmacology and the nursing process,* ed. 6, St. Louis, 2011, Mosby. From Rick Brady, Riva, MD.)

Insertion spike

Macrodrip chamber

Roller clamp

Filter

Needle adapter and protective cap

Secondary port

A

B

Outpatient centers, emergency vehicles, outpatient recovery units, home-care settings, rehabilitation units, and long-term care units are examples of places where gravity devices may be encountered.

Gravity infusions are hung on a pole approximately 36 inches above heart level of the patient. The flow rate is dependent on the flow rate control clamp adjustment, positioning of the solution, tubing patency, and the patient's position.

Intravenous Administration Sets

Intravenous tubing provides the connection between the IV solution and the patient. The nurse selects the tubing needed based on the order and the infusion equipment provided by the agency.

➤ The physician does not specify the equipment. Some tubing administration sets may be used interchangeably on infusion pumps and gravity devices. The tubing label describes the use. The containers are available in supply stations. The tubing is supplied in various widths to accommodate various flow rates and solution viscosities.

There are several types of specialized IV tubing. The main types include

- Primary (main) tubing for "main" and "maintenance" IV lines, EIDs, and gravity infusion devices (see Figure 9-3, *B*)
- Secondary, *shorter* tubing that connects to the primary tubing at a port to permit additional intermittent solutions to be added (piggybacked) without having to create a new injection site (see Figure 9-3, *B*)

- Blood administration sets with special filters and a Y connector for NS solution to prime the lines before and flush after blood transfusion or to use if the blood needs to be stopped or removed for any reason
- Extension tubings that are used when more length is needed (e.g., for ambulation)

A needle adapter with a cap, tubing, a clamp to stop and start flow, a drip chamber, and an insertion spike are included in the administration sets.

Selection of Gravity Infusion Administration Sets

For gravity devices, the nurse selects the calibration of tubing needed based on the equipment available, the flow rate ordered, and the contents of the IV solution. The DF is available on the tubing administration set. Figure 9-4, *A* illustrates a DF of 10 (10 drops per mL).

Macrodrip (large-diameter) tubing, with a DF of 10, 15, or 20, is selected for unmedicated solutions, solutions requiring faster flow rates, and solutions that have less powerful medications (Figure 9-5, *A*).

Microdrip tubing (also known as pediatric tubing) has a DF of 60 and narrow tubing that delivers tiny drops from a *needle-like* projection to achieve 60 drops/mL. Because of the projection, microdrip sets can be recognized at a glance without having to go to a supply room to check the DF (Figure 9-5, *B*).

Check agency policy for administration set selection protocols.

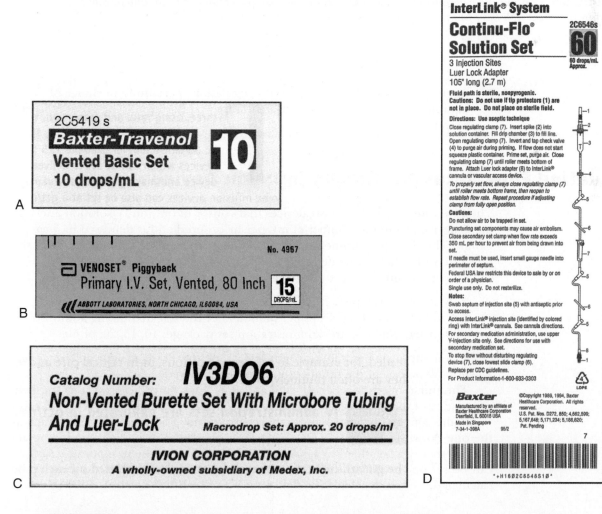

FIGURE 9-4 A, DF 10. **B,** DF 15. **C,** DF 20. **D,** DF 60. (From Gray Morris D: *Calculate with confidence,* ed. 5, St. Louis, 2010, Mosby.)

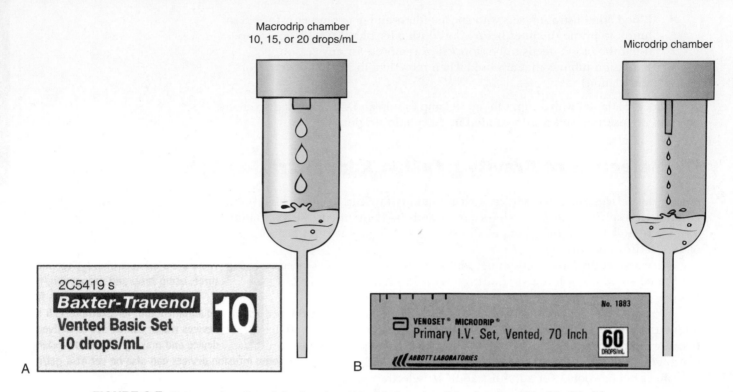

FIGURE 9-5 Contrast the macrodrip chamber (**A**) with the microdrip chamber (**B**). (Modified from Clayton BD, Stock YN: *Basic pharmacology for nurses,* ed. 15, St. Louis, 2010, Mosby.)

➤ Agency policies must be checked for regulations pertaining to choice of IV equipment. If a solution is medicated, it may be required to be on a volumetric pump.

Calculating Flow Rates for Gravity Infusion Devices

The flow rate for simple gravity devices that consist of only an IV solution and tubing is derived from the number of mL per hr ordered and is delivered in *drops per minute*. The drop-per-minute rate is calculated by the nurse. The nurse adjusts the flow rate with a hand-operated slide pinch or roller clamp (Figure 9-6).

To convert mL per hr to drops per minute, identify the following factors:

1 Number of mL per hr ordered
2 Calibration (DF, or drops per milliliter) of the selected tubing administration set, stated on the administration set package: 10, 15, 20, or 60.

When the drop-per-minute count is correct, the flow rate will deliver an *approximate equivalent* of the number of mL per hr ordered.

The nurse needs to assess IV sites and flow rates during each visit to the bedside and/or every hour or more often. Check agency policies.

Some agencies provide a flow rate control device for gravity infusions, such as the one shown in Figure 9-7. The Dial-a-Flo device is an example of an in-line apparatus that can be added to a gravity infusion set so that the number of *mL per hr* can be set on the dial and the number of drops per minute does not have to be calculated.

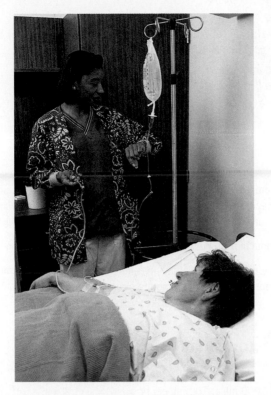

FIGURE 9-6 Nurse adjusting flow of IV infusion. (From Perry AG, Potter PA: *Clinical nursing skills and techniques,* ed. 7, St. Louis, 2010, Mosby.)

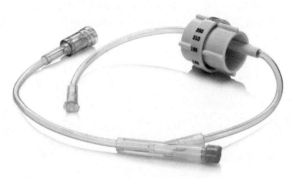

FIGURE 9-7 Dial-a-Flo® extension set with pre-pierced Y-site. (From Hospira, Inc., Lake Forest, IL.)

➤ Check calibrations on gravity flow rate devices. Dial-a-Flo provides a range from 5 to 250 mL per hr.

Calculation of gravity infusion rates

The key to accurate calculation of flow rates for gravity devices is to understand the underlying process. Once the method described in this section is thoroughly understood, faster methods will become apparent.

EXAMPLES

Ordered: IV D5W 1000 mL at 100 mL per hr or 1 L D5W q10h. How many drops per minute will the nurse set on the gravity infusion set?

- Identify the *mL per hour* to be infused: 100 mL per hr
- Identify the DF from the IV administration set.

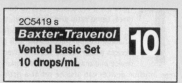

2C5419 s
Baxter-Travenol
Vented Basic Set
10 drops/mL
10

➤ Note that 10 drops per mL × 100 mL per hr ordered = 1000 drops per hr. The nurse cannot count the drops for an hour to see if the rate is correct. The nurse wants to know the count for 1 minute that would result in the desired number of drops per hour.

- Enter the data in a DA equation along with an hr to min conversion.

All the data can be entered in *one* equation (when the number of mL per hr is known) to obtain the number of drops per minute. Examine the example that follows.

Calculation of gravity infusion rates using DA

EXAMPLES

Ordered: IV D5W 1000 mL at 100 mL per hr
Drop factor (DF): 10 (10 drops per mL)
(The DF is found on the tubing administration set.)
The nurse will set the flow rate for how many drops per minute (min)?

Step 1	:	Step 2	×	Step 3	=	Answer
Desired Answer Units	:	Starting Factor	×	Given Quantity and and Conversion Factor(s)	=	Estimate, Multiply, Evaluate

$$\frac{drops}{min} : \frac{\overset{1}{\cancel{10}} \, drops}{1 \, \cancel{mL}} \times \frac{100 \, \cancel{mL}}{1 \, \cancel{hr}} \times \frac{1 \, \cancel{hr}}{\underset{6}{\cancel{60}} \, min} = \frac{100 \, drops}{6 \, min}$$

$$= 16\frac{2}{3} \text{ drops per min, rounded to 17 drops per min}$$

The final equation will be written like this:

$$\frac{drops}{min} : \frac{\overset{1}{\cancel{10}} \, drops}{1 \, \cancel{mL}} \times \frac{100 \, \cancel{mL}}{1 \, \cancel{hr}} \times \frac{1 \, \cancel{hr}}{\underset{6}{\cancel{60}} \, min} = \frac{100 \, drops}{6 \, min} = 16\frac{2}{3} \text{ rounded to 17 drops per min D5W}$$

Analysis: We need a *rate, drops* and *time* in the answer. Once again, the selected Starting Factor, the conversion factor of 10 drops in 1 mL, was the factor containing the desired answer units. The rate and time factor was 100 mL per hr. The only time available was *hour* so we used it and then converted hours to minutes. The rest of the factors were entered so that they could be canceled sequentially starting with mL. Drops has to be in a numerator and minutes has to appear in a denominator.

Evaluation: Only the desired answer units remain. Our estimate of about 1/6 of 100 is supported by the answer (Math check: 100 ÷ × 6 = 16 2/3 rounded to 17 drops per minute). The equation is balanced. Note that once again, cancellation makes the math simple.

➤ Note the 1000 mL in the order was not needed. Rate, drops, and time were already selected. If we had also added the 1000 mL somewhere in the equation, mL would have appeared 3 times and could not have been canceled. The answer would have been 17,000 mL drops per minute; however, 60 drops per minute is about as fast as the nurse can count.
➤ Be aware that some orders still use the outdated abbreviation "gtt" for drops.

FAQ | *What is the advantage of a Dial-a-Flo type rate control device (Figure 9-7, p. 275) over gravity infusion sets?*

ANSWER | The nurse does not have to calculate drops per minute. The Dial-a-Flo device takes care of that step when the precise mL per hr from the order is entered. (These devices are not always supplied.)

Calculating Flow Rates for Gravity Infusions Using DA Equations

RAPID PRACTICE 9-4

Estimated completion time: 15 minutes   Answers on page 536

Directions: *Examine the example on p. 276 and the example in problem 1. For problems 2-5, identify the number of mL per hr and the drop factor. Calculate the flow rates to the nearest whole drop per minute for the ordered solutions. Evaluate the equation. Use a calculator for long division and multiplication.*

➤ Remember that the DF is in drops per 1 mL. The DF and the number of mL per hr ordered must be entered in the equation.

1 Ordered: IV 500 mL to infuse over 4 hours on a gravity infusion. Administration set DF: 15.

   a. How many mL per hr are ordered? mL per hr = 500 ÷ 4 = 125 mL/hr
   b. How many drops per minute will be set?

   DA equation:

$$\frac{drops}{minute} : \frac{\overset{1}{\cancel{15}}\ drops}{1\ \cancel{mL}} \times \frac{125\ \cancel{mL}}{4\ \cancel{hours}} \times \frac{1\ \cancel{hour}}{\underset{4}{\cancel{60}}\ min} = 31.25,\ \text{rounded to 31 drops/min}$$

   c. Evaluation: The equation is balanced. The desired answer units are the only ones remaining. (Milliliters and hours had to be entered twice in order to be canceled). All drops per minute equations use an hour-to-minutes conversion formula.

   ➤ Note that 500 mL total volume was not needed in the equation because the mL per hr was known.) You can enter $\frac{500\ mL}{4\ hr}$ for the same result.

2 Ordered: IV 1000 mL q12h on a gravity infusion device. Administration set DF: 20.

   a. How many mL per hr are ordered? _____
   b. How many drops per minute will be set? _____

   DA equation:

   c. Evaluation: _____

3 Ordered: IV 250 mL to infuse at 75 mL per hr. Administration set DF: 10.

   a. How many mL per hr are ordered? _____
   b. How many drops per minute will be set? _____

   DA equation:

   c. Evaluation: _____

4   Ordered: IV 500 mL to infuse over 6 hours. Administration set DF: 20.

   a. How many mL per hr are ordered? _____

   b. How many drops per minute will be set? _____

   DA equation:

   c. Evaluation: _____

5   Ordered: IV 100 mL to infuse at 10 mL per hr. The drop factor is 60.

   a. How many hours will it last? _____

   b. How many drops per minute will be set? _____

   DA equation:

   c. Evaluation: _____

Estimating the number of drops per minute for a drop factor of 60

Equations must be set up for DFs of 10, 15, and 20 and can be set up for DF 60.

➤ Drop factors of 60, for microdrip pediatric administration sets, do *not* require equations *when the number of mL per hr is known.* Because a DF of 60 divided by 60 minutes provides a factor of 1, the number of mL per hr = the number of drops per minute. Study the example that follows.

EXAMPLES

Ordered: IV 50 mL to infuse over 1 hour, with a DF of 60.

$$\frac{drops}{minute} : \frac{\cancel{60}\ drops}{1\ \cancel{mL}} \times \frac{50\ \cancel{mL}}{1\ \cancel{hr}} \times \frac{1\ hr}{\cancel{60}\ minutes} = 50\ drops\ per\ minute$$

Note how the quantity 60 in the *numerator* and the quantity 60 in the *denominator* are canceled, leaving only the 50 mL per hr. Thus, 50 mL per hr = 50 drops per min.

Microdrip (60 DF) flow rate in drops per minute = mL/hr.

➤ 60 DF = mL per hr applies only to *continuous infusions* or those that are to infuse for *60 minutes* or more

Study the explanations and equation above and the example worked out in Rapid Practice 9-4, problem 1.

Q: **Ask Yourself**

A: **My Answer**

1   How many drops per minute would I estimate if the infusion was ordered for 30 mL per hr and the DF was 60?

_____

2   If the DF on the tubing administration is known to be 60 and the order is for 20 mL per hr, how many drops per minute would I estimate for the gravity device?

_____

➤ Microdrip tubing is used for low flow rates up to and including 60 drops per min (60 mL per hr). It is too difficult to count a faster drop flow than 1 drop per sec, or 60 drops per min.

➤ You will encounter the abbreviation gtt for the word drops in some written orders and printed literature.

Calculating Solution Flow Rates for EIDs and Macrodrip and Microdrip Gravity Devices Using DA-Style Equations

Estimated completion time: 20-25 minutes   Answers on page 537

Directions: *Calculate the flow rate in mL per hr or drops per minute depending on the equipment. Use a calculator when needed. Round all mL per hr and drops per minute to the nearest whole number. For credit, please label all answers in mL per hr or drops per minute, as appropriate for the equipment available.*

1   Ordered: 600 mL NS q8h to be infused continuously on an EID.

What flow rate will the nurse set? (Use simple arithmetic.) _____

2   Ordered: 500 mL D5W at 25 mL per hr. Equipment: pediatric microdrip administration set for gravity infusion with a DF 60 (60 drops per mL).

   a. What is the estimated flow rate? (Use mental calculation.) Label the answer. _____

   b. Calculated flow rate:

      DA equation:

   c. Evaluation: _____

3   Ordered: 1000 mL L/R at 80 mL per hr. Equipment: gravity infusion device with a DF of 10.

   a. Calculated flow rate:

      DA equation:

   b. Evaluation: _____

   c. Is the flow rate reasonable for counting drops per minute? (see p. 278)
      Yes or No? _____

4   Ordered: 250 mL 0.45NS at 25 mL per hr. Equipment: gravity infusion set with macrodrip tubing, DF 15.

   a. Calculated flow rate:

      DA equation:

   b. Evaluation: _____

   c. Is the flow rate reasonable for counting drops per minute?
      Yes or No? _____

5   Ordered: 1000 mL 5LR at 100 mL per hr. Equipment: gravity infusion set with macrodrip tubing, DF 20.

   a. Calculated flow rate:

      DA equation:

   b. Evaluation: _____

   c. Is the flow rate reasonable for counting drops per minute?
      Yes or No? _____

➤ Remember that calculations of IV flow rates begin with examination of the prescriber's order to be able to determine milliliters for mL per hr. IV calculations require this value, not just for further calculations, but also to evaluate flow rate at the bedside.

Q: *Ask Yourself*

A: *My Answer*

1 If a flow rate is 50 mL per hr using a microdrip (pediatric) set, how many drops per minute will I set? (Use mental arithmetic.)

_____

2 Noting that the DF denotes the number of drops per milliliter, which of three *macrodrip* sets—10, 15, and 20—would deliver the largest drop and therefore be suitable for a fastest rate of flow or more viscous fluids, such as blood products?

_____

➤ Remember that the microdrip set is selected for flow rates up to 60 drops per min.

Counting drops per minute at the bedside

The nurse counts the drops at eye level for 15 or 30 seconds or 1 minute to ensure that the IV solution is flowing at the appropriate rate (Figure 9-8). The slower the rate, the longer the needed counting period. Multiply the 15-second count by 4 and the 30-second count by 2 to obtain the drops per minute.

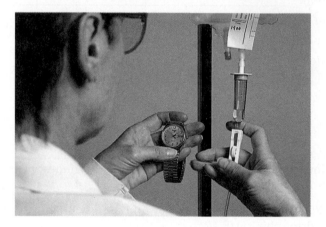

FIGURE 9-8 IV sites, flow rates, and volume infused need to be assessed during each visit to the bedside. (From Perry AG, Potter PA, Stockert PA, Hall A: *Basic nursing*, ed. 7, St. Louis, 2011, Mosby.)

RAPID PRACTICE 9-6

Gravity Infusion Rates and DA Equations

Estimated completion time: 20-25 minutes   Answers on page 538

Directions: *Use DA equations to calculate the flow rates. Remember that gravity infusion calculations include an "hour-to-minute" conversion. Use a calculator for long division and multiplication to solve the equations. Use mental calculations for continuous microdrip calculations. Refer to p. 278 for an explanation.*

1 Ordered: IV D5W (continuous) at 10 mL per hr, DF 60.

   a. What flow rate will the nurse set? (Use mental calculation.) _____

   b. Is this a macrodrip or microdrip tubing factor? _____

   c. How can the nurse tell at a glance if a tubing factor is macro- or microdrip when it is infusing? _____

2   Ordered: IV D5NS at 100 mL per hr, DF 10 administration set selected.

    a. Flow rate will be set at_____

    DA equation:

    b. Evaluation: _____

3   Ordered: IV LRS at 125 mL per hr, DF 15 administration set selected.

    a. Flow rate will be set at _____

    DA equation:

    b. Evaluation: _____

4   Ordered: IV D10W at 75 mL per hr, DF 20 administration set selected.

    a. Flow rate will be set at _____

    DA equation:

    b. Evaluation: _____

5   Ordered: IV 0.45% NaCl sol at 120 mL per hr, DF 10 administration set selected.

    a. Flow rate will be set at _____

    DA equation:

    b. Evaluation: _____

1   What does the DF on the gravity tubing mean exactly in terms of a milliliter?

    _____

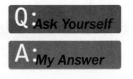

Q: *Ask Yourself*

A: *My Answer*

2   Which is the DF of the narrowest tubing that delivers the smallest drops and therefore delivers the greatest number of drops per milliliter?

    _____

Gravity Infusion Rates for Continuous IV Infusions

RAPID PRACTICE 9-7

Estimated completion time: 15 minutes   Answers on page **538**

Directions: *Use the hourly flow rate to calculate the IV flow rates. Use the simplified method for pediatric (microdrip) tubing if minutes equal 60. Verify with a DA equation.*

1   Ordered: 1000 mL D5W at 125 mL per hr, DF 10.

    a. Flow rate: _____

    DA equation:

    b. Evaluation: _____

2   Ordered: 500 mL NS at 50 mL per hr, DF 15.

   a. Flow rate: _____

   DA equation:

   b. Evaluation: _____

3   Ordered: 5RL 500 mL at 50 mL per hr, DF 20.

   a. Flow rate: _____

   DA equation:

   b. Evaluation: _____

4   Ordered: 10DW 500 mL at 75 mL per hr, DF 10.

   a. Flow rate: _____

   DA equation:

   b. Evaluation: _____

5   Ordered: 5LRS 250 mL at 40 mL per hr, DF 60.

   a. Flow rate: _____

   DA equation:

   b. Evaluation: _____

Intravenous Piggyback Solutions

For intermittent use, medicated piggyback solutions are often prepared in the pharmacy and supplied in small volumes such as 50 or 100 mL to be administered through a secondary line for 20, 30, or 60 minutes (Figure 9-9). These solutions frequently contain antibiotics that may be infused intermittently (e.g., q4h or q6h) to maintain therapeutic blood levels of the medication.

They are connected (piggybacked) to a primary line port through a shorter secondary tubing set. Most intermittent infusions will be administered over 30 or 60 minutes. However, the nurse must be prepared to know the math for 20- and 40-minute infusions.

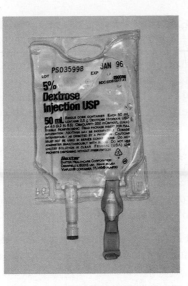

FIGURE 9-9 50 mL of solution for IVPB infusion. (From Brown M, Mulholland JL: *Drug calculations: process and problems for clinical practice,* ed. 8, St. Louis, 2008, Mosby.)

Calculating flow rates in milliliters per hour (mL per hr) for intravenous piggyback infusions to infuse in less than 1 hour

Ordered: IVPB antibiotic 50 mL in 30 minutes. How many mL per hr will be set on the EID? The equation will require a conversion formula from minutes to hours.

DA equation:

$$\frac{mL}{hr} : \frac{50\ mL}{\underset{1}{\cancel{30}\ min}} \times \frac{\overset{2}{\cancel{60}\ min}}{1\ hr} = 100\ mL\ per\ hr$$

Evaluation: The equation is balanced. It is logical that, to infuse 50 mL in 30 minutes, the rate would have to be set at 100 mL per hr (60 min). The 60 min = 1 hr conversion is needed to convert the 30-min order to an hourly rate. ($\frac{mL}{hr}$ = mL per hour)

Increasing your understanding of calculations for intermittent small-volume intravenous flow rates on electronic infusion devices

The flow rate for piggyback solutions is set in *mL per hr* for EIDs.

1 If I drink 60 mL in 60 minutes, how much fluid will I have consumed in *30 minutes* if I had been sipping at the same rate for the entire time?

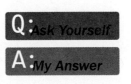

_____

2 If an IV antibiotic label states, "Infuse at 60 mL per hr for 30 minutes," what volume will have been completed in an hour if the infusion "continued" for the hour?

_____

3 If an IV is to infuse at 20 mL per *hr* for 30 minutes, how much fluid should infuse in *30 minutes?*

_____

Simplified piggyback calculations for milliliter-per-hour settings

Because small-volume intermittent piggyback infusions are usually administered over 20, 30, or 60 minutes on a secondary IV line, the nurse can perform mental calculations to obtain the flow rate in mL per hr. A simple DA equation can be employed for verification. No arithmetic is required for a 60-minute infusion.

> ➤ For 60-minute infusions, volume = milliliter-per-hour rate.
> ➤ For 30-minute infusions, *double* the amount of milliliters ordered for 30 minutes to obtain the 60-mL (hourly) rate
> ➤ For 20-minute infusions, *triple* the milliliter volume ordered for 20 minutes to obtain the 60-mL (hourly) rate.

Do not forget to check the infusion to be sure that the main IV line restarts after the 20-, 30-, or 60-minute period is completed. On some EIDs, each line is programmed separately. The nurse needs to confirm that the programming is accurate for both the primary and secondary solutions.

The IV infusion will be completed in the ordered time period. The nurse then ensures that the primary IV line resumes at its ordered rate.

> ➤ The flow rate for the IVPB line is set at what would have been the volume for 1 hour. That rate is often different from and may be faster than the primary IV infusion rate.

EXAMPLES

Primary rate: D5W continuous IV at 75 mL per hr.

Piggyback rate: 50 mL over 20 minutes, or 150 mL per hr.

Adjust the rate from 150 down to 75 mL per hr when the piggybacked solution is finished. The trend is to use EID equipment that has separate control devices for flow rates for primary and secondary lines.

FAQ | *Why are IVPB solutions given at different rates than the primary IV infusion?*

ANSWER | Effective treatment of resistant or acute conditions, such as acute infections or tumors, requires heavily concentrated infusions of drugs at periodic intervals to maintain therapeutic blood levels of the medication around the clock. These infusions must be given on time and are ordered at a specific rate to deliver the amount of drug for maximum effectiveness. It is important to change the flow rate for the medication if the order so indicates and to change the rate back to the primary rate when the intermittent infusion is completed. To do less imperils the patient's recovery. If the intermittent medicated solution is to be administered quickly and the primary solution is a maintenance IV infusion, failure to adjust the rates as required can result in fluid or medication underload or overload.

> ➤ The nurse's responsibility to adjust IV infusion flow rates is time-consuming and requires a variety of nursing skills: comprehension, calculation, organization, prioritization, vigilance, experience, and focus.

Estimated Piggyback Flow Rate for Milliliters per Hour with DA Verification

Estimated completion time: 30 minutes   Answers on page 539

Directions: *Examine the examples on p. 283 and in problem 1 below. For problems 2-5, use mental calculations to calculate the milliliters-per-hour setting on an EID for the piggy-backed solution. Verify the calculation with a DA equation.*

1   Ordered: 100 mL (IVPB) antibiotic over 30 minutes.

    a. Estimated flow rate in mL/hr: <u>100 mL × 2, or 200 mL per hr for 30 minutes</u>

    b. DA verification:

$$\frac{mL}{hr} : \frac{100\ mL}{\cancel{30\ min}_{1}} \times \frac{\cancel{60\ min}^{2}}{1\ hour} = 200\ mL\ per\ hr*$$

    c. Evaluation: <u>The equation is balanced. The estimate supports the answer.</u>

    ➤   *Recheck calculations for high-volume flow rates such as this.

2   Ordered: 80 mL anti-cancer drug (IVPB) over 30 minutes.

    a. Estimated flow rate in mL per hr: _____

    b. DA verification:

    c. Evaluation: _____

3   Ordered: 50 mL antibiotic (IVPB) over 20 minutes.

    a. Estimated flow rate in mL per hr: _____

    b. DA verification:

    c. Evaluation: _____

4   Ordered: 30 mL antibiotic (IVPB) over 20 minutes.

    a. Estimated flow rate in mL per hr: _____

    b. DA verification:

    c. Evaluation: _____

5   Ordered: 25 mL anti-cancer drug (IVPB) over 30 minutes.

    a. Estimated flow rate in mL per hr: _____

    b. DA verification:

    c. Evaluation: _____

FAQ | *Why is the DA verification needed if we can mentally calculate the flow rate for the IVPB solution?*

ANSWER | As with all other calculations, the nurse must be proficient in setting up the DA equation as a backup method in case an odd number of minutes is ordered, which would make a mental calculation difficult. Applying the DA setup to a variety of problems now and reviewing it periodically is necessary to *maintain* proficiency. Verify pharmacy calculations also.

Calculating flow rates for piggyback gravity infusions in drops per minute to infuse in less than 1 hour

Equations used to calculate IVPB infusions on *gravity* devices are very simple and *different* from other infusion equations: they do not use a milliliter-per-hour calculation.

If an IVPB order is for 50 mL over 30 minutes with a DF administration set of 10, the question to be solved by a DA equation is: *How many drops per minute will be set?*

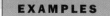

$$\frac{\text{drops}}{\text{min}} : \frac{\overset{1}{\cancel{10}}\ \text{drops}}{1\ \cancel{\text{mL}}} \times \frac{50\ \cancel{\text{mL}}}{\underset{3}{\cancel{30}}\ \text{min}} = 16.6,\ \text{rounded to 17 drops per minute}$$

Analysis: The desired answer units are drops per minute. Enter the drop factor with its accompanying milliliter unit first to match the desired answer numerator. The order to be converted is 50 mL over 30 minutes.

➤ There is *no need to enter hours* in the equation. The answer will *not* be in mL per hr. Entry of the minutes unit is postponed until the entry of the denominator of the second fraction. Seventeen drops per minute will deliver 50 mL in 30 minutes.

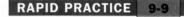

IVPB Flow Rates Practice in Milliliters per Hour and Drops per Minute for Gravity Devices

Estimated completion time: 15-25 minutes   **Answers on page 540**

Directions: *Estimate the flow rate in mL per hour. Calculate the flow rate in drops/minute to the nearest whole number for gravity devices. Use a calculator for long division and multiplication to solve the equations. Label answers.*

1 Ordered: IVPB antibiotic 50 mL over 20 minutes, DF 10.

   a. Estimated flow rate in mL per hr: _____
   b. Flow rate in drops per minute: _____

   DA equation:

   c. Evaluation: _____

2 Ordered: IVPB antibiotic 100 mL over 30 minutes, DF 15.

   a. Estimated flow rate in mL per hr: _____
   b. Flow rate in drops per minute: _____

   DA equation:

   c. Evaluation: _____

3 Ordered: IVPB anti-cancer drug 75 mL over 60 minutes, DF 20.

   a. Estimated flow rate in mL per hr: _____
   b. Flow rate in drops per minute: _____

   DA equation:

   c. Evaluation: _____

4 Ordered: IVPB anti-infective drug 30 mL over 30 minutes, DF 60.

   a. Estimated flow rate in mL per hr: _____

   b. Flow rate in drops per minute: _____

   DA equation:

   c. Evaluation: _____

5 Ordered: IVPB cortisone product 50 mL over 20 minutes, DF 10.

   a. Estimated flow rate in mL per hr: _____

   b. Flow rate in drops per minute: _____

   DA equation:

   c. Evaluation: _____

Regulating and Positioning Gravity Infusion Devices

Note the positioning of the primary and secondary IVPB solutions in Figure 9-10. The higher IV solution is currently infusing. When it is empty, the lower solution will resume infusing. At this point, the nurse must change the flow rate back to the primary flow rate if the secondary rate is different.

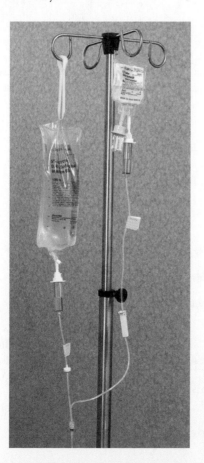

FIGURE 9-10 Gravity-flow IVPB. The IVPB is elevated above the existing IV, allowing it to infuse by gravity. (In Lilley LL, Collins SR, Harrington S, Snyder JS: *Pharmacology and the nursing process,* ed. 6, St. Louis, 2011, Mosby. From Rick Brady, Riva, MD.)

Solutions for gravity flow devices need to be 3 feet above the patient's heart level. The solution that is on "hold" is lowered *below* the solution that is to flow. A simple hanger extender device is used to accomplish this.

RAPID PRACTICE   9-10

Calculating IVPB Flow Rates for EID and Gravity Devices

Estimated completion time: 15 minutes   Answers on page 540

Directions: *Fill in the following IVPB flow rate table with the needed flow rates in the spaces provided. Examine the example provided for the first entry. Label all answers in mL per hr or drops per minute, as needed.*

IVPB Order and Equipment	Estimated Flow Rate (mL per hour)	Flow Rate Equation (in mL per hr or drops per min as needed)
1 50 mL antibiotic solution to infuse over 30 minutes on EID	100 mL per hr	$\dfrac{50 \text{ mL}}{\cancel{30 \text{ min}}_{\,1}} \times \dfrac{\cancel{60 \text{ min}}^{\,2}}{1 \text{ hr}} = 100 \text{ mL per hr}$
2 30 mL anti-cancer medication to infuse over 20 minutes on EID	_____	_____
3 20 mL antibiotic solution to infuse over 30 minutes on gravity infusion device DF 60	_____	_____
4 60 mL antibiotic solution to infuse over 40 minutes on EID	_____	_____
5 25 mL antibiotic solution over 20 minutes on gravity infusion device DF 20	_____	_____

RAPID PRACTICE   9-11

Intravenous Infusion Practice

Estimated completion time: 15 minutes   Answers on page 541

Directions: *Read the IV order and equipment available, and supply the infusion information in the spaces provided.*

Order	Equipment Available	Continuous or Intermittent	Flow Rate Equation (Label Answer)
1 1000 mL D5W q10h	IV administration set DF 10	_____	_____
2 50 mL antibiotic solution to infuse over 20 minutes	Volumetric pump	_____	_____

Order	Equipment Available	Continuous or Intermittent	Flow Rate Equation (Label Answer)
3	250 mL D5W over 4 hr	Electronic rate controller	_____	_____
4	500 mL NS every 6 hr	IV administration set DF 15	_____	_____
5	30 mL antibiotic solution to infuse over 30 minutes	Pediatric microdrip administration set	_____	_____

The nurse always needs to know the ordered flow rate and must be able to verify that rate at the bedside, whether it is being administered on a volumetric pump or any other kind of equipment.

The prescriber orders mL per hr for unmedicated solutions, not drops per minute.

Flow Rate Errors

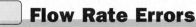

Flow rates can get behind or ahead of schedule for many reasons:

- Positional dislodgement of the needle
- Movement of the patient
- Occlusion of the entry site
- Incorrect flow rate entry
- Administration of other fluids on a secondary line
- Incorrect positioning of the IV solutions
- Equipment failure
- Temporary discontinuance for travel to the x-ray or other department
- A change in flow rate orders by the prescriber since the nurse last checked for new orders

Monitoring the Flow Rate on Infusion Devices

The nurse verifies the *ordered flow rate* by

- Reading the entry on the infusion pump
- Checking the rate controller on a gravity device
- Counting the drops on a gravity device and converting to mL per hr
- Examining the timed tape, if present, on the solution container

➤ The flow rate and site must be monitored frequently.

The patient and family need to be given a call bell, advised that the nurse will be checking in on them, and advised to call the nurse if an alarm device becomes activated. "There will be an alarm to warn us when the solution gets low," "Here is the call light," or "Call me if the solution stops dripping." It is a bad shift when an IV has to be restarted in another site because of coagulation from running dry. It is also a bad shift when the nurse finds that an IV that was supposed to infuse in 8 hours has infused in 2 hours. There is no need to warn the patient of all the malfunctions that can cause an alarm, such as air in the line and the like. If the patient has orders to leave the bed for any reason, tell the patient to call for assistance before getting out of bed until there is assurance the patient can move independently with the equipment. Remember that IV fluids will increase the need to urinate. Do not forget to ask, "Do you have any questions?"

CLINICAL RELEVANCE

➤ Each hour and during visits to the bedside, the IV site is examined and the solution is examined to ensure that the site is patent, the appropriate volume has been infused to date, and the rate is correct. Previous caretakers may have set incorrect rates. The nurse also needs to be aware that orders may be changed frequently by the prescriber.

Timed tapes

Timed tapes are placed on full IV solution containers by the nurse. The top calibration on the top of the tape is placed opposite the hanging fluid level, with the current time written next to it (Figure 9-11).

The nurse writes in the anticipated time the solution should reach the major volume calibrations based on the rate ordered. Examining a few timed tapes at the bedside provides a quick understanding of the information to be entered and the placement of the tape.

➤ A timed tape should be placed on all IV solution containers, both with electronic devices and with gravity devices, to further ensure that the volume infused matches the hourly ordered rate. The timed tape is very helpful but only if it is checked frequently as a rough gauge of fluid infused. Flow rate devices can fail. Check agency policies for timed tapes.

CLINICAL RELEVANCE

➤ The nurse must be aware of the following *warnings about flow rate adjustments.* If the flow is deemed to be infusing too slowly or quickly, beware of "catching-up." There are no hard and fast rules nor formulas about how much a flow rate can be adjusted to catch up to the ordered rate. The safety of such adjustments depends on the patient's condition and the contents of the IV solution. Guessing is dangerous. Flow rates affect major organ function. Med-

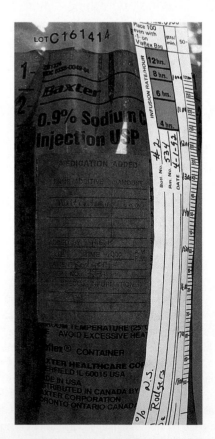

FIGURE 9-11 IV bag with timed tape. (From Potter PA, Perry AG, Stockert PA, Hall A: *Basic nursing,* ed. 7, St. Louis, 2011, Mosby.)

icated IV solutions are prescribed to deliver drugs at a therapeutic rate. It may seem safe to lower an IV rate, but if there is a medication included, slowing the infusion may cause the patient to suffer from abrupt withdrawal. Check with the prescriber about any adjustments.

➤ The best way to keep IV flow rates on target is thorough knowledge of the current ordered IV infusion rate and frequent monitoring, every hour and every visit.

➤ Check with the prescriber before speeding up an IV flow rate. Increasing the flow rate should be done gradually to ensure that the patient's condition does not suffer adverse effects.

➤ Never open up an IV line to full flow to catch up.

➤ Gravity flow rates are not stable. The tubing may become pinched; the clamp that regulates the flow may slip; or a positional change may cause a flow rate to increase, decrease, or halt. Educate the patient and family, if possible, to call for assistance if the flow rate stops or seems to be infusing too quickly. Volumetric pumps are more reliable than gravity infusion devices but not 100% reliable.

For further details, refer to the FAQ on p. 305.

There have been incidents in which a patient or family member changed the setting on an EID. Also, staff on the previous shift may have entered the wrong setting or the order may have changed.

Calculating Milliliters per Hour from Drops per Minute on Gravity Devices at the Bedside

As mentioned before, the usual *ordered* flow rate for gravity infusions is in mL per hr, not drops per minute.

When caring for patients whose IV infusions have been initiated by someone else—a previous caretaker—the currently assigned nurse must verify during each visit that the flow rate is as ordered. For example, a nurse visits the bedside and notes that a gravity device has been used. She or he will count the current drop-per-minute flow rate. At that point, the nurse has two choices for verifying that *ordered flow rate* is infusing:

1 Calculate the derived flow rate in drops per minute from the mL per hr order and compare it to the current drops-per-minute flow rate.

2 Calculate the milliliters-per-hour flow rate from the current flow.

The nurse must be able to perform both calculations. A prescriber may ask at the bedside, "What is the current flow rate?," and will want the answer in mL per hr.

By counting the current flow rate in drops/minute, the nurse can verify the flow rate in mL per hr.

An IV is infusing at 30 drops per min. The DF is 20. How many mL per hr are being infused at this rate?

EXAMPLES

$$\frac{mL}{hr} : \frac{1 \ mL}{\underset{2}{\cancel{20 \ drops}}} \times \frac{\overset{3}{\cancel{30 \ drops}}}{1 \ min} \times \frac{60 \ \cancel{min}}{1 \ hr} = \frac{180}{2} = 90 \ mL \ per \ hr$$

Analysis: The number of drops per minute and the DF are the known data. (Most agencies buy one brand of administration sets in bulk. The nurse learns the DFs for the main equipment used in the agency during orientation and initial observation of the tubing set labels.) The DF must be entered in the DA equation along with the number of drops per minute. If *hour* is needed in the *answer,* the conversion *60 minutes = 1 hour* is required in the equation to convert minutes to hours.

Evaluation: The equation is balanced. Only mL per hr remains.

RAPID PRACTICE 9-12

Calculating Flow Rates in Milliliters per Hour for Gravity Infusions

Estimated completion time: 20-30 minutes   **Answers on page 541**

Directions: *Calculate mL per hr from the drops per minute flowing on the gravity device. Use a calculator for long division and multiplication to solve the equations. Label all answers.*

	Drops per Sec Counted at Bedside	Drops per Min (Mental Calculation)	Administration Set DF	Flow Rate Equation
1	10 drops per 15 sec	40 (10 × 4)	20	$\dfrac{mL}{hr} : \dfrac{1\ mL}{\underset{1}{\cancel{20\ drops}}} \times \dfrac{40\ \cancel{drops}}{1\ \cancel{min}} \times \dfrac{\overset{3}{\cancel{60\ min}}}{1\ hr} = 120$ mL per hr
2	8 drops per 30 sec	_____	10	
3	6 drops per 15 sec	_____	60	
4	12 drops per 30 sec	_____	15	
5	15 drops per 30 sec	_____	60	

Setting the Alarm for Electronic Intravenous Equipment

EIDs have a variety of safety alarm settings, depending on the sophistication of the device. In addition to setting the flow rate in mL per hr, the nurse programs the volume that will generate an alarm to give notice that the current infusion is almost finished. This warning serves several functions:

- The nurse has warning time to prepare a subsequent solution, if ordered.
- The IV line is prevented from running dry.
- The entry site will maintain patency and will not become coagulated.
- The patient will not have to be subjected to another injection for a new site because of clot formation.
- Medications and fluids will be delivered at the scheduled time.

Maintaining patency means safety and comfort for the patient, on-time delivery of fluids and medications, and time saved for the nurse.

Calculating the Volume for a "Volume to Be Infused" Alarm

Setting the advance warning alarm time is simple. Usually, the nurse programs the alarm to sound based on three criteria:

- How many hours will the IV solution be infused and at what rate?
- How much notice does the nurse need or want in order bring the next infusion container and equipment, such as new tubing, that may be needed?
- How many milliliters will have been infused by the time the nurse wants the alarm to sound?

➤ The nurse does not enter the entire volume to be infused. That would prevent advance warning time.

A rough guideline for determining the volume at which the alarm should sound is to subtract 50 mL from the total volume in the bag for faster infusion rates and 25 mL for slower flow rates. This guideline should be adjusted for other volumes, for low volumes or very slow volumes, or for very rapid rates. Experience, preference, and work load help the nurse to determine how much warning is needed.

EXAMPLES

For a total IV infusion volume of 1000 mL:

Infusion Rate	Amount to Subtract from Total Volume	Volume to Be Infused for Alarm to Sound
150 mL per hr	50 mL	950 mL
75 mL per hr	25 mL	975 mL

➤ With or without an alarm, the nurse needs to develop a reminder for the anticipated time at which to prepare the next container. Some nurses tune out alarms because they sound too often from various rooms.

1 If the flow rate was very rapid, would I want the alarm to sound earlier or later than average?

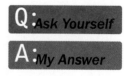

_____

➤ Disposal of IV tubing, needles, and sponges according to the guidelines and policies of the clinical agency and the federal Occupational Safety and Health Administration is a critical safety issue. Special hazardous waste containers must be used, and special care must be taken to avoid leaving any contaminated equipment at or in the bedside furnishings. Doing so could cause a needle-stick injury or bodily fluid exposure to a staff member at bedside or during transport for disposal.

Intravenous Infusion Review

RAPID PRACTICE 9-13

Estimated completion time: 10-20 minutes **Answers on page 542**

Directions: *Study the previous material and supply the requested information pertaining to basic IV infusions:*

1 Basic intravenous flow rates are usually ordered in which of the following terms: _____

   1. Drops per hour   **3.** Liters per minute

   2. mL per hr   **4.** Liters per hour

2 How does the nurse determine the number of drops per milliliter for a gravity IV infusion line? _____

    1. Refer to relevant IV pharmacology references.

    2. Call the agency pharmacist or consult a wall chart on the unit.

    3. Ask an experienced nurse on the unit.

    4. Read the DF on the IV administration set container.

3 An example of an order indicating that a continuous IV infusion solution is to be started on a patient would be _____

    1. Ampicillin 2 g IVPB q6h   **3.** 5DW 1 L q8h at 50 mL per hr

    2. Pantoprazole 40 mg IV push daily   **4.** Lorazepam 1 mg IV push

4 An IV device that permits the patient to control and administer an intermittent medicated (analgesic) solution for pain relief is called _____

    1. IV push   **3.** IV piggyback

    2. PCA   **4.** TKO

5 A reasonable short-term IV maintenance rate for an NPO adult patient in good health would be _____

    1. 300 mL per hr   **3.** 75-125 mL per hr

    2. 150-200 mL per hr   **4.** 10-20 mL per hr

RAPID PRACTICE 9-14   *Gravity Device Flow Rate Practice*

Estimated completion time: 20-25 minutes   **Answers on page 542**

Directions: *Assume that all the continuous IV infusions ordered in problems 1-5 are to be administered with gravity equipment. Calculate the flow rates as requested. Use a calculator for long division and multiplication.*

1   Ordered: IV D5W 1000 mL at 150 mL per hr

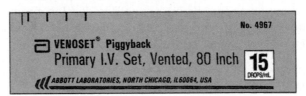

    a. Macrodrip or microdrip: _____

    b. mL per hr flow rate: _____

    c. Flow rate in drops per minute: _____

    DA equation:

    d. Evaluation: _____

    e. Infusion duration in hours (and minutes if applicable):

    _____

2 Ordered: IV D5LR 500 mL q10h

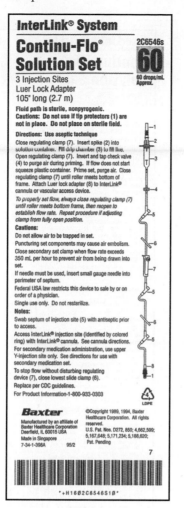

a. Macrodrip or microdrip: _____

b. Estimated flow rate in drops per minute: _____

DA equation:

c. Evaluation: _____

3 Ordered: IV D5NS 1000 mL q8h

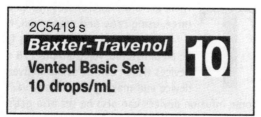

a. Macrodrip or microdrip: _____

b. Flow rate in drops per minute: _____

DA equation:

c. Evaluation: _____

4 Ordered: medicated IVPB of 40 mL to infuse in 1 hour (an intermittent IV)

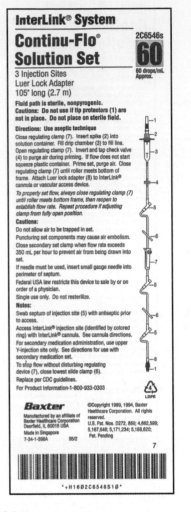

a. Macrodrip or microdrip: _____

b. Flow rate in drops per minute: _____

DA equation:

c. Evaluation: _____

5 Ordered: medicated IVPB of 100 mL to infuse in 1 hour (60 minutes)

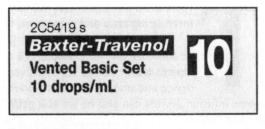

a. Macrodrip or microdrip: _____

b. Flow rate in drops per minute: _____

DA equation:

c. Evaluation: _____

1 Can I write the four drop factors for gravity infusions, starting with the microdrip?

_____

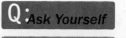

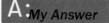

Distinguishing Flow Rates for Infusion Pumps and Microdrip-Macrodrip Gravity Infusion Devices

RAPID PRACTICE 9-15

Estimated completion time: 25 minutes   **Answers on page 543**

Directions: *Notice the type of equipment that will be used: pump or gravity infusion device. Calculate the flow rate in mL per hr or drops per minute, whichever is needed. Round the answer to nearest whole number. Label all answers in mL per hr or drops per minute, as appropriate.*

1 Ordered: 1000 mL D5LR q12h. Equipment: gravity device with tubing DF 15.

   a. The nurse will set and monitor the flow rate at _____

   DA equation:

   b. Evaluation: _____

2 Ordered: 500 mL L/R q4h. Equipment: infusion pump.

   a. The nurse will set and monitor the flow rate at _____

   DA equation:

   b. Evaluation: _____

3 Ordered: 1000 mL D5W q8h. Equipment: gravity device with tubing DF 10 and Dial-a-Flo device. (Refer to Figure 9-7, p. 275)

   a. The nurse will set and monitor the flow rate in mL per hr at _____

   DA equation:

   b. Evaluation: _____

4 Ordered: 250 mL NS q6h. Equipment: gravity device with tubing DF 20.

   a. The nurse will set and monitor the flow rate at _____

   DA equation:

   b. Evaluation: _____

5 Ordered 1 L $\frac{1}{2}$ NS q24h. Equipment: gravity device with tubing DF 60.

   a. The nurse will set and monitor the flow rate at _____

   DA equation:

   b. Evaluation: _____

"To Keep Open" Flow Rates

The order "To keep open" (TKO) indicates the slowest rate that can be infused on the available equipment when the goal is to have a patent's line available for potential future use. A TKO flow rate can be 10 to 15 mL per hr. Defer to facility policies. More frequently, prescribers order an indwelling injection port known as an "IV lock," "med-lock," or "heplock." Infusions, syringes, and long, straight infusion lines can be connected to an indwelling capped cannula or needle only when needed. The lock is flushed with saline solution* to prevent clotting. It is accessed for IV solutions when needed. The IV lock provides convenience and more mobility for the patient.

Calculating Grams of Solute in Intravenous Solutions

➤ As stated in Chapter 1, % means "per 100."

Using 5% DW as an example, the percentage of dextrose in solution means 5 g dextrose per 100 mL.

Calculating total grams of solute in a solution

➤ To determine total grams of solute in a solution, given the percentage, change the percentage value to grams per 100 mL and multiply that fraction form by the total volume in milliliters.

Formula: g in solution = number of $\dfrac{g}{100 \text{ mL}}$ × total volume in mL = g in total volume.

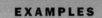

EXAMPLES

Question: How many grams of dextrose are in the following solution: 5% DW in 1000 mL?

$$\text{g dextrose}: \dfrac{5 \text{ g dextrose}}{\dfrac{100 \text{ mL}}{1}} \times \dfrac{\overset{10}{\cancel{1000 \text{ mL}}}}{1} = 50 \text{ g dextrose}$$

Analysis: The starting factor matches the desired answer.
Evaluation: The equation is balanced. The equation eliminates milliliters so that only grams remain.

EXAMPLES

Question: How many grams of sodium chloride (NaCl) are in the following solution: 1000 mL NS solution (0.9%NaCl)?

$$\text{g sodium chloride}: \dfrac{0.9 \text{ g NaCl}}{\dfrac{100 \text{ mL}}{1}} \times \dfrac{\overset{10}{\cancel{1000 \text{ mL}}}}{1} = 0.9 \times 10 = 9 \text{ g sodium chloride}$$

Analysis: The starting factor matches the desired answer.
Evaluation: Equation is balanced. Only grams remain.

➤ Note that 0.9 is *less than* 1%. NaCl contains sodium *and* chloride. A liter of NS contains 9 g of NaCl and 3.6 g of sodium.

➤ Remember to make the decimal points prominent so they are not missed in calculations.

---

*Occasionally heparin is used for a flush.

Calculating Grams of Dextrose and Sodium in IV Solutions · RAPID PRACTICE 9-16

Estimated completion time: 10 minutes   Answers on page 543

Directions: *Calculate the total number of grams of solute in the IV solution supplied. Mentally change L to mL for the equation. Verify your answer using a calculator.*

1   Solution: 1 L of 10% DW

   a. What is the total number of grams of dextrose? <u>100 g dextrose</u>

   DA equation:

$$\text{g dextrose: } \frac{10 \text{ g}}{\cancel{100 \text{ mL}}_1} \times \frac{\cancel{1000 \text{ mL}}^{10}}{1} = 100 \text{ g dextrose}$$

   b. Evaluation: <u>Equation is balanced. Only g remain.</u>

2   Solution: 1.5 L of 5% D/RL.

   a. What is the total number of grams of dextrose? _____

   DA equation:

   b. Evaluation: _____

3   Solution: 1.5 L of NS.

   a. What is the total number of grams of sodium chloride (NaCl)? _____

   DA equation:

   b. Evaluation: _____

4   Solution: 2 L 10% D/RL.

   a. What is the total number of grams of dextrose? _____

   DA equation:

   b. Evaluation: _____

5   Solution: 0.5 L $\frac{1}{2}$ NS.

   a. What is the total number of grams of sodium chloride (NaCl)? _____

   DA equation:

   b. Evaluation: _____

1   Which one of the IV solutions in Rapid Practice 9-17 is a hypotonic solution?

_____

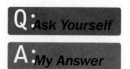

⚑ A Word about Potassium Chloride

Potassium chloride (KCl) is ordered to be added to many primary IV solutions, particularly for patients who are NPO. It has been identified by the Institute for Safe Medication Practices as a high-risk medication, meaning that it has high potential to cause adverse effects. For safety reasons, many agencies do not carry KCl ampules on the units. The pharmacy prepares the solution, or a premixed (diluted) solution is used. (Reminder: The red flag icon indicates a high-alert drug.)

➤ Consult agency and TJC guidelines regarding IV potassium administration. Following are some of the key considerations the nurse should keep in mind:

- The *amount* ordered
- The *concentration* ordered
- The *SDR* and *dilutions* recommended in the literature
- The *rate* ordered and the *rate* recommended in the literature
- Results of the patient's most recent *serum potassium* levels
- Results and implications of the patient's most recent *renal function* tests, including serum creatinine and BUN
- Results and implications of physical assessment for side effects of too little (hypokalemia) or too much potassium (hyperkalemia)

➤ Potassium is never administered undiluted in an IV. Even if it is to be added to a large-volume IV, measures must be taken to ensure that it is well mixed with the IV fluid before it gets into the tubing.

If added by the nurse, it is usually added to a full bag of the main IV solution after the main solution is *removed* from the IV pole with the tubing temporarily clamped. It is then thoroughly mixed with the main solution so that the KCI does not proceed undiluted into the IV tubing. Do not inject directly into a *hanging* solution. Monitor the flow rate very closely.

➤ If KCI is administered undiluted, it can cause tissue necrosis, vessel damage, and cardiac arrest. Too rapid a flow of diluted KCl can also cause cardiac arrest.
➤ Administering KCI preparations safely requires further study, supervision, and experience.
➤ You must be able to distinguish mEq from mg and mL on the label.*

Intravenous Intermittent Solution Delivery Systems

Intermittent solutions, usually medicated, may be delivered in five ways: (1) IV piggyback solutions, which have already been studied, (2) volume-control devices, (3) IV (direct) push with a syringe, (4) syringe pumps, or (5) PCA pumps.

There is a trend toward using more manufacturer-prepared IV medication systems. An example of a pre-prepared piggyback IV solution container and medication is the Hospira Add-Vantage® with a drug vial of vancomycin (Figure 9-12) and the Hospira Add-Vantage® System (Figure 9-13).

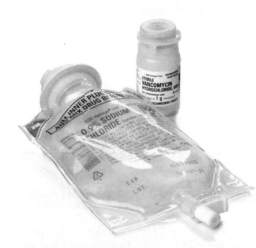

FIGURE 9-12 Hospira ADD-Vantage® with a drug vial of vancomycin. (From Hospira, Inc., Lake Forest, IL.)

*Refer to Chapter 3, Figure 3-2 (p. 80).

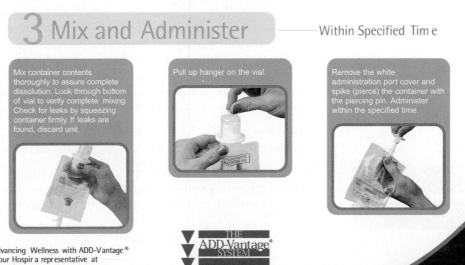

ADD-Vantage® System
As Easy as 1, 2, 3

1 Assemble ———— Use Aseptic Technique

Swing the pull ring over the top of the vial and pull down far enough to start the opening. Then pull straight up to remove the cap. Avoid touching the rubber stopper and vial threads.

Hold diluent container and gently grasp the tab on the pull ring. Pull up to break the tie membrane. Pull back to remove the cover. Avoid touching the inside of the vial port.

Screw the vial into the vial port until it will go no further. Recheck the vial to assure that it is tight. Label appropriately.

2 Activate — Pull Plug/Stopper to Mix Drug with Diluent

Hold the vial as shown. Push the drug vial down into container and grasp the inner cap of the vial through the walls of the container.

Pull the inner plug from the drug vial: allow drug to fall into diluent container for fast mixing. Do not force stopper by pushing on one side of inner cap at a time.

Verify that the plug and rubber stopper have been removed from the vial. The floating stopper is an indication that the system has been activated.

3 Mix and Administer — Within Specified Time

Mix container contents thoroughly to assure complete dissolution. Look through bottom of vial to verify complete mixing. Check for leaks by squeezing container firmly. If leaks are found, discard unit.

Pull up hanger on the vial.

Remove the white administration port cover and spike (pierce) the container with the piercing pin. Administer within the specified time.

For more information on Advancing Wellness with ADD-Vantage® family of devices, contact your Hospira representative at 1-877-9467(1-877-9Hospira) or visit www.Hospira.com

©Hospira, Inc. -275 North Field Drive, Lake Forest, IL 60045   6-131-1-Nov. 04

THE ADD-Vantage® SYSTEM

FIGURE 9-13 Hospira ADD-Vantage® System. (From Hospira, Inc., Lake Forest, IL.)

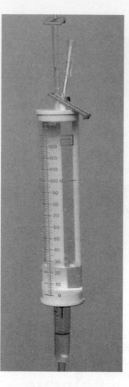

FIGURE 9-14 Volume-control device. (From Perry AG, Potter PA, Stockert PA, Hall A: *Basic nursing,* ed. 7, St. Louis, 2011, Mosby.)

Volume-control device (calibrated burette chamber)

When there is a need to protect the patient from a possible *fluid or medication overload,* a simple volume-control device may be placed between the main IV container and the drip chamber (Figure 9-14). If the volume-control device is being used for medication administration, the solutions in the primary bag and the medication must be checked for compatibility.

The calibrated chamber, which usually holds 100 to 150 mL, will be filled with a limited specific amount of the primary IV solution or with a medication. A *clamp above the chamber* to the main IV line *will be closed.* This system may be used for pediatric and other at-risk patients. Burettes have a DF of 60, so 1 mL = 1 drop.

➤ Agencies specify the *maximum amount* of fluid that may be placed in the burette at any one time: *1 to 2 hours' worth at the ordered flow rate.* Medications placed in the burette will need to be diluted according to the manufacturer's guidelines for IV infusion. Flushing procedures before and after administering medications with the device must be followed according to policy, and comprehensive labels stating date, time, medication contents, and flow rate need to be employed. The nurse opens the clamp to refill the calibrated chamber as needed.

➤ The nurse must have a system in place for the timing of the refill. If the chamber empties and the clamp to the primary bag is closed, the IV site will coagulate.

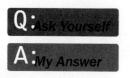

1　If the ordered flow rate is 15 mL per hr for a baby and the agency policy is a limit of 2 hours' worth of volume in the volume-control device, what is the maximum number of milliliters that may be placed in the device?

Intravenous (direct) push

IV push medications are very small-volume medications administered one time only or intermittently with a syringe directly into an infusion line or port closest to a vein (Figure 9-15). Many of these medications must be diluted in a small volume of a

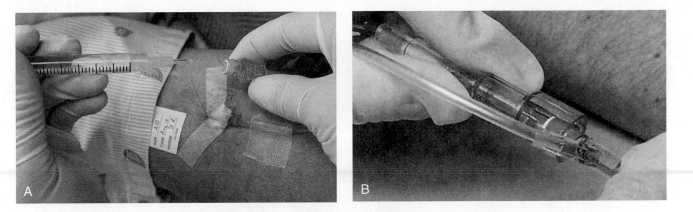

FIGURE 9-15 A, IV push with needleless syringe. **B,** Needleless connection into port. (**A,** From Elkin MK, Perry AG, Potter PA: *Nursing interventions and clinical skills,* ed. 4, St. Louis, 2007, Mosby.)

specific diluent, and all must be administered at a controlled rate. In large agencies, the pharmacy will specify these instructions. If they are not available, the nurse must check with an appropriate pharmacology reference or the pharmacist for dilution and rate instructions. The trend is to use needleless systems to prevent injury. IV push calculations are covered in more detail in Chapter 10.

➤ Do not abbreviate *IV push. IVP* refers to a kidney function test.

Syringe pump

Syringe pumps are manual, electronic, or battery-operated devices that use positive pressure and a plunger to deliver a specific programmed amount of a smaller-volume medicated or unmedicated IV solution over a specific period of time. Tubing from the syringe is connected to an access device, such as a port (Figure 9-16).

Patient-Controlled Analgesia (PCA) Pump A PCA pump is an IV infusion syringe pump device connected to an indwelling line and programmed by the nurse to deliver pain medication in prescribed small increments at programmed intervals with lockout periods to prevent overdoses (Figure 9-17). These often deliver controlled drugs and require narcotic counts.

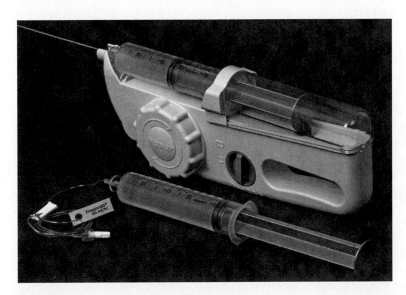

FIGURE 9-16 Freedom 60 syringe infusion pump system. (From Repro-Med Systems, Inc., Chester, NY.)

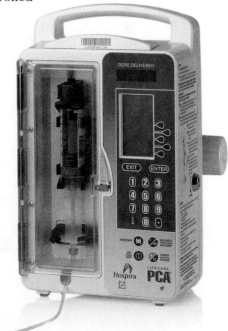

FIGURE 9-17 LifeCare® PCA 3 Infusion System. (From Hospira, Inc., Lake Forest, IL.)

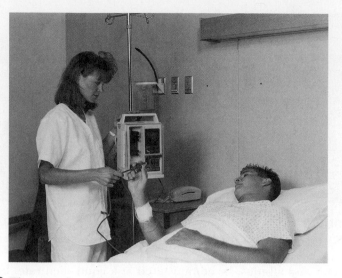

FIGURE 9-18 The nurse instructs the patient on the use of a PCA pump remote-controlled device. (From Lilley LL, Collins SR, Harrington S, Snyder JS: *Pharmacology and the nursing process,* ed. 6, St. Louis, 2011, Mosby.)

The patient pushes a button on a small remote control device that releases boluses of medication into the established I.V. line. A small basal (continuous) rate of the medication *may* be programmed to be administered continuously between boluses (Figure 9-18).

A sample order for a programmed dose regimen for a patient with pain would be:

> *Initial bolus: morphine 2 mg*
> *Incremental dose: morphine 1 mg*
> *Lockout (delay time) interval: 15 minutes*
> *Basal rate: 0 mg per hr*
> *One-hour limit: 4-6 mg (permits prn bolus)*
> *PRN bolus: 2 mg q4h*

The pharmacy provides a prefilled syringe with the analgesic. The nurse places the pump on an established continuous-flow IV line with a compatible solution, inserts the syringe in the pump, programs the orders, and monitors the use and effectiveness of the dose.

The PCA pump gives control of pain to the patient, relieves anxiety about having to wait for medication, provides a steadier degree of pain relief, and is thought to result in overall reduced total usage of analgesics. Assessments of the pump readouts of the number of attempts made, amounts used, and relief obtained are usually recorded hourly.

The nurse replaces the prefilled syringe cartridges as needed.

Administration of Blood
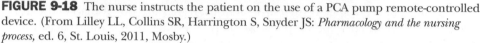

- There are many steps in the protocols for blood administration. The agency procedures must be followed scrupulously by a registered nurse to avoid a potentially very serious adverse event.
- Blood is administered only after a primary line is established with NS solution on Y tubing with a blood administration set for a pump or a gravity device (Figures 9-19 and 9-20).

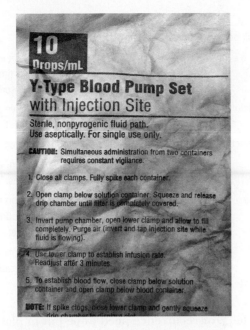

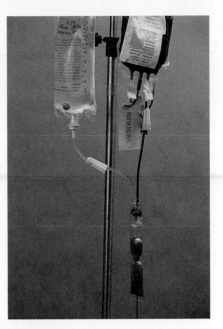

FIGURE 9-19 Y-type blood administration pump set: 10 drops/mL. (From Macklin D, Chernecky C, Infortuna H: *Math for clinical practice*, ed. 2, St. Louis, 2011, Mosby.)

FIGURE 9-20 Blood administration gravity setup with Y-tubing and NS solution. (From Perry AG, Potter PA: *Clinical nursing skills and techniques*, ed. 7, St. Louis, 2010, Mosby.)

➤ The usual initial flow rate for a unit of blood is 2 mL per min for the first 15 to 30 minutes. Check agency policies. The nurse is required to be present for the initial part of the transfusion for a specified time period in case of adverse reaction.

A unit of whole blood is often administered without the plasma. Without plasma, the unit "packed cells" contains about 250 mL. With plasma, the amount will be closer to 500 mL.

➤ Agency protocols must be consulted for patient identification, patient care, blood storage and administration, disposal of used blood transfusion equipment, and actions to take should a suspected adverse event occur.

FAQ | *What should I do if ordered IV fluids are delayed, behind schedule, or have been infusing too fast?*

ANSWER | It takes a lot of nursing experience to make safe adjustments. Unfortunately, there is neither a simple answer nor a magic formula. Guidelines that state that the remaining fluid needs to be recalculated to make the IV finish on time are unsafe if taken at face value. IV infusions need to be monitored hourly or more often. Inexperienced nurses and those with any doubts should always consult with the prescriber. Study the following considerations.

Question	Some Considerations
Is there medication in the solution?	Adjustments need to be made in consultation with the prescriber. There may be adverse consequences for underdose or sudden overdose and a need for remedial orders.
Has there been a significant drop or increase in percentage of IV infused? Over what time period? Was the ordered flow rate, slow or rapid?	Consult with the prescriber. When the ordered flow rate is particularly slow or rapid, there is a medical reason that will make it necessary to consult with the prescriber for adjustment.
How much time remains in the IV schedule?	Can a loss possibly be corrected gradually with the next infusion?

Question	Some Considerations
Is this an at-risk patient? Dehydrated, frail, poor heart, lung, or renal function?	Consult the prescriber.
When was volume infused last monitored?	A significant change over an unknown time period requires consultation with the prescriber.
What was the purpose of the solution? Maintenance? Replacement?	These issues affect urgency of corrective actions (e.g., hydration status of the patient).
Have intake and output been adversely affected?	Assess and then consult with the prescriber.
Is the site patent?	The line may have to be changed before any decision is made about fluid rate changes.
Is there a positional problem with a gravity infusion?	This can be adjusted and calls attention to the need for more frequent monitoring in addition to patient or family teaching, if applicable.
Is anyone tampering with the flow rate?	Not a frequent occurrence but can happen and will need to be documented and reported.

Measures to prevent a flow rate error recurrence need to be put in place. The nurse cannot legally prescribe medications and flow rates unless the physician writes an order to titrate the drug.

➤ Above all, the nurse cannot "open up" the infusion line to try to catch up the flow rate in a few minutes at the bedside. This is a totally unsafe practice that has potentially dire consequences for the patient.

An adult patient with good cardiac, lung, and renal function receiving an unmedicated IV infusion of 75-125 mL per hr can probably tolerate a small increase in rate without difficulty. If it is considered necessary by the prescriber to have the infusion complete on time, the calculation is very basic: Divide the remaining solution by the remaining number of hours as if it were a new IV infusion. Evaluate the difference in rate between the order and the new rate.

EXAMPLES

Ordered: 1000 mL D5W at 100 mL per hr. Total duration: 10 hr. Start time: 1200. Scheduled end time: 2200.
Evaluation: At 1800 hrs, there should be 400 mL remaining.

Remaining mL at 1800 Hours	Remaining Hours	New Flow Rate per Prescriber
600 mL	÷ 4 hr	= 150 mL per hr

Do not forget to document the assessments and actions.

CLINICAL RELEVANCE

Obtaining an order to change from 100 to 150 mL per hr would be mandatory. Increases in rate need to be gradual to reduce physiological stress on the patient. Slowing down medicated IV infusions also often needs to be gradual. Remember the 75 to 125 mL per hr average figure for average healthy adults cited at the beginning of the chapter. During the infusion and on completion, assess the patient for signs of fluid overload—shortness of breath, bounding pulse, moist lung sounds, and complaints of discomfort—and document the findings.

Calculating Catch-up Flow Rates

Estimated completion time: 25 minutes   Answers on page 544

Directions: *Calculate the new flow rate to the nearest mL based on the remaining number of milliliters of infusion to the nearest whole number and the remaining hours to be infused. Assume that the solutions are unmedicated and that the prescriber has confirmed the catch-up or slowdown.*

Note: *The timed tape on the solution bag is useful.*

1   Started at 0700 hrs: 500 mL at 50 mL per hr. Observed at 1000 hrs: 250 mL remains.

   a. Total hours to infuse: ___10 hr___
   b. Hours elapsed: _____3 hr_____
   c. Amount infused: _250 mL_   Amount that should have infused: _150 mL_
   d. Ahead of schedule, behind, or on time: ____Ahead of schedule____
   e. Hours remaining: _7 hr_   mL remaining: _250 mL_
   f. Adjusted flow rate: ___250 ÷ 7 = 36 mL per hr___

2   Started at 1500 hrs: 1000 mL at 100 mL per hr. Observed at 2200 hrs: 100 mL remains.

   a. Total hours to infuse: _____
   b. Hours elapsed: _____
   c. Amount infused: _____   Amount that should have infused: _____
   d. Ahead of schedule, behind, or on time: _____
   e. Hours remaining: _____   mL remaining: _____
   f. Adjusted flow rate: _____

3   Started at 2300 hrs: 250 mL NS at 50 mL per hr. Observed at 0100 hrs: 200 mL remains.

   a. Total hours to infuse: _____
   b. Hours elapsed: _____
   c. Amount infused: _____   Amount that should have infused: _____
   d. Ahead of schedule, behind, or on time: _____
   e. Hours remaining: _____   mL remaining: _____
   f. Adjusted flow rate: _____

4   Started at 1100 hrs: 500 mL D5RL 125 mL per hr. Observed at 1300 hrs: 100 mL remains.

   a. Total hours to infuse: _____
   b. Hours elapsed: _____
   c. Amount infused: _____   Amount that should have infused: _____
   d. Ahead of schedule, behind, or on time: _____
   e. Hours remaining: _____   mL remaining: _____
   f. Adjusted flow rate: _____

5   Started at 1700 hrs: 250 mL RLS at 25 mL per hr. Observed at 1900 hrs: 200 mL remains.

   a. Total hours to infuse: _____
   b. Hours elapsed: _____
   c. Amount infused: _____   Amount that should have infused: _____
   d. Ahead of schedule, behind, or on time: _____
   e. Hours remaining: _____   mL remaining: _____
   f. Adjusted flow rate: _____

CHAPTER 9 MULTIPLE-CHOICE REVIEW

Estimated completion time: 30 minutes   **Answers on page 544**

Directions: *Analyze the IV-related questions and select the best answer using the available equipment.*

1 Ordered: 500 mL D5W, an isotonic fluid maintenance solution to infuse over 12 hr. Equipment available: infusion pump. The nurse will set the flow rate at _____.

   1. 41 mL per hr   **3.** 43 mL per hr
   2. 41.7 mL per hr   **4.** 42.5 drops per min

2 The average maintenance flow rate for a healthy adult who is NPO is _____.

   1. 10-15 mL per hr   **3.** 75-125 mL per hr
   2. 25 mL per hr   **4.** 150-250 mL per hr

3 An isotonic electrolyte solution used for IV infusions is _____.

   1. 5DW   **3.** D5LR
   2. 10DW   **4.** 2.5% DW

4 Ordered: NS 500 mL q4h. Equipment available: gravity device with rate controller. The nurse will set the flow rate at _____.

   1. 100 drops per min   **3.** 125 mL per hr
   2. 125 drops per min   **4.** 150 mL per hr

5 Ordered: RLS 1000 mL q8h. Equipment available: gravity device, DF 20. The nurse will set the flow rate at _____.

   1. 20 mL per hr   **3.** 42 mL per hr
   2. 42 drops per min   **4.** 125 mL per hr

6 Ordered: 50 mL antibiotic IVPB q6h infused over 30 minutes. Equipment available: gravity device, DF 15. The nurse will set the flow rate at _____.

   1. 25 drops per min   **3.** 25 mL per hr
   2. 12.5 drops per min   **4.** 100 mL per hr

7 Ordered: 30 mL antibiotic IVPB q4h infused over 30 minutes. Equipment available: infusion pump. The nurse will set the flow rate at _____.

   1. 25 mL per hr   **3.** 60 mL per hr
   2. 50 drops per min   **4.** 200 mL per hr

8 Ordered: 1000 mL 5D/NS q24h. Equipment available: Pediatric microdrip administration set. The nurse will set the flow rate at _____.

   1. 41 drops per min   **3.** 42 drops per min
   2. $41\frac{2}{3}$ mL per hr   **4.** 42 mL per hr

9 Ordered: 1 unit of blood (250 mL) to be infused over 2 hours. Equipment available: an infusion pump. After initial slow flow, the nurse will set the flow rate at _____.

   1. 125 mL per hr   **3.** 12.5 mL per hr
   2. 125 drops per min   **4.** 12.5 drops per min

10 D10W 1000 mL contains _____ grams of dextrose.

   1. 15   **3.** 50
   2. 25   **4.** 100

CHAPTER 9 FINAL PRACTICE

Estimated completion time: 1 hour   Answers on page 545

Directions: *Show work, label answers. Calculate with a DA equation when requested. Use a calculator for long division and multiplication. All flow rates must be labeled drops per min or mL per hr.*

1 Name the three purposes of IV therapy:

_____ _____

_____

2 State the names of three isotonic IV solutions commonly ordered:

_____

_____

_____

3 Select the type of administration set that would be selected for an IVPB solution: *primary* or *secondary?* (Circle one)

4 State the meaning of DF of 10 on a gravity infusion administration set.

_____

5 a. State the DF for a microdrip, or pediatric, infusion administration step.

_____

   b. State the flow rate limit for infusions using microdrip sets. _____

6 Ordered: 250 mL NS q4h. Equipment available: gravity device with DF 10.

   a. State the grams of sodium in the solution: _____

   DA equation:

   b. Evaluation: _____

   c. State the flow rate that would be set: _____

   DA equation:

   d. Evaluation: _____

7 Ordered: 250 mL 5DW at 50 mL per hr.

   a. How long will the IV infusion last? _____

   b. If an alarm is set for $\frac{1}{2}$ hour before the solution will be completely infused, how much volume to be infused would be entered for the alarm to sound?

   _____

8 Ordered: 500 mL RLS q8h. Equipment available: EID

   a. State the flow rate that would be set to nearest 0.5 mL: _____

   b. If the IV infusion started at 1200, at what time (military time) would the nurse prepare the next solution to have it at the bedside $\frac{1}{2}$ hour before the container would be empty? _____

9 What is a nursing responsibility pertaining to flow rate when a secondary infusion or IVPB has been completed and the primary IV resumes flow?

_____

10 State the most serious adverse effect of an error with overdose or over-concentration during KCl IV administration: _____

11 Ordered: whole blood to be infused initially at 2 mL per min for the first 15 minutes. Equipment available: infusion pump for blood and blood administration pump set.

State the flow rate in mL per hr that the nurse would set on the pump for the first 15 minutes: _____

12 Ordered: 250 mL whole blood to be infused over 2 hours. Equipment available: gravity blood administration set, DF 10

   a. Calculate the flow rate with a DA equation:

   b. Evaluation: _____

13 Ordered: 3 L D5RLS q24h. Equipment available: gravity administration set with DF 15.

   a. Calculate the flow rate with a DA equation:

   b. Evaluation: _____

14 Ordered: 500 mL D5W q8h. Equipment available: gravity infusion device with DF 20.

   a. Calculate the flow rate with a DA equation:

   b. Evaluation: _____

15 Ordered: 50 mL 50% dextrose solution for a diabetic patient in insulin shock.

   a. How many grams of dextrose are contained in the solution? _____

   DA equation:

   b. Evaluation: _____

16 a. What type of device would the nurse connect between an IV solution and tubing to protect a patient from a fluid or medication overload? _____

   b. What are the usual guidelines or criteria for the amount of fluid placed in this device? _____

17 An IV of 1000 mL D5W at 100 mL per hr is ordered and started at 0800. At 1200, the nurse observes that 800 mL remain. The prescriber wants the IV completed on time.

   a. Amount that should remain at 1200: _____

   b. Hour at which ordered IV should be completed: _____

   c. Remaining number of hours that ordered solution needs to be completed: _____

   d. Flow rate for remaining IV fluid on an infusion pump that delivers to the nearest tenth of a mL: _____

18 An IVPB of 50 mL is ordered to be infused over 30 minutes. Estimate the flow rate on an infusion pump: _____

19 An IVPB of 20 mL is ordered to be infused over 20 minutes.

   a. Estimate the flow rate on a microdrip device. _____

   DA equation:

   b. Evaluation: _____

20 State five considerations that need to be kept in mind when an IV flow rate is behind schedule:

   _____

   _____

   _____

   _____

   _____

   _____

Suggestions for Further Reading

Gahart BL, Nazareno AR: *2009 Intravenous medications: a handbook for nurses and health professionals,* ed. 27, St. Louis, 2011, Mosby.

www.baxter.com
www.cc.nih.gov/nursing
www.ismp.org
www.jointcommission.org
www.ccforpatientsafety.org

ⓔvolve Additional practice problems can be found in the Intravenous Calculations section of the Student Companion on Evolve.

Chapter 10 covers advanced IV infusion calculations using this chapter as a foundation. Note the high-alert drugs.

"I have no great talent. I am just passionately curious."

—ALBERT EINSTEIN

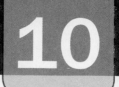
10

Advanced Intravenous Calculations

OBJECTIVES

- Calculate infusion flow rates for the following units of measurement: mg per mL, mg per hr, mg per min, mcg per mL, mcg per hr, mcg per min, mcg per kg, mcg per kg per hr, mcg per kg per min, mg per kg, mg per kg per hr, mg per kg per min, and mEq per hr.
- Confirm IV medication orders with safe dose range (SDR) criteria.
- Calculate schedules for manual IV direct push medications.
- Calculate the parameters of flow rates for titrated IV infusions.
- State the difference between central venous lines and peripheral venous lines.
- Calculate the calories in selected IV solutions.
- State the general purpose, contents, and types of hyperalimentation (PN) infusions.
- Identify patient safety issues for the administration of IV medications, including PN infusions.

Essential Prior Knowledge

- Mastery of Chapters 1-9
- Review of Chapter 9, Basic Intravenous Calculations, highly recommended

Essential Equipment

- Calculator
- IV equipment for laboratory and clinical observation, when available

Estimated Time To Complete Chapter

- 2-3 hours

Introduction

Chapter 9 focused on prepared IV solutions that required simple flow rate calculations. This chapter emphasizes more complex dose-based flow rate calculations for a variety of medicated IV solutions for peripheral access sites. The principles of the equation setup are the same as in earlier chapters.

Although D5W, NS, and 5% L/R solutions are vehicles for many IV medications, certain medications require a specific solution. The trend for safety purposes is to have pharmacy-prepared IV mixtures.

➤ The nurse must always check for compatibilities *and incompatibilities* before mixing and or administering medications and solutions. It must be assumed that IV solutions and medications, including diluents, are incompatible unless the literature states otherwise. With the great increase in available medications, the responsibility to protect the patient increases.

Intravenous medications ordered for the treatment of at-risk patients, such as the acutely ill and frail young and elderly, may require calculation and adjustment of dosage (titration), depending on the patient's response to the medication. Many

312

Filters	Used in some IV medication lines to prevent contaminants, particles, and clots from reaching patient circulation. Liquids can pass through the filter. Specific guidelines for use and nonuse and filter size must be checked with agency and manufacturer guidelines prior to administration of medications. The smaller the size filter, the finer the filter. Blood administration sets are supplied with a clot filter, and other filters may be added for specific purposes, depending on the age of the blood product. Filters are not routinely used for IV infusions.
Parenteral Nutrition (PN) (AKA, "Hyperalimentation," "Hyperal")	*Parenteral nutrition* (PN) refers to an IV caloric infusion of nutrients, vitamins, minerals, and electrolytes through a central (CPN) or peripheral (PPN) venous line. Contents and amounts are prescribed on an individual basis.
Infusion Access Sites: Central and Peripheral Venous	Central venous sites are large blood volume sites (such as the superior vena cava and right atrium) that can be accessed by catheter from large veins (such as the jugular) or surgically accessed chest veins. They can also be accessed from peripherally inserted central catheters (PICC), which are less invasive and threaded to the superior vena cava–right atrial junction from a peripheral vein. The central venous sites provide rapid dilution of concentrated solutions such as TPN and medications and are more suitable for longer term therapy and more concentrated solutions than smaller peripheral veins.
IV Flush (SAS) (SASH)	Technique that maintains patency of IV sites used before and after infusion of medications and for periodic maintenance. Saline solution or less frequently, low-dose heparin solution is injected through infusion ports in accordance with agency protocols for milliliter amounts for each type of flush solution and the equipment being flushed. The longer the line, the more solution must be used. Also used to clear lines of solutions before administering a potentially incompatible solution. *SAS* means "saline, administer drug, saline flush." *SASH* means "saline, administer drug, saline, heparin flush."
Kilocalorie (Kcal)	Metric measurement, unit of energy, necessary to raise the temperature of 1 kg of water by 1° C. Commonly described as "calorie," even though there are 1000 calories in a *kilo*calorie, as the metric prefix indicates. The "Calories" on food labels are actually kilocalories.
Peak and Trough Levels	Serum levels of drugs derived from blood samples drawn 30 minutes before the next dose is due (trough) and 30 minutes after administration (peak) for IV drugs and 1-2 hours after oral drugs (peak). Guides the prescriber for effective dosing and avoidance of toxicity or damage to renal function. Nurse must label specimen with peak or trough, exact time drawn, and time and dose of last medication infusion. Certain drugs, such as aminophylline, the IV bronchodilator used for severe asthma, have widely varying rates of individual absorption and necessitate peak and trough measurements.
Titrated Medication	Flexible drug order for dose adjustments to achieve desired therapeutic result, such as a specific urinary output, systolic or diastolic blood pressure, or glucose level (e.g., "dobutamine 2-8 mg per kg per min IV infusion. Increase or lower by 1-2 mg every 30 minutes to achieve/maintain systolic pressure between 90 and 110 degrees). Administered and adjusted by experienced registered nurses.
Vascular Implanted Devices Vascular Access Devices (VAD)	Surgically implanted subcutaneous self-access sealing injection ports that can tolerate repeated injections with a special Huber needle. The port is attached to a catheter threaded to the target site, most commonly the subclavian vein. Saves the patient the discomfort of multiple injections.

of the math skills mastered in earlier chapters will be reviewed and employed: analysis of the problem, basic multiplication and division, conversion among metric units of measurement, calculation of weight in kilograms, DA-style equations set-ups, and flow rate calculations.

RAPID PRACTICE 10-1 | *Vocabulary Review*

Estimated completion time: 10 minutes   **Answers on page 546**

Directions: *Read the introduction and the essential vocabulary. Identify the terms.*

1 Intravenous infusion access sites are generally divided into which two major areas: _____

   1. Hyperalimentation and IV push
   2. Peripheral and central
   3. Peaks and troughs
   4. Flushes and implantable vascular access ports

2 The term for IV nutritional infusions is _____

   1. Central venous line
   2. Drug titrations
   3. Parenteral nutrition
   4. Nutritional kilocalories

3 Which of the following statements is true about infusion line filters? _____

   1. One size can be used for all infusions.
   2. All IV infusions must use filters.
   3. Blood administration sets are always supplied with a filter.
   4. The larger the filter size, the smaller the pores of the filter.

4 Flushes are used before and after administration of many medicated IV solutions for the following purpose: _____

   1. To prevent drug and solution incompatibility and site coagulation
   2. To provide a higher intake for the patient who may be dehydrated
   3. To test the patient's ability to tolerate an IV solution over a prolonged period
   4. To provide medication before and after an infusion

5 An example of a titrated IV drug order would be _____

   1. Give clindamycin phosphate 1 g IV every 6 hours over 60 minutes for 72 hrs.
   2. Give ampicillin 25 mg IV stat and q8h for 72 hours.
   3. Alternate 1000 mL D5W q8h with 1000 mL lactated Ringer's solution.
   4. Give nitroprusside sodium 0.1-5 mcg per kg per min to maintain systolic blood pressure below 160.

Equation Setups for Advanced Intravenous Calculations

It will be helpful to practice a few exercises in preparation for setting up and understanding medicated IV calculations.

RAPID PRACTICE 10-2 | *Basic Intravenous Calculations Review*

Estimated completion time: 20-25 minutes   **Answers on page 546**

Directions: *Estimate and calculate the requested IV infusion as shown. Use a calculator for long division and multiplication to solve equations.*

1 Ordered: 2 mL per min. Need to know: mL per hr.

   a. Estimated answer: $2 \times 60 = 120$ mL per hr.

     DA equation:

$$\frac{mL}{hr} : \frac{2\ mL}{1\ \cancel{min}} \times \frac{60\ \cancel{min}}{1\ hr} = 120\ mL\ per\ hr$$

   b. Evaluation: Equation is balanced. Only mL/ hr remain.

2 Ordered: 120 mL per hr. Need to know: mL per min to nearest tenth of a mL.

   a. Estimated mL per min: _____

      DA equation:

   b. Evaluation: _____

3 Ordered: 4 mg per min. Need to know: mg per hr.

   a. Estimated mg per hr: _____

      DA equation:

   b. Evaluation: _____

4 Ordered: 60 mg per hr. Need to know: mg per minute.

   a. Estimated mg per min: _____

      DA equation:

   b. Evaluation: _____

5 Ordered: 2 mg per kg per min. Weight: 10 kg. Need to know: mg per minute.

   a. Estimated mg per min: _____

      DA equation:

   b. Evaluation: _____

   c. Estimated mg per hr: _____

      DA equation:

   d. Evaluation: _____

Conversion Factors That May Be Needed for Intravenous Infusion Calculations

One or more conversion factors may be required to complete IV infusion calculations. Refer back to these as you work through the chapter.

Conversion Factors	Purpose
60 minutes = 1 hour	Often needed to obtain milliliters or medication dose per hour, this formula also may be needed to verify how much drug per minute or volume per minute is being infused. For example: **Ordered:** Drug Y, 1 mg per min. Question: How many milligrams or milliliters per hour will be infused?
1000 mg = 1 g 1000 mcg = 1 mg	Needed for conversion when the drug units supplied do not match the drug units ordered. For example: **Ordered:** Drug Y, 2 mcg per min. Supplied: Drug Y, 500 mg.
1000 mL = 1 L	Needed to convert liters to milliliters for IV flow rate calculations. IV flow rates are delivered in milliliters. Ordered: 1 L q8h. 1 L = 1000 mL. 1000 mL ÷ 8 = 125 mL per hr.
2.2 lb = 1 kg	Occasionally needed to calculate the dose ordered when the dose is based on weight and the weight in pounds is known and that in kilograms is not. For example: **Ordered:** Drug Y, 2 mg per kg per min. Weight: 50 lb.

*Kg weight-based dosing is recommended by several agencies.

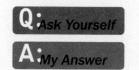

1 What are four conversion factors that may be needed for IV infusion calculations? (Give a brief answer.)

Calculating Medicated Intravenous Flow Rates That Require One Conversion Factor

Intravenous flow rates are usually calculated in milliliters per hour (mL per hr) but may be ordered in units of a drug to be infused per hour or per minute. Following are some examples of how the amount of a drug to be given per a unit of time may be expressed in medication orders:

2 mg per min	5 mcg per min	3 units per min
4 mg per hr	3 mcg per hr	10 mEq per hr
0.3 mg per kg per min	1 mcg per kg per min	0.5 milliUnits per min

Orders for powerful drugs may be written for a drug dose per minute or per hour. Following are some examples of drug concentrations supplied in IV solutions:

250 mg drug per 500 mL D5W	500 mg drug per 250 mL NS	100 mg drug per 250 mL D5W
250 mg drug per 1000 mL NS	100 mg drug per 50 mL NS	1 g drug per 1000 mL D5W

EXAMPLES

Ordered: Drug Y, 5 mg per min. Available: Drug Y, 400 mg per 200 mL. Question: The flow rate must be set at how many mL per hr to deliver 5 mg per min?

Three factors must be entered in the medication equation to determine mL per hour flow rates:

1 Ordered medication amount and time frame to be infused
2 Available drug concentration
3 Needed conversion factors

$$\frac{mL}{hr} = \frac{\overset{1}{\cancel{200}}\ mL}{\underset{\underset{1}{2}}{\cancel{400}}\ \cancel{mg}} \times \frac{5\ \cancel{mg}}{1\ \cancel{min}} \times \frac{\overset{30}{\cancel{60}}\ \cancel{min}}{1\ hr} = 150\ mL\ per\ hr$$

Analysis: The data with mL will be entered *in the first numerator*. Milligrams will need to be canceled. The order is in mg, and that quantity ordered is entered next to cancel the mg in the drug concentration. Hr is entered in the last *denominator* with the required min to hr conversion. Note the progression for canceling undesired units from one denominator to the next numerator—mg to mg and min to min—as in prior DA equations.

Evaluation: The equation is balanced. Only mL per hr remain.

➤ *One* conversion factor is needed. Because the drug ordered and the drug supplied are in the *same terms, milligrams,* a minutes to hours conversion is the *only* factor needed.
➤ The drug concentration is entered as one factor. Reduction and cancellation makes the math easy.
➤ If the drug ordered was ordered in mg, and the amount supplied in g, a conversion formula from mg to g would have to be entered.

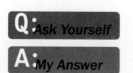

1 What are three factors that need to be entered in the equation in order to calculate medicated IV infusion rates in mL per hr? (Use one- or two-word answers.)

Converting IV Flow Rates from Milligrams per Minute to Milliliters per Hour

Estimated completion time: 20 minutes   Answers on page 547

Directions: *For each problem, determine which conversion formula will be needed. Calculate the mL/hr flow rate as shown in the preceding example. Cancel units before doing the math. Use a calculator for long division and multiplication. Label answers.*

TEST TIP: After cancellation of units in the equation, it often simplifies the math to reduce the available drug concentration fraction if it can be reduced.

1 Ordered: Drug Y, 2 mg per minute. Available: 1000 mg Drug Y in 1000 mL D5W.

    a. mL per hr flow rate?

       DA equation:

    b. Evaluation: _____

2 Ordered: Drug Y, 1 mg per minute. Available: 500 mg Drug Y in 1000 mL LRS.

    a. mL per hr flow rate?

       DA equation:

    b. Evaluation: _____

3 Ordered: Drug Y, 0.5 mg per minute. Available: 500 mg per 250 mL 0.45 NS.

    a. mL per hr flow rate?

       DA equation:

    b. Evaluation: _____

4 Ordered: Drug Y, 0.2 mg per minute. Available: 100 mg per 100 mL D5W.

    a. mL per hr flow rate?

       DA equation:

    b. Evaluation: _____

5 Ordered: Drug Y, 0.4 mg per minute. Available: 250 mg in 1 L D5W.

    a. mL per hr flow rate?

       DA equation:

    b. Evaluation: _____

Calculating Intravenous Flow Rates That Require Two Conversion Factors

A nurse who knows how to calculate flow rates no matter how they are ordered provides critical patient safety. The nurse is liable for any medication administration errors regardless of whether they may be computer, prescriber, or pharmacy errors.

➤ If a drug is ordered in mcg per min but supplied in mg per ml **or** ordered in mg per min but supplied in g per ml, two conversion factors must be included in the equation as shown in the example which follows:

➤ The drug ordered and the drug supplied must be converted to the same terms.

EXAMPLES

Ordered: Drug Y, 100 mcg per min. Available: Drug Y, 400 mg per 250 mL.

What flow rate will be set?

Conversion factors available: 1000 mcg = 1 mg, 1000 mg = 1 g, 60 minutes = 1 hour, and 1000 mL = 1 L.

$$\frac{mL}{hr} : \frac{\overset{5}{\cancel{250}}\,mL}{\underset{8}{\cancel{400}}\,mg} \times \frac{1\,\cancel{mg}}{\underset{\underset{1}{10}}{\cancel{1000}}\,\cancel{mcg}} \times \frac{\overset{1}{\cancel{100}}\,\cancel{mcg}}{1\,\cancel{min}} \times \frac{\overset{6}{\cancel{60}}\,\cancel{min}}{1\,hr} = \frac{30}{8} = 3.75, \text{ rounded to 4 mL per hr*}$$

Analysis: Drug concentration was entered first because it contained mL for the desired answer. In addition to the drug order, two conversion formulas will be needed: mg to mcg to cancel mg in the first denominator and to cancel mcg in the drug order. Finally, the min to hr conversion formula was entered to provide hr for the desired answer. Stop before doing the math. Do only the desired answer units remain? Answer: Yes.

Evaluation: The equation is balanced. Only mL per hr remain.

➤ Note how sequential cancellation guides the setup.

*Many IV pumps can deliver tenths of a mL such as 3.8 mL per hr (rounded from 3.75). The equipment determines the nearest measurable flow rate.

RAPID PRACTICE 10-4

Calculating IV Flow Rates That Require Two Conversion Factors

Estimated completion time: 20-25 minutes   **Answers on page 548**

Directions: *Analyze the preceding example and worked-out problem 1. Determine how many conversion factors are needed. Calculate using needed conversion factors. Conversion factors: 60 minutes = 1 hour, 1000 mcg = 1 mg, and 1000 mg = 1 g. Use a calculator for long division and multiplication.*

1 Ordered: Drug Y, IV infusion 200 mcg per min. Available: Drug Y, 250 mg per 1000 mL D5W.

   a. What will the flow rate be in mL per hr?

   DA equation:

$$\frac{mL}{hr} : \frac{\overset{4}{\cancel{1000}}\,mL}{\underset{1}{\cancel{250}}\,mg} \times \frac{1\,\cancel{mg}}{\underset{5}{\cancel{1000}}\,\cancel{mcg}} \times \frac{\overset{1}{\cancel{200}}\,\cancel{mcg}}{1\,\cancel{min}} \times \frac{\overset{12}{\cancel{60}}\,\cancel{min}}{1\,hr} = 48\,\frac{mL}{hr}$$

   b. Evaluation: Equation is balanced. Only mL per hr remain.

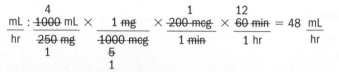

2   Ordered: Drug Y, IV infusion 75 mcg per min. Available: Drug Y, 10 mg per 100 mL NS.*

    a. What will the flow rate be in mL per hr?

      DA equation:

    b. Evaluation: _____

3   Ordered: Drug Y, IV infusion 5 mg per min. Available: Drug Y, 1 g per 200 mL LRS.

    a. What will the flow rate be in mL per hr? _____

      DA equation:

    b. Evaluation: _____

4   Ordered: Drug Y, IV infusion 200 mcg per min. Available: Drug Y, 500 mg per 250 mL D5W.

    a. What will the flow rate be in mL per hr? _____

      DA equation:

    b. Evaluation: _____

5   Ordered: Drug Y, IV infusion 1.5 mg per min. Available: Drug Y, 2 g per 200 mL NS.

    a. What will the flow rate be in mL per hr? _____

      DA equation:

    b. Evaluation: _____

1   Why are two conversion factors needed in problems 1 and 2? Which factors are they?

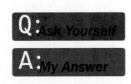

_____

Calculating Flow Rates for Weight-Based Doses

An order for a continuous IV infusion may read: dopamine 2 mcg per kg per min. The solution available may be: dopamine 200 mg per 250 mL D5W. How many ml per hr will be set? The patient weight today is 50 kg.

    1 Identify the desired answer units.
    2 Calculate the ordered dose based on the requested units of weight.
    3 Enter the drug concentration available, the ordered dose, and any needed conversion formulas in a DA equation to obtain the desired answer.

---

*NS solution is 0.9% NaCl solution. Refer to Chapter 9. Any concentration other than 0.9% is stated, e.g., 0.45% NaCl ($\frac{1}{2}$ NS).

As stated earlier, the dose ordered must always be entered in the medication equation along with the concentration available and the conversion factors.

➤ Step 2, calculating the ordered dose based on weight, is the only additional step compared to the problems in Rapid Practice 10-4.

➤ The desired answer is a ml per hr flow rate.

Calculating the total dose ordered for weight-based orders: micrograms and milligrams per kilogram

Calculate the *total drug ordered* using the patient's body weight in kilograms.

EXAMPLES

Ordered: dopamine 2 mcg per kg per min IV. Patient's weight: 50 kg.
How many total micrograms per minute are ordered?
Estimated dose in micrograms: (2 mcg × 50 kg) = 100 mcg total dose per minute.

Step 1	:	Step 2	×	Step 3	=	Answer
Desired Answer Units	:	Starting Factor	×	Given Quantity and and Conversion Factor(s)	=	Estimate, Multiply, Evaluate
$\dfrac{mcg}{min}$	:	$\dfrac{2\ mcg}{1\ kg \times min*}$	×	$\dfrac{50\ kg}{1}$	=	$\dfrac{100\ mcg}{min}$

The final equation will be written like this:

$$\frac{mcg}{min} : \frac{2\ mcg}{1\ kg \times min} \times \frac{50\ kg}{1} = 100\ mcg\ per\ minute$$

Analysis: ➤ Note how the 2 mcg per kg per minute will always set up with the kg per minute(s) in the accompanying denominator in this kind of order that contains 3 units (e.g., 5 mg per kg per hour or 10 mcg per kg per hr).

If the patient's weight is 110 lb and the weight in kilograms is not known, just enter one more conversation factor for pounds to kilograms (1 kg = 2.2 lb).

$$\frac{mcg}{min} \times \frac{2\ mcg}{1\ kg\ per\ minute} \times \frac{1\ kg}{2.2\ lb} \times \frac{110\ lb}{1} = 100\ mcg\ per\ minute$$

➤ $\dfrac{100\ mcg}{min}$ can be written as 100 mcg per minute.

➤ Many IV medications are high-alert medications.

FAQ | *Why are kilograms not retained in the answer for milligrams-per-kilogram problems?*

ANSWER | The desired answer is in *micrograms per minute.* The dose is *based on the patient's weight:* 2 mcg for *each* kilogram of weight. After factoring in the kilogram weight by multiplying micrograms by kilograms, the kilogram units *are eliminated* from the answer.

If you were asked how many cups of water you drink during the day, you might respond, "I drink about 1 cup *per hour,* so I drink 8 cups a day." The desired units in the answer are *cups per day.* Hours were only factored in to get the total amount, just as kilograms of body weight are factored in only to get a total amount of milligrams. Hours would be eliminated from the final answer, as are kilograms.

Calculating the flow rate in milliliters per hour (mL per hr) for weight-based orders

The example that follows illustrates a one-step equation for IV weight-based orders.

Ordered: Dopamine 2 mcg per kg per min. On hand: An IV of Dopamine 200 mg in 250 mL of D5W. Patient's weight: 60 kg.

What flow rate will be set on the IV pump the nearest tenth of a mL?

Conversion factors: 60 minutes = 1 hr; 1000 mcg = 1 mg.

Step 1 :
Step 1
Starting
Factor = Answer

$$\frac{mL}{hr} : \frac{\overset{1}{\cancel{\underset{4}{\cancel{5}}}\,\cancel{250}\,mL}}{\cancel{200}\,mg} \times \frac{1\,\cancel{mg}}{\underset{\underset{1}{100}}{\cancel{\underset{200}{1000}}}\,\cancel{mcg}} \times \frac{\overset{1}{\cancel{2}}\,\cancel{mcg}}{\cancel{kg} \times \cancel{min}} \times \frac{\cancel{60}\,\cancel{kg}}{1} \times \frac{\cancel{60}\,\cancel{min}}{1\,hr} = 9\,\frac{mL}{hr}$$

➤ Remember to cancel units to verify the setup *before* doing the math cancellations.

Analysis: Each denominator leads to the placement of the next numerator for cancellation of unwanted units. Note how the math is greatly simplified with the reduction of the IV starting factor as well as cancellation of zeros. In these problems, the medicated IV concentration becomes the starting factor because it contains the needed mL. Concentrations can be inverted to be placed correctly to match the desired answer.

➤ Note that the trend is for pharmacy to prepare and supply premixed IV medicated solutions. They also usually supply the ordered flow rate. Verify the rate.

FAQ | *Why do medication infusion orders sometimes specify a range for drug dose or flow rate?*

ANSWER | A range allows the nurse to titrate the dose or rate, starting with the lowest dose, until the desired response is achieved (e.g., a pulse over 60, or to maintain a minimum urinary output etc., Based on intervals of time and dose specified in the order, the rate or dose is increased at a specified interval or gradually until the desired response is achieved and maintained. This may require many adjustments if the patient's condition is unstable.

The order may read: Drug Y at 10-20 mcg per min to maintain a systolic pressure of 90 to 100 or a minimum urinary output of 30 mL per hr. May be increased by 2 mcg per min every hr. The calculations are performed separately for each amount in a range.

FAQ | *If pharmacy supplies medicated IV solutions, does the nurse still have to do the calculations?*

ANSWER | Mistakes have been made in physicians' orders and calculations and by pharmacies as well. The nurse needs to double check the current order, the SDR references, the contents, and the flow rates in order to protect the patient.

FAQ | *Can the weight-based ordered dose calculation (2 mcg per kg per min = 60 mcg per minute or 3600 mcg per hr or 3.6 mg per hr) be calculated separately and then entered in the equation to shorten it?*

ANSWER | You have the option of entering all of the data in one equation or breaking it up into two steps. One step makes a very long equation as shown in the preceding example. There are two considerations: The more steps in the process, the more likelihood of making an error. But, as shown, the longer one step equation can be greatly simplified with reduction and cancellation. The one step equation also reveals that all the needed data are entered.

RAPID PRACTICE **10-5** *Calculating IV Infusion Rates for Weight-Based Orders*

Estimated completion time: 25 minutes **Answers on page 548**

Directions: *Study the preceding example and the following worked-out problem 1. Identify the desired answer units. Identify and calculate the dose ordered. Calculate the desired flow rate with a DA equation. Remember that reducing the drug concentration fraction after cancellation of units simplifies the math. Use a calculator for long division and multiplication.*

▶ **1** Ordered: dobutamine hydrochloride IV infusion 0.5 mcg per kg per min for 24 hours for a patient with cardiac decompensation. Available: dobutamine 250 mg per 250 mL D5W. Patient's weight: 100 kg.

    a. DA equation to calculate mL per hr:

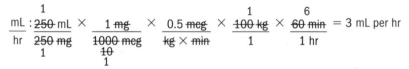

$$\frac{\text{mL}}{\text{hr}} : \frac{\overset{1}{\cancel{250}} \text{ mL}}{\underset{1}{250 \text{ mg}}} \times \frac{1 \cancel{\text{mg}}}{\underset{\underset{1}{10}}{1000 \cancel{\text{mcg}}}} \times \frac{0.5 \cancel{\text{mcg}}}{\cancel{\text{kg}} \times \cancel{\text{min}}} \times \frac{\overset{1}{\cancel{100} \cancel{\text{kg}}}}{1} \times \frac{\overset{6}{\cancel{60} \cancel{\text{min}}}}{1 \text{ hr}} = 3 \text{ mL per hr}$$

    b. Evaluation: <u>Equation is balanced. Only mL per hr remain.</u>

2 Ordered: aminophylline IV infusion 0.5 mg per kg per hr for a patient with asthma. Available: aminophylline 500 mg in 250 mL D5W. Patient's weight: 80 kg.

   a. DA equation to calculate mL per hr:

   b. Evaluation: _____

3 Ordered: isoproterenol hydrochloride IV infusion 0.1 mcg per kg per min for 8 hours for a patient with severe asthma. Available: isoproterenol hydrochloride 1 mg in 250 mL D5W. Patient's weight: 40 kg (88 lb).

   a. DA equation to calculate mL per hr:

   b. Evaluation: _____

4 Ordered: dopamine hydrochloride IV infusion 3 mcg per kg per min for 24 hours for a patient to maintain blood pressure. Available: dopamine hydrochloride 400 mg in 500 mL D5W. Patient's weight: 70 kg.

   a. DA equation to calculate mL per hr to nearest tenth:

   b. Evaluation: _____

5 Ordered: bretylium tosylate IV infusion 2 mg per min for a patient with a ventricular arrhythmia. Available: 1 g bretylium tosylate in 1 L NS.

   a. DA equation to calculate mL per hr to nearest tenth:

   b. Evaluation: _____

Equipment for Medicated Intravenous Solutions

The patient's safety is never more important than when administering IV medications. The trend of providing more prepackaged IV medications in a variety of doses and concentrations, needleless medication systems, and infusion pumps that calculate dose rates reflects the effort to reduce medication errors. Infusion pumps, unlike gravity devices, do not need secondary infusions to be hung at a higher level.

Remember that it is preferable to infuse medicated solutions on electronic volumetric pumps. EIDs can be very sophisticated. Figure 10-1 shows an example of an infusion pump used in intensive care units that can regulate four simultaneous infusions for one patient. This device frees space at the bedside. The nurse must ensure that each programmed rate is for the appropriate infusion solution.

This EID can be programmed by the nurse for the dose ordered, drug, concentration, and patient's weight. The pump calculates the flow rate. The nurse then confirms all the data (Figure 10-2).

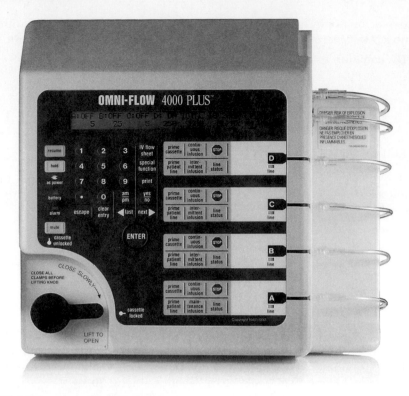

FIGURE 10-1 Omni-Flow® 4000 Plus Medication Management System 4-Channel IV Pump. (From Hospira, Inc., Lake Forest, IL.)

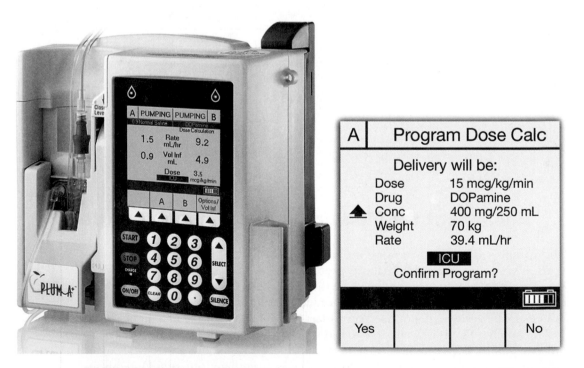

FIGURE 10-2 Plum A+® Drug Confirmation Screen. (From Hospira, Inc., Lake Forest, IL.)

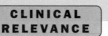

CLINICAL RELEVANCE

Be aware that the more flexibility high technology equipment offers, such as IV pumps that can be used for any medication dose on a patient of any age, the more chances for serious programming errors that can result in ADE, including fatalities. What if a decimal point is entered as a 0?

New IV pumps are being developed called *smart pumps,* which have input from multiple sources for the designated clinical area, target patient population, and usual doses to provide alarms and alerts. For instance, they can alarm if someone programs a dose for mg per kg per minute *instead of* mcg per kg per minute (an error of 1000 times the ordered dose). The alarm or alert would sound or occur if the nurse entered pound weight instead of kilogram weight (a 2.2 times overdose) because the pump was programmed for the usual dose parameters for that population. Keep in mind that there can be errors programmed into a smart pump. Refer to the website at the end of the chapter.

➤ Remember that there is a 1000-fold difference between a microgram and a milligram. Be scrupulous about entering the correct units of measurement when programming doses. Sentinel events have occurred from confusing units of measurement, such as mcg and mg.

➤ Note that the flow rate in Figure 10-2 is in tenths of a mL.

If an infusion pump is unavailable and a gravity device must be used, a microdrip pediatric set may be used for medicated infusions. The flow rate would be in drops per minute equal to the mL per hr calculated flow rate. Review the material in Chapter 9 on microdrip gravity infusions, if needed.

➤ Powerful medications are often given at low flow rates. Careful attention must be given to dilution directions.

Calculating Flow Rates for Medicated Infusions

RAPID PRACTICE 10-6

Estimated completion time: 15-20 minutes   **Answers on page 549**

Directions: *Identify the desired answer units and conversion factors needed. Calculate the ordered dose if it is weight based. Enter the critical factors and cancel unwanted units so that only the desired answer units of mL per hr remain. Use a calculator for long division and multiplication. Calculate to the nearest tenth of a mL per hr. Label answers.*

1   Ordered: Infuse Drug Y at 0.1 mg per min. Available: Drug Y, 200 mg per 250 mL NS.

   a. What flow rate should be set on the infusion pump?

   DA equation:

   b. Evaluation: _____

2   Ordered: Infuse Drug Y at the rate of 2 mL per min.

   a. What flow rate should be set on the infusion pump?

   DA equation:

   b. Evaluation: _____
   c. Would this flow rate be suitable for a gravity microdrip device? _____

3 Ordered: Infuse Drug Y at 5 mg per min. Available: Drug Y, 1 g per 250 mL D5W.

    a. What flow rate should be set on the infusion pump?

      DA equation:

    b. Evaluation: _____

4 Ordered: Titrate Drug Y at 8 to 10 mcg per kg per min to maintain a heart rate over 60. Available: Drug Y, 500 mg per 1 L LRS. Patient's weight: 44 kg.

    a. Initial total dose to be infused per minute:

      DA equation:

    b. What flow rate (to the nearest tenth of a mL) should be set on an infusion pump?

      DA equation:

    c. Evaluation: _____

5 Ordered: Increase the drug dose in problem 4 to 10 mcg per kg per min.

    a. Total dose to be infused per minute:

      DA equation:

    b. What flow rate (to the nearest tenth of a mL) should be set on the infusion pump?

      DA equation:

    c. Evaluation: _____

Q: Ask Yourself

A: My Answer

1 If the flow rate is 10 mL per hr on a pump for a medicated infusion, how would you set the rate on a pediatric microdrip set?

_____

Calculating Milligrams per Milliliter (mg per mL) from Available Drug Concentration

The nurse needs to be able to calculate the number of mg per mL contained in any IV solution.

Some IV solutions offer multiple dilution directions. The concentration of mg per mL will have specified limits for various routes; for example:

"For IV infusion: do not exceed a concentration of 1 mg per mL."
"For IV push: do not exceed a concentration of 10 mg per mL."

The *greater the amount* of drug per milliliter, the more concentrated the solution. (Think of 1 teaspoon of lemon juice in a glass of water versus 10 teaspoons of lemon juice.) This is a very basic calculation: think of *per* as a division line.

➤ To obtain mg per mL, divide the total number of milligrams of drug by the total number of mL of solution.

For example, if the available concentration is 500 mg of drug in a 250-mL solution, the number of mg per mL is obtained as follows:

$$\frac{mg}{mL} : \frac{\overset{2}{\cancel{500}} \ mg}{\underset{1}{\cancel{250}} \ mL} = \frac{2 \ mg}{mL}$$

Evaluation: Equation is balanced. Only mg per mL remain.

1 Which is *less* concentrated: Drug Y, 100 mg per mL or Drug Y, 250 mg per mL?

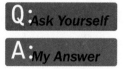

Q: Ask Yourself

A: My Answer

_____

Deriving Infusion Dose from Existing Flow Rate and Available Solution

The nurse may be asked how many milligrams or micrograms of a drug a patient is currently receiving per minute at the existing flow rate.

An IV solution labeled Drug Y, 500 mg per 250 mL, is infusing at 15 mL per hr. How many mg per min are being delivered? The equation setup begins with the same rule as for other equations: identify the desired answer units.

EXAMPLES

Two factors are known:
- Drug concentration ratio of the prepared solution: 500 mg per 250 mL
- Current flow rate: 15 mL per hr

$$\frac{mg}{min} : \frac{\overset{2}{\cancel{500}} \ mg}{\underset{1}{\cancel{250}} \ \cancel{mL}} \times \frac{\overset{1}{\cancel{15}} \ \cancel{mL}}{1 \ \cancel{hr}} \times \frac{1 \ \cancel{hr}}{\underset{4}{\cancel{60}} \ min} = \frac{2}{4} = \frac{0.5 \ mg}{min}$$

Evaluation: Equation is balanced. Only mg per min remain.

Analysis: The three primary factors in IV infusion calculations are the dose ordered, the drug concentration, and the flow rate. When *any two of the three* are known, the third can be obtained. Earlier equations calculated the flow rate from the drug concentration and dose ordered. Any relevant conversion factors, such as minutes to hours or hours to minutes, must also be entered in the equation.

RAPID PRACTICE 10-7

Calculating Infusion Rates in Milligrams per Minute and Micrograms per Minute

Estimated completion time: 20-25 minutes   **Answers on page 550**

Directions: *Identify the desired answer units and conversion formulas. Calculate the number of milligrams per milliliter and milligrams per minute to the nearest hundredth as shown in the preceding examples and problem 1. Evaluate the equation. Label answers. Use a calculator for long division and multiplication.*

TEST TIP: Take a moment to decide which of the conversion formulas will be needed for the equation: metric and minutes per hours.

1   Available: Drug Y, 500 mg per 1000 mL. Existing flow rate: 20 mL per hr.

    a. mg per mL concentration: $\underline{0.5\text{ mg per }1\text{ mL }(\frac{500\text{ mg}}{1000\text{ mL}})}$

    b. mg per min flow rate:

       DA equation:

$$\frac{\text{mg}}{\text{min}} : \frac{\overset{1}{\cancel{500}}\text{ mg}}{\underset{2}{\cancel{1000}\text{ mL}}} \times \frac{\overset{1}{\cancel{20}\text{ mL}}}{1\,\cancel{\text{hr}}} \times \frac{1\,\cancel{\text{hr}}}{\underset{3}{\cancel{60}}\text{ min}} = \frac{1}{6} = 0.166, \text{ rounded to } 0.17 \text{ mg per min}$$

    c. Evaluation: <u>Equation is balanced. Only mg per min remain.</u>

2   Available: Drug Y, 250 mg per 1000 mL. Existing flow rate: 30 mL per hr.

    a. mg per mL concentration: _____

    b. mcg per min flow rate: _____

       DA equation:

    c. Evaluation: _____

3   Available: Drug Y, 500 mg per 250 mL. Existing flow rate: 25 mL per hr.

    a. mg per mL concentration: _____

    b. mg per min flow rate: _____

       DA equation:

    c. Evaluation: _____

4   Available: Drug Y, 1 g per 250 mL. Existing flow rate: 10 mL per hr.

    a. mg per mL concentration: _____

    b. mg per min flow rate: _____

       DA equation:

    c. Evaluation: _____

5   Available: Drug Y, 500 mg per 500 mL. Existing flow rate: 12 mL per hr.

    a. mg per mL concentration: _____

    b. mg per min flow rate: _____

       DA equation:

    c. Evaluation: _____

Dilutions: When the Nurse Prepares the Drug for the Intravenous Solution

If the pharmacy does not prepare the drug in solution and if it is not available pre-prepared by a manufacturer, the nurse may need to prepare a drug and add it to the appropriate IV infusion. For the initial drug dose ordered, preparation is exactly the same as for all injectables.

Medications for IV infusion often call for two dilutions:

- The first dilution is to reconstitute the drug with a specific diluent, such as SW or sterile saline solution for injection. A small amount of diluent is added according to manufacturer directions, usually just enough so that the ordered dose can be withdrawn. This preparation is often too *concentrated* to administer to the patient.
- The second dilution, if required, provides a safe concentration for IV administration.

EXAMPLES

Ordered: ampicillin 1.2 g over 30 min. Available: ampicillin 500 mg powder. Directions: Each 500-mg ampule is to be reconstituted with 5 mL of SW for injection. May be further diluted in 50 mL or more of NS, D5W, or LR and given as an infusion over not more than 4 hours. Final concentration should not exceed 30 mg per mL. May be added to the last 100 mL of a compatible IV solution.

1. *First dilution.* Prepare the drug so that the precise dose *ordered* may be withdrawn from the total amount in the vial. This is the same preparation as for any injectable. Three ampules will have to be reconstituted to have enough for 1200 mg of ampicillin. Fifteen milliliters of SW for injection will be used to reconstitute the 1500 mg. From that amount, the nurse will calculate the number of mL needed for the 1200 mg ordered.

$$\frac{mL}{dose} : \frac{\overset{1}{\cancel{15}} \, mL}{\underset{1}{\cancel{1500} \, mg}} \times \frac{\cancel{1200} \, mg}{dose} = \frac{12 \, mL}{dose}$$

After reconstitution, there may be *more* than 12 mL because the powder will displace some of the solution. Read the label for that information.

Evaluation: Is the answer reasonable? Yes, because the answer has to be slightly less than 15 mL, which contained 1500 mg.

2. *Second dilution.* This dilution is for safe IV infusion. If 50 mL of IV solution is used, will the concentration be *less than* the 30 mg per mL safe maximum limit stated on the label?

$$50 \, mL \text{ plus } 12 \, mL = 62 \, mL$$

$$\frac{mg}{mL} : \frac{1200 \, mg}{62 \, mL} = 19.35, \text{ or } \frac{19 \, mg}{mL}$$

The 19 mg per mL is *less* concentrated than 30 mg per mL, so it is safe to use 50 mL of diluent. It also would be safe to dilute "to 50 mL" because the concentration would still be below 30 mg per mL (1200 per 50 = 24 mg per mL).

3. *Flow rate.* The order is to infuse 62 mL over 30 minutes. Calculate as for any infusion.
   Mental estimate: 62 mL over 30 minutes = 124 mL per hr.

$$\frac{mL}{hr} : \frac{62 \, mL}{\underset{1}{\cancel{30} \, min}} \times \frac{\overset{2}{\cancel{60} \, min}}{1 \, hr} = \frac{124 \, mL}{hr}$$

Evaluation: The equation is balanced. Only mL per hr remain.

Set the flow rate at 124 mL per hr. The 62 mL will have infused in 30 minutes. The infusion pump is preferred for medicated solutions.

➤ The fact that more medications are being supplied in various concentrations imposes a greater burden for verification. Was a 10, 20, or 50% dextrose solution ordered? Was 100 mcg or 100 mg ordered? Was 1 mg given IV instead of 0.1 mg because a decimal was not seen? Was there a leading zero that indicated a decimal would follow? Was the medication supposed to be diluted once or twice?

➤ Always check the manufacturer's literature or a current IV drug reference for preparation including dilution directions. Don't hesitate to call pharmacy for assistance.

FAQ | *What is the difference between "dilute in" 100 mL and "dilute to" 100 mL?*

ANSWER | "Dilute in" means add the drug, whether it is powder or liquid, to the specified amount of diluent. This is often written for the *first* dilution of a drug so that the dose ordered may be withdrawn. Dilute 25 mg in 5 mL of SW means add the 25 mg to 5 mL water. This will result in more than 5 mL. The label will state the concentration after dilution. "Dilute to" means that the drug plus the diluent will add up to the specified amount. Dilute 25 mg of the drug to 5 mL (total) of SW or "further dilute" to 50 mL (total). This is often written when there is to be a second dilution of the medication in an IV infusion solution. The nurse can remove excess diluent before mixing the medication to obtain the desired total amount.

EXAMPLES

Ordered: Drug Y 100 mg in IV infusion. **Available:** Drug Y, 100 mg powder. **Directions:** Dilute each 100 mg in 3 mL of SW. Further dilute to 50 mL with IV solution. The nurse prepares the ordered amount first by reconstituting it with 3 mL SW. After that is gently and thoroughly mixed, it will be added to 47 mL of the IV solution.

Intravenous Direct Push Medications

IV push medications are usually diluted in 1 to 50 mL. They may be administered over a minute to 30 minutes or more. A 5-mL minimum volume facilitates administration and titration rates.

The equipment selected depends on the amount of solution and duration of administration. If the injection is to be given through a distal port or an infusion line, agency flushing procedures must be followed. Current IV drug references must be consulted for safe dose ranges, dilutions, rates, and compatibility with the infusing solution.

Small amounts of some drugs usually are to be given over a period of 1 to 5 minutes and may be administered manually and slowly by the nurse with a syringe directly into an infusion line or a port closest to the patient. Larger amounts of solutions to be administered over a longer period of time may be administered using a syringe pump or a volume-control device.

➤ As with all IV medications—and this is even more urgent for patients receiving rapid concentrated doses—the patient needs to be assessed before, during, and after the medication is administered. The assessments include mental status, vital signs, and specific drug-related reactions and side effects.

Many agencies now supply IV tubing with an adapter so that needles are unnecessary for direct IV injections. The syringe connects to the adapter. This prevents needle-stick injuries. Figure 10-3 shows an example of medication being administered by IV push into an infusion line.

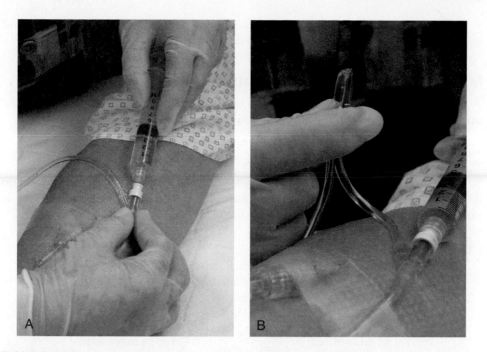

FIGURE 10-3 IV push (bolus) into existing infusion line using blunt cannula needleless equipment. (From Perry AG, Potter PA: *Clinical nursing skills and techniques*, ed. 7, St. Louis, 2010, Mosby.)

Intravenous Direct Push Calculations

A direct IV push is given over a *specified* period of time. A reliable drug reference must be consulted for the administration time. It is important to focus, use a watch, and record the time started and time to be finished so that the patient does not receive the medication too quickly. There are many distractions in the work place that may contribute to a rate error, and the medication is often concentrated and powerful.

The schedule is based on two factors:

1 Total number of mL in the *prepared* syringe after dilution
2 Total number of minutes and/or seconds to be injected

➤ A 10-mL or larger syringe needs to be used for all IV push medications.
➤ Using less than a 10-mL (wide-diameter) syringe can place excessive pressure on the vascular access device, whether it is peripheral or central.

Method 1: milliliters per minute

The drug is *first prepared* according to directions and then diluted according to current IV drug references for IV push medications and the manufacturer's guidelines. If the amount of mL per min to be injected is a whole number, this method works easily.

Prepare the drug dose ordered, and then dilute according to directions. Determine the number of mL per min (total mL in syringe ÷ total minutes to be given).

Treat "per" as a dividing line.

4 mL *prepared* to be given over 4 minutes: <u>1 mL per min</u>

4 mL *prepared* to be given over 2 minutes: <u>2 mL per min</u>

$$\frac{mL}{min} : \frac{4\ mL}{4\ min} = 1\ mL\ per\ min \qquad \frac{mL}{min} = \frac{\overset{2}{4}\ mL}{\underset{1}{\cancel{2}}\ min} = 2\ mL\ per\ min$$

EXAMPLES

Decide on a time to start and the exact stop time. Start when the second hand is on 12. Inject slowly and steadily. Avoid all distractions.

Method 2: seconds per calibration

Two factors are needed to calculate the infusion rate of an IV push based on the number of seconds needed to inject a solution per calibration mark on a syringe:

1 Number of calibrations occupied by the *prepared, diluted* drug in solution
2 Number of total seconds the drug is to be administered*

The syringe is examined for the number of calibrated lines the medication and diluent occupy. The total number of minutes for the injection is converted to seconds. How many seconds per calibration?

EXAMPLES

Ordered: morphine 4 mg direct IV push. Available: morphine sulfate 10 mg per mL. Literature: May be given undiluted, but it is appropriate to further *dilute* to 5 mL with SW, NS, or other compatible solutions. "Current drug reference": Administer over 5 minutes.

$$\text{mL prepared dose}: \frac{1 \text{ mL}}{\cancel{10 \text{ mg}}^{5}} \times \frac{\overset{2}{\cancel{4 \text{ mg}}}}{\text{dose}} = 0.4 \text{ mL to be administered}$$

Preparation: Withdraw ordered dose, 0.4 mL of morphine sulfate in a 10-mL syringe, and add 4.6 mL SW. This will make a total prepared volume of 5 mL.

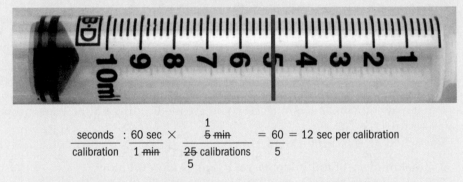

$$\frac{\text{seconds}}{\text{calibration}} : \frac{60 \text{ sec}}{1 \text{ min}} \times \frac{\overset{1}{\cancel{5 \text{ min}}}}{\underset{5}{\cancel{25} \text{ calibrations}}} = \frac{60}{5} = 12 \text{ sec per calibration}$$

➤ Note that the calibrations replace the mL volume in this type of equation.

➤ Prepare the precise ordered dose before adding diluent. The total amount in the syringe is the prepared precise ordered dose plus the specified diluent. The total volume of the two solutions is used to calculate the schedule.

The nurse uses a watch to count 12 seconds while pushing each increment on the syringe. It is important *not to exceed* the prescribed rate of injection. The drugs may be powerful enough to cause severe adverse effects from too rapid injection.

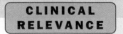

Q: *Ask Yourself*
A: *My Answer*

1 When the seconds per calibration method is used to calculate rate of injection, why aren't the total mL needed in the equation? What data replace the total mL?

_____

CLINICAL RELEVANCE

Any site to be used for IV administration needs to first be checked for patency. If using a med-lock IV port device to administer the medication, patency can be assessed by slight withdrawal of the syringe plunger to observe a blood return, followed by a flush injection of a 2- or 3-mL of sterile NS solution, with observation for swelling or discomfort. Neither method guarantees patency.

_____

*Consult a current drug reference for the exact time limits for the push.

IV Push Calculations

Estimated completion time: 20-25 minutes   **Answers on page 551**

Directions: *Calculate the medication dose. Using the directions for administration rate, examine the syringe for the calibrations occupied by the medication volume. Calculate the number of mL per min and seconds per calibration. Use a calculator for long division and multiplication. Label answers. Evaluate your own equations.*

1 Atropine 0.8 mg IV, for bradyarrhythmia. Directions: Dilute in up to 10 mL of SW. The nurse adds enough SW to the prepared medication to make 5 mL. Inject 1 mg or less over 1 minute.

> NDC 0641-2210-43
> 10 X 20 mL Multiple Dose Vials
> **ATROPINE**
> SULFATE INJECTION, USP
> **400 mcg/mL**
> (0.4 mg/mL)
> FOR SC, IM OR IV USE
>
> Each mL contains atropine sulfate 400 mcg (0.4 mg), sodium chloride 9 mg and benzyl alcohol 0.015 mL in Water for Injection. pH 3.0-6.5; sulfuric acid added, if needed, for pH adjustment.
> **POISON**
> USUAL DOSE: See package insert.
> Store at controlled room temperature 15°-30°C (59°-86°F).
> Caution: Federal law prohibits dispensing without prescription.
> Product Code
> 2210-43   B-32210
>
> ELKINS-SINN, INC. Cherry Hill, NJ 08003-4099
> *A subsidiary of A. H. Robins Company*

a. Total amount of prepared medication in mL: _____

   DA equation:

b. Total amount of diluted medication in mL (if applicable): _____
c. Total minutes to administer: _____
d. mL per min to be administered: _____
e. Total calibrations for the diluted medication: _____

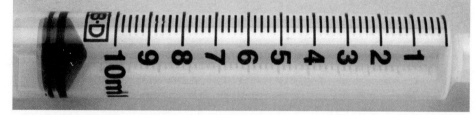

f. Total seconds to administer: _____
g. seconds per calibration: _____

   DA equation:

h. Evaluation: _____

2 Ordered: diazepam 10 mg IV push. Directions: Give undiluted. Rate: Inject at rate of 5 mg per min.

> 10 mL
> 5 mL
> FOR INVENTORY ONLY SAMPLE - NOT FOR DISTRIBUTION
> **10 mL** Multiple Dose Vial
> NDC 0641-2289-41
> 6505-01-240-6894
> **DIAZEPAM** CIV
> INJECTION, USP
> **5 mg/mL**
> FOR INTRAMUSCULAR or INTRAVENOUS USE
> Each mL contains diazepam 5 mg, propylene glycol 0.4 mL, ethyl alcohol 0.1 mL, benzyl alcohol 0.015 mL and sodium benzoate/benzoic acid, a total of 50 mg, in Water for Injection, pH 6.2-6.9. Sealed under nitrogen.
> USUAL DOSAGE: See package insert for complete prescribing information.
> NOTE: Solution may appear colorless to light yellow.
> Store at controlled room temperature 15°-30°C (59°-86°F).
> Caution: Federal law prohibits dispensing without prescription.
> Product Code
> 2289-41
> LOT   EXP.
> A-2289c
> ELKINS-SINN, INC. Cherry Hill, NJ 08003
> *A subsidiary of A. H. Robins Company*

a. Total amount of ordered medication in mL: _____

DA equation:

b. Total amount of diluted medication in mL (if applicable): _____

c. Total minutes to administer: _____

d. mL per min to be administered: _____

e. Total calibrations for the diluted medication: _____

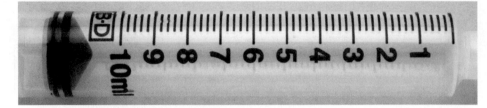

f. Total seconds to administer: _____

g. seconds per calibration: _____

DA equation:

h. Evaluation: _____

3 Ordered: phenobarbital 90 mg IV push, for a patient with seizures. Follow directions on label for dilution and rate of injection. For IV use, dilute to 3 mL of SW for injection. Do not exceed injection rate of 1 mL per min. Do not use if solution is not clear.

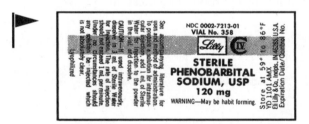

a. Total amount of prepared medication in mL to the nearest tenth: _____

DA equation:

b. Total amount of diluted medication in mL (if applicable): _____

c. Total minutes to administer: _____

d. mL per min to be administered: _____

e. Total calibrations for the diluted medication: _____

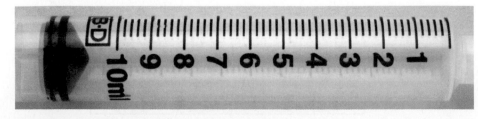

f. Total seconds to administer: _____

g. seconds per calibration: _____

   DA equation:

h. Evaluation: _____

4   Ordered: Drug Y, 60 mg IV push. Dilute to 5 mL of SW or NS. Give over
     5 minutes. Available: Drug Y, 75 mg per mL.

   a. Total amount of prepared medication in mL to the nearest hundredth:

   _____

      DA equation:

   b. Total amount of diluted medication in mL (if applicable): _____
   c. Total minutes to administer: _____
   d. mL per min to be administered: _____
   e. Total calibrations for the diluted medication: _____

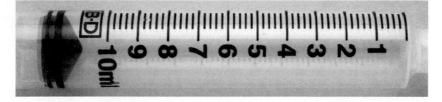

5   Ordered: furosemide 40 mg IV push, for an anuric patient. Directions: Should
     be infused in anuric patients at a rate of 4 mg per min. May be given undiluted.

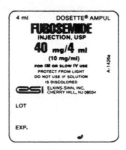

Communication about patient condition and needs at change of shift when giving the "hand-off"
report from one nurse to the next must include priority medication-related information, particularly patient allergies, high-alert medications, IVs, new or changed orders, and medications that
are due to be given soon after shift change, as well as any new symptoms that might indicate a
possible reaction to a medication. This is part of TJC patient safety goals to reduce ADE. Check
your agency's policies. Also refer to Appendix C.

**CLINICAL
RELEVANCE**

a. Total amount of prepared medication in mL: _____

b. Total amount of diluted medication in mL (if applicable): _____

c. Total minutes to administer: _____

d. mL per min to be administered: _____

e. Total calibrations for the medication: _____

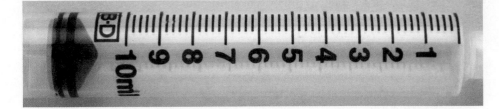

f. Total seconds to administer: _____

g. seconds per calibration: _____

DA equation:

h. Evaluation: _____

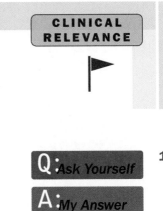

➤ Existing lines must be flushed before and after medication injection according to agency procedure. Such procedures are written for flushes of med-locks and infusion lines. Any existing site for IV administration needs to be checked for patency. IV medication injections can cause adverse reactions (e.g., sudden changes in mental status, blood pressure, and pulse). Assess the patient before, during, and after the procedure.

Q: Ask Yourself

1 Why is it suggested that the nurse start the push count with the second hand of the watch on the 12 o'clock mark?

A: My Answer

_____

Hyperalimentation: Parenteral Nutrition

➤ All total parenteral solutions are on the ISMP List of high-alert medications (see Appendix B).

Hyperalimentation (*hyperal,* for short) provides high-calorie IV nutrition. Also known as parenteral nutrition (PN), it can provide up to 1 kcal per mL with amino acids, dextrose, electrolytes, vitamins, and minerals to meet total nutritional needs. About 10% or 20% lipid emulsions can also be delivered intravenously as part of the PN order. Lipids may be added intermittently to provide needed calories (Figure 10-4). Insulin, a high-alert medication is ordered as an additive to normalize glucose levels based upon the results of frequently drawn glucose tests and prescriber's orders.

Ordinary IV fluids such as D5W only supply 5 g dextrose per 100 mL of solution, or 50 g dextrose (200 kcal) per 1000 mL. Three L per day would supply the

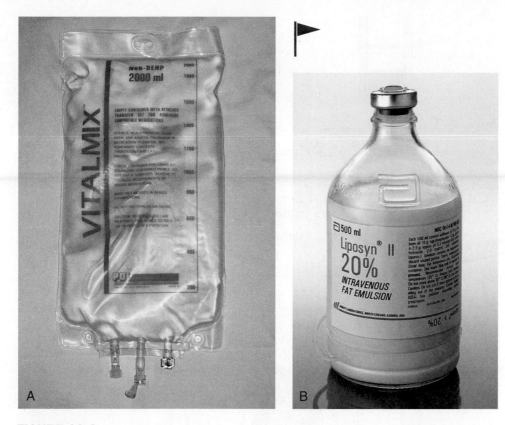

FIGURE 10-4 **A,** Amino acid. **B,** Liposyn. (**A** from Brown M, Mulholland JL: *Drug calculations: process and problems for clinical practice,* ed. 8, St. Louis, 2008, Mosby. **B** from Abbott Laboratories, Abbott Park, IL.)

patient with only 600 kcal per day, a starvation diet. Adults usually consume between 1500 and 2500 or more kcal per day of protein, carbohydrate, and fat to meet nutritional needs and maintain health and energy levels.

Solutions' contents are customized by the prescriber and prepared by the pharmacy based on frequent current laboratory tests and patient condition.

How many Calories do you consume on an average day?

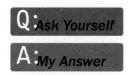

_____

For long-term therapy and high solution concentrations, PN can be administered into the vena cava via a centrally inserted catheter; this is known as *central parenteral nutrition* (CPN). The vena cava provides rapid dilution of stronger solutions (Figure 10-5). A peripherally inserted central catheter (PICC) (Figure 10-6) may also be threaded into the vena cava from a large peripheral vein, usually for short or intermediate periods.

For short-term therapy, large peripheral veins can be used; this is known as *peripheral parenteral nutrition* (PPN). PPN uses nore dilute solutions than CPN to protect the peripheral vein wall from irritation. PPN is not threaded into the vena cava.

1   Is the PN solution for the home infusion order on p. 339 (Figure 10-7) isotonic, hypotonic, or hypertonic?

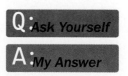

_____

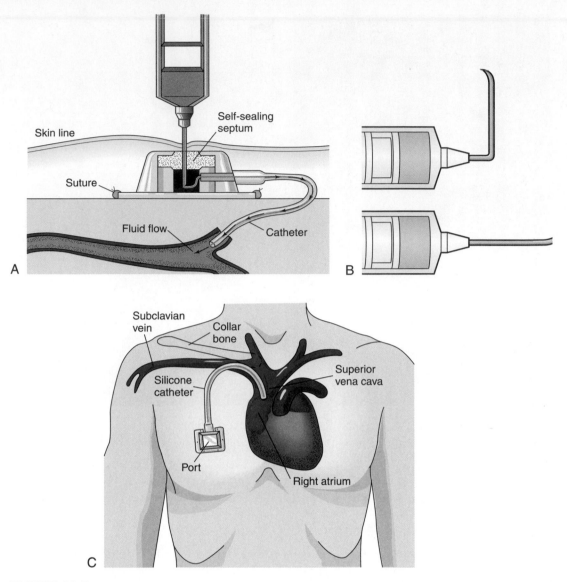

FIGURE 10-5 **A,** Implantable infusion port. **B,** Assortment of Huber needles. **C,** Infusion port placed in subcutaneous pocket with centrally inserted catheter. (From Perry AG, Potter PA: *Clinical nursing skills and techniques,* ed. 7, St. Louis, 2010, Mosby.)

2 What are two main differences between CPN and PPN?

_____

3 Which components provide (a) protein, (b) carbohydrate, and (c) fat (see Figure 10-7)?

_____

4 Which high-risk medication must be added just before infusion (see Figure 10-7)?

_____

CHAPTER 10

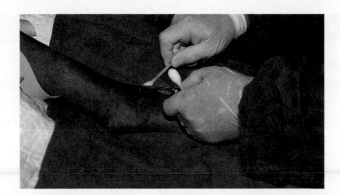

FIGURE 10-6 Prepping peripherally inserted central catheter (PICC) site. (From Perry AG, Potter PA: *Clinical nursing skills and techniques,* ed. 5, St. Louis, 2004, Mosby.)

```
     HOME  INFUSION  PHARMACY
▬▬▬▬▬▬▬▬▬▬▬▬▬▬▬▬▬▬▬▬▬▬▬▬▬▬▬
 RX#37856   ▬▬▬▬▬▬▬▬▬▬▬
▬▬▬▬▬▬▬▬▬

 AMINO*ACIDS 10%=425ML DEXTROSE*10%=357ML
 STER*WATER=341ML LIPIDS*20%=125ML
 MVI=10ML/DAY *ADDITIVES PER LITER*
 SOD*CHLOR=35mEq POT*PHOS=15mM CALCIUM=5mEq
 MAGNESIUM=5mEq

 QTY#      TPN 40-51GM PROTEIN+LIPIDS
 INFUSE NIGHTLY 8PM TO 8AM THRU IV PICC LINE
 VIA SIGMA PUMP. *****ADD 10 UNITS
 HUMULIN-R TO EACH BAG JUST PRIOR TO
 INFUSION***** **NOTE:CONTAINS PN
 SOLN+LIPIDS:RATE ADJUSTED** SETTINGS:
 RATE=104ML/HR VOLUME=1248ML

       *** REFRIGERATE ***


 EXPIRATION DATE:01/06/13
```

Amino acids provide protein. Lipids provide fat and calories. Dextrose provides carbohydrate.
MVI = Multivitamins. Additives per liter in this order are electrolytes.

FIGURE 10-7 PN bag label for home infusion therapy. (From Brown M, Mulholland JL: *Drug calculations: process and problems for clinical practice,* ed. 8, St. Louis, 2008, Mosby.)

➤ The nurse must compare the label contents and percentage of each PN solution with the prescriber's current order. Orders may be changed daily.
➤ PN is a lifeline and administered on a protected dedicated IV line. The sites cannot be used for the administration of medications, blood, or many other products. Check agency protocols.
➤ CPN and PPN are administered ONLY on an infusion pump.

The solution decomposes quickly. Keep refrigerated and check expiration dates.

CLINICAL RELEVANCE

➤ To preserve the line, and avoid the risk of infection, air emboli, incompatibilities, precipitation, coagulation, hyperglycemia and hypoglycemia, and so on, familiarize yourself with the procedures, including changes of tubing, aseptic technique for site care, flushing protocols, and equipment permitted for approved compatible additives (e.g., Y tubing). Following the assessment protocols for weight, signs of infection, and laboratory tests permits early detection of complications.

Estimated completion time: 30 minutes   Answers on page 552

Directions: *Select the correct intravenous-related response. Verify answers with a DA equation. Use a calculator for long division and multiplication.*

1 An IV flow rate of 2 mL per min of 5% L/R would be set at which flow rate on an infusion pump?

    1. 60 drops per min   **3.** 120 drops per min
    2. 60 mL per hr   **4.** 120 mL per hr

2 Ordered: IV of 500 mL D5 NS with KCl 40 mEq, for a patient with hypokalemia, at 10 mEq per hr. Check serum potassium level when completed. Continue until serum potassium level greater than 4, then discontinue. The nurse will set the flow rate at:

    1. 10 mL per hr for 4 hours   **3.** 50 mL per hr for 4 hours
    2. 40 mL per hr for 10 hours   **4.** 125 mL per hr for 4 hours

Direct injection of concentrated KCl can cause cardiac arrest.

3 An available IV solution contains 1g in 250 mL. How many milligrams per milliliter are contained in the solution? (Use mental arithmetic.)

    1. 4   **3.** 25
    2. 0.25   **4.** 100

4 How many kilocalories of dextrose are contained in a central PN solution of 1 L that contains 25% dextrose? (Conversion factor: 4 kcal = 1 g of dextrose.)

    1. 25   **3.** 250
    2. 100   **4.** 1000

5 Ordered: IVPB antibiotic of 30 mL to infuse in 30 minutes. What will the flow rate be set on a gravity device with a microdrip set? (Use mental arithmetic.)

    1. 30 mL per hr   **3.** 90 drops per min
    2. 60 drops per min   **4.** 100 drops per min

6 Ordered: morphine sulfate 3 mg IV push, for a patient in pain. Drug reference directions for IV direct injection: Dilute to 5 mL with SW. Available: morphine sulfate 10 mg per mL. Directions: Administer over 5 minutes. How many mL per min will the medication deliver?

    1. 1   **3.** 10
    2. 5   **4.** 50

7 The recommendation for adjusting medicated IV infusions that are behind the ordered schedule for the amount infused is

    1. Adjust up to 25% more than the ordered rate.
    2. Adjust up to 10% more than the ordered rate.
    3. Let the rate stay behind the ordered rate for the remainder of the infusion.
    4. Assess the patient condition and consult with the licensed prescriber.

8 An existing unmedicated IV solution is flowing at 100 mL per hr when the nurse arrives to care for the patient. 500 out of 1000 mL have been infused in 5 hours. The order reads: 1000 mL q8h. The patient is NPO 1 day postoperatively and has good heart, lung, and renal function. The urinary output appears concentrated. The nurse's assessment is that it would be safe to adjust the IV to complete it on time. The adjustment would be:

    1. The flow rate needs adjustment to 125 mL per hr.
    2. The flow rate needs adjustment to 167 mL per hour.
    3. The flow rate needs to be opened up until it is on target for the current time and then adjusted to 125 mL per hr.
    4. The flow rate should be adjusted to 155 mL per hr until completed.

9 Which of the following is the most concentrated IV solution?

1. 250 mg per 1000 mL

3. 100 mg per 100 mL

2. 250 mg per 500 mL

4. 50 mg per 100 mL

10 An order of 500 mg of a drug in 1000 mL is being infused at 10 mL per hr. The hourly amount of drug infused is

1. 2 mg per hr

3. 10 mg per hr

2. 5 mg per hr

4. 15 mg per hr

CHAPTER 10 FINAL PRACTICE

Estimated completion time: 1-2 hours   **Answers on page 553**

Directions: *Calculate the advanced intravenous problems. Verify your answers with a DA equation. Label answers. Use a calculator for long division and multiplication. Evaluate your equations.*

1 Ordered: furosemide 30 mg IV push, for a patient with anuria, at 4 mg per min. Directions: May be given undiluted.

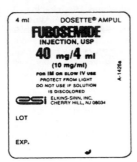

a. Total mL to inject: _____

DA equation:

Evaluation: _____

b. Calibrations occupied by the medication:

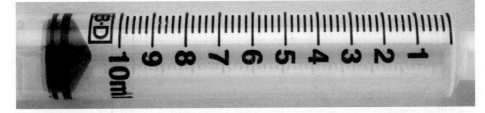

c. Total seconds for injection: _____

DA equation:

Evaluation: _____

d. Seconds per calibration for injection: _____

DA equation:

Evaluation: _____

2 Ordered: aminophylline IV infusion for a patient with acute asthma. Titrate: 0.3 to 0.6 mg per kg per hr. Patient's weight: 75 kg. Directions: Dilute in 250 mL NS. Consult the label for drug amount placed in the IV. The nurse will withdraw 20 mL of NS before adding the aminophylline.

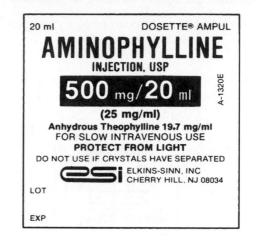

a. What flow rate, to the nearest tenth of a mL, will be set on the infusion pump for 0.3 mg per kg per hr? _____

DA equation:

Evaluation: _____

b. The patient's respiratory status does not improve. The theophylline serum levels are still within normal levels. The nurse increases the flow rate to 0.4 per mg per kg per hr. What will the flow rate be adjusted to?

Evaluation: _____

3 Ordered: Nitropress IV infusion. Start at 0.3 mcg per kg per min, for a patient with severe hypertension. Titrate to keep systolic blood pressure below 160 and diastolic pressure below 90. Directions: Dilute 50 mg in 250 mL D5W. The nurse will use 250 mL as the total amount of solution for calculation purposes. Patient weight: 60 kg.

> **Protect from light.**
> Exp.
> Lot
> ▭ **2 mL** Single-dose Fliptop Vial   NDC 0074-3024-01
> **NITROPRESS®**
> **Sodium Nitroprusside Injection**
> 50 mg / 2 mL Vial **(25 mg/mL)**
> **FOR I.V. INFUSION ONLY.**
> Monitor blood pressure before and during administration.   06-7378-2/R2-12/93
> *ABBOTT LABS, NORTH CHICAGO, IL 60064, USA*

a. mg per mL concentration in the final solution: _____

DA equation:

Evaluation: _____

b. The nurse will set the flow rate on the infusion pump at (nearest tenth of a mL)_____.

Evaluation: _____

4 Ordered: dobutamine 2.5 mcg per kg per min. Directions: Dilute in 500 mL D5W. The nurse will withdraw 20 mL of the D5W, discard it, and use 480 mL of the D5W plus 20 mL of the dobutamine solution to make a 500-mL medicated solution. Patient weight: 64 kg.

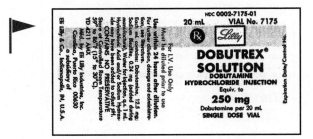

a. mg per mL concentration in the final solution: _____
b. The nurse will set the flow rate on the infusion pump at: _____

DA equation:

Evaluation: _____

5 Ordered: KCl 10 mEq per hr, for a patient with hypokalemia. Available: KCl 40 mEq per 500 mL D5 $\frac{1}{2}$ NS. The nurse will set the flow rate on the infusion pump at: _____

DA equation:

Evaluation: _____

6 Ordered: dopamine HCl infusion 3 mcg per kg per min. Patient's weight: 82 kg. Flow rate when the nurse begins the shift: dopamine HCl at 15 mL per hr.

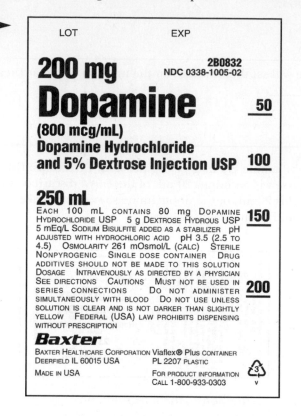

a. How many milligrams per hour are ordered to the nearest whole number?

_____

DA equation:

Evaluation: _____

b. What is the ordered flow rate to the nearest tenth of a mL? _____

DA equation:

Evaluation: _____

7 Ordered: atropine sulfate 1 mg bolus IV push, for a patient with bradyarrhythmia. Directions: Dilute to 10 mL SW for injection (total amount) and give over 1 minute.

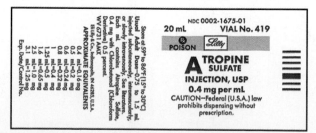

a. How many mL of atropine will the nurse prepare? _____

DA equation:

Evaluation: _____

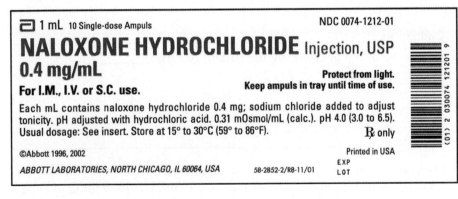

b. After dilution, how many seconds per mL will the atropine be injected?

_____

DA equation:

Evaluation: _____

8 Ordered: naloxone infusion, to wean a patient with narcotic depression, to be infused over 6 hours at 0.03 mg per hr. Directions: Dilute 2 mg in 500 mL NS or D5W.

1 mL 10 Single-dose Ampuls	NDC 0074-1212-01

NALOXONE HYDROCHLORIDE Injection, USP
0.4 mg/mL
For I.M., I.V. or S.C. use.

Protect from light.
Keep ampuls in tray until time of use.

Each mL contains naloxone hydrochloride 0.4 mg; sodium chloride added to adjust tonicity. pH adjusted with hydrochloric acid. 0.31 mOsmol/mL (calc.). pH 4.0 (3.0 to 6.5). Usual dosage: See insert. Store at 15° to 30°C (59° to 86°F).   ℞ only

©Abbott 1996, 2002

ABBOTT LABORATORIES, NORTH CHICAGO, IL 60064, USA   58-2852-2/R8-11/01

Printed in USA
EXP
LOT

(01) 2 030074 121201 9

a. How many mL of naloxone will be added to the 500 mL? _____

DA equation:

Evaluation: _____

b. The nurse will set the flow rate on the infusion pump at (round to the nearest tenth of a mL): _____

DA equation:

Evaluation: _____

9 Ordered: magnesium sulfate 2.5 mL per min IV infusion, for a patient with convulsions. Directions: Dilute 4 g in 250 mL of D5W. The label states 500 mg per mL. Prepare 4 g.*

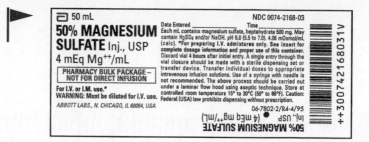

*Note the confusing abbreviation Mg for magnesium. **Do not use.** It may be confused with mg (milligram).

a. How many mL of magnesium sulfate will the nurse prepare for the infusion?

_____

DA equation:

Evaluation: _____

The nurse will remove an amount of D5W equal to the amount of medication being added so that the IV solution remains 250 mL.

b. Following the ordered rate, what will be the flow rate on the infusion pump?

_____

DA equation:

Evaluation: _____

c. How many mg per min will the patient receive? _____

DA equation:

Evaluation: _____

10 Ordered for an NPO patient: Potassium chloride* continuous infusion of 5 mEq per hr. Supplied by pharmacy: KCl 40 mEq in 1000 mEQ of D5W.

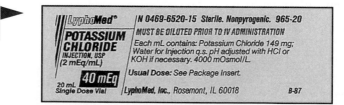

*➤ Potassium chloride is a common additive to IV solutions and is usually prepared by the pharmacy. Concentrated KCl can cause arrhythmias and cardiac arrest if given undiluted. After dilution, the IV bag must be gently rotated several times before hanging to ensure that the potassium is dispersed *throughout* the bag. It is preferably administered via an infusion pump. It *must be administered* via an infusion pump in stronger concentrations. Notify the prescriber if by chance the infusion is administered at a rate that exceeds the order. A timed tape is helpful for monitoring volume infused even when a pump is being used.

a. Is potassium chloride compatible with D5W (using a current drug reference)? _____

b. What flow rate will be set on the infusion pump? _____

DA equation:

Evaluation: _____

c. How long will the infusion last (using mental arithmetic)? _____

Suggestions for Further Reading

Gahart BL, Nazareno AR: *2011 Intravenous medications: a handbook for nurses and health professionals*, ed. 27, St. Louis, 2011, Mosby.

Lilley LL, Collins SR, Harrington S, Snyder JS: *Pharmacology and the nursing process*, ed. 6, St. Louis, 2011, Mosby.

Perry AG, Potter PA: *Clinical nursing skills and techniques*, ed. 7, St. Louis, 2010, Mosby.

www.baxter.com
www.globalrph.com/tpn.htm
www.hospira.com
www.safemedication.com
www.apsf.org/resource_center/newsletter/2003/spring/smartpump.htm

⊝volve   Additional practice problems can be found in the Advanced Intravenous Calculations section of the Student Companion on Evolve.

Now that you have mastered the principles and contents of this chapter, you will be on the road to safer practice and will also find Chapter 11, Antidiabetic Agents, and subsequent chapters relatively easy to learn.

PART V

Oral and Injectable Hormone Medications

300 mg
20 ML
0.9%
1000 g = 1 kg
>400 m
0.4 mg/mL

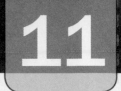

Antidiabetic Agents

OBJECTIVES

- Define terms related to tests and treatment for patients receiving medications for type 1 and type 2 diabetes.
- Identify risks of look-alike generic oral antidiabetic products.
- Contrast the various insulin products by onset of activity.
- Calculate and titrate subcutaneous and IV insulin dosages based on blood glucose levels.
- Evaluate blood glucose levels for prescribed insulin administration.
- Select the appropriate syringe and measure syringe doses for subcutaneous insulin administration.
- Identify the most common adverse effect of insulin therapy.
- Define *hypoglycemia* and *hyperglycemia*.
- Identify causes of, risks of, and nutrients needed for hypoglycemia.
- Identify critical patient safety issues related to antidiabetic medications and blood glucose levels.

Essential Prior Knowledge

- Mastery of Chapters 1-10

Essential Equipment

- The learner will benefit from further practice preparing and administering various types and mixtures of insulin under clinical supervision using insulin syringes.

Estimated Time To Complete Chapter

- 2-2½ hours

Introduction

Diabetes is an epidemic that is increasing at an alarming rate and has generated many new medicines for treatment. According to the International Diabetic Federation (IDF), the highest rate of diabetes prevalence in 2009 was in North America, where it was thought to be 10.2% of the population. In 2010, the Centers for Disease Control and Prevention (CDC) estimated that 1 out of 3 adults might have diabetes by 2050. Worldwide prevalence, if left unchecked, was projected by the CDC to be 433 million by 2030.

Measuring an ordered insulin dose in a syringe for subcutaneous administration is a basic skill that does not require math. However, IV insulin administration does require math calculations. To administer antidiabetic agents *safely,* the nurse must understand frequently encountered terms, know how to interpret orders and labels, differentiate blood glucose laboratory levels, distinguish the various pharmacological products ordered for treatment, identify manifestations

➤ If blood glucose levels are reported by a laboratory in millimoles per liter, *multiply* by 18 to convert to milligrams per deciliter. Divide milligrams per deciliter by 18 to obtain the equivalent millimoles per liter.

Vocabulary Review

RAPID PRACTICE 11-1

Estimated completion time: 10-15 minutes   **Answers on page 555**

Directions: *Study the vocabulary and laboratory terminology. Answer the following questions with brief, one- or two-word answers.*

1 What are the main *differences* in measurement among the following tests: stat BG, FBS, 2-hour postprandial, fructosamine, and HbA1c?

_____

_____

_____

2 What four-letter *abbreviation* does a nurse write if the patient reports results of self-monitored sugar level? _____

3 What is a normal fasting blood sugar level range? _____

4 What does insulin do in the body to blood glucose? (State answer in a few words.)

_____

5 Contrast in one or two words the difference between insulin shock and diabetic ketoacidosis (DKA) in terms of blood glucose levels and the main drug administered for treatment.

Insulin shock: _____

DKA: _____

Oral and Injectable Non-Insulin Antidiabetic Agents

➤ All hypoglycemic agents are ISMP high-alert medications (see Appendix B).

Oral and injectable non-insulin antidiabetic medications are a growing number of hypoglycemic agents with varying pharmacologic properties that target specific problems of glucose metabolism for patients with type 2 diabetes mellitus. Many are available in more than one concentration. Some examples of these agents follow:

Class: biguanides
    Metformin (glucophage,
       glucophage XR)
Class: meglitinides
    Prandin (repaglinide)
    Starlix (nateglitinide)
Class: sulfonylurea
    Diabeta (glyburide)
    Amaryl (glimepiride)
    Glucotrol (glipizide)
Class: DPP-4 inhibitors
    Onglyza (saxaglipten)
    Januvia (sitaglipten phosphate)
Class: alpha-glucosidase inhibitors
    Precose (Acarbose)

Injectable Non-Insulin Products
Class: Incretin mimetics
    Byetta (exenatide) (given for
      type 2 diabetes as an
      injection)

Class: Amylinomimetics
    Symlin (pramlintide acetate)
      (given for type 2 and type 1
      diabetes as an injection)

➤ Note carefully the similarities of generic names. Confusion of look-alike drug names has resulted in medication errors.

Some of these drugs are available in several doses. They may be combined with other drugs to enhance the effectiveness of treatment. Refer to the PrandiMet label. Metaglip is a combination of glipizide and metformin.

➤

NDC 0169-0093-01
List 009301

PrandiMet®
(repaglinide/metformin HCl) Tablets
1 mg/500 mg

100 Tablets

Rx only

novo nordisk®

Do not store above 25°C (77°F).
Tablets for oral use.
Each tablet contains
1 mg repaglinide and
500 mg metformin HCl.
See accompanying package insert
for full prescribing information.
Keep all prescription drugs out
of reach of children.
Protect from moisture.
Keep bottle tightly closed.

(01) 103 0169 0093 01 1

Manufactured for Novo Nordisk Inc.
Princeton, NJ 08540
by Recipharm Stockholm AB, Sweden

Exp. Date/ Lot:

8-1733-31-201-1

EXAMPLES

Following are some examples of prescribers' orders for oral antidiabetics, along with the drug labels:
Glucophage 500 mg PO tid with meals

➤

N 3 0087-6060-10 9

Each tablet contains 500 mg of metformin hydrochloride.
See enclosed package insert for dosage information.
Caution: Federal law prohibits
dispensing without prescription.
Store between 15°–30° C (59°–86° F).
Dispense in light resistant container.
Glucophage is a registered trademark of LIPHA s.a.
Licensed to Bristol-Myers Squibb Company.
Distributed by
Bristol-Myers Squibb Company
Princeton, NJ 08543 USA

606010DRL-2
34-007102-01

500 Tablets   NDC 0087-**6060-10**

GLUCOPHAGE®
(metformin hydrochloride
tablets)

500
mg

✳ Bristol-Myers Squibb Company

Prandin 1 mg PO tid 30 minutes ac

➤

Prandin® (repaglinide) Tablets   NDC 0169-0081-81
List 008181
0.5 mg   100 tablets
Do not store above 77°F (25°C).

(01) 103 0169 0081 81 0

Marketed by:
Novo Nordisk Inc.
Princeton, NJ 08540

8-1767-31-201-5

Exp./
Control:

➤

Prandin® (repaglinide) Tablets   NDC 0169-0082-81
List 008281
1 mg   100 tablets
Do not store above 77°F (25°C).

(01) 103 0169 0082 81 7

Marketed by:
Novo Nordisk Inc.
Princeton, NJ 08540

8-1777-31-201-5

Exp./
Control:

➤

Prandin® (repaglinide) Tablets   NDC 0169-0084-81
List 008481
2 mg   100 tablets
Do not store above 77°F (25°C).

(01) 103 0169 0084 81 1

Marketed by:
Novo Nordisk Inc.
Princeton, NJ 08540

8-1787-31-201-5

Exp./
Control:

CHAPTER 11

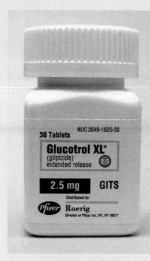

Glucotrol XL 2.5 mg daily with breakfast ⚑

➤ Match the prescriber's order, drug name, drug dose, and labels carefully. Do not try to guess the product contents from the name. The math is simple for the oral medications. The doses are available as ordered or in multiples of the amount ordered. They must be given at the prescribed time to control potential mealtime-generated elevations of glucose levels.

Parenteral Antidiabetic Agents: Insulin Products

➤ All insulin products are ISMP-identified high-alert medications.

The hormone insulin is supplied in rapid-onset, intermediate-acting, and long-acting forms in standardized units.

- It is supplied in two concentrations: U-100 (100 units per mL) and U-500 (500 units per mL; Figure 11-1).
- U 100 is the most commonly ordered concentration.

➤ The U-500 concentration is ordered for the **rare** patient who needs very high doses.

- Insulin types are related to the product source as well as to the onset and duration of action. Recombinant DNA (rDNA) insulin, a highly purified version of human insulin, is similar in structure and function to human insulin.
- Insulin is most often prescribed and administered subcutaneously. The IV route is reserved for specific acute-care situations.

➤ Do not confuse U-100 with the total amount in the vial. U-100 refers to the concentration per milliliter (100 units per mL).

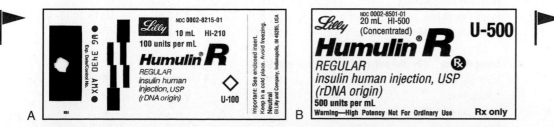

FIGURE 11-1 **A,** U-100 (100 units per mL) insulin. **B,** U-500 (500 units per mL) insulin.

> The most common adverse effect of insulin therapy is *hypoglycemia*.
> Spell out "units" even though the abbreviation U may be seen in some orders and preprinted MARs. It can be mistaken for zero and is on the "Do Not Use" list of the TJC (p. 101).
> Warning: Insulin activity varies among individuals. Monitor blood glucose levels closely.
> Prescribed timing of insulin administration and timing of meals are linked to the time of onset of the insulin activity. *Hypoglycemic* reactions may occur at any time, but insulin onset and peak activity times warrant close observation for potential hypoglycemic reactions.
> Consult manufacturer literature re: mixing with other insulins and oral antidiabetic products. There are important differences and interactions among the products.

Examine the insulin activity chart in Table 11-1. Insulin fixed-combination mixes are supplied for patients who experience patterns of mealtime elevations.

TABLE 11-1	Insulin Activity Chart for Subcutaneous Administration, in Order of Activity Onset*			
Type	**Brand Name**	**Onset of Subcutaneous Route**	**Peak**	**Duration**
Short and Rapid Acting				
Insulin aspart	Novolog	10-20 min	1-3 hr	3-5 hr
Insulin lispro	Humalog	15 min	1 hr	3.5-4.5 hr
Insulin glusiline	Apidra	20-30 min	1-1.5 hr	less than 6 hr
Short and Intermediate Acting				
70% insulin aspart protamine suspension + 30% insulin aspart (fixed premix)	Novolog Mix 70/30	10-20 min	2.4 hr	24 hr
75% insulin lispro protamine + 25% insulin lispro (fixed premix)	Humalog Mix 75/25 Humalog Mix 50/50	15 min	30-90 min	24 hr
Insulin injection regular	Novolin R	30 min	2.5-5 hr	8 hr
	Humulin R	30 min	2-4 hr	6-8 hr
	Iletin II Regular (pork source)	30 min	2-4 hr	4 hr
Insulin isophane suspension (NPH) + regular insulin combination	Novolin 70/30	30 min	2-12 hr	24 hr
	Humulin 70/30	30 min	2-12 hr	24 hr
	Humulin 50/50	30 min	3-5 hr	24 hr
Intermediate Acting				
Insulin isophane suspension (NPH)	Novolin N	1.5 hr	4-12 hr	Up to 24 hr
	Humulin N	1-2 hr	6-12 hr	18-24 hr
Long Acting (➤ do not mix with other insulins)				
Insulin glargine	Lantus	1 hr	None	24 hr or more
Insulin zinc suspension (L)		1-3 hr	6-12 hr	18-26 hr
Insulin detemir	Levemir	0.8-2 hr	None	24 hr

The mixes contain rapid-acting insulin mixed with longer-, slower-acting insulin, which reduces the fluctuations and elevations in blood glucose patterns. The intermediate- and longer-acting insulins contain additives that extend the action but render them unsuitable for IV administration.

1 What are the five column headings in Table 11-1 that reveal key pieces of information that the nurse must understand about each type of insulin?

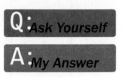

2 Which type of insulin does not have a peak?

FAQ | *How are insulin types and amounts selected?*

ANSWER | Types and amounts are selected on the basis of patterns in the patient's recent blood glucose levels, including the timing of elevations, particularly related to mealtime and activity patterns. The patient's motivation and compliance are also factored into insulin prescriptions.

CLINICAL RELEVANCE

- If the patient is hospitalized with extremely high levels of blood glucose, a rapid-acting insulin may be administered subcutaneously or intravenously to stabilize the patient.
- Some patients exhibit elevations only after meals, some have nighttime or early-morning spikes, and others have constant elevations.
- A small amount, **basal** (slow, low, continuous release) dose of long-acting insulin, such as insulin glargine, may be ordered with weekly dose adjustments. This amount does not cover mealtime elevations. The dose will be low enough to avoid *hypo*glycemic reactions. **Bolus** (single, concentrated) doses of insulin aspart and lispro, or regular insulins, may be ordered and administered separately to cover mealtime and/or other elevations.
- When a pattern of blood glucose levels in relation to meals emerges, the type and amount of insulin can be customized.
- Insulin mixes may be ordered twice a day to cover a patient's basal needs and mealtime elevations when a pattern is known.
- Intermediate- and long-acting insulins are *not* used to treat *acute hyper*glycemia.

1 What is a basal dose of insulin?

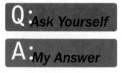

2 What are two reasons that bolus doses would be added to basal doses?

Insulin Labels

Take a few minutes to examine the insulin product labels and identify the following:

- Name
- Type
- Concentration: U-100 or U-500 (U-500 rarely ordered)
- Product source: rDNA
- Storage of insulin products, opened and unopened, is controversial. Some say refrigerate all. Others say current bottle can be at room temperature and unopened bottles must be refrigerated. Read the **product insert and label** information for **each** bottle used regarding room temperature storage and refrigeration storage and respective expiration dates. The nurse writes the date opened on the label and discards the bottle according to the manufacturer guidelines, usually a month. Insulin may not be effective after expiration dates of 28 days.
- Expiration date

Short- and Rapid-Acting Insulins

There are several types and brands of short- or rapid-acting insulins on the market. Short- and rapid-acting insulins are administered to treat a current blood glucose elevation or an anticipated elevation in the near future, such as after the next meal. Figures 11-2 to 11-5 illustrate product labels of various short-acting insulins.

Humalog and Novolog insulin are to be given 10 to 15 minutes *before* a meal or with the meal, whereas Humulin R and Novolin R must be given 30 minutes before a meal (see Figures 11-2 to 11-4).

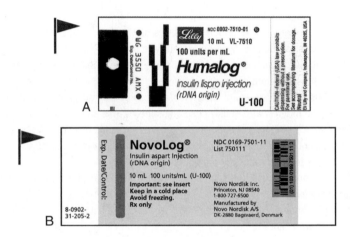

FIGURE 11-2 **A,** Humalog insulin. **B,** NovoLog insulin. (**B,** From Novo Nordisk Inc., Princeton, NJ.)

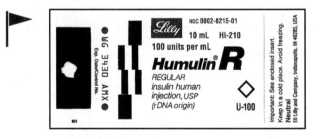

FIGURE 11-3 Humulin R insulin.

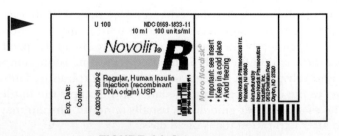

FIGURE 11-4 Novolin R insulin.

➤ If there is any chance that mealtime may be delayed, such as might occur in a hospital, do *not* give Humalog or Novolog until the meal arrives.

1 What does U-100 on the label of the insulin vial mean?

_____

2 What is the most common adverse effect of insulin therapy?

_____

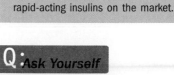

✳ **Mnemonic**

Humalog and Novolog, described as "mealtime" insulins, are analogs of human insulin and, when administered, "log" in faster than regular rapid-acting insulins on the market.

➤ Avoid giving diet beverages or artificially sweetened foods, such as sugar alcohols and aspartame, for suspected *hypo*glycemic reactions. Follow prescriber and agency policies for insulin reactions. *Dextrose* (glucose) is the ingredient needed to raise the blood glucose level promptly. Dextrose administration is usually followed by a complex carbohydrate-containing meal to sustain a higher blood glucose level.

Q: Ask Yourself

A: My Answer

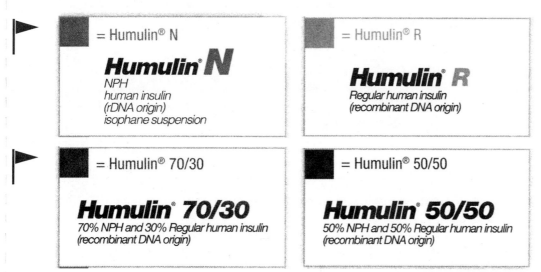

= Humulin® N

Humulin® N
NPH
human insulin
(rDNA origin)
isophane suspension

= Humulin® R

Humulin® R
Regular human insulin
(recombinant DNA origin)

= Humulin® 70/30

Humulin® 70/30
70% NPH and 30% Regular human insulin
(recombinant DNA origin)

= Humulin® 50/50

Humulin® 50/50
50% NPH and 50% Regular human insulin
(recombinant DNA origin)

1 What is the difference among each of these four types of Humulin insulin? Which are fast acting, intermediate, or both?

_____

2 When reading two different numbers on the mixes, which number is the fast acting: the first or the second?

_____

Q: Ask Yourself

A: My Answer

Rapid- and Short-Acting Insulin Label Interpretation

RAPID PRACTICE 11-2

Estimated completion time: 10-15 minutes   **Answers on page 556**

Directions: *Read the information presented in the previous sections, examine the short-acting insulin labels on p. 358, and answer the questions briefly.*

1 If there is a chance that a meal will be delayed, which two of the fast-acting insulins should be held and given *with* the meal?

_____

2 **a.** What is the concentration of insulin on the labels? _____

   b. How many total units of insulin are contained in each vial? _____

3 What is the name of the ingredient needed to raise blood sugar levels promptly? _____

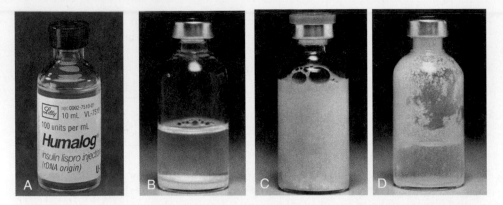

FIGURE 11-5 A, Humalog insulin should always look clear. **B,** Insulin at the bottom of the bottle. Do not use if insulin stays on the bottom of the bottle after gentle rolling. **C,** Clumps of insulin. Do not use if there are clumps of insulin in the liquid or on the bottom of the vial. **D,** Bottle appears frosted. Do not use if particles of insulin are on the bottom or sides of the bottle and give it a frosty appearance. (Copyright Eli Lilly and Company. All rights reserved. Used with permission.)

4   If the patient is experiencing a *hypo*glycemic episode, why should diet beverages and sugar alcohols not be given?

_____

_____

5   Which two of these insulins must be given 30 minutes before a meal?
  a. Novolin R
  b. Novolog (insulin aspart)
  c. Humulin R
  d. Humalog (insulin lispro)

➤ Only regular (R) insulins, insulin aspart (Novolog), and insulin glulisine (Apidra) can be administered *intravenously as well as subcutaneously.* They must be *clear,* without precipitates, for IV administration. They do not need to be rolled or shaken because they are not suspensions (see Figure 11-5).

➤ Humalog is clear but is not approved for IV use. Always check the label for the permitted routes of administration.

As with all multiuse vials, the nurse needs to write the *date and time opened* and her or his initials on the label. Discard the opened vial according to the product insert directions, after approximately a month. Consult product labels and inserts for more detailed information about storage, activity, expiration dates, and incompatibilities.

➤ Some of the labels say "Human Insulin" injection. They are not made from human pancreas. They are identical in structure to human insulin but are of rDNA origin.

➤ Do not confuse the capital letter *R* for *Regular* insulin with the small superscript ® indicating a registered product.

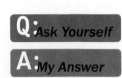

1   What would be expected to happen to the patient's blood sugar levels if Humulin R, Novolin R, insulin lispro, or insulin aspart were given and the meal was delayed?

_____

Intermediate-Acting Insulins

Usually patients receiving intermediate-acting products, including mixes, receive *two* injections a day—one in the morning and one in the evening—plus a bed-time snack of complex carbohydrate, such as a half a cheese sandwich or milk, to cover a potential hypoglycemic reaction from overlapping duration. Mixes are usually prescribed for specified periods of time before breakfast and dinner. Some are ordered AM and PM without time specification.

➤ Clarify AM and PM orders with the prescriber as to precise time desired.

Isophane Insulin Human (abbreviated as NPH or N) is a modified insulin suspension that provides delayed basal insulin release. It has a longer duration than the short-acting insulins. The additives that extend the action make the solutions cloudy, rendering them inappropriate for IV administration. Suspension label directions call for either rolling or gentle shaking of the vial to mix the ingredients before drawing up in a syringe. Read the manufacturer label.

They then must be given promptly. The additives extend the duration of coverage up to 26 hours, depending on the preparation (Figure 11-6).

1 What would happen to the solution in the syringe if there were a delay between drawing up the suspension and administering it?

_____

2 Why might people whose employment regularly or irregularly requires second- or third-shift hours need special assistance with their antidiabetic medication schedule?

_____

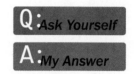

Q:*Ask Yourself*

A:*My Answer*

Intermediate-Acting Insulin Suspensions

RAPID PRACTICE 11-3

Estimated completion time: 5-10 minutes   **Answers on page 556**

Directions: *Read the foregoing material pertaining to intermediate-acting insulin products and answer the questions with brief phrases:*

1 How many injections of intermediate-acting insulins per day do people usually receive?_____

2 Can a suspension be administered intravenously in an emergency?

_____

3 What is the units per mL concentration on each intermediate product label in Figure 11-6?

_____

4 Would these intermediate-acting products be clear or cloudy?

_____

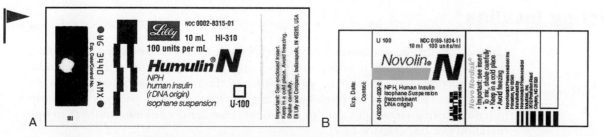

FIGURE 11-6 Intermediate-acting modified insulin suspensions.

5   Why do patients on insulin mixes and bedtime short-acting insulins require a bedtime snack of a complex carbohydrate? What potential adverse effect are they trying to avoid?

_____

_____

Short- and Intermediate-Acting Insulins: Insulin Fixed-Combination Mixes

Various insulin mixes combine rapid-acting with slower acting insulin that can help control insulin and glucose levels through the fluctuations that follow two meals and reduce the number of injections the patient takes. Fixed-combination premixes, such as those shown below, spare the patient from having to self-prepare two types of insulin separately and then combine them. The concentration of mix selected depends on the patient's usual blood glucose patterns and levels. Patients with unstable levels and patterns cannot use premixed insulins. They must adjust their insulin doses to a current blood glucose test for better glycemic control. Most patients take a larger amount of intermediate-acting (slower release) insulin and _less_ of the short rapid-acting, thus the 75/25 and 70/30 premixes.

Mixed insulins are taken twice a day at a _specific_ number of minutes before the morning and evening meal so that the short-acting part covers the first meal. Each injection covers two meals (or one meal and a bedtime controlled balanced snack.).

➤ The timing of the injection depends upon the type and specific onset of the _short-acting_ insulin.

➤ The intermediate- and long-acting insulins contain additives that make them unsuitable for IV administration.

= Humalog® Mix75/25™

Humalog mix **75/25**™

75% insulin lispro protamine suspension
25% insulin lispro injection (rDNA origin)

= Humalog® Mix50/50™

Humalog mix **50/50**™

50% insulin lispro protamine suspension
50% insulin lispro injection (rDNA origin)

= Humulin® 70/30

Humulin® 70/30
70% NPH and 30% Regular human insulin
(recombinant DNA origin)

Long-Acting Insulins

Long-acting insulin contains additives that cause it to be released more slowly than the fast- and intermediate-acting insulins. Long-acting insulin products are administered _subcutaneously_ to patients with type 1 or 2 diabetes whose blood glucose levels are unresponsive to intermediate-acting insulins, such as patients with early-morning fasting elevations, and/or to patients who cannot tolerate more than one injection per day (Figure 11-7).

➤ Long-acting insulins cannot be given IV because they contain additives to extend the action. These additives are not suitable for IV use.

Insulin glargine (Lantus) and insulin detemir (Levemir) are clear. They do *not* have a peak. They provide a steady release of insulin throughout the duration of 24-26 hours. For this reason, they are known as *basal* long-acting insulins.

➤ Insulin glargine and insulin detemir *cannot* be mixed with any other insulin even though they are clear solutions. They may be given at any hour but must be given at the *same* time each day to provide a steady release of basal (low-dose) insulin for 24 hours without a peak. If additional short-acting insulin is needed, it is administered subcutaneously as a bolus in a *separate* syringe.

Read the instructions on the Lantus label to the right.

➤ It is safest to assume that insulin products cannot *be mixed* until you read the drug literature for each order. New products are emerging on the market. Some may be mixed, and others may not. Nurses who frequently work with diabetic patients can integrate the capabilities of new products. Nurses who do not regularly work with diabetic patients cannot rely on memory. It is best to make a habit of always checking compatibilities with current drug literature and/or the pharmacy.

➤ Patients on evening fast-acting or any intermediate- or long-acting insulin should have a bedtime snack.

➤ There are no intermediate- or long-acting forms of Humalog or Novolog.

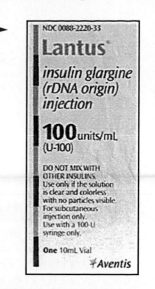

FIGURE 11-7 Lantus insulin.

Mnemonic

Lantus begins with an *L* and has a Long duration.

Long-Acting Insulin

RAPID PRACTICE **11-4**

Estimated completion time: 5-10 minutes   **Answers on page 556**

Directions: *Read the foregoing information about long-acting insulin products and answer the following questions in two- or three-word phrases.*

1 What is the generic name for Lantus insulin? _____

2 What is a unique feature of insulin glargine and insulin detemir?

_____

3 Can long-acting insulins be administered intravenously?

4 What is the concentration of the insulin glargine label shown above?

_____

5 Can insulin glargine or insulin detemir be mixed with any other insulin?

_____

Steps to Prepare Doses for Insulin Syringes

1 Obtain and/or interpret the current blood glucose value. Follow the prescriber's directions for blood glucose values. Withhold insulin if the blood glucose level is low according to the prescriber's directions and agency policy. Contact the prescriber promptly if directions for low values are not written in the orders, and document the verification.

2 Read the order for name, type, dose, time, and route. If you are using an opened bottle, check the discard date, as with all multidose vials.

3 Select the appropriate insulin and an insulin syringe that is calibrated for the *same* concentration (e.g., 100 units per mL).

4 Examine all medication vials for clumps and precipitates. Insulin may develop precipitates if the temperature is too warm, if the vial has been contaminated, or if it has passed the expiration date.

5 If the insulin is a suspension, *gently roll or* shake it to disperse the contents, according to the manufacturer's current recommendations. Rough shaking will cause air bubbles, which will alter the dose. Draw the appropriate amount of units in the insulin syringe using the technique learned for withdrawal of injectables from a vial.

Calculations are not needed for single insulin injections.

➤ Some agencies require two nurses for the *entire* preparation of all orders for insulin and other high-risk medications. They must cosign the MAR indicating that each step of the preparation of the ordered insulin dose is correct. Check agency policy. Refer to independent nurse check, p. 376.

Matching Insulin Concentration and Syringes

➤ The insulin syringe matches the number of units per mL on the label of the insulin bottle; for example, U-100 and 100 units per mL on the insulin bottle label and 100 units per mL on the syringe label. This is the most commonly used concentration in the United States.

Examine the following order: Give Novolin R 10 units subcut stat.

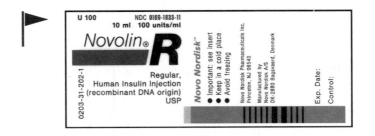

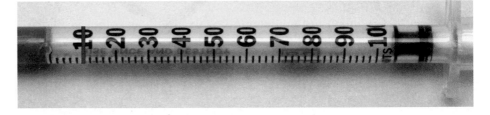

Examine the label. What is the brand name? *Novolin* R

What is the type (action)? *Short-acting (regular)*

Are there any terms not understood? Check current references and call the pharmacy if necessary.

How many total milliliters are there in the vial? *10 mL*

What is the concentration of drug to solution? *100 units per mL (U-100)*

How many total units in the vial? *10 mL × 100 units = 1000 units, a multidose vial*

Does this type of insulin need to be mixed or rolled? *No, because it is not a suspension.*

➤ Prepare insulin with an insulin syringe only.

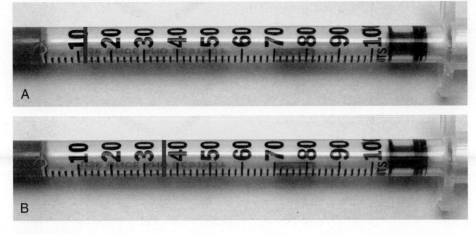

FIGURE 11-8 A, 100-unit insulin syringe marked at 12 units. **B,** 100-unit insulin syringe marked at 36 units.

Reading Units on Insulin Syringes

Insulin is manufactured, prescribed, and administered in units. The insulin syringe is calibrated in units.

Examine the syringes in Figure 11-8. The calibrations are for even amounts of insulin. Always note the total capacity of the syringe (1 mL, 100 units for this syringe), then ensure that the syringe calibrations are units, and finally note the number of calibrations between the markings. Reading the calibrated units on the insulin syringe is straightforward.

Each calibration represents *two* units on these 100 unit per 1 mL syringes.

Even- and Odd-Numbered Scales on Insulin Syringes

Syringes are available with calibrations in even numbers on one side and odd numbers on the other. There are also syringes available with either even or odd calibrations (Figure 11-9).

The dose administered must be in the *precise* number of units ordered. Each calibration is worth *2* units on the even- and on the odd-numbered scale.

➤ The standard insulin syringe calibrated in units, designed for a concentration of 100 units per mL, must be distinguished from the tuberculin syringe, which is also a 1-mL syringe calibrated in 0.01 mL (Figure 11-10).

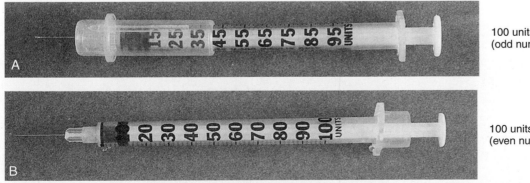

100 units per mL
(odd numbers)

100 units per mL
(even numbers)

FIGURE 11-9 A, Insulin Safety-Lok syringe calibrated in 100 units per mL with odd number markings up to 95 units. **B,** Insulin syringe calibrated in 100 units per mL with even number markings up to 100 units. (Used with permission from Becton, Dickinson and Company. Copyright 2003.)

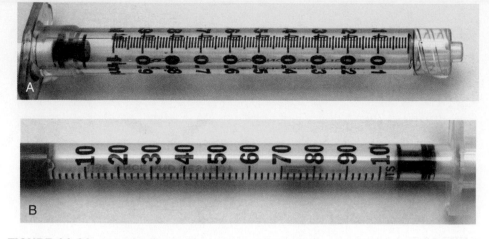

FIGURE 11-10 **A,** 1-mL tuberculin syringe calibrated in hundredths of a mL. **B,** 1-mL 100 units per mL insulin syringe calibrated in 2-unit increments.

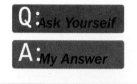

Q: *Ask Yourself*

A: *My Answer*

1 How will you know the difference between an insulin syringe and a tuberculin syringe?

_____

CLINICAL RELEVANCE

Several drugs, but not all, must be given at very precise times.

➤ Insulin is one of those drugs that must be *prioritized* to be given on time. Check insulin orders one or two times per shift. The orders change rapidly with the patient's response to treatment. Always know the patient's most recent blood glucose level.

Lo-Dose Syringes

Aging populations and patients with complications of diabetes often have diminished vision. Lo-Dose syringes are designed for persons with special visual needs. They allow for better visualization of the smaller doses.

➤ The Lo-Dose syringe is calibrated in 1-unit increments.

The syringe volume occupies 30 or 50 units and can be used by patients who are taking up to 30 or 50 units of insulin per dose (Figures 11-11 and 11-12).

➤ They are calibrated for U-100 insulin (100 units per mL).

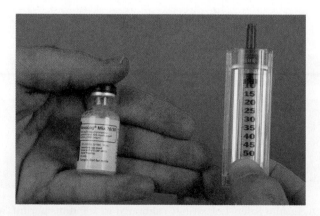

FIGURE 11-11 50-unit Lo-Dose insulin syringe with magnifier. (From Perry AG, Potter PA: *Clinical nursing skills and techniques,* ed. 5, St. Louis, 2004, Mosby.)

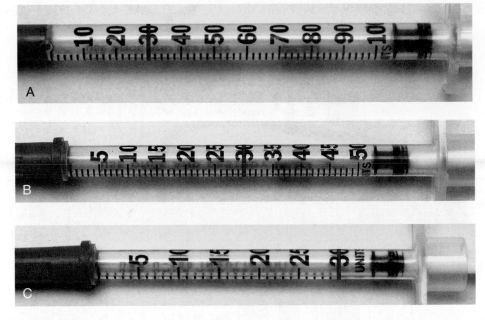

FIGURE 11-12 A, 30 units marked in a U-100 100-unit insulin syringe. **B,** 30 units marked in a U-100 50-unit Lo-Dose insulin syringe. **C,** 30 units drawn in a U-100 30-unit Lo-Dose insulin syringe.

1 What is the difference between the calibration of units on the 1-mL insulin syringe and that on the Lo-Dose syringe?

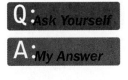

Q: *Ask Yourself*

A: *My Answer*

_____

Note the difference in visualization of 30 units of insulin drawn in each of the syringes in Figure 11-12.

Reading Units on an Insulin Syringe

RAPID PRACTICE 11-5

Estimated completion time: 10 minutes   Answers on page 556

Directions: *Read the syringe dose measurement in units and write the number of units in the space supplied for problems 1 and 2. For problems 3-5, mark the syringe with the ordered number of units. All of the syringes are calibrated for U-100 insulin.*

1 _____ units

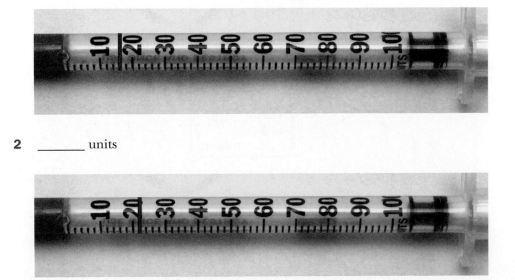

2 _____ units

3 Ordered: Humulin R insulin 7 units subcut ac breakfast. Mark the dose ordered.

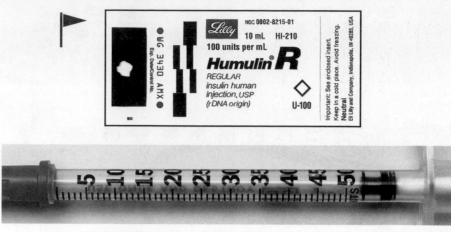

4 Ordered: Humulin N insulin 28 units subcut AM and PM. Mark the dose ordered.

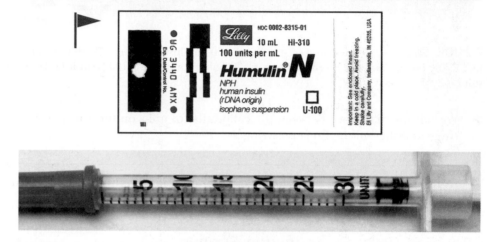

5 Ordered: insulin glargine 32 units subcut at bedtime daily. Mark the dose ordered.

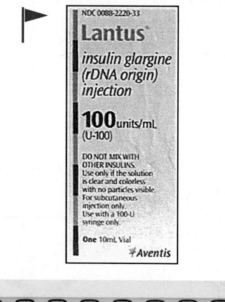

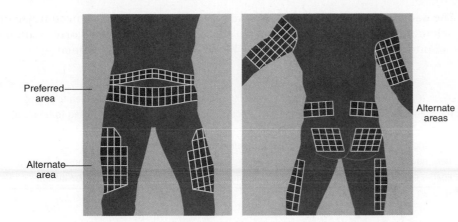

FIGURE 11-13 Insulin injection areas. (Copyright Eli Lilly and Company. All rights reserved. Used with permission.)

✱ Communication

"Which sites do you usually use for injection at home?"

➤ Use and rotate sites that the patient does not use at home (Figure 11-13). Document the site on the MAR.

Sites for Insulin Injection

Insulin may be administered subcutaneously in the fatty tissue of the abdomen in a radius 2 *inches away from the umbilicus,* in the thigh, in the fatty tissue of the posterior upper arm, or in the fatty tissue of the buttocks.

Sliding-Scale Insulin (SSI)

Sliding-scale short-acting insulins are titrated to *patients' current blood glucose* levels. They are usually ordered q6h for hospitalized patients on continuous liquid gastrointestinal tube feedings, or TPN.

They may also be ordered ac and bedtime to cover meal and bedtime glucose elevations for newly diagnosed patients until the patient can be stabilized on longer-acting insulins. The insulin dose "slides," or changes, with the most recent glucose levels. The scale is customized for each patient. Patterns of glucose elevations usually emerge.

Patients who experience difficult control of blood glucose levels may continue to cover elevated levels at mealtime on a sliding scale with bolus doses of short-acting insulin orders at home in addition to the longer-acting variety. The term *brittle diabetic* has been used to describe a patient who experiences poorly controlled blood glucose levels despite insulin therapy.

Examples of hand-held glucose monitors for bedside and home finger-stick draws of capillary blood are shown in Figure 11-14.

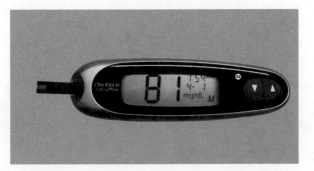

FIGURE 11-14 Life Scan One Touch® Ultra Mini®. Hand-held blood glucose monitor for finger or forearm stick with 50 test result memory.

The patient may draw blood under the supervision of an experienced nurse or may self-monitor and report the result to the nurse (SMBG). The correct sliding scale amount is drawn promptly after the blood glucose level is obtained.

CLINICAL RELEVANCE

Recheck a very low or high blood glucose level with a different monitoring device before acting on the reading. Examine the insulin bottle for discoloration if the product is supposed to be clear, and check it for particles. Ensure that a bottle that is supposed to be clear (Regular, insulin detemir, or insulin glargine) is clear, not cloudy. Suspensions will be cloudy.

There have been some cases where hospitalized patients who self-administered insulin had inexplicable elevations of blood glucose and were finally observed to be discarding the insulin rather than taking it. Observe patients' technique when they are self-administering.

EXAMPLES

Examine the following sample sliding scale for a hospitalized patient.

Ordered: Humulin R subcut per sliding scale q6h, for a patient on TPN.

Sliding Scale for Subcutaneous Short-Acting Insulin Administration

Blood Sugar (mg per dL)	Insulin Amount
70-150	0 units
151-200	4 units
201–250	6 units
251-300	10 units
301-350	12 units (Recheck blood glucose level 1 hr after administration.)
351-400	15 units (Recheck blood glucose level 1 hr after administration.)
>400	Call physician and draw plasma blood glucose.

Monitor the results. Blood glucose levels are checked by the nurse with the handheld device at the bedside unless a serum blood glucose lab test is ordered. This may be done to verify abnormal BG levels.

➤ Note the *small amounts* of fast-acting insulin to be given.

➤ The trend is to replace SSI with customized bolus-basal weight-based doses.

RAPID PRACTICE **11-6**

Interpreting Sliding-Scale Orders

Estimated completion time: 10 minutes   **Answers on page 557**

Directions: *Read the sliding scale in the example above and answer the questions with brief phrases.*

1 If a morning capillary BGM test reveals a level of 300 mg per dL, place an arrow on the syringe with the pointer touching the line for the amount of insulin you would prepare.

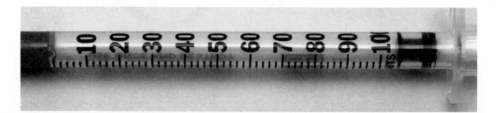

✳ Communication

"Mr. Y, your blood glucose is 180. Your physician has ordered 2 units of Novalin R for this blood glucose level." Always keep your patient informed about BG levels and type and dose of insulin. This is not only a teaching mechanism, it may prevent administration of a type or dose with which the patient has had an adverse event.

2   If the bedtime capillary BGM level was 330 mg per dL, what two actions would you take?*

_____

_____

3   If a BGM test before dinner indicated a blood glucose level >400 mg per dL, what two actions would you take?

_____

_____

4   What might be a reason that a plasma blood glucose test would be ordered from the laboratory instead of another capillary blood glucose test using the monitor at the bedside?

_____

5   If the sliding-scale blood glucose level was 140 mg per mL, what would the nurse do?

_____

_____

1   If the sliding scale was written 70-150, 150-200, 201-250, 250-300, 300-350, how much insulin would you give if the patient's blood glucose level was 150 mg per dL? With whom would you clarify this entire scale?

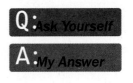

Q: *Ask Yourself*

A: *My Answer*

_____

➤   Separate flow sheets are usually maintained on the MAR for insulin administration. Table 11-2 provides examples of the information that may be contained on such a record.

FAQ | *Why is insulin not given for all blood glucose levels that are above normal?*

ANSWER | Smaller elevations may not be treated with insulin to avoid hypoglycemic reactions. Dietary and lifestyle adjustments may be ordered to control lower elevations.

---

*➤ Take care if the abbreviation HS (bedtime) is encountered. It has been mistaken for half strength.

TABLE 11-2	Subcutaneous Insulin Administration Flow Sheet

GENERAL HOSPITAL

John Doe
#528995

Date	Test Time	Test Result	Type of Test (BGM; SMBG; serum)	Insulin Type/Dose	Route/Location	Signature/ Title
1/1/11	0630	195	BGM	Novolog 4 units	subcut LA	Mark Smith, RN
1/1/11	1100	95	SMBG	0	N/A	Mark Smith, RN
1/1/11	1700	210	BGM	Novolog 5 units	subcut RA	Jan Carter, RN
1/1/11	2100	90	BGM /	0	N/A	Jan Carter, RN
1/2/11	0630	200	Serum FBS	Novolog 4 units	LT	Cal Pace, RN

BGM blood glucose monitor (capillary sample) performed by nurse
SMBG self blood glucose monitoring (by patient) (capillary sample)
Serum FBS fasting blood sugar (by lab or RN) (venous [serum] sample)

RAPID PRACTICE 11-7	*Interpreting Insulin Orders*

Estimated completion time: 10-15 minutes   **Answers on page 557**

Directions: *Examine the answers given to problem 1. Read and interpret the insulin orders in problems 2-5 as requested. Refer to the vocabulary list and the insulin activity chart in Table 11-1 if needed. Mark the syringes with the dose ordered if appropriate.*

1   Ordered: Humalog insulin lispro 6 units subcut tid 15 minutes ac for a patient with DM type 1.

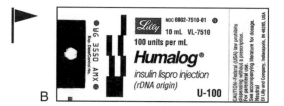

a. What is the recommended time to administer this dose in the hospital? <u>With the arrival of the meals.</u>
b. Why is this time recommended? <u>Because it is difficult to ensure the meal delivery within a 15-minute time frame.</u>
c. What is the concentration of the product as shown on the label? <u>U-100, 100 units per mL.</u>
d. Will the solution be clear or cloudy? <u>Clear.</u>
e. Which of the following syringes is shaded to the correct amount? <u>Syringe number 1.</u>

1.

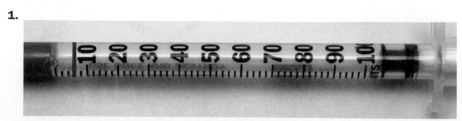

2.

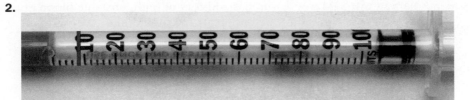

2 Ordered: Humulin N (NPH) 28 units subcut in AM daily for a patient with DM type 1.

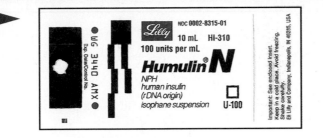

a. Is this a rapid- or intermediate-acting product? _____
b. Is it clear, or is it a suspension? _____
c. Does it need to be agitated before being withdrawn from the vial? _____
d. In how many hours will it peak? _____
e. By what route will it be administered? _____
f. Mark the syringe with the ordered dose.

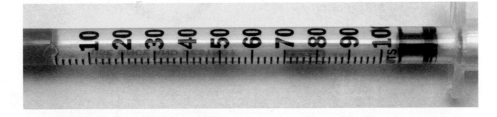

3 Ordered: Novolin R 10 units tid subcut ac, for a patient with a severe infection who has type 2 diabetes and poor vision. The nurse plans to assess the patient's ability to visualize the calibrations on a Lo-Dose syringe.

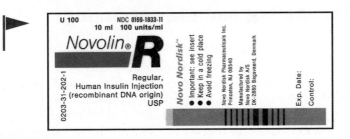

a. How long after administration will the action of this insulin action begin (onset)? _____
b. When will the action peak? _____
c. How long will it last? _____
d. Mark the syringe with the ordered dose.

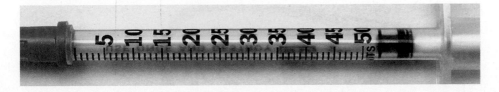

4 A patient with DM type 1 who has a history of high, unstable blood glucose levels is taking Humulin R before meals and at bedtime.

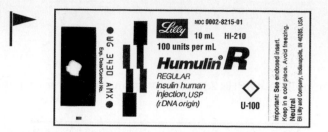

a. According to the label, how many total units of insulin are contained in the vial? _____

b. Is this a rapid- or intermediate-acting product? _____

c. What is the concentration? _____

5 Ordered: Novolin N 42 units subcut AM daily for a patient with DM type 1 maintenance.

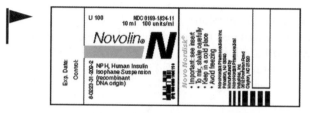

a. What route will be used to administer this order?

b. Mark the syringe with the ordered amount.

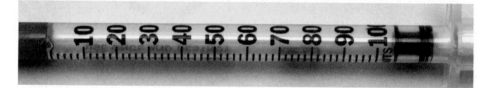

Mixing Insulins: Short Fast-Acting and Slower-Acting Intermediate Mixes

Mixed insulins provide blood glucose coverage for meals with a small amount of short-acting insulin and between-meal coverage with an added amount of slower-release, intermediate-acting insulin. They are administered subcutaneously. Insulin mixes may be ordered twice a day for patients until their blood glucose pattern is established or to provide additional coverage for postprandial blood glucose elevations.

As with all insulins, initial orders for intermediate mixes are conservative to prevent hypoglycemic episodes.

The trend is to prescribe one of the *fixed premixed* combinations available on the market.

Fixed premixed intermediate- and short-acting combination insulins

The *first* number of a fixed combination insulin mix indicates the *percentage* of slower-, *intermediate*-acting insulin. The second number indicates the *percentage* of short-, or *rapid*-acting insulin. The product label in Figure 11-15 illustrates this information.

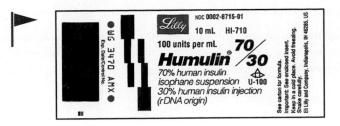

FIGURE 11-15 Humulin 70/30 insulin.

➤ If the order is for *10* units, 7 units (70% of 10 units) would contain NPH, the intermediate-acting insulin, and 3 units (30% of 10 units) would contain the fast-acting insulin.

These mixes are offered as a safe and convenient method for patients who would have difficulty drawing up injectable mixtures in a syringe. The amounts are small, and an error of even 1 unit can make a difference. In addition to ease of preparation, the premixed combinations reduce chance of error and save time. Most patients receive a larger amount of intermediate-acting insulin and a smaller amount of short-, rapid-acting insulin. Some patients need a 50/50 mix because of very high mealtime blood glucose elevations.

A premix order specifies the number of units based on the patient's need for each type. For example:

Humulin Mix 50/50, 10 units subcut 30 minutes ac breakfast and dinner.

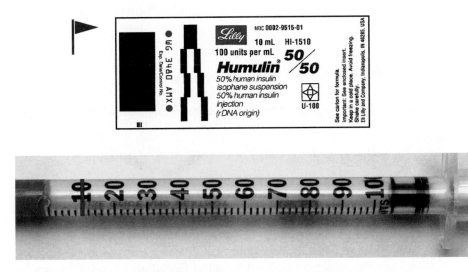

Novolin Mix 70/30, 18 units subcut 30 minutes ac breakfast and dinner.

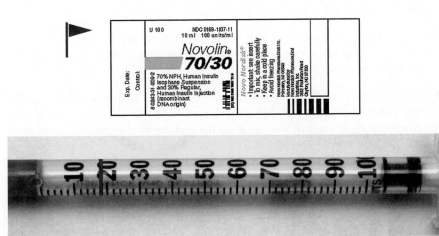

➤ Note that the order for a premixed insulin mix is in *total* number of units.

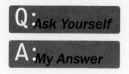

1 If you were giving 8 units of Humulin 50/50 insulin, how many units would contain intermediate-acting NPH insulin and how many units would contain fast-acting insulin?

_____

➤ ISMP recommends that two nurses do an independent check of drug and dose for all high risk medications *before* administration.

When the Mix Must Be Prepared by the Nurse

Occasionally, the nurse must prepare an insulin mix, drawing up two different insulins in one syringe. Regular and intermediate-acting insulins are the most common combination. They are bracketed or designated "Mix" in the order:

Humulin R 6 units
Humulin N 20 units ⎫ subcut bid AM and PM 30 minutes ac

Read both product labels to be sure they are compatible. Not all insulin brands can be mixed with others.

➤ Do not confuse Humulin products with Humalog.

Like the intermediate suspensions, the mixes need to be rolled or shaken gently but adequately until well mixed, according to the manufacturer's directions. Too vigorous shaking will result in extensive air bubble formation, making the dose inaccurate. The dose is less than 1 mL.

Technique for Preparing Insulin Mixes

The technique for preparing a mix requires practice and supervision under the direction of an instructor or experienced nurse. Prepare a mix according to the following text:

Check the order and compatibility of the two types of insulin.

1 Identify the vials, verify the orders, and place them in a meaningful order in front of you. Shake the intermediate suspension gently. Clean the tops of each vial with an alcohol swab.

2 Measure and insert air *equal* to the amount of ordered insulin into each vial, the intermediate-acting insulin *first,* followed by the short-acting insulin, with the syringe to be used for administration. Keep the bottles on the counter to insert the air into the air at the top of the vial. Inserting air into the liquid will create air bubbles.

3 ➤ Always withdraw the clear, short-acting insulin *first* to protect the vial from contamination. A very small amount of intermediate-acting insulin can alter the action of the short-acting insulin. Verify the amount.

4 After withdrawing the ordered amount of regular insulin, gently mix the suspension according to label directions and withdraw exactly the amount ordered. Gently tap out any air bubbles and verify the precise combined amount. If the total amount is incorrect, discard the syringe and start over. One extra unit is 1 unit too much.

➤ Protect the short-acting insulin vials from contamination by withdrawing from them first. Do not allow distractions during this procedure (Figure 11-16).

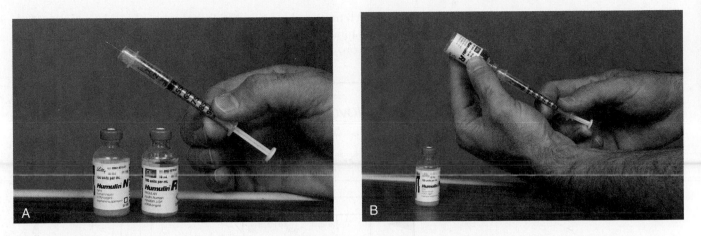

FIGURE 11-16 A, Vials of intermediate- or long-acting insulin and rapid- or short-acting insulin and syringe with air aspirated. **B,** Withdrawal of regular insulin. Always withdraw the regular insulin first after the vials have been prepared. (From Perry AG, Potter PA: *Clinical nursing skills and techniques,* ed. 7, St. Louis, 2010, Mosby.)

In addition to verifying labels, it may be helpful to remember the sequence with the following table, keeping in mind that *cloudy* refers to intermediate suspension preparations and *clear* refers to short-acting preparations:

Step 1	Step 2	Step 3	Step 4
Air in	Air in	Withdraw short-acting	Withdraw intermediate-acting
Cloudy	Clear	Clear	Cloudy

This sequence permits the nurse to proceed from step 2 to step 3 with the short-acting preparation without removing the needle from the vial.

The following is an example of a mixture of 24 units of Humulin N plus 6 units of Humulin R, for a total dose of 30 units.

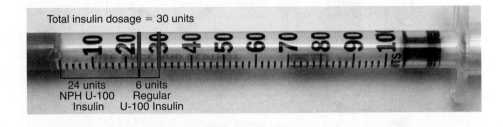

Total insulin dosage = 30 units

24 units
NPH U-100
Insulin

6 units
Regular
U-100 Insulin

FAQ | *How can I remember which insulin products can be mixed and which cannot?*

ANSWER | ➤ Always read the product label and inserts. Consult the pharmacy if necessary. Do not rely solely on the prescriber's order. In general, remember that a mix consists of a short-acting and an intermediate-acting insulin of the same brand and that the long-acting insulin glargine and insulin detemir cannot be mixed with any other insulin.

Short- and Intermediate-Acting Insulin Mixes

RAPID PRACTICE 11-8

Estimated completion time: 15 minutes   **Answers on page 558**

Directions: *Read the explanation of short-acting and intermediate-acting insulin mixes on p. 374 and study the illustrations. Examine the answers provided for problem 1 and complete problems 2-5 in a similar manner.*

1   Ordered: Novolin R 6 units and Novolin N 20 units subcut bid AM and PM. Mark the syringe with the total amount. Place an arrow touching the intermediate-acting dose calibration.

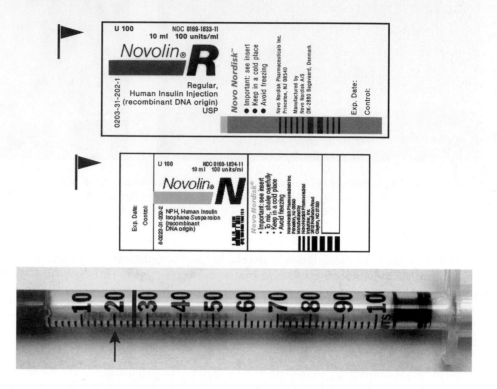

2   Ordered: Humulin N 30 units and Humulin R 4 units subcut bid AM and PM. Mark the syringe with the total amount. Place an arrow touching the intermediate-acting dose calibration.

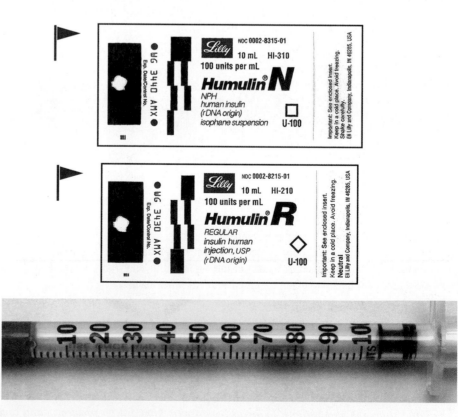

3   Ordered: Novolin R 2 units and Novolin N 16 units subcut AM and PM. Mark the syringe with the total amount. Place an arrow touching the intermediate-acting dose calibration.

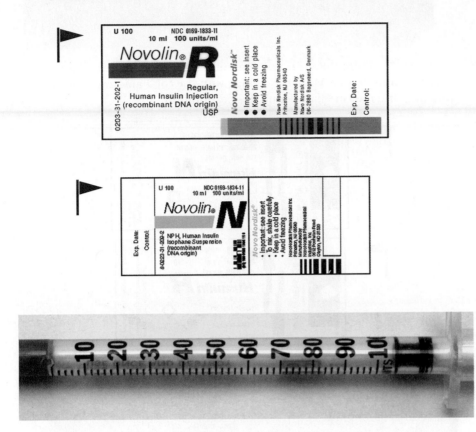

4   Ordered: Novolin R 10 units and Novolin N 42 units subcut 30 min ac breakfast and dinner. Mark the syringe with the total amount. Place an arrow touching the intermediate-acting dose calibration.

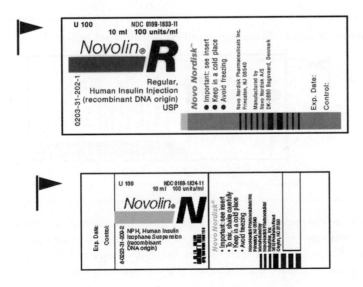

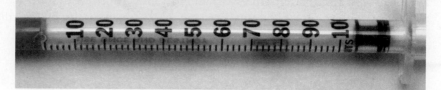

5 Ordered: Humulin R 8 units and Humulin N 24 units subcut 30 minutes ac breakfast and dinner. Mark the syringe with the total amount. Place an arrow touching the intermediate-acting dose calibration.

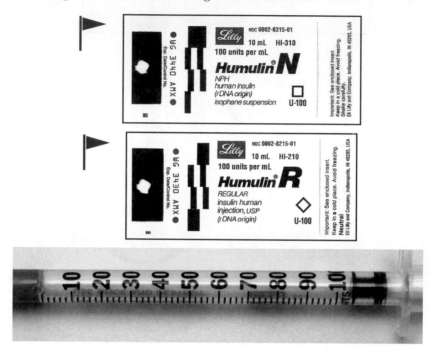

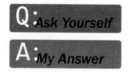

1 How many units per mL are supplied in the labels shown above?

2 How many units per milliliter are supplied in the label below?

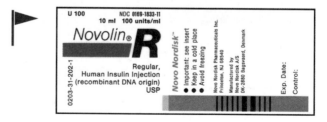

A few patients with severe DM type 1 who must have very large amounts of insulin, over 100 units per dose, may be prescribed U-500 insulin (500 units per mL) to reduce the volume of the injections and spare the injection sites. This is not a common order and is usually administered only in the hospital.

Intravenous Insulin Infusions

Insulin infusions are administered in the hospital for acute hyperglycemia. Many agencies publish their own standard for the concentration of an insulin infusion, either 1 unit per mL or 0.5 unit per mL, in 0.9% NaCl solution.

➤ Use a fresh, unopened bottle of Regular or Humalog insulin, whichever is ordered, to prepare the infusion.

A label with the number of units and concentration needs to be attached to the IV solution, as with all other medicated IV solutions. Insulin should be administered on its own separate line.

When the concentration is 100 units in 100 mL of 0.9% NaCl (1 unit per mL) or 50 units in 100 mL of 0.9% NaCl (0.5 unit per mL), it is *very helpful* to estimate the flow rate in milliliters per hour using mental arithmetic. Remember that the flow rate cannot be calculated until the concentration of the solution in units per milliliter is known. Verify the estimate with a DA equation.

Infuse	Concentration	Flow Rate
0.5 units per hr	100 units per 100 mL, or 1 unit per 1 mL	0.5 mL per hr
3 units per hr	100 units per 100 mL, or 1 unit per 1 mL	3 mL per hr
1 unit per hr	50 units per 100 mL, or 0.5 unit per 1 mL	2 mL per hr
3 units per hr	50 units per 100 mL, or 0.5 unit per 1 mL	6 mL per hr

EXAMPLES

The flow rates are very low, and with a 1:1 (1 unit to 1 mL, or 100 units to 100 mL) concentration, the number of units ordered per hour is equal to the mL per hr flow rate.

➤ Use an IV pump for IV insulin administration.

Ordered: Humulin R IV infusion 5 units per hr, recheck BG 1 hr and call office.

$$\frac{mL}{hr} = \frac{\cancel{100}\ mL}{\cancel{100\ units}} \times \frac{5\ \cancel{units}}{1\ hr} = 5\ mL\ per\ hr$$

EXAMPLES

➤ Check orders frequently for changes. Changes are common in acute-care situations. Monitor blood glucose levels at least every hour or more often, according to agency protocol. Report low and high blood glucose levels and unusual changes promptly. Follow the prescriber's and agency's directions for treatment. Document the instructions. Know where a 50% dextrose injection and/or a glucagon injection is available for hypoglycemic emergencies (Figure 11-17).

CLINICAL RELEVANCE

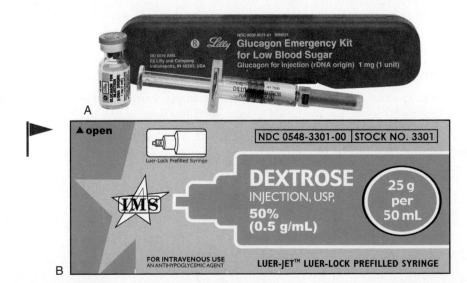

A

B

FIGURE 11-17 A, Glucagon emergency kit. **B,** Dextrose 50%. (**A,** Copyright Eli Lilly and Company. All rights reserved. Used with permission.)

Communication

Nurse to readmitted diabetic patient with very high glucose levels:
"Mrs. Evans, What has been the hardest part about managing your diabetes? (Listen) What has worked for you in the past to bring the glucose levels down? What hasn't worked? (spares giving unneeded nontherapeutic advice) What sort of changes might work for you after you go home? (Do they have a plan?)

RAPID PRACTICE **11-9** *IV Infusions*

Estimated completion time: 20 minutes   Answers on page 558

Directions: *Study the foregoing examples. Calculate the flow rate with mental arithmetic if possible and verify with a written DA equation. Use a calculator for long division and multiplication. Label answers.*

1 Ordered: Humulin R insulin IV at 3 units per hr. Available: Humulin R insulin 100 units in 100-mL 0.9% NaCl solution.

   a. Estimated flow rate in mL per hr? _____
   b. Ordered flow rate in mL per hr? _____

     DA equation:

   c. Evaluation: _____

2 Ordered: IV at 4 units per hr, for a patient with a glucose level of 325 mg per dL. Available: 50 units Novolin R insulin in 100 mL 0.9% NaCl solution.

   a. Estimated flow rate in mL per hr? _____
   b. Ordered flow rate in mL per hr? _____

     DA equation:

   c. Evaluation: _____

3 Ordered: Humulin R insulin IV at 6 units per hr, for a patient with a glucose level of 400 mg per dL. Draw a plasma glucose test stat to verify the capillary monitor level and recheck in 1 hour. Available: 50 units Humulin R insulin in 100 mL 0.9% NaCl solution.

   a. Estimated flow rate in mL per hr? _____
   b. Ordered flow rate in mL per hr? _____

     DA equation:

   c. Evaluation: _____

4 Ordered: to wean the patient (refer to example in problem 3) and reduce the flow rate by 50% because the blood glucose level has dropped to 185 mg per dL.

   a. Estimated flow rate in mL per hr? _____
   b. Ordered flow rate in mL per hr? _____

     DA equation:

   c. Evaluation: _____

5 Ordered: Novolin R insulin IV at 2 units per hr. Infusing: IV of D5W 100 mL with 50 units Novolin II R insulin added. It is flowing at 2 mL per hr.

   a. Estimated flow rate ordered: _____

   b. Ordered flow rate in mL per hr? _____

     DA equation:

   c. Evaluation: _____

   d. What nursing actions, if any, should be taken? _____

Insulin Differences

Estimated completion time: 10-15 minutes   **Answers on page 559**

Directions: *Answer the questions pertaining to the differences among the insulin solutions available.*

1 **a.** Which are the only types of insulin that may be given intravenously?

    _____

   b. Are they clear or cloudy in the bottle? _____

2 Which two types of insulin within the same brand are most frequently given in mixed combination: short-, intermediate-, or long-acting?

   _____

3 **a.** What are the two concentrations of insulin supplied? _____

   b. Of the two, which one is more commonly used? _____

4 Are there intermediate- or long-acting forms of Humalog or Novolog?

   _____

5 **a.** When short- and intermediate-acting insulin are combined, which of the two is usually given in the larger dose? _____

   b. Why do you think this is so? _____

Insulin Administration Devices

New products on the market are developed to make insulin administration more convenient, easier, and less painful.

- Finer needles are being developed to reduce the discomfort of injections (Figure 11-18).

Prefilled pens

Prefilled insulin pens contain regular insulin, intermediate-acting insulin, and mixtures of the two for ease of use by patients who have difficulty manipulating syringe equipment. They are also used for low-vision patients. The dose can be dialed easily. Pens are less noticeable than are syringes for injection in public places (Figure 11-19).

   The InnoLet is a hand-held device used with either the NovoFine® 30G or NovoFine® 31G needles to administer subcutaneous insulin. Prefilled with 300 units available in two types of insulin, the large dial permits easy visualization of the number of units to administer. A window provides an estimate of how much insulin remains. This device eliminates the need to prepare an individual syringe for administration (Figure 11-20).

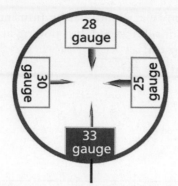

BD Ultra-Fine™ 33 Lancet (magnified)

FIGURE 11-18 BD Ultra-Fine™ 33 Lancet. Prefilled pens are convenient for work and travel. They are also used for patients with poor vision. (From Becton, Dickinson and Company, Franklin Lakes, NJ.)

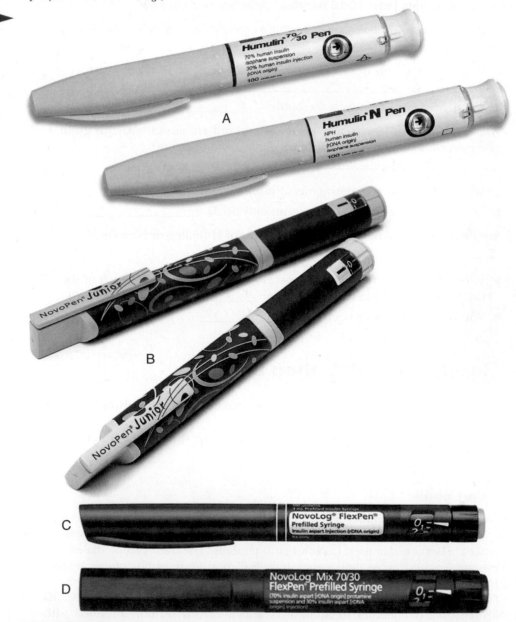

FIGURE 11-19 **A,** Humulin® 70/30 and Humulin® N insulin pens. **B,** NovoPen® Junior. **C,** NovoLog® FlexPen®. **D,** NovoLog® Mix 70/30 FlexPen®. (**A,** Copyright Eli Lilly and Company. All rights reserved. Used with permission. **B, C,** and **D,** From Novo Nordisk Inc., Princeton, NJ.)

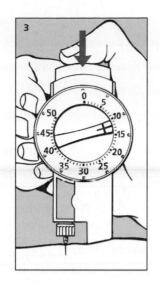

FIGURE 11-20 InnoLet®. (From Novo Nordisk Inc., Princeton, NJ.)

Teaching patients about diabetes is a challenge. Consider all the content in this chapter, which is limited to medication administration only. The diabetic patient has a great deal more to learn about the disease than just medication administration. The patient most often is not a health-care professional. Usually it is helpful to plan the teaching around the reason for hospitalization: is this a newly diagnosed patient, or did illness, travel, or noncompliance with the medication regimen cause the hospitalization in a person who has had diabetes for a long time? What is the patient's assessment of the reason for hospitalization?

CLINICAL RELEVANCE

Insulin pumps

Insulin pumps are devices worn by patients who are unresponsive to intermittent sub-cutaneous injections and need more frequent administration to maintain control of glucose levels (Figure 11-21). Two types are available: implantable and portable. A programmed, continuous, subcutaneously injected basal (flat, low, continuous) dose of fast-acting insulin is delivered through a subcutaneous access site throughout the day and night. The basal dose does not cover mealtime needs or other elevations. Added boluses are administered on the pump to cover meals and glucose elevations.

➤ Only short-acting insulins are used in insulin pumps. Frequent blood glucose monitoring is recommended for these patients to normalize their glucose levels. A continuous monitoring device is now on the market. This allows rapid dosage adjustments for better glucose control.

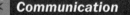
✳ Communication

"What brought you to the hospital?" "Has this happened before?" "What has been the most difficult part of this disease for you?" "What parts of the diet are difficult?" Be prepared to listen to the patient's answers to these questions. Then, assess the teaching needs and formulate a prioritized practical teaching plan that takes into account what the patient already knows and urgently needs to know.

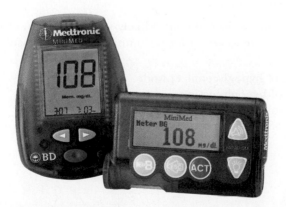

FIGURE 11-21 Paradigm Link® blood glucose monitor and Paradigm® 515 insulin pump. (From Medtronic, Minneapolis, MN.)

CHAPTER 11 MULTIPLE-CHOICE REVIEW

Estimated completion time: 30 minutes   Answers on page 559

Directions: *Select the best answer for the following questions.*

1 Which insulin must never be mixed with any other? _____

    1. Humulin N

    2. Humalog

    3. Novolin R

    4. glargine (Lantus)

2 Which route is most commonly prescribed for administering insulin?

_____

    1. Intradermal

    2. Subcutaneous

    3. Intramuscular

    4. Intravenous

3 Which types of insulin should be clear? _____

    1. Regular, insulin glargine, and insulin detemir

    2. Humulin N

    3. All insulin preparations

    4. Novolin N

4 At which level of blood glucose may a patient be likely to experience symptoms of hypoglycemia? _____

    1. >400 mg per dL

    2. 100-200 mg per dL

    3. 100 mg per dL

    4. <70 mg per dL

5 How may a nurse's action be *most likely* to cause a hypoglycemic episode for a patient? _____

    1. Administer too low a dose of insulin for a patient of a particular weight.

    2. Give a dextrose-containing beverage to a patient.

    3. Administer a dose of regular or fast-acting insulin that is not followed by a meal.

    4. Set up an insulin pump for a patient with the prescribed basal dose.

6 What does a prepared insulin mix such as Humulin N 70/30 contain?

_____

    1. Lower doses than if each insulin was administered separately

    2. 70% fast-acting insulin and 30% intermediate-acting insulin

    3. 100% Humulin N

    4. 70% intermediate-acting insulin and 30% fast-acting insulin

7 Which insulin schedule requires a bedtime snack? _____

    1. Regular insulin in the morning and before lunch

    2. Short-acting insulin before lunch

    3. Intermediate-, long-acting, and any evening insulins

    4. Insulin lispro before lunch

8 Which explanation reflects the most likely serious and unwelcome result of reversing the dosage for an order for 6 units of Regular Insulin and 30 units of NPH? _____

    1. Early onset of hypoglycemic episode

    2. Late onset of hypoglycemic episode

    3. Early onset of hyperglycemic episode

    4. Late onset of hyperglycemic episode

9 What expectation is reasonable for nurses to have about most prescribed doses of fast-acting insulin? _____

    1. They are usually high doses.
    2. They are usually low doses.
    3. They are always combined with intermediate-acting insulins.
    4. They contain additives to extend their action.

10 Which word best describes the major effect of insulin overdose? _____

    1. Hypotension
    2. Hyperglycemia
    3. Hypoglycemia
    4. Polyuria

CHAPTER 11 FINAL PRACTICE

Estimated completion time: 1-1½ hours   **Answers on page 559**

Directions: *Answer the following questions using DA equations to verify doses and flow rates. Use a calculator for long division and multiplication. Label answers.*

1 a. What is the most common concentration of insulin preparations? _____

    b. When preparing an insulin mix, which insulin must be protected and withdrawn first from the vial? _____

    c. Why? _____

2 Ordered: Novolin N 30 units subcut AM and PM, 30 minutes before meals. Select the appropriate syringe. Draw an arrow touching the calibration for the correct dose.

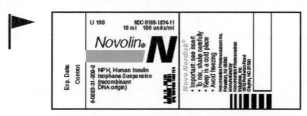

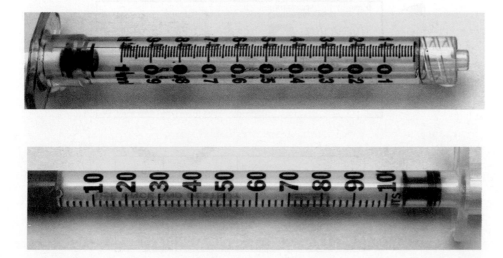

3 Ordered:

Humulin R 10 units
Humulin N 44 units } subcut 30 minutes before breakfast and dinner.

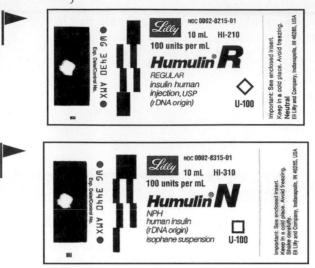

a. Which insulin will you withdraw first? _____
b. Mark the syringe to the total dose. Place an arrow touching the calibration for the amount of intermediate-acting insulin.

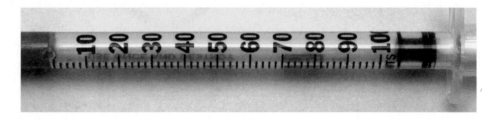

4 Ordered:

Novolin R 6 units
Novolin N 20 units } subcut 30 minutes before breakfast and dinner.

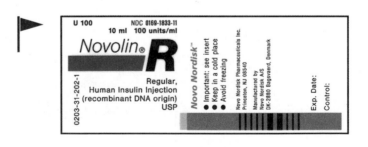

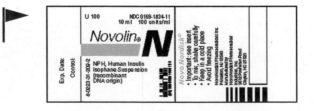

a. Which insulin will you withdraw first? _____

b. Mark the syringe to the total dose. Place an arrow touching the calibration for the amount of intermediate-acting insulin.

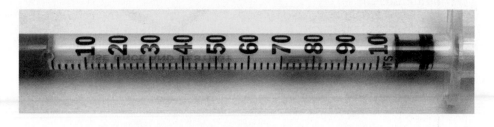

5 Ordered: insulin lispro 6 units tid 10 minutes before meals.

a. Is this a rapid-, intermediate-, or long-acting insulin?

_____

b. Place an arrow touching the calibration for the amount of the insulin.

Problems 6-9 refer to the patient in problem 6.

6 Ordered: Humulin Regular insulin IV infusion in 0.9% NaCl to start at rate of 5 units per hr, for a patient with a blood level glucose >400 mg per dL. Available: Humulin Regular 100 units per 100 mL of 0.9% NaCl solution. Obtain BGM test results every hour. Discontinue any other insulin orders.

a. How many units per mL are contained in the available solution?

_____

b. Estimate the flow rate with mental arithmetic and verify with a DA equation. _____

DA equation:

c. Evaluation: _____

d. Should the infusion be administered on a electronic infusion pump?

_____

7 The patient referred to in problem 6 has a blood glucose level of 325 mg per dL.

   a. Using the sliding scale below, what flow rate in milliliters per hour will be administered? _____

Blood Glucose Level (mg per dL)	Infusion Rate (units per hr)
151-200	1
201-250	2
251-300	3
301-400	4
>400	5

   b. Use a DA equation to back up mental arithmetic flow rate estimate. _____

   DA equation:

   c. Evaluation: _____

8 The physician also orders an IV of D5W at 100 mL per hr to avoid hypoglycemia while on insulin infusion. This IV solution has a small amount of glucose in it.

   a. How many grams of glucose are contained in a 1000-mL container of D5W?

   DA equation:

   b. Evaluation: _____

9 The next blood glucose level obtained for the patient in problem 7 is 210 mg per dL. The order calls for decreasing the flow rate by 50%. Refer to problem 7 flow rate sliding scale.

   a. Estimate the rate the nurse will set on the pump and verify with a DA equation. _____

   DA equation:

   b. Evaluation: _____

10 a. What are the three major types of exogenous insulin available in terms of onset of insulin activity in the body?

   _____

   b. What type of nutrient will the nurse promptly administer if the patient is conscious, is symptomatic, and can swallow and the blood glucose level falls below 70 mg per dL?

   _____

Suggestions for Further Reading

www.bd.com
www.diabetes.niddk.nih.gov/dm
www.diabetes.org
www.diabetes.org/diabetes-statistics/prevalence.jsp
www.hospira.com
www.ismp.org
www.jointcommission.org
www.joslin.org
www.lillydiabetes.com
www.medtronic.com
www.revolutionhealth.com/conditions/diabetes
www.novonordisk-us.com

 Additional practice problems can be found in the Advanced Calculations section of the Student Companion on Evolve.

Chapter 12 focuses on anticoagulants, high-alert drugs that are also delivered in units. Many of the principles learned in this chapter can be applied to Chapter 12.

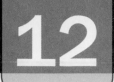

> *"Our greatest weakness lies in giving up. The most certain way to succeed is to try just one more time."*
>
> —THOMAS EDISON

⚑ Anticoagulant Agents

OBJECTIVES

- Differentiate oral and parenteral anticoagulant agents and related tests.
- Calculate doses for oral and parenteral anticoagulant agents.
- Evaluate and titrate anticoagulant doses based upon relevant laboratory tests.
- Identify antidotes for anticoagulant therapy.
- Identify critical patient safety issues related to anticoagulant therapy.

Essential Prior Knowledge

- Mastery of Chapters 1-11

Essential Equipment

- None needed

Estimated Time To Complete Chapter

- 1-2 hours

☐ Introduction

As noted with the prior chapter on antidiabetic agents, safe administration of these high-alert anticoagulants requires comprehension of the underlying theory of action of the medications, the differences, the antidotes, related pathophysiologic conditions, and relevant clinical assessments including interpretation of laboratory results. There have been many preventable adverse drug events (ADE)/sentinel events with anticoagulants. The calculations are relatively simple but, due to variations in patients' dose response, the dose must be carefully titrated based on results of frequent patient-based laboratory testing. The goal is to extend clotting time sufficiently to prevent adverse clotting events. Normal clotting time poses a risk of thromboembolic events for a variety of conditions.

Anticoagulants are now prescribed for many conditions, for example:

- Prolonged immobility
- Pre-, intra-, and postoperative lower extremity orthopedic surgery
- Potential, intra-, and post-cardiac events, such as arrhythmias, myocardial infarcts, and cardiac surgery
- Intra- and post-pelvic surgery
- History of thromboembolic conditions, such as deep vein thromboses, pulmonary emboli, and stroke
- Maintenance of patency of selected IV lines

Nurses are expected to evaluate and administer oral, subcutaneous, and IV anticoagulants. These medications may be encountered in the hospital, clinic, office, and home settings.

Students need to consult pharmacology, pathophysiology, and medical surgical nursing texts, as well as clinical skills texts, for complete understanding of anticoagulant therapy. Clinical mentors are required for supervised experience and practice of the skills required for safe anticoagulation therapy.

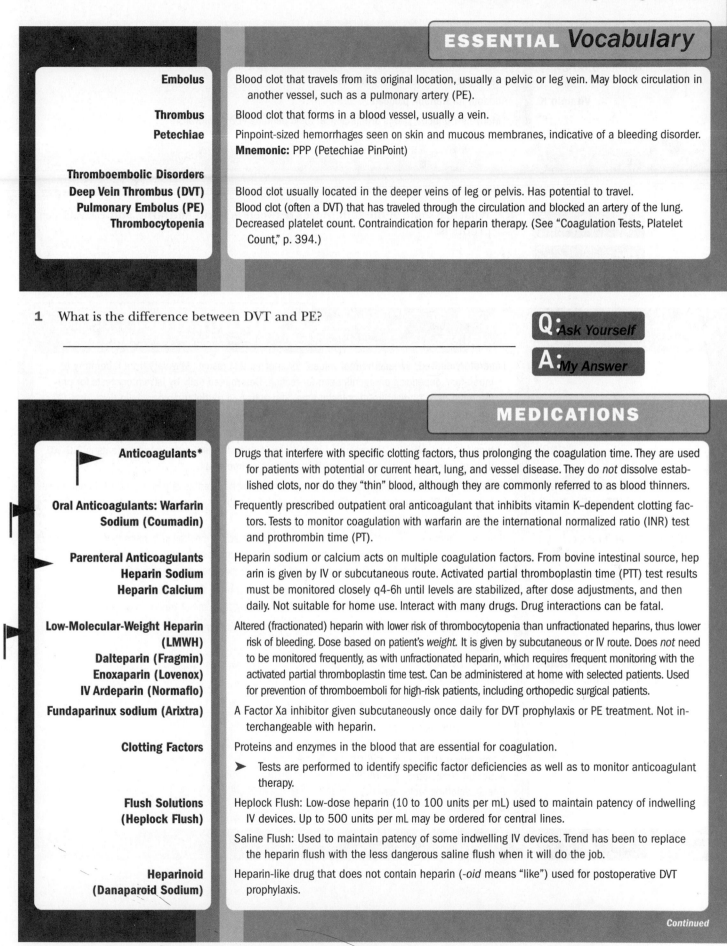

ESSENTIAL *Vocabulary*

Embolus	Blood clot that travels from its original location, usually a pelvic or leg vein. May block circulation in another vessel, such as a pulmonary artery (PE).
Thrombus	Blood clot that forms in a blood vessel, usually a vein.
Petechiae	Pinpoint-sized hemorrhages seen on skin and mucous membranes, indicative of a bleeding disorder. **Mnemonic:** PPP (Petechiae PinPoint)
Thromboembolic Disorders	
Deep Vein Thrombus (DVT)	Blood clot usually located in the deeper veins of leg or pelvis. Has potential to travel.
Pulmonary Embolus (PE)	Blood clot (often a DVT) that has traveled through the circulation and blocked an artery of the lung.
Thrombocytopenia	Decreased platelet count. Contraindication for heparin therapy. (See "Coagulation Tests, Platelet Count," p. 394.)

1   What is the difference between DVT and PE?

_____

Q: *Ask Yourself*

A: *My Answer*

MEDICATIONS

⚑ **Anticoagulants***	Drugs that interfere with specific clotting factors, thus prolonging the coagulation time. They are used for patients with potential or current heart, lung, and vessel disease. They do *not* dissolve established clots, nor do they "thin" blood, although they are commonly referred to as blood thinners.
⚑ **Oral Anticoagulants: Warfarin Sodium (Coumadin)**	Frequently prescribed outpatient oral anticoagulant that inhibits vitamin K–dependent clotting factors. Tests to monitor coagulation with warfarin are the international normalized ratio (INR) test and prothrombin time (PT).
⚑ **Parenteral Anticoagulants Heparin Sodium Heparin Calcium**	Heparin sodium or calcium acts on multiple coagulation factors. From bovine intestinal source, heparin is given by IV or subcutaneous route. Activated partial thromboplastin time (PTT) test results must be monitored closely q4-6h until levels are stabilized, after dose adjustments, and then daily. Not suitable for home use. Interact with many drugs. Drug interactions can be fatal.
⚑ **Low-Molecular-Weight Heparin (LMWH) Dalteparin (Fragmin) Enoxaparin (Lovenox) IV Ardeparin (Normaflo)**	Altered (fractionated) heparin with lower risk of thrombocytopenia than unfractionated heparins, thus lower risk of bleeding. Dose based on patient's *weight.* It is given by subcutaneous or IV route. Does *not* need to be monitored frequently, as with unfractionated heparin, which requires frequent monitoring with the activated partial thromboplastin time test. Can be administered at home with selected patients. Used for prevention of thromboemboli for high-risk patients, including orthopedic surgical patients.
Fundaparinux sodium (Arixtra)	A Factor Xa inhibitor given subcutaneously once daily for DVT prophylaxis or PE treatment. Not interchangeable with heparin.
Clotting Factors	Proteins and enzymes in the blood that are essential for coagulation.
	➤ Tests are performed to identify specific factor deficiencies as well as to monitor anticoagulant therapy.
Flush Solutions (Heplock Flush)	Heplock Flush: Low-dose heparin (10 to 100 units per mL) used to maintain patency of indwelling IV devices. Up to 500 units per mL may be ordered for central lines.
	Saline Flush: Used to maintain patency of some indwelling IV devices. Trend has been to replace the heparin flush with the less dangerous saline flush when it will do the job.
Heparinoid (Danaparoid Sodium)	Heparin-like drug that does not contain heparin (*-oid* means "like") used for postoperative DVT prophylaxis.

Continued

Protamine Sulfate	Antidote for heparin and heparinoid drugs.
Thrombolytic Agents	Drugs that "lyse," or dissolve, clots if given within a specified amount of time. Used for patients with acute stroke or pulmonary embolism.
Vitamin K	Antidote for warfarin products.
	*Many new anticoagulants are in clinical trials pending FDA approval.

Q: *Ask Yourself*

A: *My Answer*

1 What are some of the differences between heparin, warfarin, and LMWH products?

_____

COAGULATION *Tests*

Control Values	Laboratory derived "average normal values" for specific test results. May vary from laboratory to laboratory, depending on agents used for testing. Determined daily by laboratory tests for prothrombin time, partial thromboplastin time, and activated partial thromboplastin time tests to ensure efficacy of agents used for each batch of tests for accurate measurement.
International Normalized Ratio (INR)	Standardized formula-derived laboratory value *preferred* for monitoring *warfarin* therapy. Normal blood has an INR of 1. Therapeutic target range for blood of anti-coagulated patients is 2.0-3.0 INR value, derived from patient-specific prothrombin time value.
Prothrombin Time (PT, or Pro Time)	Formerly used for monitoring warfarin therapy, it now may be used as adjunct to INR. It is not as reliable as INR. Normal control values in *uncoagulated* patients vary from laboratory to laboratory by from 11 to 15 seconds.
Activated Partial Thromboplastin Time (aPTT)	*Shortened* form of the PT test with activators added, *preferred* for monitoring *heparin* therapy, *not* to be confused with PT test for warfarin or the longer partial thromboplastin time (PTT) test. "Normal" control aPTT time is about 30-40 seconds (about $\frac{1}{2}$ minute), depending on test agents used.
Platelet Count	Actual count of number of thrombocytes in blood (normal adult value, 150,000-400,000 per mcL). Less than 50,000 per mcL poses risk of bleeding from minor trauma and surgery.
	Less than *20,000* per mcL poses *great risk* of spontaneous hemorrhage.
Other Tests that May Be Ordered for Patients Receiving Anticoagulant Therapy or Those with Coagulation Disorders	Bleeding time Hematocrit (Hct) Hemoglobin (Hgb) Stool test for occult blood Urine test for blood Liver function tests (LFTs) Renal function tests Whole blood clotting time (WBCT) Activated coagulation time (ACT) Specific clotting factor assays D-dimer test

1 What is the preferred test for patients receiving heparin products, as opposed to the test for those receiving warfarin products?

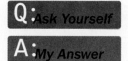

_____

2 What is the main risk for patients who have thrombocytopenia?

_____

FAQ | *What is the difference between a normal (control) value for a PT or an aPTT and a therapeutic level?*

ANSWER | The normal control value is the coagulation time in seconds for a specific test, such as the aPTT, for a person who is *not* receiving anticoagulants. It varies from test to test and laboratory to laboratory, depending on the agents used for the test.

When patients receive anticoagulants, they receive a *"therapeutic amount"* of drug that will *extend* their coagulation time to reduce their risk of having a thromboembolic event. Anticoagulant doses are individualized for each patient, or "patient-specific," based on the patient's test results.

The therapeutic level is based on the laboratory daily control value. It is the desired *target* coagulation range in seconds that prevents clot formation in patients who are at risk. It is *longer than* the normal control finding for an aPTT coagulation test, which is 30-40 seconds for a person who is *not* receiving heparin.

The therapeutic level for an aPTT test is within *1.5 to 2.5 times the control value in seconds* (45-100 seconds), a narrow therapeutic range that will prolong clot formation but not be excessive enough to cause bleeding.

To evaluate a patient-specific coagulation test result:
- Obtain the therapeutic target range by multiplying the control value by the desired factors for the range.
- Compare the patient's test result to see if it falls within the range.

EXAMPLES

1/1/11, Control value for aPTT tests: 30 seconds

Therapeutic target range: 1.5 to 2.5 times the control value (45 to 100 seconds)

aPTT results for Patient X, a patient receiving heparin: 130 seconds

Decision: Hold the anticoagulant. It is not within the desired therapeutic range. Notify the prescriber promptly. Obtain orders. Document. Monitor the patient for bleeding events.

Analysis: Patient's aPTT coagulation time has been *extended* too long with recent doses of anticoagulants. Patient is at risk for bleeding. Antidote may be prescribed.

Note that if the value was *below* the therapeutic range, the patient would be at risk for a thromboembolic event.

CLINICAL RELEVANCE

➤ Assess clients on anticoagulants for bleeding gums, bruises pinpoint and large, and prolonged bleeding after injections. Always check current coagulation test results.

---

1 If a *control value* for a coagulation test is 12 seconds and the *therapeutic range* is 1.5 to 2.5 times the control value, would the patient's test result be within therapeutic range if it was *24 seconds*? (Use simple arithmetic with or without a calculator.)

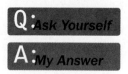

_____

RAPID PRACTICE 12-1

Vocabulary Review: Anticoagulants and Tests

Estimated completion time: 5-10 minutes   Answers on page 561

Directions: *Study the Introduction and Essential Vocabulary list. Select the correct response.*

TEST TIP: Quickly place a single line through the incorrect responses to narrow your choices.

1   Anticoagulants are used for the following purposes: _____
   1. To dissolve well-established clots in high-risk patients
   2. To decrease coagulation time
   3. To treat hemorrhage
   4. To prevent thrombi and emboli formation

2   An oral anticoagulant that is ordered for outpatient use is _____
   1. Warfarin sodium (Coumadin, Sofarin, Warfilone)
   2. Enoxaparin (Lovenox)
   3. Streptokinase and alteplase
   4. Danaparoid sodium

3   The standardized relevant laboratory test for monitoring therapeutic levels of warfarin is called _____
   1. INR   **3.** Vitamin K level
   2. PTT   **4.** aPTT

4   The most commonly used laboratory test to monitor therapeutic levels of heparin is _____
   1. aPTT   **3.** INR
   2. PT   **4.** Vitamin K level

5   The main danger of *excessive* anticoagulant therapy is _____
   1. DVT formation   **3.** Hemorrhage
   2. PE   **4.** Increased platelet count

RAPID PRACTICE 12-2

Anticoagulant Agents and Antidotes

Estimated completion time: 5-10 minutes   Answers on page 561

Directions: *Identify the correct agent, term, purpose, or antidote for anticoagulant therapy.*

1   The drug antidote for warfarin excess is _____
   1. Blood transfusion   **3.** Vitamin K (phytonadione)
   2. Iron   **4.** Protamine sulfate

2   The drug antidote for heparin excess is _____
   1. Blood transfusion   **3.** Vitamin K (phytonadione)
   2. Iron   **4.** Protamine sulfate

3   Intravenous flush solutions are used for which purpose? _____
   1. Occult blood in stool and hematuria   **3.** Petechiae and ecchymoses
   2. Epistaxis   **4.** Patency of IV access devices

4   The difference between a control value and a therapeutic value for a specific anticoagulant test is _____
   1. The control value is the extended blood coagulation time in seconds needed to prevent clots, whereas the therapeutic desired value is the normal coagulation time in seconds for a patient not receiving anticoagulants.
   2. The control value is the level that the prescriber orders for the patient to control his or her blood coagulation. The therapeutic coagulation levels or range is less time in seconds than the control value.

3. The control value is the laboratory-derived normal coagulation time in seconds for a particular test for a patient who is not receiving anticoagulants. The therapeutic value is the desired extended time in seconds for the patient receiving a specific anticoagulant.

4. The control value and the therapeutic time in seconds for coagulation are the same for all patients receiving a specific anticoagulant.

5 Drugs that dissolve clots are classified as _____

   1. Anticoagulants   **3.** Thrombolytic enzyme agents
   2. Hormones   **4.** Salicylates

FAQ | *What is the relationship between the PT value and the INR value?*

ANSWER | A current INR standardized test value introduced by the World Health Organization in 1983 is required to adjust or titrate warfarin doses. The patient's therapeutic INR range is determined daily by the individual laboratory based in part on the PT value. The INR is not a separate test. It is a formula-derived value:

$$INR = \frac{\text{Patient's PT Value}}{\text{Mean Normal PT Value*}} \Bigg\} ISI$$

The INR value is used to evaluate the patient's response to treatment. Some prescribers also require the PT to be reported with the INR.

*ISI: International Sensitivity Index, a value assigned to the thromboplastin reagent by the manufacturer of the specific laboratory test material.

FAQ | *How can I remember the differences between heparin therapy and warfarin therapy?*

ANSWER | Write out a brief outline of the differences. Be able to reproduce this critical information. Following is one suggested format that emphasizes the differences.

➤ All anticoagulant products are high-alert medications.

Comparison of Anticoagulant Products

	Warfarin	Heparin (Unfractionated)	Low Molecular Weight Heparin (LMWH)
Name	Coumadin	Heparin	dalteparin (Fragmin) enoxaparin (Lovenox) ardeparin (Normaflow)
Route	Oral	Subcutaneous or IV	Subcutaneous or IV
Tests	INR usual test; also PT	Frequently aPTT	aPTT infrequently needed
Action	Interferes with extrinsic (tissue injury site) vitamin K–dependent clotting mechanisms	Interferes with intrinsic (within vessel) clotting mechanisms	Interferes with intrinsic and extrinsic clotting mechanisms Less chance for bleeding than unfractionated heparin
Drug antidote	Vitamin K	Protamine sulfate	Protamine sulfate

➤ Heparin and LMWH doses are *not* interchangeable.
➤ Do not confuse PT with PTT.
➤ Plasma, plasma expanders, and blood also may be needed to counteract loss of blood from overdoses of anticoagulants.
➤ Examine the drug labels as you work through the chapter.
➤ Keep abreast of new anticoagulant products.

Interpreting INR and PT Results for Patients Receiving Warfarin Therapy

Estimated completion time: 20 minutes   Answers on page 561

Directions: *Study the Essential Vocabulary, Coagulation Tests, and explanations on pp. 393-394. Examine the test results supplied in the problems. Provide the requested answers.*

1 A patient, Mr. X, was discharged post–myocardial infarction on Coumadin 5 mg PO bedtime daily. The patient has been requested to return to the office twice a week for INR test follow-up to ensure that the Coumadin dose is within therapeutic range. The medication is prescribed at bedtime so that, if the following morning laboratory test result requires dose adjustment, it can be made the same evening.

A prescription was given for warfarin 5 mg #60 pills. "Take 5 mg at bedtime as directed." The tablets are scored so that, if the dose needs to be reduced, the patient can take 2.5 mg if prescribed without purchasing another prescription.

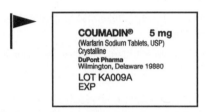

COUMADIN® 5 mg
(Warfarin Sodium Tablets, USP)
Crystalline
DuPont Pharma
Wilmington, Delaware 19880
LOT KA009A
EXP

CLINICAL RELEVANCE

Patient discharge teaching needs to be comprehensive, including the many foods which contain vitamin K, limitations on alcohol intake, (prescriber recommended) need to "regularize" food patterns to stabilize test results, not to omit doses, need for frequent follow-up lab testing, signs and symptoms of problems, and when to call the physician. Information on OTC medicines to avoid is critical. Written instructions should also be provided.

The normal therapeutic range of INR for Mr. X on anticoagulant therapy is 2 to 3. For the first laboratory test in the office, the INR value was 2.6. What is the expected decision for Mr. X? (Circle one.)

a. Continue on 5-mg per day dose and return to office in 3 days for next INR.
b. Hold the Coumadin. Come in for vitamin K (phytonadione) injection.
c. Increase the Coumadin dose to 7.5 mg per day.
d. Order an aPTT test.

2 Mr. X, named in problem 1, has a PT test ordered in addition to the INR. PT was reported at 25 seconds. The laboratory control PT value was 11.5 seconds.

➤ The therapeutic PT time for an anticoagulated patient such as Mr. X is 2 to 2.5 times the laboratory control value.

What is the desired PT range for Mr. X in seconds? _____

3 What is the nurse's evaluation of Mr. X's PT time (25 seconds)? (Circle one.)

a. 25 seconds is within the desired range for extended coagulation for Mr. X.
b. Mr. X needs a higher dose of anticoagulant and is at risk for thrombus or embolus formation.
c. Mr. X is receiving too much anticoagulant.
d. Mr. X's PT value should be 11.5 seconds.

4 A few weeks later, Mr. X's INR result is 7, and he is complaining of bleeding when he brushes his teeth as well as dark-colored urine and stools, which test positive for presence of blood. The PT value is 49 seconds. The therapeutic INR value is 2 to 3 for Mr. X. The control PT is 12 seconds.

   a. What is the nurse's evaluation of the laboratory results? (Circle one.)
     1. Mr. X is in danger of forming thrombi or emboli.
     2. Mr. X is in danger of bleeding from excessive anticoagulation.
     3. Mr. X's results are within normal limits for anticoagulation.

The physician orders vitamin K 2 mg subcut stat to reverse the warfarin and lower the INR.

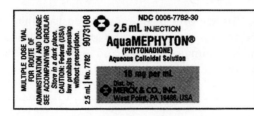

   b. How many mL of vitamin K will the nurse prepare for injection after the dilution? Use mental arithmetic, and verify with a DA equation. _____

DA equation:

Evaluation: _____

Mr. X is instructed to hold the Coumadin dosage until results of his next INR test.

5 Three days later, Mr. X's INR is 3. The physician lowers the Coumadin dose to 2.5 mg per day. Mr. X's tablets are scored. He is instructed to buy a pill cutter at a local pharmacy and to keep a record of when he takes his nightly Coumadin dose. His next few laboratory tests will be scheduled weekly.

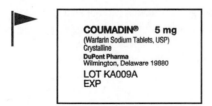

   a. How many pills will Mr. X take daily? _____
   b. Which of the following Coumadin doses would be safest for Mr. X to have prescribed for his next prescription, assuming that his INR remains stable?

_____

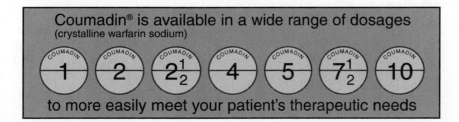

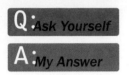
Communication

"Mr. X, how do you keep track of your anticoagulant medications when you take them at home?"

Q: *Ask Yourself*

A: *My Answer*

➤ Noncompliance with anticoagulant therapy can be fatal. Forgetting to take a medication or doubling up is not a rare occurrence, even in the most alert patient population. Remember that there is a difference between what is taught and what is learned. Communication for teaching need not be formal. For example, the patient will have little interest in learning the chain of physiologic clotting mechanisms from a flow chart.

1 Take a minute to browse your most comprehensive current pharmacology text for drug and food interactions with Coumadin. Besides aspirin, other nonsteroidal anti-inflammatory drugs, and antibiotics, what other medications do you recognize on the list? What effect do they have on the anticoagulant?

_____

2 Does the length of the list illustrate the need to check the medications each patient is currently receiving? (While you are in that section of the text, browse the side effects also.)

_____

CLINICAL RELEVANCE

Teaching of outpatients receiving anticoagulants is critical. One example of a preventable tragedy was a patient who suffered lacerations in a relatively minor automobile accident and who died from loss of blood. The patient did not carry a wallet card with information about the medication (warfarin) nor the dose, nor did the patient wear an identification bracelet. Another example is illustrated by the case of a patient on anticoagulants who became seasick on a cruise and had several episodes of hematemesis. He stayed in bed and sent his wife to the cruise ship front desk for oral pills for seasickness for 2 days but could not keep them down. Eventually, he sought care from the ship's physician. Units of blood had to be delivered by helicopter to save the patient's life.

CLINICAL RELEVANCE

➤ A responsible family member must have all the priority information about the anticoagulant dose, timing, testing, and follow-up visits. Patients need to be reminded to carry a list of their medicines and doses on their person.

Injectable Anticoagulants

The prototypical parenteral anticoagulant is heparin sodium, which must be administered IV in the hospital because of its short half-life and the need for frequent titration to laboratory results. Subcutaneous heparin is also only administered by nurses. Derived from pork and bovine intestinal mucosa, it interacts with many drugs. The nurse must check the medications the patient is receiving against the lengthy drug interaction list for heparin.

➤ If ordered IV, heparin must be administered on an infusion pump with an IV line dedicated for heparin administration only. Check institutional policies. If this is not feasible, a saline flush must be administered before and after using an existing line.

Take a moment to examine some examples of the varied doses of heparin available. It helps to have a general understanding of the purpose of the range of doses because the selection of the correct concentration is a critical nursing decision.

➤ As with most liquid injectables for adults, drug amounts in mL are usually rounded to the nearest tenth of a mL.

➤ Check agency policies re: requirements for an independent nurse check of anticoagulants before each dose administration.

Low-Dose Heparin Concentrations Used to Maintain Patency of Intravenous Devices (Flushes)

Flushes of very low-dose heparin are administered to maintain the patency of venous access sites. They are *not* given to anticoagulate a patient (Figure 12-1).

➤ The flush solution—saline or heparin—is selected according to agency protocol.
➤ Saline solution may be preferred as a flush for certain venous access devices.

The prescriber does not write the volume in milliliters of the flush to be used. The volume of the flush depends on the fluid capacity of the indwelling device and institutional policy. The longer the catheter, the more volume will be needed to "flush" the line.

➤ There have been tragic consequences when the wrong dose has been used for a heparin flush.
➤ Consult agency guidelines and equipment literature for precise concentrations and volumes for each type of flush.
➤ Know the difference when you see these acronyms:

SASH, acronym for heparin flush: Saline, Administer (drug), Saline, Heparin
SAS, acronym for saline flush: Saline, Administer (drug), Saline

1   As I check my pharmacology reference for heparin drug interactions, why do I realize it would be critical to flush IV lines with saline solution *before* and *after* administering heparin?

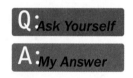

_____

2   Which incompatible drug is one I have most frequently seen or heard about?

_____

3   Why must IV heparin have a separate IV line and be administered using an infusion pump?

_____

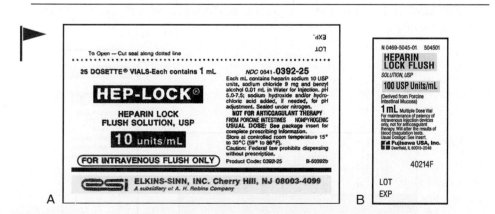

FIGURE 12-1 **A,** Hep-Lock 10 units per mL. **B,** Heparin Lock Flush 100 units per mL. Note the different concentrations.

Heparin Concentrations Used for Subcutaneous Administration and Bolus Intravenous Doses

Like many other drugs, heparin is supplied in several concentrations. Refer to Figures 12-2 and 12-3.

➤ These concentrations should *not* be used for flushes.

➤ Heparin has been identified as a high-alert drug by the Institute for Safe Medication Practices (ISMP) (see Appendix B). It is critical to select the correct ordered concentration of a powerful drug such as heparin.

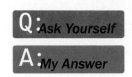

Q: *Ask Yourself*

A: *My Answer*

1 What is the difference in the heparin product concentrations shown in Figures 12-2 and 12-3?

_____

_____

_____

• A dose of 5000 units per 1 mL is 5 times more concentrated than 1000 units per mL. A dose of 10,000 units per 1 mL is 10 times more concentrated than 1000 units per mL.

• The more concentrated the dose, the greater the anticoagulant effect and the greater the risk of bleeding.

• Adding or subtracting a zero from an order or misreading a *U* as a zero must be avoided.

• Many at-risk patients receive a standard dose of 5000 units of heparin subcutaneously q12h for DVT prevention. This dose does not require aPTT monitoring. Platelet counts may be ordered every few days.

• Injection sites are rotated. Refer to Sites for Insulin Injection in Chapter 11 (p. 369).

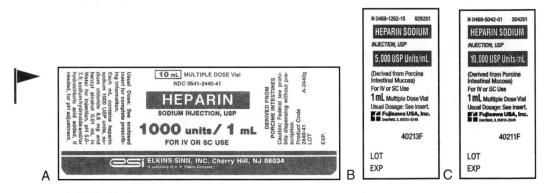

FIGURE 12-2 **A,** Heparin 1000 units per mL. **B,** Heparin 5,000 units per mL. **C,** Heparin 10,000 units/mL.

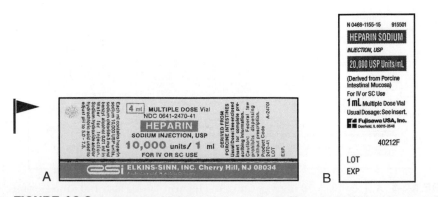

FIGURE 12-3 **A,** Heparin 10,000 units per mL. **B,** Heparin 20,000 units per mL.

- Heparin injections are not aspirated before administration.
- Avoid massaging the site.
- Needle angle depends on patient size.
- A bolus of low-dose heparin, 5000 units, may be given as a loading dose (fast startup) and/or as a test for reactions such as allergies before an IV infusion.
- Heparin is never given via the IM route.
- When a label such as a heparin label states the concentration as 1:1000 or 1:10,000, it is interpreted as g per mL. Thus, 1:1000 means 1 g per 1000 mL, which is 10 times stronger than a solution of 1 g per 10,000 mL.

➤ Check agency policies for rounding heparin doses. They may vary from the nearest 50 to 100 units.

Heparin Concentrations Used for Intravenous Infusions

The general guidelines for continuous heparin infusions are 20,000 to 40,000 units every 24 hours, depending on the patient's condition and test results.

Although in some settings, nurses may prepare and mix IV heparin solutions, the trend is to use premixed preparations to ensure the patient's safety.

There are also premixed preparations of heparin of 12,500 units per 250 mL NS and 25,000 to 40,000 units in 250 or 500 mL NS in vials and ampules. Heparin is also available premixed in ADD-Vantage vials to accompany ADD-Vantage IV solution containers. Refer to Chapter 9 for a review of ADD-Vantage® System.

Heparin Preparations and Preventing Errors

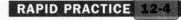

RAPID PRACTICE 12-4

Estimated completion time: 10 minutes   Answers on page 562

Directions: *Examine the preceding information about heparin and the labels on pp. 403 and 404, and review the vocabulary to answer the following questions 1-10.*

Contrast the concentration on the label below and the last label on p. 404. Three infants died in one agency as a result of being given a dose from the 10,000 units per mL label instead of the 10 units per mL label. Notice the similarity of appearance among three of the labels on p. 404.

Most medicines today have more than one form and more than one concentration, whether oral or injectable. Companies have been asked to avoid look-alike labels.

CLINICAL RELEVANCE

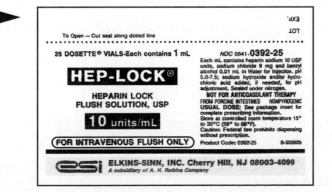

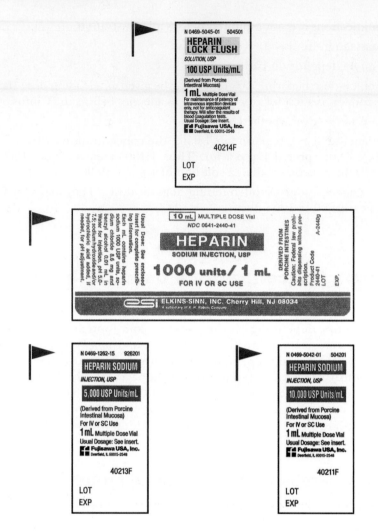

1 The volume for the heparin solutions shown on the labels is _____.

2 Which is the *lowest* concentration of solution provided on the labels above?

_____

3 The purpose of a flush solution is _____.

4 The key difference between SASH and SAS is

_____.

5 Which is more concentrated: 1000 units per mL or 10,000 units per mL?

_____

6 Which is more concentrated: a 1:1000 solution or a 1:10,000 solution? _____

7 Which is more concentrated: 5,000 units per mL or 10,000 units per mL?

_____

8 If a *U* for *units* was misread as a zero, the kind of adverse consequence to the patient receiving the heparin dose could be _____.

9 The maximum dose of IV heparin units over a 24-hour period is about (can be exceeded, depending on patient's condition) _____.

10 Heparin solutions must be isolated from other IV medications a patient is receiving because _____.

1 What is the general difference among heparin solution doses used for flush versus prophylaxis versus therapeutic administration? (Answer in brief phrases.)

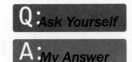

Q: Ask Yourself

A: My Answer

_____

2 Which heparin solution shown on p. 404 has the *highest* concentration?

_____

Calculating Heparin Flow Rates in Milliliters per Hour (mL per hr) and Units per Hour Using DA-Style Equations

Calculations are the same as for any other DA-style equation.

Determining mL per hr From a Weight-Based Order of Units per kg per hr

Weight-based orders based on kg weight are recommended by TJC for all drugs to reduce dosing errors. In addition, it is recommended that the prescriber calculate the dose and show the calculations. The nurse still has to do an independent math check of the flow rate based on the order and the IV solution (label) even if the flow rate was supplied by prescriber, pharmacy or the IV pump computer.

EXAMPLES

Ordered: heparin 24 units per kg per hr. Patient weight is 50 kg.
Available: heparin 25,000 units in 500 mL D5W (500 mL per 25,000 units)
How many milliliters per hour (to the nearest tenth of a mL per hr) should be administered?

Step 1	:	Step 2	×	Step 3	=	Answer
Desired Answer Units	:	Starting Factor	×	Given Quantity and Conversion Factor(s)* *as needed	=	Estimate, Multiply, Evaluate

$$\frac{mL}{hr} : \frac{\dfrac{\cancel{500}\ mL}{\cancel{25{,}000}\ units}}{\dfrac{50}{1}} \times \frac{24\ \cancel{units}}{\cancel{kg} \times 1\ hr} \times \frac{\dfrac{1}{\cancel{50}\ \cancel{kg}}}{1} = 24\ mL\ per\ hr$$

The final equation will be written like this:

$$\frac{mL}{hr} : \frac{\dfrac{\cancel{500}\ mL}{\cancel{25{,}000}\ units}}{\dfrac{50}{1}} \times \frac{24\ \cancel{units}}{\cancel{kg} \times 1\ hr} \times \frac{\dfrac{1}{\cancel{50}\ \cancel{kg}}}{1} = \frac{24\ mL}{hr}$$

Analysis: This equation has a required numerator and denominator containing the desired answer units. The selected starting factor is positioned with mL in the numerator. Hr appear in the denominator of step 3. Reduction and cancellation before multiplication simplifies the math.

Evaluation: The answer matches the desired answer. The order of 1200 units per hr is within the recommended heparin continuous adult infusion rate of 20,000 to 40,000 units per 24 hrs. My estimate after all the data are entered is that the flow rate will be low—about 1/50 of 1200 (500 divided by 25,000 = 1/50) (1200 ÷ 50 = 24). The estimate supports the answer.

➤ Remember that IVs for high-alert drugs must be administered on an infusion pump.

Determining Units Per hr Being Infused on an Existing Infusion

The nurse often comes on shift duty to find IVs infusing. The nursing responsibility is to ensure that each flow rate is correct for the dose ordered and solution concentration (label) provided, and to be able to report how many units per hr are infusing. Are the units per hr being administered the same as ordered by the prescriber? Is the dose within adult SDR (20,000 to 40,000 units) for continous IV for 24 hrs? If not, why not?

➤ A standard heparin solution concentration on many units is 25,000 units in 250 mL of D5W.

➤ Contrast the mL per hr flow rate with the number of heparin units per hr.

EXAMPLES

Existing infusion: heparin flowing at 10 mL per hr

Infusion labeled 25,000 units heparin in 250 mL D5W

How many units per hour (to the nearest 100 units per hour) are being administered?

Step 1	:	Step 2	×	Step 3	=	Answer
Desired Answer Units	:	Starting Factor	×	Given Quantity and Conversion Factor(s)* *as needed	=	Estimate, Multiply, Evaluate

$$\frac{units}{hr} : \frac{\frac{100}{25{,}000 \text{ units}}}{\frac{250 \text{ mL}}{1}} \times \frac{10 \text{ mL}}{1 \text{ hr}} = 1000 \frac{units}{hr}$$

The final equation will be written like this:

$$\frac{units}{hr} : \frac{\frac{100}{25{,}000 \text{ units}}}{\frac{250 \text{ mL}}{1}} \times \frac{10 \text{ mL}}{1 \text{ hr}} = \frac{1000 \text{ units}}{1 \text{ hr}} = 1000 \frac{units}{hr} \text{ of heparin}$$

Analysis: Convert the flow rate from volume per hr (mL per hr) to medication per hr (units per hr). *The selected starting factor, obtained from the labels on the IV bottle, permitted a match with units, one of the two desired answers. The flow rate provided a match with the second desired answer unit, hr, in the denominator (hr must appear in the denominator under the dividing line). Reduction and cancellation make the math easy in this simple equation.

Evaluation: My estimate after the data are entered in the equation is 50 × 20, and the estimate supports the answer. The equation is balanced. 1000 units per hr is within the recommended continuous heparin infusion rate of 20,000 to 40,000 units per 24 hours.

RAPID PRACTICE 12-5

Titrating Heparin Doses to aPTT Values

Estimated completion time: 20-30 minutes   Answers on page 562

Directions: *Read the following case history information for the patient on heparin therapy. Calculate the doses and provide the requested nursing evaluations. Round all doses to the nearest 100 units. Label all work. Use a calculator for long division and multiplication.*

Mr. Y has been hospitalized with arterial fibrillation, a condition that predisposes him to thromboembolus formation. The physician has ordered a complete blood screening for clotting and bleeding times, including a baseline platelet count and aPTT. Mr. Y's baseline aPTT is 30 seconds. He is not receiving anticoagulants yet.

The platelet count is: 250,000 per microliter.

Because both of Mr. Y's values are within the normal range, the physician institutes heparin therapy to extend coagulation time.

> Initial order for Mr. Y: heparin 5000-unit bolus loading test dose IV slowly. Pharmacology references state to infuse the first 1000 units over 1 minute, then give the rest of the IV loading dose before starting a continuous infusion. Follow with continuous infusion at 1000 units per hr. Obtain an aPTT in 4 hours.

Thus, the slow bolus test dose is ordered.

```
N 0469-1262-15    926201

HEPARIN SODIUM
INJECTION, USP

5,000 USP Units/mL

(Derived from Porcine
Intestinal Mucosa)
For IV or SC Use

1 mL Multiple Dose Vial
Usual Dosage: See Insert.

Lyphomed™
Fujisawa USA, Inc.
Deerfield, IL 60015
40213D
```

1 Why is thrombocytopenia, as measured by a platelet count under 100,000 per microliter, a contraindication to the institution of heparin therapy? Refer to Essential Vocabulary if necessary. (Give a brief answer.)

_____

2 The physician leaves the following order: Start infusion at 1000 units per hr. Available: heparin 25,000 units per 250 mL of NS. Heparin infusions are administered on infusion pumps.

a. The nurse will set the flow rate at how many mL per hr?

DA equation:

b. Evaluation: _____

Prescriber orders IV heparin schedule for Mr. Y, whose weight is 80 kg. Titrate (adjust) heparin q4h to maintain aPTT. Up to **44 seconds**, increase infusion by 1 unit per kg per hr. **45 to 75** seconds: no adjustment. **76 to 80** seconds: decrease infusion by 1 unit per kg per hr. aPTT greater than **80 seconds**: hold infusion. Call physician for orders. All rates are to be rounded to the nearest 100 units per hr.

3 Mr. Y's next aPTT is 50 seconds. Control is 30 seconds. Desired aPTT for patient receiving heparin anticoagulant therapy is 1.5 to 2.5 times control.

a. Desired therapeutic range in seconds for Mr. Y: _____

b. Is Mr. Y's current result within the aPTT therapeutic range? (Yes/No)

_____

c. Does an adjustment need to be made in IV heparin units per hr and IV flow rate based upon the aPTT result and the titration schedule? (Use brief phrases.)

_____

_____

DA equation if applicable:

d. Evaluation: _____

4 Mr. Y's next aPTT is 76 seconds. Control is 30 seconds.* Desired aPTT for patient receiving anticoagulant therapy is 1.5 to 2.5 times control.

    a. What is the desired therapeutic aPTT range in seconds for Mr. Y? _____

    b. Is it within the desired therapeutic range? _____

    c. Will an adjustment in units per hr be needed based on the aPTT result and the titration schedule ordered in problem 2? (Answer briefly.)

    _____

    d. If so, how many units per hr should Mr. Y receive? Round answer to nearest 100 units per hr.

    DA equation:

    e. Will there be an adjustment needed in Mr. Y's IV flow rate? _____

    f. If so, how many mL per hr should he receive?

    DA equation:

5 The orders for a new patient read: Heparin infusion: 32 units per kg per hr. The nurse on the oncoming shift sees that the existing flow rate is 32 mL per hr. Patient wt is 50 kg.

    a. How many units per hr to the nearest 100 units is the patient receiving based on the existing concentration of heparin 12,500 units per 250 mL of NS? _____

    DA equation:

    b. Evaluation: (Is the flow rate correct or incorrect for the order?)

    _____

    c. Is this amount within the usual recommended 24-hour range of 20,000 to 40,000 units per hr for IV heparin infusions? (Yes/No) _____

Communication

Nurse to patient and responsible family member (a patient's memory may be impaired at time of transfer): "Mrs. Jones, What medications do you take at home?" (dose, time, frequency). "What sort of medications do you buy without a prescription—vitamins, minerals, painkillers?"* (OTC medications). "I'm asking because some of these may interfere with the medicines the doctor has ordered for you." "Do you go to any other doctors beside Dr. X?" "Have they prescribed medications for you?" "How often do you take them?" "Here is the list I have. Have I left anything out?" "Have you ever had a problem with any of these medications? Rash, breathing or brusing or bleeding problems, diarrhea, dizziness?" (Follow-up with when, what happened, etc.) "How do you remember to take all these medications each day?" "Do you carry a current list in your wallet?" "What sorts of foods and medications do you avoid when you are taking anticoagulants?"

CLINICAL RELEVANCE

Medication resolution is never more critical than for high-alert drugs. Deficient transfer information has resulted in sentinel events (injury and death) particularly with high-alert drugs such as anticoagulants and insulin. Physician, pharmacist, patient, family and current and past medical records need to be consulted to provide medication resolution for transfer. The nurse who admits, transfers, or discharges the patient plays a major role in medication resolution (refer to TJC and ISMP websites).

*Think of a *half-minute* as a rough, approximate normal aPTT. The normal range is about 20 to 35 seconds. Use the precise range supplied by the individual laboratory for heparin administration.

Heparin and Heparinoid Preparations

Estimated completion time: 20 minutes   Answers on page 563

Directions: *Read each patient's history. Calculate the doses using a DA equation and a calculator for long division and multiplication.*

1 Mr. M is receiving heparin continuous infusion of 12 units per kg per hr. Available: premixed heparin 25,000 units in 500 mL. Mr. M's weight is 90 kg.

   a. How many units per hour of heparin should Mr. M receive to the nearest 100 units? _____

   b. What rate will the nurse set on the infusion pump to the nearest mL?

   DA equation:

   c. Evaluation: _____

2 Mr. M.'s aPTT exceeds 90 seconds. The control aPTT is 35 seconds. The physician orders laboratory tests, including a platelet count, and protamine sulfate 1 mg IV for every 100 units of half the *hourly heparin dose administered in the past hour.*

   a. Is Mr. M. at risk of thrombi or bleeding? (Circle one.)

   b. Number of units of heparin administered in the past hour rounded to the nearest 100 units per hr: _____

   c. Half the amount of units of heparin administered in the past hour (to the nearest 100 units): _____

   d. Number of milligrams of protamine sulfate to be administered based on the order: _____

   DA equation:

   e. Evaluation: _____

3 A current drug reference states to administer the protamine sulfate IV ordered in problem 2 *slowly over 1 to 3 minutes.* ➤ Too-rapid administration can result in anaphylaxis, severe hypotension, hypertension, bradycardia, and dyspnea.

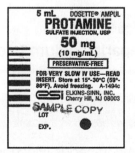

   a. How many mL (to the nearest tenth) of protamine sulfate IV will be administered to Mr. M (problem 2)? _____

   DA equation:

   b. Evaluation:

4   Mrs. J is scheduled for a hip replacement. She is placed on prophylactic anti-coagulation with a LMWH agent, dalteparin (Fragmin):

2500 international units subcut 2 hours before surgery
2500 international units subcut 8 hours after surgery
5000 international units subcut daily for 14 days postoperatively in the hospital and at home

Periodic complete blood count, platelet count, and stool test for occult blood were ordered.

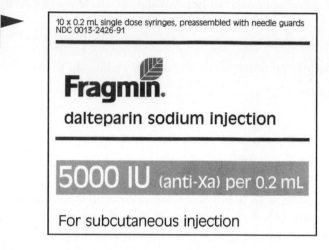

10 x 0.2 mL single dose syringes, preassembled with needle guards
NDC 0013-2426-91

Fragmin®

dalteparin sodium injection

5000 IU (anti-Xa) per 0.2 mL

For subcutaneous injection

How many mL will Mrs. J need to receive preoperatively (to the nearest tenth of a mL)?

a. Estimated dose:

b. DA verification:

c. Evaluation _____

5   Fragmin 80 international units per kg is ordered prophylactically q12h subcut for Mrs. V, a patient with unstable angina. Mrs. V weighs 110 lb.

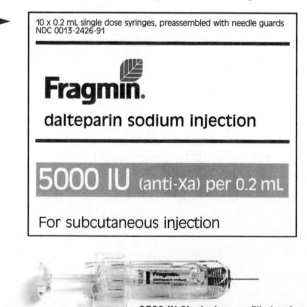

10 x 0.2 mL single dose syringes, preassembled with needle guards
NDC 0013-2426-91

Fragmin®

dalteparin sodium injection

5000 IU (anti-Xa) per 0.2 mL

For subcutaneous injection

2500 IU Single-dose prefilled syringe

What is Mrs. V's weight in kg?

a. Estimate:

DA equation:

b. Evaluation: _____

c. How many units will the nurse prepare for Mrs. V.?

DA equation:

d. Evaluation: _____

e. How many mL will the nurse prepare to the nearest hundredth of a mL?

f. Estimate:

DA equation:

g. Evaluation: _____

➤ Do *not* interchange units with milligrams for dose. Check the order and label, and compare units ordered to units supplied.

CHAPTER 12 MULTIPLE-CHOICE REVIEW

Estimated completion time: 20-30 minutes   **Answers on page 563**

Directions: *Select the correct answer.*

1 Which of the following medications require(s) INR testing? _____

  1. Streptokinase

  2. Heparinoids

  3. Heparin sodium or calcium

  4. Warfarin products

2 Which medication is given orally? _____

  1. Warfarin

  2. Heparinoids

  3. Heparin sodium

  4. Heparin calcium

3 Which bests describes the "control value" for aPTT and PT testing? _____

  1. It reflects the patient's current laboratory value before treatment.

  2. It is a measure of therapeutic response to anticoagulation.

  3. It reflects the current laboratory norm based on the batch of materials used for testing that day.

  4. It is the general range of norms for all patients receiving anticoagulants.

4 The general recommended flow rate for initial continuous heparin infusions for adults, which can vary widely depending on the patient's condition and test results, is approximately _____

  1. 1000 to 1700 units per hr

  2. 5 to 10 units per hr

  3. 5000 units per hr

  4. 25,000 units per hr

5 The main reason unwanted amounts of medicine need to be discarded from prefilled syringes before administering the prescribed volume to the patient is _____

   1. Remainders are to be discarded from all prefilled syringes.

   2. The nurse might inadvertently administer more than the ordered amount.

   3. There is risk of undermedication and a potential thromboembolic event.

   4. It is usually hospital policy.

6 Which of the following statements is true about the relationship between international units and milligrams? _____

   1. Milligrams are a measure of weight, and international units are a standardized amount that produces a particular biologic effect.

   2. Milligrams and corresponding units can be determined by the nurse using a standard formula for all drugs.

   3. The effect of 1 mg is equal to the effect of 1 international unit of the same product.

   4. Milligrams, milliliters, and international units can be used interchangeably.

7 When may a physician have to consider the danger of prescribing anticoagulants for a patient? _____

   1. The patient is at high risk for DVT.

   2. The patient is at very high risk for developing clots.

   3. The patient is noncompliant with medication and test regimens.

   4. The patient is elderly and lives with children.

8 The preferred test for monitoring heparin therapy is _____

   1. PT

   2. aPTT

   3. PTT

   4. INR

9 Which of the following dose concentrations are commonly used if a heparin flush is ordered? _____

   1. 10 to 25,000 units per 250 mL   **3.** 5000 to 10,000 units per mL

   2. 10 to 100 units per mL   **4.** 1000 to 5000 units per mL

10 Which antidote should be on hand for patients receiving heparin therapy? _____

   1. Activated charcoal   **3.** Potassium chloride

   2. Vitamin K   **4.** Protamine sulfate

CHAPTER 12 FINAL PRACTICE

Estimated completion time: 1-2 hours   **Answers on page 564**

Directions: *Answer the anticoagulant-related questions. Use a calculator for long division and multiplication. Evaluate your equations. Label all answers.*

1 Ordered: Coumadin (warfarin sodium) 5 mg at bedtime for an elderly patient for discharge post–myocardial infarction. INR values are ordered twice weekly for the first month. The target therapeutic INR is 2 to 3 for this patient. The laboratory reports the patient's INR result at 5.

   a. What will the physician probably do regarding the dosage of Coumadin—rise it or lower it? (Circle one.)

   b. If the patient has several different strengths of Coumadin at home because of dosage adjustments, what sort of advice would be advisable to give the patient regarding drug storage?

2 Ordered: heparin infusion of 2000 units per hr based on patient's weight. A heparin infusion of 25,000 units in 250 mL is being administered at 20 mL per hr.

a. How many *units per hour,* to nearest 100 units, are being infused?

DA equation:

b. Evaluation: _____

3 Ordered: heparin 18 units per kg per hr in a continuous infusion. Available: heparin 25,000 units in 500 mL D5W. Patient's weight: 70 kg

a. How many units per hr are ordered:

DA equation:

b. Evaluation: _____
c. The nurse will set the flow rate at how many mL per hr: _____

DA equation:

d. Evaluation: _____

4 Ordered: heparin infusion of 1500 units per hr based on an order of 20 units per kg per hr for a patient weighing 75 kg. Available: heparin 25,000 units per 500 mL NS. The IV is infusing at 20 mL per hr when the nurse arrives on the shift.

a. Is the existing flow rate correct? If not, what should it be?

DA equation:

b. Evaluation: _____

5 Ordered: Lovenox 30 mg subcut daily at bedtime: It is supplied in a prefilled syringe.

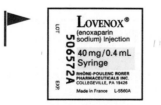

a. What type of drug is Lovenox: heparin, LMWH, warfarin, or thrombolytic derivative? _____
b. How many mL will the nurse prepare?

DA equation:

c. Evaluation: _____

6 Ordered: continuous heparin infusion to maintain the aPTT between 60 and 70 seconds, for a patient with atrial fibrillation. After the initial slow bolus loading dose of 5000 units IV, draw a stat aPTT and begin the infusion at 1000 units per hr. Obtain the aPTT q6h. Patient weight is 70 kg. The following sliding scale is given to titrate the heparin infusion:

aPTT	Action
30-45 seconds	Increase the drip by 3 units per kg per hr.
46-70 seconds	No change.
71-85 seconds	Reduce the drip by 2 units per kg per hr.
Over 85 seconds	Hold the infusion for 1 hr. Call the physician for orders.

Available: 25,000 units of heparin in 250 mL D5W. The first aPTT drawn is 40 seconds.

a. Initial flow rate in mL per hr at 1000 units per hr should be set at:

DA equation:

b. Evaluation: _____

c. Nurse's evaluation of the first aPTT. (Give a brief answer.)

_____

d. Adjusted number of units per hr if applicable:

DA equation:

e. Evaluation: _____

f. Adjusted number of mL per hr if applicable: _____

DA equation:

g. Evaluation: _____

7 The patient described in problem 6 has another aPTT drawn 6 hours later. The result is 65 seconds.

a. Adjustment in mL per hr if applicable. _____

DA equation:

b. Evaluation: _____

8 A nurse checks an infusion of heparin 25,000 units per 500 mL Ringer's solution. It is flowing at 40 mL per hr.

a. How many units of heparin per hour are being delivered?

DA equation:

b. Evaluation: _____

c. Is this order within the recommended 24-hour dose for heparin infusions?

_____

9 The order for the infusion solution in problem 8 is for 1200 units per hr based on kg weight.

   a. For how many mL per hr will the nurse set the infusion?

   DA equation:

   b. What adverse effect will the nurse monitor for, in addition to obtaining another aPTT? _____

10 a. What does "extended coagulation time" mean to you? _____

   b. Why should a heparin infusion be administered on an infusion pump?
   _____

Suggestions for Further Reading

http://clotcare.com/clotcare/search.aspx?by=med
www.ahrq.gov/downloads/pub/advances/vol3/Harder.pdf
www.cdc.gov/mmwr
www.ehow.com/way_5588472_heparin-levels-guidelines-heparin.html
www.ismp.org
www.ncbi.nPm.nih.gov
www.nlm.nih.gov/medlineplus/druginformation.html
\www.jointcommission.org/sentinelevents/sentineleventalert/sea_35.htm
\www.psqh.com/january-february-2009/202-heparin-improving-treatment-and-
   reducing-risk-of-harm.html

℮volve Additional practice problems can be found in the Advanced Calculations section of the Student Companion on Evolve.

Chapter 13 focuses on pediatric dose calculations. These determinations are often multi-step calculations of fractional doses of medications using the familiar techniques of dimensional analysis.

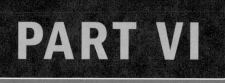

PART VI

Medications for Infants and Children

CHAPTER 13 Pediatric Medication Calculations

300 mg
20 ML

0.9%
1000 g = 1 kg
>400 m
0.4 mg/mL

"*Children have neither past nor future; they enjoy the present,
which very few of us do.*"
—JEAN DE LA BRUYERE

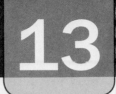

Pediatric Medication Calculations

OBJECTIVES

- Distinguish the milligram (mg), microgram (mcg), gram (g), and square meter (m2) units of measurement.
- Evaluate orders for minimum and maximum pediatric SDR doses.
- Calculate pediatric weight-based doses for oral and parenteral routes.
- Calculate pediatric doses based on body surface area.
- Calculate flow rates for IV volume-control devices.
- State measures to prevent medication errors for pediatric patients.

Essential Prior Knowledge

- Chapters 1-12

Essential Equipment

- A calculator is useful for converting pounds to kilograms and calculating SDR.

Estimated Time To Complete Chapter

- 2-2½ hours

Introduction

To have therapeutic value and to avoid injury, medication doses must be highly individualized for pediatric populations. The requirements for body fluid and electrolyte balance in infants and children, as well as immature renal and liver function, dictate a need for great care with fluid and medication administration. The necessary departures from average adult unit doses have resulted in medication errors for a vulnerable population.

Medications for children may be referred to as *"fractional doses"* if they consist of a partial dose of the amount supplied. Doses for children are usually based on *weight*—micrograms, milligrams, or grams per kilogram of body weight—or on *surface area:* micrograms or milligrams per square meter of body surface area. Therapeutic doses for children are included in most current medication references. The trend is for the pharmacy to supply more pediatric-specific pre-prepared medications to reduce the chance of calculation error.

➤ Occasionally, young patients receive a higher-than-usual adult dose because of the severity of illness, the threat to life, or the lack of response to lower doses and other medications. The particular emphases for safe medication administration with pediatric populations, beyond the selection of appropriate equipment and sites for the medications, are:

1 Verifying that the order is within the SDR for the target population
2 Distinguishing microgram, milligram, and square meter units of measurement
3 Calculating accurate fractional doses and fluid needs for all routes
4 Identifying the correct patient when the patient cannot speak
5 Assessing side effects and complications in nonverbal patients

418

The nurse has extra responsibilities to protect the safety of the pediatric patient.

➤ Pediatric patients cannot protect themselves from medication errors. Many cannot identify themselves and are not in a position to question medications and medication orders or to verbalize physical complaints. In addition to using printed identification bracelets, bar codes, and other methods, the nurse should have a family member verify the identity of a pediatric patient.

➤ Pediatric patients suffer a much higher rate of medication errors than adults.

The preceding chapters provide a considerable foundation for mastering the calculations in this chapter. Weight-based orders and safe dose ranges for adults have been covered in Chapters 5 and 10.

▲ **Cultural Note**

Cultural awareness of naming practices is important in avoiding misidentification of a patient who is to receive medications and treatments. When identifying a pediatric patient, keep in mind that naming practices of parents and children vary widely among cultures. Family members may have different last names, based on particular paternal and maternal naming practices.

ESSENTIAL *Vocabulary*

Body Surface Area (BSA)	Area covered by the skin measured in square meters. Used for accurate dosing of powerful drugs and for adult and pediatric at-risk populations.
Square Meter (m²)	Metric unit of area measurement. Powerful medications, particularly anti-cancer medications, may be based on square meters of BSA.
Milligrams per Kilogram (mg per kg)	Drug amount in milligrams based on kilograms of body weight. The most common unit of measurement for prescribed doses of medications for pediatric and frail patients and for powerful drugs.
Nomogram	Graphic representation of numerical relationships. A BSA nomogram is used to estimate square meters of body surface area.
Safe Dose Range (SDR)	Minimum-to-maximum therapeutic dose range for a target population: adult, child, infant, neonate, or elderly.

Vocabulary Review

RAPID PRACTICE 13-1

Estimated completion time: 5 minutes   Answers on page 565

Directions: *Read the vocabulary and introductory material to provide the answers to the questions.*

1 Medication dose that is less than the usual adult dose:

_____

2 Abbreviation for the minimum-to-maximum therapeutic dose range cited by manufacturers:

_____

3 The most common measurement used for determining the dose for pediatric patients:

_____

4 Units of measurement that may be used to calculate doses for pediatric populations:

_____

5 Which metric unit is used to measure BSA?

_____

Comparing Adult and Pediatric Medication Doses and Schedules

➤ Examine the selected examples in Table 13-1, and note the differences in dosing and units of measurement for adults and children.

There may be many more subclassifications of drug dose based on precise age groups of neonates, infants, and children and on various conditions for which one drug may be prescribed.

Q: *Ask Yourself*

A: *My Answer*

1   Which of the recommended SDRs for amoxicillin is weight-based: the adult or the child? (Refer to Table 13-1)

_____

➤ Taking 2 or 3 minutes to verify a safe dose order with a current pediatric drug reference and/or pharmacy may prevent a tragic error.

TABLE 13-1 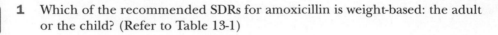 **IV Dose Comparison by Age Group for Selected Drugs**

Name of Drug	Dose Comparison
Potassium Chloride (KCl)*	SDR, **Adult,** Individualized: IV 20-60 mEq q24h
	200 mEq per 24 hr for hypokalemia is usually not exceeded. 40 mEq dilution per liter preferred
	SDR, **Child,** Individualized: IV 1-4 mEq per kg of body weight per 24 hr
	OR
	10 mEq per hr, whichever is <u>less</u>, not to exceed 40 mEq per 24 hr. Must be at least 40 mEq dilution per liter.
	Monitor serum potassium levels.
	Contact prescriber if patient is fluid-restricted.
	Monitor ECG for symptoms of hypokalemia and hyperkalemia.
	Pediatrics: KCl must be infused on electronic infusion pump. Obtain written order for *each* infusion.
Morphine Sulfate	
Pain relief	**Adult,** IV: 2.5-15 mg q4h
Postoperative analgesia	**Child,** IV: 0.01-0.04 mg per kg per hr
	Neonate, IV: 0.015-0.02 mg per kg per hr*
Severe chronic cancer pain	**Child,** IV: 0.025-2.6 mg per kg per hr
Prazosin HCl	**Adult,** PO: 1 mg at bedtime to start
	Child, PO: 5 mcg per kg q6h to start
Amoxicillin	**Adult,** PO: 250-500 mg q8h
	Child, PO: 25-50 mg per kg per d (max 60-80 mg per kg per d divided q8h)
Digoxin IV Injection	Initial loading (digitalizing dose)
	Premature: 15-25 mcg per kg; **2-5 yrs:** 25-35 mcg per kg;
	over 10 years: 8-12 mcg per kg

*A neonate refers to an infant in the first 4 weeks of life. Consult drug references for child age-related dose guidelines. They vary.
➤ Slashes (/) will be seen in printed drug references. Write out "per" for slashes to avoid misinterpretation and medication errors.

Medication Dosing Differences for Children and Adults

Estimated completion time: 10-15 minutes   Answers on page 565

Directions: *Examine Table 13-1 to answer the questions pertaining to SDR guidelines.*

1   What is the difference in the drug *unit of measurement* for adults and children for the antihypertensive drug prazosin? (How many mcg are there in a mg?)

_____

2   What is the difference in the initial *frequency schedules* for the antihypertensive drug prazosin for adults and children?

_____

3   What is the difference in the *maximum* doses of morphine sulfate for a child with postoperative pain and a child with severe chronic cancer pain?

_____

4   What is the *maximum* recommended initial loading dose of Digoxin IV injection for a child over 10 yrs? _____; a premature infant? _____

5   What action must be taken if a patient is fluid restricted and potassium is ordered?

_____

Calculating Kilograms to the Nearest Tenth from Pounds and Ounces

A patient's body weight in pounds or kilograms is usually calculated to the nearest tenth for determining pediatric doses.

➤   It is important to note that ounces must be converted to tenths of a pound *before* kilograms are calculated. 5 lb 4 oz is *not* equal to 5.4 lb.

How many kilograms are equivalent to 5 lb 4 oz?

First: Convert 5 lb 4 oz to pounds.
Conversion factor: 16 oz = 1 lb

EXAMPLES

➤   Ounces must be converted to tenths of a pound *before* kilograms are calculated. 5 lb 4 oz is *not* equal to 5.4 pounds.

Step 1	:	Step 2	$\times$	Step 3	=	Answer
Desired Answer Units	:	Starting Factor	$\times$	Given Quantity and Conversion Factor(s)	=	Estimate, Multiply, Evaluate
lb	:	$\dfrac{1\text{ lb}}{\cancel{16\text{ oz}}_{4}}$	$\times$	$\dfrac{\cancel{4\text{ oz}}^{1}}{1}$	=	$\dfrac{1}{4} = 0.25$ lb, rounded to 0.3 lb

The equation to convert ounces to pounds will be written like this:

$$\text{lb} : \dfrac{1\text{ lb}}{\cancel{16\text{ oz}}_{4}} \times \dfrac{\cancel{4\text{ oz}}^{1}}{1} = 0.25 \text{ lb, rounded to 0.3 lb}$$

Total pounds = 5 lb + .3 lb = 5.3 lb.

Next: Convert 5.3 lb to kilograms.
Conversion factor: 2.2 lb = 1 kg.

Step 1	:	Step 2	×	Step 3	=	Answer
Desired Answer Units	:	Starting Factor	×	Given Quantity and Conversion Factor(s)	=	Estimate, Multiply, Evaluate
kg	:	$\dfrac{1 \text{ kg}}{2.2 \text{ lb}}$	×	$\dfrac{5.3 \text{ lb}}{1}$	=	2.4 kg

The final equation will be written like this:

$$kg : \frac{1 \text{ kg}}{2.2 \text{ lb}} \times \frac{5.3 \text{ lb}}{1} = 2.4 \text{ kg}$$

Analysis: Two simple conversion equations were used for this problem. Ounces needed to be changed to lb and then added to the 5 lb.

Evaluation: The answer unit is correct: kg. A rough estimate of (lb ÷ 2) supports the answer. (Math check: 5.3 ÷ 2.2 = 2.4). The equation is balanced.

➤ Estimates can alert you to major math errors. Always verify your estimates.
  ➤ The nurse must know how to set up a DA equation to calculate doses in case a functioning calculator is not available.

RAPID PRACTICE 13-3

Converting Pounds to Kilograms

Estimated completion time: 20-25 minutes   Answers on page 566

Directions: *Estimate and calculate the weight in kg. Calculate the weight in kg to the nearest tenth of a kilogram using DA-style equations. Verify the result with a calculator. Remember to change ounces to pounds if necessary.*

1 12 lb 3 oz
  a. Estimated kg wt: _____
  b. Actual wt in kg:

    DA equation:

    c. Evaluation: _____

2 20 lb 6 oz
  a. Estimated kg wt: _____
  b. Actual wt in kg:

    DA equation:

    c. Evaluation: _____

3 4 lb 8 oz
  a. Estimated kg wt: _____
  b. Actual wt in kg:

DA equation:

  c. Evaluation: _____

4 25 lb 9 oz
  a. Estimated kg wt: _____
  b. Actual wt in kg:

    DA equation:

  c. Evaluation: _____

5 18 lb 12 oz
  a. Estimated kg wt: _____
  b. Actual wt in kg:

    DA equation:

  c. Evaluation: _____

Sequence for Calculating Safe Dose Range (SDR)

➤ Review the logic and example of the multi-step process for evaluating an order for safe dose. A calculator is helpful.

STEPS

  1 Obtain the total body weight in the desired terms.
  2 Calculate the SDR.
  3 Compare and evaluate the order with the SDR. Contact the prescriber if the order is not within the SDR.
➤ **4** If the order is safe, estimate, calculate, and evaluate the dose.

Ordered: Drug Y, 60 mg PO per day in AM   **Patient's wt:** 26 lb 6oz
SDR: 5-10 mg per kg per day in a single dose
Supplied: Drug Y, 100 mg per 5 mL
Conversion factors: 16 oz = 1 lb and 2.2 lb = 1 kg

EXAMPLES

Steps

1. **Total lb:** $\dfrac{1 \text{ lb}}{16 \text{ oz}} \times \dfrac{6 \text{ oz}}{1} = 0.375$, rounded to 0.4 lb.

    26 + 0.4 lb = 26.4 total lb

Total kg: *(not needed for order; total lb to kg will be entered within SDR equation)**

2. **SDR for this child:**

$$\frac{\text{mg}}{\text{day}} : \frac{5 \text{ mg}}{\text{kg} \times \text{day}} \times \frac{1 \text{ kg}}{2.2 \text{ lb}} \times \frac{26.4 \text{ lb}}{1} = 60 \text{ mg per day low safe dose}$$

$$\frac{\text{mg}}{\text{day}} : \frac{10 \text{ mg}}{\text{kg} \times \text{day}} \times \frac{1 \text{ kg}}{2.2 \text{ lb}} \times \frac{26.4 \text{ lb}}{1} = 120 \text{ mg per day high safe dose}$$

3. **Evaluation:** It can be seen at a glance that the dose ordered is within the SDR for the total amount and the schedule. Medication is safe to give.

4. Dose Calculation:

Estimate: Will be giving less than 5 mL

$$\frac{mL}{dose} : \frac{\frac{1}{\cancel{5}\ mL}}{\frac{\cancel{100\ mg}}{2}} \times \frac{\cancel{60\ mg}}{dose} = 3\ mL\ per\ dose$$

Analysis and evaluation: The equation is balanced. This is a reasonable dose because the order was for slightly more than one-half the number of mg supplied in 5 mL.

*Had the order been for mg per kg or mcg per kg, the lb to kg conversion would have been done separately first.

- Note that once the *total number of pounds* is determined, it is entered in the SDR equations with the conversion formula to kilograms.

➤ Do not confuse the SDR doses with the order.

Q: Ask Yourself

A: My Answer

1 What are the four main steps in the sequence for evaluating and calculating the recommended safe dose? (State your answer using 1 to 3 key words for each step.)

_____

CLINICAL RELEVANCE

Please take time to read TJC discussion and recommendations to prevent pediatric medication errors in their Sentinel Event Alert #39 at http://www.jointcommission.org/sentinelevents/sentineleventalerts/sea_39.htm.

RAPID PRACTICE 13-4

Evaluating Pediatric Medication Orders in Terms of SDR

Estimated completion time: 25 minutes   Answers on page 566

Directions: *Obtain total lb and change to kg if needed. Calculate the SDR. Compare the ordered dose with the SDR in same units of measurement (compare mcg to mcg, mg to mg, and g to g using metric conversion formulas). Evaluate the order for safe dose. Use a calculator for long division and multiplication.*

1 Ordered: Drug Y, 500 mcg IV per hr. SDR for children: 10-20 mcg per kg per hr. Patient's weight: 66 lb.

   a. Estimated kg wt: _____ Actual kg wt: _____
   b. SDR for this child: _____

   DA equation:

   c. Evaluation: *Safe to give* or *Hold and clarify promptly with prescriber?* (Circle one.)

2 Ordered: Drug Y, 5 mg IV q8h. SDR for children: 200-500 mcg per kg per day in 3 divided doses. Patient's weight: 12 lb.

   a. Estimated kg wt: _____ Actual kg wt: _____
   b. SDR for this child: _____

   DA equation:

   c. Evaluation: *Safe to give* or *Hold and clarify promptly with prescriber.* (Circle one.)

3 Ordered: Drug Y, 250 mg PO 4 times daily. SDR for children: 1-1.5 g per day in 4 divided doses.

   a. SDR for children: _____

   b. Evaluation of order: _____

   c. Evaluation: *Safe to give* or *Hold and clarify promptly with prescriber?* (Circle one.)

4 Ordered: Drug Y, 2 mg PO q6h. SDR for children: 500-800 mcg per kg per day in 4-6 divided doses. Patient's weight: 22 lb.

   a. Estimated kg wt: _____ Actual kg wt: _____

   b. SDR for this child: _____

    DA equation:

   c. Evaluation: *Safe to give* or *Hold and clarify promptly with prescriber?* (Circle one.)

5 Ordered: Drug Y, 35 mg IM stat

   SDR for children: 1-3 mg per kg q4-6h

   Patient wt: 20 lb 4 oz

   a. Estimated kg wt: _____ Actual kg wt: _____

   b. SDR for this child: _____

    DA equation:

   c. Evaluation: *Safe to give* or *Hold and clarify promptly with prescriber?* (Circle one.)

Body Surface Area (BSA)

The weight-based medication orders for mg per kg and mcg per kg are the most frequently encountered units of measurement found in medication orders for children. Occasionally, the nurse will encounter an order for a child or adult based on body surface area (BSA) in square meters (m^2) of skin. BSA-based dosing is considered superior to weight-based dosing for specific medications.

Most medications ordered in square meters of BSA are calculated by the pharmacist or prescriber and frequently are antineoplastic drugs administered by a nurse who has chemotherapy certification. Square meters of BSA may also be used for the SDR of drugs other than anticancer agents, particularly for infants, children, and geriatric patients. In addition, BSA may be used for calculating fluid and ventilation requirements.

➤ The nurse is expected to be able to define BSA, identify square meters, and, *most important*, distinguish among m^2 and mg and mcg metric measurements when reading orders, medication records, and current drug references and when calculating SDR. The nurse rarely calculates the BSA. Pharmacy usually supplies it.

The BSA is derived from formulas based on weight and height. There are two BSA formulas, one for the metric system and one for the English system.

Metric Formula

$$\sqrt{\frac{\text{weight (kg)} \times \text{height (cm)}}{3600}} = \text{BSA (m}^2)$$

English Formula

$$\sqrt{\frac{\text{weight (lb)} \times \text{height (in)}}{3131}} = \text{BSA (m}^2)$$

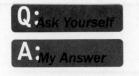

1   A meter is just a little larger than a yard (1 meter = 1.09 yard). If you estimated your BSA in square yards, would you expect the amount to be very small?

2   What is my BSA? Use your weight and a calculator to apply one of the BSA formulas. Multiply the numerators, divide by the denominator, and then enter the square root sign. Does the term *square meters* provide a clue as to size of the result?

Reading body surface area in square meters on a nomogram

The BSA nomogram is an *estimation* of BSA and is faster to use than the formulas. Figure 13-1 is an example of a nomogram of a BSA-derived medication dose.

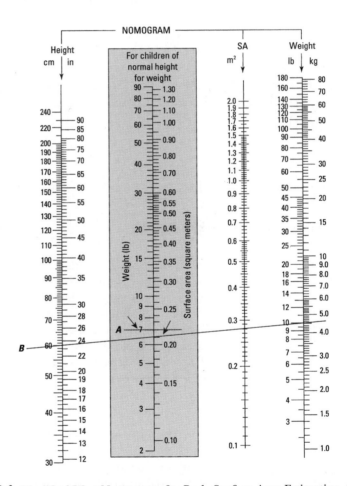

FIGURE 13-1 Modified West Nomogram for Body Surface Area Estimation. The red line denoted by arrow *A* in the highlighted column, "Children of Normal Height for Weight," illustrates a BSA of 0.7 m² for a child weighing 7 pounds. Calculations for children who are *not* at normal height for weight as determined by pediatric standard growth charts will have a different BSA for their weight. The outside columns are used to plot their height and weight. The BSA is read at the intersection as indicated by the red arrow over line *B* on the column titled "*SA*" by connecting the two plotted measurements with a straight line *B*. There are additional nomograms for adults. (Nomogram modified with data from Kliegman RM, Behrman RE, Jenson HB, Stanton BF (editors): *Nelson textbook of pediatrics*, ed. 18, Philadelphia, 2007, Saunders.)

Calculating milligrams per square meter (mg per m²)

In calculating the mg per m² of BSA, the sequence is the same as that used in mcg- and mg-based SDR calculations.

➤ The calculation of milligrams per square meter is performed using a DA-style equation or simple multiplication, just as it is for calculating milligrams per kilogram (e.g., 2 mg per m² means "2 milligrams of medicine for each square meter of body surface area").

Examine the following example.

Ordered: Drug Y, 4 mg PO qid

Patient's BSA: 0.8 m². SDR: 20 mg per m² daily in 4 divided doses.

$$\frac{mg}{day} = \frac{20\ mg}{m^2\ day} \times \frac{0.8\ m^2}{1} = 16\ mg\ per\ day\ (\div\ 4 = 4\ mg\ per\ dose)$$

SDR: 16 mg total per day divided in 4 doses

Order: 16 mg total per day, 4 mg per dose

Evaluation: The total dose and the frequency schedule are in accordance with the SDR. Give 4 mg.

EXAMPLES

➤ Pay close attention to the placement of decimal points. Square meters of BSA are *very small amounts*. A missing decimal point would result in a tenfold dose error.

➤ Pediatric doses are calculated to the *nearest hundredth* of a mL. Check agency policies.

FAQ | *Where will the staff nurse find the BSA of the patient?*

ANSWER | The pharmacy usually provides the BSA and the dose on a MAR or a separate chemotherapy medication sheet. The nurse uses the pharmacy-provided BSA calculation to check the SDR obtained from a current pharmacology reference or drug package insert. If the BSA is not available and a nomogram for the appropriate age group is not available, the pharmacy can be contacted.

Evaluating Pediatric SDR

RAPID PRACTICE 13-5

Estimated completion time: 15-20 minutes **Answers on page 567**

Directions: *Evaluate the following orders. For BSA in square meters, read the nomogram in Figure 13-1 and calculate the safe dose. Set up a DA equation, and verify your answer with a calculator. State reason for giving or withholding the medication.*

1 Ordered: An IV infusion of heparin 225 units per hr for a baby of normal height for weight weighing 10 lb.

SDR: 20,000 units per m² q24h continues IV infusion
a. BSA for this child: _____
b. SDR for this patient: _____

DA equation:

c. Evaluation: *Safe to give* or *Hold and clarify promptly with prescriber?* (Circle one and state reason.) _____

2 Ordered: vincristine 1 mg IV once a week, for a child with Hodgkin's disease of normal height for weight weighing 30 lb. SDR: 1.5-2 mg per m² per week.
a. BSA for this child: _____

    b. SDR for this patient: _____

    DA equation:

    c. Evaluation: *Safe to give* or *Hold and clarify promptly with prescriber?* (Circle one and state reason.) _____

3 Ordered: methotrexate 15 mg PO daily, for a child with leukemia of normal height for weight weighing 70 lb. SDR: 3.3 mg per m² per day.

    a. BSA for this child: _____
    b. SDR for this patient: _____

    DA equation:

    c. Evaluation: *Safe to give* or *Hold and clarify promptly with prescriber?* (Circle one and state reason.) _____

4 Ordered: gentamicin 125 mg every 8 hours IV, for a child with severe infection weighing 50 kg. SDR: 2-2.5 mg per kg q8h.

    a. Is BSA needed? Why or why not? _____
    b. SDR for this patient: _____

    DA equation:

    c. Evaluation: *Safe to give* or *Hold and clarify promptly with prescriber?* (Circle one and state reason.) _____

5 Ordered: dopamine 20 mcg per min IV, for an infant with respiratory distress syndrome weighing 5 kg. SDR: starting dose 1-5 mcg per kg per min.

    a. Is BSA needed? Why or why not? _____
    b. SDR for this patient: _____

    DA equation:

    c. Evaluation: *Safe to give* or *Hold and clarify promptly with prescriber?* (Circle one and state reason.) _____

➤ There may be a good reason for a very high dose order, such as severity of illness or nonresponsiveness to a lower dose. The nurse must clarify and document the response from the prescriber, as in the following example:

"4/25/11, 1800: High dose of Drug Y, 5 mg per hr IV for 22-kg child, verified with prescriber per TC. John Smith, R.N. "

Equipment for Medication Administration to Pediatric Patients and Patients Unable to Chew Tablets and Pills

In addition to dose modifications, the equipment used to deliver medication to a child may be different from that used for the average adult. Droppers, bottle nipples, measuring teaspoons, special oral syringes, and regular syringes *with the needle removed,* with or without a short tubing extension, may be used.

CLINICAL RELEVANCE

The medications may be administered with pleasant-tasting, nonessential foods to disguise an unfamiliar or unwelcome taste. A pill-crushing device or mortar and pestle may be needed to grind and mix non–enteric-coated pills, if permitted (Figure 13-2). Water, applesauce, or sherbet may be used to mix the medication or formula to follow the medication, depending on diet orders, swallowing ability, and age. Popsicles may be permitted immediately after a medicine to offset the taste. Some children prefer to drink from a 1-oz medicine cup.

➤ If a nipple is used to deliver medication, rinse the nipple with water first so that the medicine will flow rather than stick to the nipple.

➤ Follow the medicine with water or formula *within the fluid limitations* permitted for the patient (Figure 13-3).

When family members are present, they can be very helpful by holding the child and/or giving the oral medication and something more pleasant-tasting to follow.

Remember that medications can be measured accurately with a syringe and transferred to another device.

➤ Do NOT mix medicines in milk or formula. An off-taste in an essential food is very undesirable.
➤ Take extra measures to assess swallowing ability before attempting to give any medications by mouth to at-risk populations. This may include checking the gag reflex with a tongue blade.
➤ The presence of a gag reflex alone is not enough to assume swallowing ability. Follow up with a test of swallowing some sips of water. Do not assume that a baby can always drink from a bottle. Infants and children can have swallowing problems, just as adults can.

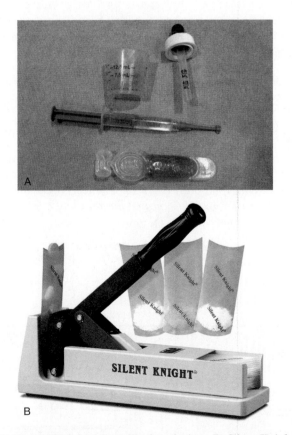

FIGURE 13-2 **A,** Pediatric liquid oral medication devices. **B,** Silent Knight® Tablet Crushing System. A pill crusher that contains disposable pouches for the tablet to prevent cross-contamination with prior crushed medications. (**B,** Used with permission from Links Medical Products, Inc., Irvine, CA.)

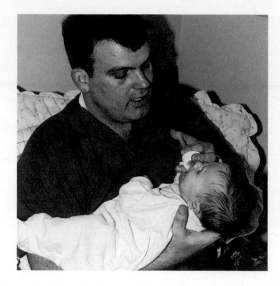

FIGURE 13-3 Using a nipple to deliver medication. (From Clayton BD, Stock YN, Cooper S: *Basic pharmacology for nurses,* ed. 15, St. Louis, 2010, Mosby.)

➤ Reminder: Never cut unscored tablets. Never crush enteric-coated, E-R, S-R, or gel coated medications. Do not crush capsules. Check with pharmacy and/or prescriber if it is deemed necessary to alter the ordered form of medication.

CLINICAL RELEVANCE

Giving medications to pediatric patients can be a challenge. Some nurses have the intuitive skills necessary to obtain cooperation, and others acquire skills through experience. It helps the pediatric nursing student to shadow an experienced pediatric nurse. The records and report should provide clues as to the child's behaviors and preferences. Clinical experience in pediatric units is often limited, and there may not be enough time to have several successes.

RAPID PRACTICE 13-6

Pediatric Oral Medications

Estimated completion time: 30-60 minutes   Answers on page 568

Directions: *Determine the patient's weight in kg to the nearest tenth if needed. Calculate SDR, and evaluate the order for appropriate dose and schedule. Use a calculator for long division and multiplication. If the order is safe to administer, calculate liquid doses to nearest tenth and doses less than 1 mL to nearest hundredth of a mL. If the drug is to be held, state the reason but do not calculate the dose.*

1 Ordered: Keflex (cephalexin for oral suspension) 150 mg PO qid for a child with a mild upper respiratory infection.

Read the label to obtain the SDR.

Patient's weight: 36 lb

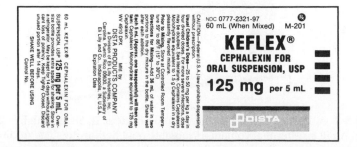

a. SDR for this child: _____

DA equation:

b. Evaluation: *Safe to give* or *Hold and clarify promptly with prescriber?* (Circle one and state reason.) _____

c. Total number of mg in container: _____

d. Dilution directions (use brief phrases):

_____

e. Volume to be administered if safe dose: _____

2   Ordered: leucovorin 20 mg PO 6 hr after administration of the antineoplastic methotrexate today to prevent toxicity.

SDR: 10 mg per m^2 per dose

Patient's weight: 70 lb (31.8 kg). BSA: 1.10 m^2*

Each tablet contains:
Leucovorin Calcium
USP, (equivalent to
5 mg Leucovorin).

Usual Dosage:
See package outsert.
Dispense with child-
resistant closure in a
tight, light-resistant
container as defined
in the USP/NF.
Store at controlled
room temperature
15°-30°C (59°-86°F).
PROTECT FROM LIGHT
BARR LABORATORIES, INC.
Pomona, NY 10970
R6-91

BARR LABORATORIES, INC.

b

**Leucovorin
Calcium
Tablets**

5 mg

Caution: Federal law prohibits
dispensing without prescription.

100 Tablets

NDC 0555-0484-02
NSN 6505-01-176-2543

0555-0484-02   SAMPLE

Exp. Date:

Lot No.:

a. SDR for this child: _____

DA equation:

b. Evaluation: *Safe to give* or *Hold and clarify promptly with prescriber?* (Circle one and state reason.) _____

c. Amount to be administered if safe dose: _____

DA equation:

d. Evaluation: _____

1   What amount would have been administered if the nurse was unfamiliar with square meters and used the weight in kilograms or pounds instead of square meters in problem 2 to calculate the dose?

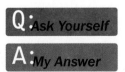

_____

3   Ordered: Biaxin (clarithromycin oral suspension) 150 mg PO bid, for a child with otitis media.

SDR for this child: 15 mg per kg per day in 2 divided doses

_____

*Trailing zeros (e.g., 1.10 m^2) are not permitted (per TJC) in patient medication-related documents. They are encountered in printed laboratory, drug, and scientific references and are appropriate for BSA nomograms.

Patient's weight: 44 lb

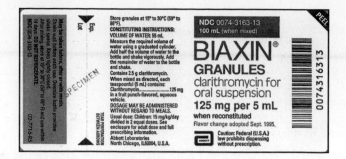

    a. SDR for this child: _____

    DA equation:

    b. Evaluation: *Safe to give* or *Hold and clarify promptly with prescriber?* (Circle one
    and state reason.) _____

    c. Dilution directions: _____

    d. Amount to be administered if safe dose: _____

4   Ordered: Lanoxin (digoxin) elixir 0.1 mg PO bid maintenance dose, for a
4-year-old child with congestive heart failure who has already received a loading dose

SDR for children >2 years: loading dose 0.02-0.04 mg per kg divided q8h
over 24 hr; maintenance dose 0.006-0.012 mg per kg in divided doses q12h

Patient's weight: 18 kg

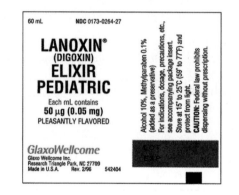

    a. SDR for this child to nearest tenth of a mg: _____

    DA equation:

    b. Evaluation: *Safe to give* or *Hold and clarify promptly with prescriber* (Circle one
    and state reason.) _____

    c. Amount to be administered if safe dose:

    Estimated dose: _____

    DA equation:

    d. How many mcg per mL are provided in the medication container?

    _____

5   Ordered: Epivir solution (lamivudine), an antiviral agent, 18 mg PO tid for a baby with HIV infection

SDR for children <50 kg: 2 mg per kg per day in divided doses q8h with zidovudine

Patient's weight: 20 lb

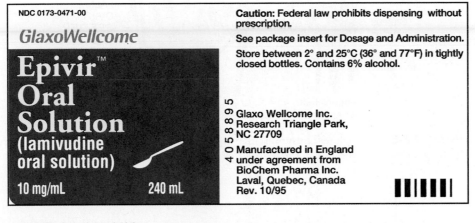

a. SDR for this child: _____

DA equation:

b. Evaluation: *Safe to give* or *Hold and clarify promptly with prescriber?* (Circle one.)
c. Amount to be administered if safe dose: _____

Injection Sites for Pediatric Patients

Injections are traumatic for pediatric patients. IV Med-lock ports are often used to administer medications.

Check agency policies regarding injection sites. With all injections, the potential site must be fully visible and carefully assessed.

The vastus lateralis muscle can be used from birth to adulthood but is a *preferred injection site* for babies younger than 7 months of age (Figure 13-4).

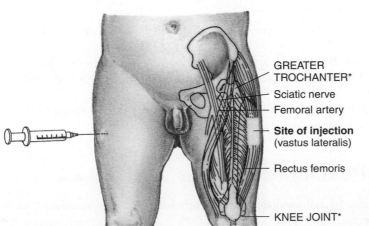

FIGURE 13-4 Vastus lateralis injection site. (From Wilson D, Hockenberry MJ: *Wong's clinical manual of pediatric nursing,* ed. 7, St. Louis, 2008, Mosby.)

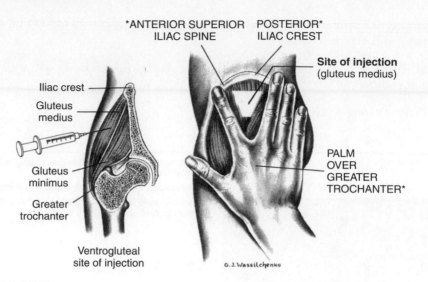

FIGURE 13-5 Ventrogluteal intramuscular injection site. (From Wilson D, Hockenberry MJ: *Wong's clinical manual of pediatric nursing,* ed. 7, St. Louis, 2008, Mosby.)

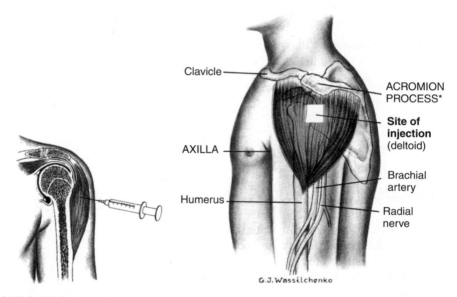

FIGURE 13-6 Deltoid injection site. (From Wilson D, Hockenberry MJ: *Wong's clinical manual of pediatric nursing,* ed. 7, St. Louis, 2008, Mosby.)

➤ The ventrogluteal muscle is an *alternate site* for children over 7 months of age and adults (Figure 13-5).
➤ The deltoid site may be used for small-volume, non-irritating medications (0.5 to 1 mL) in older children and adults with well-developed deltoid muscles (Figure 13-6).
➤ The dorsogluteal site is not a recommended injection site due to danger of damaging the sciatic nerve and striking blood vessels.

Injection Volumes for Pediatric Populations

Injection volumes must be adjusted downward, depending on the size and condition of the area to be injected.

➤ 0.5 mL is the maximum for subcutaneous injections in infants and small children.

➤ 1 mL is the maximum for IM injections in children *<2 years*. Assess the potential sites for older children before making a decision to increase the volume per site.

As with adults, subcutaneous and IM medications in children must be administered with the correct size and angle of needle for the area being injected. A angle may be needed for IM injections for underweight patients.

The syringe is selected based on the volume of the medication. A 1-mL syringe may be used for medication doses of <1 mL. This syringe permits administration to the *nearest hundredth* of a milliliter.

Supervised practice and reference to current clinical skills textbooks are needed to develop these injection skills.

Subcutaneous and Intramuscular Injections for Children   RAPID PRACTICE 13-7

Estimated completion time: 25-30 minutes   Answers on page 569

Directions: *Evaluate the following orders. If the dose is safe to administer, calculate the dose. Evaluate all your equations. Indicate the nearest measurable dose with an arrow on the syringe provided. Use a calculator for long division and multiplication.*

1 Ordered: atropine sulfate 0.2 mg subcut on call to the operating room, as prophylaxis for excess secretions and salivation during anesthesia.

SDR for children: 0.01 mg per kg subcut per dose

Patient's weight: 22.9 kg

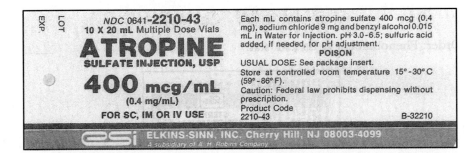

a. SDR for this child: _____

DA equation:

b. Evaluation: *Safe to give* or *Hold and clarify promptly with prescriber?* (Circle one and state reason.) _____

c. Amount to be administered if safe to give:

DA equation:

d. Evaluation: _____

Draw an arrow pointing to the dose on the syringe.

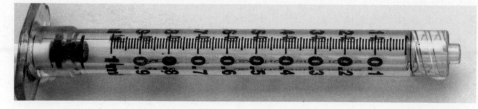

2 Ordered: AquaMEPHYTON (phytonadione) 4 mg IM once a week prophylactically for hypothrombinemia, for a child on prolonged TPN therapy who has not walked in several months.

SDR for children: 2-5 mg once weekly IM

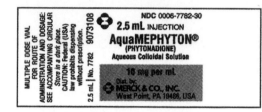

a. SDR for this child: _____

b. Evaluation: *Safe to give* or *Hold and clarify promptly with prescriber*? (Circle one and state reason.) _____

c. Amount to be administered if safe to give:

DA equation:

d. Evaluation: _____

Draw an arrow pointing to the dose on the syringe.

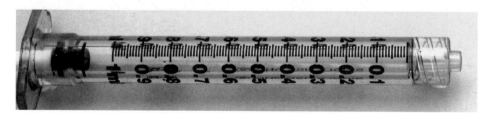

3 Ordered: Humalog insulin 3 units subcut 4 times daily ac and at bedtime, for a newly diagnosed 10-year-old child with diabetes type 1.

SDR for children: initial 2-4 units subcut 4 times daily ac and at bedtime

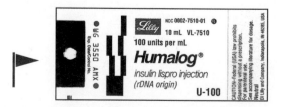

a. SDR for this child: _____

b. Evaluation: *Safe to give* or *Hold and clarify promptly with prescriber?* (Circle one and state reason.) _____

c. Draw an arrow pointing to the dose on the syringe that would be easier to read for this dose.

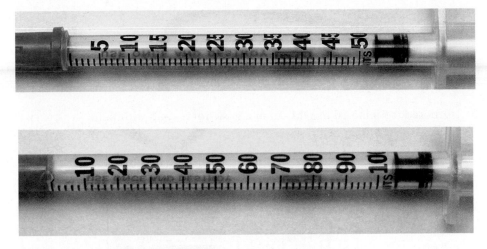

d. Would a bedtime snack be needed? If so, why?

_____

➤ Remember that you may encounter *SC* and *HS* as abbreviations for "subcutaneous" and "bedtime." Do not write these abbreviations because they can be misinterpreted.

4 Ordered: adrenaline HCl 1:1000 (epinephrine injection) 1.2 mg subcut stat, a bronchodilator for a child with asthma.

SDR for children: IM or SC 0.01-0.03 mg per kg q5min if needed

Patient's weight: 66 lb.

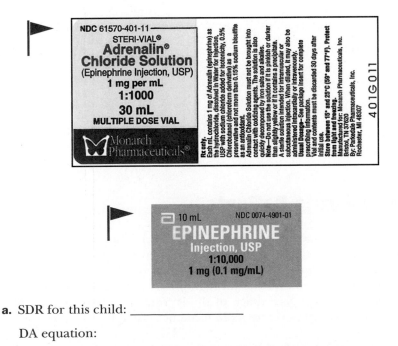

a. SDR for this child: _____

DA equation:

    b. Evaluation: *Safe to give* or *Hold and clarify promptly with prescriber?* (Circle one and state reason.) _____

    c. What is the amount of difference in concentration between the two labels?

    _____

    d. Which of the two labels is more concentrated? _____

    e. Amount to be administered if safe to give:

        DA equation:

    f. Evaluation:

5   Ordered: codeine 10 mg IM, an analgesic for a child with pain

    SDR for children: IM 0.5 mg per kg q4-6h

    Patient's weight: 44 lb.

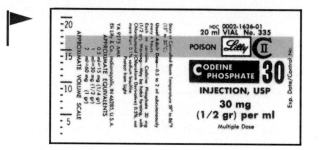

    a. SDR for this child (kg to nearest tenth; mg to nearest whole number):

        DA equation:

    b. Evaluation: *Safe to give* or *Hold and clarify promptly with prescriber?* (Circle one and state reason.) _____

    c. Amount to be administered if safe to give to nearest hundredth of a mL:

        DA equation:

    d. Evaluation:

    e. Which unit of measurement on the label is an apothecary unit?

    _____

Fluid Requirements for Pediatric Patients

Volume needs vary and need to be adjusted for the weight and age of the child. Infants have a larger percentage of fluid volume as a percentage of body weight than do older children and adults. They also have a greater BSA in relation to body mass, which causes them to lose more water through the skin than do older children and adults. They lose a higher percentage of fluids from the lungs because of their more rapid respirations and excrete more urine because it is less concentrated.

➤ Overhydration and dehydration can present a grave risk to pediatric patients. There are several formulas for calculating fluid requirements. They are adjusted for maintenance and replacement as well as for conditions requiring

TABLE 13-2	Fluid Requirements of Healthy Children and Adults				
				Average Fluid Intake Requirement	
Weight	**Normal Fluid Volume Need**	**Sample Weight (kg)**	**Daily**	**Hourly**	
Neonate	90 mL per kg per 24 hr	3 kg	270 mL	11 mL	
Up to 10 kg	120 mL per kg per 24 hr after age 7 days	8 kg	960 mL	40 mL	
11-20 kg	1000 mL + 50 mL per kg over 10 kg	15 kg	1250 mL	52 mL	
Over 20 kg	1500 mL + 20 mL per kg over 20 kg	25 kg	1600 mL	67 mL	
Average adult	2-3 liters per day	68 kg	2000-3000 mL	125 mL	

fluid restrictions. Some formulas are based on caloric metabolism and others on BSA. Keep these concepts and the data in Table 13-2, which follows, in mind when administering any kind of fluids and oral or parenteral medications to pediatric patients.

Table 13-2 illustrates the average fluid requirements of *healthy* adults, babies, and children of various weights.

1 What would be the normal 24-hr fluid intake requirement for a baby weighing 8 kg (17.6 lb) compared with an adult weighing 68 kg?

Q: *Ask Yourself*

A: *My Answer*

➤ A child with cardiac, respiratory, or renal dysfunction may have severe fluid restrictions imposed. Such restrictions would affect the amount of fluid to be administered with medications as well as IV solution flow rates.

➤ If a pediatric patient is receiving fluids from other sources, such as bottles and cups, the IV volume must be adjusted downward accordingly. This is also the case with adults.

CLINICAL RELEVANCE

Intravenous Injections for Infants and Children

➤ Infusion volumes for infants and children are much *smaller* and infusion rates *slower* than for average adults. Use of a volumetric infusion pump for IV fluids and medications is preferred for pediatric patients. Check agency policies.

Using a volume-control device

The use of a volume-control device protects patients from accidental fluid and drug overload if the flow rate is programmed correctly (Figure 13-7). Volume-control devices may be used for two purposes:

1 They protect from possible fluid overload from the main IV line. This is achieved by opening the clamp from the main IV line to fill the chamber with 1 or 2 hours worth of IV fluid, according to agency policy.

2 The medication may be added to the solution from the main IV bag or to a separate solution placed in the volume-control device. This would be an alternative to attaching a piggyback medicated solution to a port on a primary IV line. (Refer also to Ch 9.)

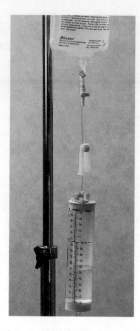

FIGURE 13-7 Volume-control device. (From Perry AG, Potter PA: *Clinical nursing skills and techniques,* ed. 7, St. Louis, 2010, Mosby.)

Using Volume-Control Chambers to Protect Patients from Fluid and Drug Overload*

EXAMPLES

Ordered: Drug Y in a continuous IV infusion at 1.5 mg per kg per hr

Available: 100 mg in 100 mL NS

Patient's weight: 8 kg

SDR: maximum 6 mg per kg per hr

Agency policy: 1 hour's worth of fluid volume is maximum amount permitted in volume control chamber.

$$\frac{mg}{hr} = \frac{1.5\ mg}{1\ \cancel{kg}} \times \frac{8\ \cancel{kg}}{hr} = 12\ mg\ per\ hr$$

To calculate the volume in mL per hr needed to deliver 12 mg per hr,

$$\frac{mL}{hr} = \frac{\overset{1}{\cancel{100}\ mL}}{\underset{1}{\cancel{100\ mg}}} \times \frac{12\ \cancel{mg}}{1\ hr} = 12\ mL\ per\ hr$$

The nurse opens the clamp on the main IV line, puts 1 hour's worth of medicated fluid (12 mL) in the volume-control device, and shuts the clamp to the main IV line (Figure 13-8). An alarm will be set off to alert staff to a need for chamber refill.

➤ Agency flush procedures must be followed.

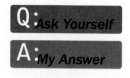

1 An IV infusion contains 100 mg of drug in 250 mL of solution. What is the maximum amount of fluid and medicine that can flow into the patient very rapidly if the main IV line malfunctions (assuming there is no volume-control device in place)?

Using a Volume-Control Device to Administer Intravenous Medication The medication dose may be added with a syringe through the port to the chamber after the IV diluent is placed in the volume-control device (Figure 13-8).

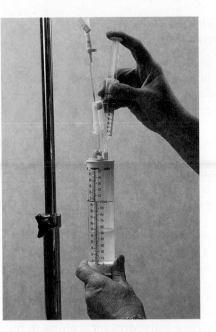

FIGURE 13-8 Adding medication to a volume-control device. (From Perry AG, Potter PA: *Clinical nursing skills and techniques,* ed. 7, St. Louis, 2010, Mosby.)

➤ If a *different medication* than that shown on the label of the main IV fluid is added to a volume-control device, a medication label must be attached to the volume-control device.

For example, with a main IV solution of potassium in D5W and an ordered antibiotic of amikacin to be infused over 30 minutes, a label such as the following would be attached to the volume-control device:

> MEDICATION ADDED
>
> 1/01/11, 1800, amikacin sulfate 50 mg per 50 mL
> D5W. Flow rate: 25 mL per hr.
>
> John Smith, R.N.

This label will alert the staff that a *flush* and possible flow rate change will be necessary after the medication infusion is completed.

Flushing a volume-control device

The volume-control device and tubing must be cleared of medication residue with a "flush" *before* and *after* the medication has been infused. If the flush solution is different from the main IV solution, a new label must be placed on the volume-control device to alert the staff that a flush is taking place. The label alerts the staff to *wait before* adding another medication to the system.

> FLUSH
>
> 1/01/11, 1830, 15 mL D5W infusing
>
> John Smith, R.N.

Check agency policies for types and amounts of flushes. A flush may be indicated before and after a medication is administered and may consist of 5-10 mL or more of solution. It should be of an amount sufficient to clear the volume-control device and the rest of the IV line to the venous entry site.

Calculating the medicated fluid amount for a volume-control device

- Calculate the *total amount of fluid* for the dose and diluent (e.g., 5 mL antibiotic to be diluted to 30 mL with NS) as stated in the drug insert or pediatric drug reference.
- Shut the clamp to the main IV line. Flush line according to agency policy. Place the diluent *minus* the amount of medicine in the calibrated chamber of the volume-control device (e.g., 30 mL − 5 mL medicine = 25 mL NS).
- Add the medicine and gently mix the medicine and diluent in the calibrated chamber.
- Administer the medicine at the ordered flow rate. Label the volume-control device.
- Flush the volume-control device with the needed amount and type of flush solution. Label the volume-control device for the flush. Reset the flow rate as needed.

➤ If an infusion pump is not available, a microdrip pediatric administration set with a DF of 60 is used with a volume-control device. Recall that the hourly drop/min flow rate for a microdrip set is equal to the number of mL/hr ordered (Figure 13-9).

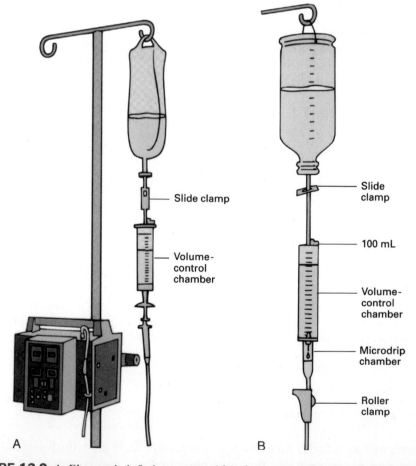

FIGURE 13-9 A, Electronic infusion pump with volume-control device. **B,** Gravity infusion with volume-control device and microdrip tubing. (From Brown M, Mulholland JL: *Drug calculations: process and problems for clinical practice,* ed. 8, St. Louis, 2008, Mosby.)

Volume-Control Device Flow Rates

Estimated completion time: 10 minutes   Answers on page 570

Directions: *Examine the example in problem 1. Calculate the amount of medicine and flush to be administered. Refer to Intravenous Piggyback Solutions in Chapter 9 (p. 282) for review if necessary.*

1 Ordered: 2 mL medicine to be diluted to 25 mL D5W in a volume-control device on a volumetric pump and infused over 30 minutes.

   a. Amount of diluent to place in volume-control device:
     25 mL − 2 mL = 23 mL diluent

   b. Amount of medicine to place in volume-control device: 2 mL medicine

   c. IV flow rate to set on the pump: 50 mL per hr

   DA equation:

$$\frac{mL}{hr} = \frac{25 \text{ mL}}{\cancel{30 \text{ min}}_{1}} \times \frac{\cancel{60 \text{ min}}^{2}}{1 \text{ hr}} = 50 \text{ mL per hr}$$

   d. Evaluation: The equation is balanced. An IV flow rate of 50 mL over 60 minutes will deliver 25 mL in 30 minutes.

Follow the medication with a 5- to 10-mL flush. Check agency policy for content and volume of flush.

2 Ordered: 10 mL medicine to be diluted to 20 mL NS in a volume-control device on a volumetric infusion pump and infused over 30 minutes.

   a. Amount of diluent to place in volume-control device: _____

   b. Amount of medicine to place in volume-control device: _____

   c. IV flow rate to set on pump: _____

   DA equation:

   d. Evaluation: _____

Follow the medication with a 5- to 10-mL flush. Check agency policy.

3 Ordered: 25 mL of medicine to be diluted to 50 mL in NS in a volume-control device attached to a gravity infusion device with a pediatric microdrip tubing set to be administered over 1 hour. (Refer to Chapter 9 for a review of flow rate calculations for microdrip sets).

   a. Amount of diluent to place in volume-control device: _____

   b. Amount of medicine to place in volume-control device: _____

   c. Flow rate to set on microdrip pediatric set: _____ drops per min

Follow the medication with a 5- to 10-mL saline flush. Check agency policy.

4 Ordered: 15 mL of medication to be diluted to 30 mL in D5W on a volumetric infusion pump to be administered over 20 minutes.

   a. Amount of diluent to place in volume-control device: _____

   b. Amount of medicine to place in volume-control device: _____

   c. Flow rate to set on infusion pump: _____

Follow the medication with a 5- to 10-mL flush. Check agency policy.

5 Ordered: 3 mL of medication to be diluted to 15 mL in NS in a volume-control device on gravity infusion with microdrip tubing to be administered over 30 minutes.

   a. Amount of medicine to prepare for volume-control device: _____

   b. Flow rate to set on microdrip pediatric set: _____ drops per min

   DA equation:

   c. Evaluation: _____

Follow the medication with a 5- to 10-mL flush. Check agency policy.

Syringe pump infusers

A syringe pump system may be used to deliver *small-volume intermittent* infusions, which can also protect the patient from fluid and drug overload if the flow rate is programmed correctly. Syringe pump infusers can now be programmed for flow rates and alarms (Figure 13-10). Syringe pump devices are convenient for administration of small-volume infusions for pediatric patients.

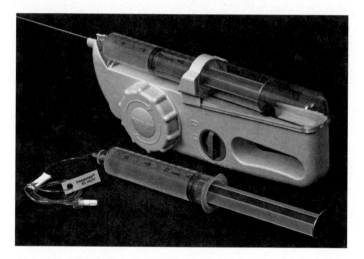

FIGURE 13-10 Freedom 60 syringe infusion pump system. (From Repro-Med Systems, Inc., Chester, NY.)

➤ To reduce errors, multiple national agencies are recommending independent double checks of high-risk drugs for pediatric and adult patients for EACH dose of the medication. Check your agency's policies also. Consult the pharmacist and/or prescriber if questions arise about the order.

Calculating medicated intravenous infusion rates review

EXAMPLES

If the ordered dose is within the SDR, the nurse calculates the flow rate in mL per hr to the nearest measurable amount on the equipment.

Ordered: Drug Y continuous infusion at 30 mcg per hr

Patient's weight: 66 lb, or 30 kg

SDR for children: 20-35 mcg/kg per 24 hr in IV infusion

Available: 2 mg ampule in 250 mL.

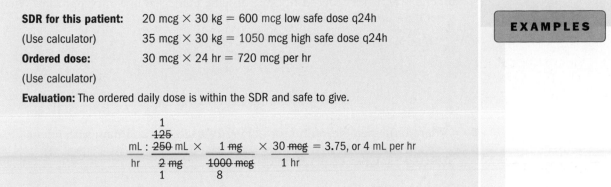

SDR for this patient: 20 mcg × 30 kg = 600 mcg low safe dose q24h

(Use calculator)   35 mcg × 30 kg = 1050 mcg high safe dose q24h

Ordered dose: 30 mcg × 24 hr = 720 mcg per hr

(Use calculator)

Evaluation: The ordered daily dose is within the SDR and safe to give.

$$\frac{mL}{hr} : \frac{\overset{1}{\cancel{125}}}{\cancel{250}\ mL} \times \frac{1\ \cancel{mg}}{\underset{8}{\cancel{1000\ mcg}}} \times \frac{30\ \cancel{mcg}}{1\ hr} = 3.75,\ or\ 4\ mL\ per\ hr$$

Administer at 4 mL per hour.

➤ When using a calculator, always repeat the calculation twice.

EXAMPLES

Comparing Safe Dose Range and Order

➤ Remember to compare the SDR and the ordered dose in the *same* units of measurement and for the same time frame: mg to mg, mcg to mcg, and hours to hours. Do not confuse the SDR and the order when performing the comparisons. When an underdose or overdose has been ordered, contact the prescriber promptly.

Intravenous Medication Calculations

RAPID PRACTICE 13-9

Estimated completion time: 30 minutes-1 hour   Answers on page 571

Directions: *Examine the example shown above. Solve the IV problems using DA equations and a calculator for long division and multiplication.*

1 Ordered: Trisenox (arsenic trioxide) IV infusion for a child with leukemia to flow at 5 mcg per min daily.

Available: Trisenox 10 mg per 250 mL NS
a. How many mcg per hr are ordered? _____
b. How many total mcg are in the available infusion? _____
c. How many mcg per mL are in the total available solution?

DA equation:

d. Evaluation: _____
e. What flow rate, to the nearest mL per hr, should be set?

DA equation:

f. Evaluation: _____

2 Use the information from problem 1. The agency has a policy that a volume-control device must be used. Agency policy states that a maximum of 2 hours' worth of volume can be placed in the device.

a. How many mL will be placed in the volume-control device? _____

b. The prescriber ordered that the dose be increased by 3 mcg per min. What will the new flow rate be?

DA equation:

c. Evaluation: _____

3 Ordered: furosemide, a diuretic, 25 mg IV q12h, for an infant with edema

SDR: 0.5-2 mg per kg per dose q6-12h

Patient's weight: 9 kg

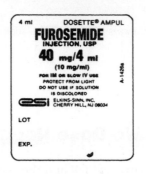

a. SDR for this infant: _____
b. Evaluation: *Safe to give* or *Hold and clarify promptly with prescriber?* (Circle one and state reason.) _____
c. Dose in mL to be administered if the order is safe to give:

DA equation:

d. Evaluation: _____

4 Ordered: KCl IV infusion 0.1 mEq per kg per hr in 100 mL D5W, ordered for a child with hypokalemia

Available from pharmacy: KCl 10 mEq per 100 mL D5W

SDR for children: up to 3 mEq per kg per 24 hr, not to exceed 40 mEq per 24 hr

Patient's weight: 8 kg

Directions in reference: Must be administered on infusion pump. Monitor electrocardiogram. Obtain order for subsequent infusion. Infuse using volume-control device with no more than 1 hour's worth of ordered fluid amount. Check potassium level every 2 hours.

a. SDR for this infant: _____
b. Amount ordered for 24 hours: _____
c. Evaluation: *Safe to give* or *Hold and clarify promptly with prescriber?* (Circle one and state reason.)_____
d. Hourly flow rate:

DA equation:

e. Evaluation:

5 Ordered: phenobarbital sodium 50 mg IV stat, for preoperative sedation of a child. SDR for children: 1-3 mg per kg per 24 hr 60-90 minutes before procedure. Patient's weight: 14 lb 8 oz. Available: phenobarbital sodium for injection 120 mg per mL.

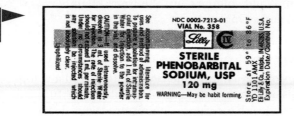

    a. Patient's weight in kg to nearest tenth: _____

    b. SDR for this child: _____

    DA equation:

    c. Evaluation: *Safe to give* or *Hold and clarify promptly with prescriber?* (Circle one and state reason.) _____

    d. Dose to be administered if the order is safe to give:

    DA equation:

    e. Evaluation:

CHAPTER 13 MULTIPLE-CHOICE REVIEW

Estimated completion time: 30-60 minutes   **Answers on page 572**

Directions: *Select the best answer. Use a calculator for long division and multiplication. Calculate kg to the nearest tenth. Calculate medications to nearest hundredth of a milliliter if less than 1 mL or to the nearest tenth if more than 1 mL.*

1 The nurse should avoid mixing medicines for an infant or toddler in which product: ____

    1. Applesauce   **3.** Water

    2. Sherbet   **4.** Milk

2 Which statement about body fluid volume in infants is true? ____

    1. Infants have a smaller amount of total body water as a percentage of body weight than do adults and therefore receive less fluid per kg than do adults.

    2. Infants and adults have approximately the same amount of total body water as a percentage of body weight.

    3. Infants have a greater fluid volume as a percentage of body weight than do adults and are subject to grave injury from dehydration.

    4. Infants are immune from body fluid deficits because of reduced intake needs.

3 The first suggested step for safe dose calculations for unfamiliar medications after reading the medication order and relevant laboratory tests is _____

    1. Call the prescriber.

    2. Calculate the SDR.

    3. Calculate the dose.

    4. Visit the parents and explain what you plan to do.

4 Two devices used in pediatric settings to help prevent drug or fluid volume overload for IV orders are _____

1. Add-Vantage systems and premixed medications
2. Gravity infusion sets and macrodrip tubing
3. Syringe pumps and volume-control burette chambers
4. PCA pumps and syringe pumps

5 If an electronic pump is not available to deliver a continuous infusion to a pediatric patient, which infusion device would be the best choice? _____

1. Gravity infusion device with microdrip tubing and a volume-control device
2. Gravity infusion device with macrodrip tubing DF 10
3. Direct injection with a syringe administered very slowly
4. PCA pump

6 An IV solution of 100 mL containing 10 mg of a drug is to be infused at 20 mcg per min. The mL per hr flow rate should be set at ____

1. 12   **3.** 100
2. 20   **4.** 120

7 An IV solution of 250 mL with 250 mg of drug is to be infused at 8 mL/ hr. The number of mg per hr to be delivered is _____

1. 1   **3.** 10
2. 8   **4.** 20

8 Ordered: 0.05 mg of a drug for a child. Available: 0.5 mg per 10 mL. How many mL will you administer? ____

1. 15   **3.** 5
2. 10   **4.** 1

9 A continuous IV of D5W at 15 mL per hr is ordered for a toddler. In the absence of an electronic infusion device, what is the correct action by the nurse? _____

1. Infuse the IV solution using a gravity device, macrodrip DF 15, at 4 mL per hr.
2. Infuse the IV solution using a gravity device, microdrip DF 60, at 15 drops per min.
3. Infuse the IV solution using a gravity device, DF 10, at 3 mL per hr.
4. Wait for an electronic infusion device to become available.

10 Ordered: phenobarbital sodium 80 mg IM for a 40-kg child who needs sedation. SDR: 6 mg per kg per day in 3 divided doses. Available: phenobarbital sodium for injection 120 mg per mL.

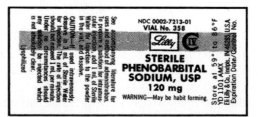

Which amount would you prepare?

1. 0.66 mL   **3.** 0.8 mL
2. 0.67 mL   **4.** Hold drug and contact prescriber.

CHAPTER 13 FINAL PRACTICE

Estimated completion time: 1-2 hours   Answers on page 572

Directions: *Use a calculator for long division and multiplication of weights and SDR. Label all answers.*

1 Ordered: diphenhydramine HCl (Benadryl Children's Liquid) 12.5 mg, for a 10-year-old child who has developed hives from an antibiotic. He is on a regular diet.

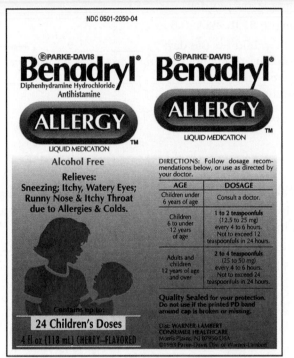

    a. How many mL will you administer? _____

    b. What might you offer to follow the dose if the child does not like the taste of the medicine? _____

2 Ordered: Augmentin oral suspension 1 gram bid, for a 5-year-old child with tonsillitis. Pt weight: 38 kg.

    SDR: 20-40 mg per kg per day in 3-4 divided doses.

    a. SDR for this child: _____

    b. Evaluation: *Safe to give* or *Hold and clarify promptly with prescriber?* (Circle one and state reason(s). _____

    c. Calculate the dose if safe.

    DA equation:

    d. Evaluation: _____

3 Ordered: cytarabine, an antineoplastic drug, 0.1 g per day IV to be infused in NS over 4 hours.

SDR: 100 mg per m^2 per day

Patient's weight: 31 lb. BSA: 0.6 m^2.

    a. SDR for this child for the day: _____

    b. Evaluation: *Safe to give* or *Hold and clarify promptly with prescriber?* (Circle one and state reason.) _____

    c. Calculate the dose if safe.

    DA equation:

    d. Evaluation: _____

4 Ordered: Mycostatin (nystatin) oral syrup 250,000 units for a 4-month-old infant with thrush (oral candidiasis).

SDR for children and infants >3 months: 250,000-500,000 units per day

Directions: Place half the dose in either side of the mouth.

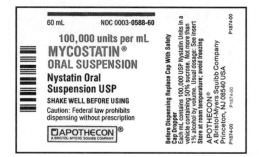

    a. If order is safe, how many mL will you prepare? _____

    DA equation:

    b. Evaluation: _____

    c. What device among those on p. 428 might be appropriate to administer this order to an infant of this age? _____

    d. How many mL will you administer on each side of the mouth of the child? _____

5 Ordered: Infants' acetaminophen 160 mg PO for a 2½-year-old child. Patient's weight: 12 kg.

Label A

Label B

Drug Facts (continued)
- use only enclosed dosing cup designed for use with this product. Do not use any other dosing device.
- if needed, repeat dose every 4 hours while symptoms last
- do not give more than 5 times in 24 hours
- do not give for more than 5 days unless directed by a doctor
- this product does not contain directions or complete warnings for adult use

Weight (lb)	Age (yr)	Dose (tsp or mL)
under 24	under 2 years	ask a doctor
24-35	2-3 years	1 tsp or 5 mL
36-47	4-5 years	1 1/2 tsp or 7.5 mL
48-59	6-8 years	2 tsp or 10 mL
60-71	9-10 years	2 1/2 tsp or 12.5 mL
72-95	11 years	3 tsp or 15 mL

Attention: use only enclosed dosing cup specifically designed for use with this product. Do not use any other dosing device.

Other information
- each teaspoon contains: sodium 3 mg
- store at 20°-25°C (68°-77°F)
- do not use if printed neckband is broken or missing

Inactive ingredients anhydrous citric acid, butylparaben, carboxymethylcellulose sodium, carrageenan, D&C red no. 33, FD&C blue no. 1, flavor, glycerin, high fructose corn syrup, hydroxyethyl cellulose, microcrystalline cellulose, propylene glycol, purified water, sodium benzoate, sorbitol solution

Questions? Call 1-800-910-6874

*This product is not manufactured or distributed by the Tylenol Company, owner of the registered trademark Tylenol®.

094 01 0137 ID209441
Distributed by Target Corporation
Minneapolis, MN 55403
© 2009 Target Brands, Inc.
All Rights Reserved Shop Target.com

NDC 11673-130-26
children's acetaminophen
oral suspension
80 mg per ½ teaspoon
(160 mg per 5 mL)
fever reducer/pain reliever

Compare to active ingredient in Children's Tylenol® Oral Suspension*

see new warnings information

alcohol free
ibuprofen free
aspirin free

up&up
grape flavor
AGE 2-11 YEARS
4 FL OZ (118 mL)

Drug Facts (continued)
- dispense liquid slowly into child's mouth, toward inner cheek
- if needed, repeat dose every 4 hours while symptoms last
- do not give more than 5 times in 24 hours
- do not give for more than 5 days unless directed by a doctor
- replace dropper tightly to maintain child resistance
- this product does not contain directions or complete warnings for adult use

Dosing Chart

Weight (lb)	Age (yr)	Dose (mL)
under 24	under 2 years	ask a doctor
24-35	2-3 years	1.6 mL (0.8 + 0.8 mL)

Attention: use only enclosed dropper specifically designed for use with this product. Do not use any other dosing device.

Other information
- store at 20°-25°C (68°-77°F)
- do not use if printed bottle wrap is broken or missing

IMPORTANT:
Concentrated Infants' Drops contains more medicine per drop than Children's Liquid. Use enclosed dropper **ONLY**. **DO NOT USE** other cups or spoons.

NDC 11673-289-05
infants' acetaminophen
concentrated drops
80 mg per 0.0 mL
fever reducer/pain reliever

Compare to active ingredient in Concentrated Tylenol® Infants' Drops*

see new warnings information

use only with enclosed dropper

up&up
grape flavor
AGE 2-3 YEARS
0.5 FL OZ (15 mL)

a. Which label would you select?_____ With which device would you administer the medication? _____

b. Is the order safe? How many mL would you prepare? _____

c. What is the concentration, in mg per mL, of children's acetaminophen susp? With which device would you administer the medication?

_____

d. What is the concentration in mg per mL, of infants' acetaminophen?

_____

e. Which is more concentrated, infants' or children's acetaminophen preparation? _____

CLINICAL RELEVANCE

These products have been confused by nurses as well as consumers. The labels are very clearly marked. However, the uninformed think that the concentrated drops are interchangeable with the children's suspension and are safe to give to children in the dose prescribed for the suspension. The infant drops are much more concentrated in order to achieve a very low volume of medication for infants. This has caused fatal errors.

Parents have also overdosed their children at home by giving too much of the over-the-counter product either by using household utensils or by giving it more often than the label states. Keep this in mind when teaching parents.

➤ Aspirin and aspirin-containing products (salicylates) should **never** be given to children under the age of 19 because of the association with Reye's syndrome, a potentially fatal neurologic disorder.

➤ Aspirin (acetylsalicylic acid) is not given to infants, children, and teenagers under *19 years* of age who have fever due to flu or viral symptoms. Aspirin has been associated with Reye's syndrome in those age groups.

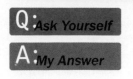

Q: *Ask Yourself*

A: *My Answer*

1 What is the difference in unit dose between the concentrated drops and children's suspension acetaminophen?

_____

2 Would it be safer always to clarify orders that specify only mL and do not state the total dose desired, such as 80 or 160 mg?

_____

6 Ordered: codeine 20 mg IM stat, for analgesia.

SDR for children: 0.5-1 mg per kg q4-6h

Patient's weight: 88 lb

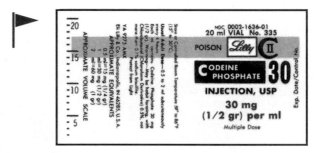

a. SDR for this child: _____

DA equation:

b. Evaluation: *Safe to give* or *Hold and clarify promptly with prescriber*? (Circle one.)

c. If safe, will you give more or less than the unit dose on hand?

DA equation:

d. What is the nearest measurable dose you will prepare for the available syringe?

DA equation:

e. Evaluation: _____

Draw a vertical line through the calibrated line on the syringe to indicate the nearest measurable dose.

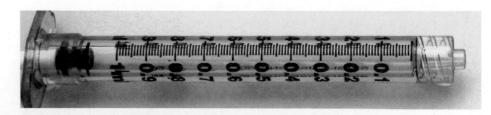

7 Ordered: KCl 10 mEq per hr for 3 hrs as an intermittent infusion, for a child with hypokalemia. Check potassium levels every 4 hours and call physician.

Available: 30 mEq KCl in 100 mL D5W

SDR for child with hypokalemia: 0.5 to 1 mEq per kg per dose not to exceed 40 mEq per 24 hr

Safe flow rate: maximum: 1 mEq per kg per hr. Patient's weight: 42 lb.

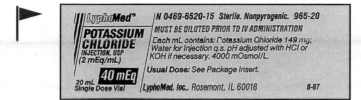

   a. Weight in kg to the nearest tenth: _____

   b. SDR for this child: _____

   c. Ordered dose for this child: _____

   d. Evaluation: *Safe to give* or *Hold and clarify promptly with prescriber?* (Circle one and state reason.) _____

   e. If safe, what should the flow rate on the infusion pump be? _____

     DA equation:

   f. Evaluation: _____

8 Ordered: atropine sulfate 0.5 mg IV, for a 5 year-old-child with bradyarrhythmia. SDR for child with bradyarrhythmia: 0.01-0.03 mg per kg to achieve pulse rate >60 beats per minute. Maximum dose for child: 500 mcg. Patient's weight: 44 lb.

   a. Weight in kg to the nearest tenth: _____

   b. SDR for this child: _____

     DA equation:

   c. Ordered dose for this child in mcg: _____

   d. Evaluation: *Safe to give* or *Hold and clarify promptly with prescriber?* (Circle one and give reason.) _____

   e. If safe, will you give more or less than the unit dose on hand? _____

   f. How many mL will you give?

     DA equation:

   g. Evaluation: _____

9 Ordered: Vancocin (vancomycin hydrochloride) 500 mg IVPB infusion q4h for a 12-year-old child with a staphylococcus infection. Directions: Dilute with 10 mL SW to withdraw from vial. Further dilute to 500 mL with D5W and infuse over 60 minutes. Patient's weight: 35 kg.

SDR IV for children: 40 mg per kg per day divided q6-12 hr not to exceed 2 g per day.

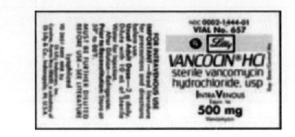

a. SDR: _____

DA equation:

b. Evaluation: _____

c. If safe, what flow rate would you set on the IV pump? _____

10 Ordered: digoxin 0.5 mg IV, for an 18 month old child with congestive heart failure

SDR: 7.5-12 mcg per kg divided in two q 12 h doses for child up to 2 years. Patient's weight 24 lb 6 oz

Directions: Administer IV over 5-10 minutes. Safe to give undiluted. If needed, dilute each mL of drug in 4 mL SW (to permit small amounts of drug to be infused over time). Use a calculator to determine SDR.

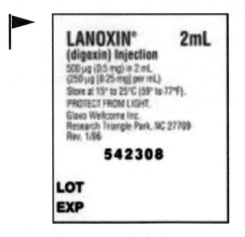

a. Weight in kg to the nearest tenth: _____

b. SDR for this child to the nearest tenth mg: _____

DA equation:

c. Ordered dose for this child: _____

d. Evaluation: *Safe to give* or *Hold and clarify promptly with prescriber?* (Circle one and state reason.) _____

e. How many mL of digoxin will you prepare before dilution? _____

Suggestions for Further Reading

> ➤ To access many Internet references on rates and types of medication errors in pediatrics, type "children's medication errors" in your favorite search engine.

Gahart BL, Nazareno AR: *2011 Intravenous medications: a handbook for nurses and health professionals,* ed. 27, St. Louis, 2011, Mosby

Taketomo, Carol K, et al: Pediatric dosage handbook, ed 15, Hudson, Ohio, 2011, Lexi-Comp

http://jalinpharm.highwire.org/cgi/content/abstract/34/11/1043
www.childrenshospital.org
www.hopkinschildrens.org/Managing-Anticoagulation-in-Pediatric-Patients.aspx
www.ismp.org/pressroom/PR20020606.pdf
www.jointcommission.org
www.medlineplus.gov
www.pedseducation.org/online_education/index.cfm
www.wo-pub2.med.cornell.edu/cgi-bin/WebObjects/PublicPediatrics.woa

Ⓔvolve   Additional practice problems can be found in the Pediatric Calculations section of the Student Companion on Evolve.

Directions: *Select the correct response for the following questions. Estimate a reasonable answer whenever you can; use a calculator for weights and safe dose ranges, and use DA for verification of doses. Evaluate your answer. Do not "guess" the answer. Put a checkmark to the right of questions that need review. After completion of the rest of the test, review any checkmarked question(s).*

1 The metric equivalent of 1500 mg is:

1. 0.015 g   **3.** 1.5 g

2. 0.15 g   **4.** 15 g

2 The metric equivalent of 0.75 g is:

1. 0.75 mg   **3.** 75 mg

2. 7.5 mg   **4.** 750 mg

3 The metric equivalent of 5000 mcg is:

1. 0.5 g   **3.** 50 mg

2. 5 mg   **4.** 500 mg

4 A patient weighs 150 lb. How many kilograms does the patient weigh (to the nearest tenth)?

1. 330 kg   **3.** 75.5 kg

2. 150 kg   **4.** 68.2 kg

Did your estimate support the answer?

5 Tetracycline 0.5 g PO four times daily is ordered for a patient with an infection. Tetracycline 250 mg per capsule is available. How many capsules will you prepare?

1. ½ capsule   **3.** 2 capsules

2. 1 capsule   **4.** 4 capsules

Did your estimate support the answer?

6 Digoxin 0.0625 mg PO daily is ordered for a patient with heart failure.

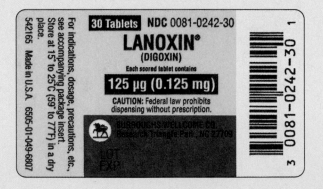

How many tablets will you prepare?

1. 4 tablets   **3.** 1 tablet

2. 2 tablets   **4.** 0.5 tablet

Did your estimate support the answer?

7 Ordered: amoxicillin capsules. 0.5 g PO four times daily for 7 days.

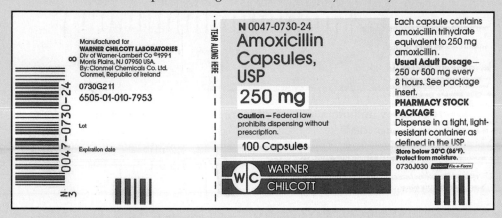

How many capsules will you prepare?

1. ½ capsule   **3.** 2 capsules

2. 1 capsule   **4.** 4 capsules

Did your estimate support the answer?

8 Ordered: amoxicillin 0.2 g PO four times a day for a patient with an infection.

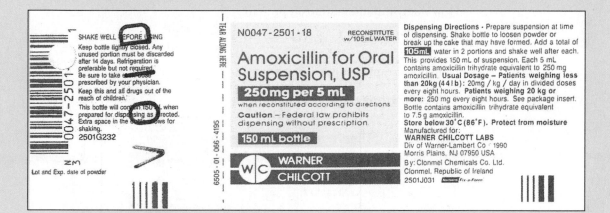

How many milliliters will you prepare?

1. 15 mL   **3.** 8 mL

2. 12 mL   **4.** 4 mL

Did your estimate support the answer?

9 Ordered: Stadol 1.2 mg IM stat for a patient with pain.

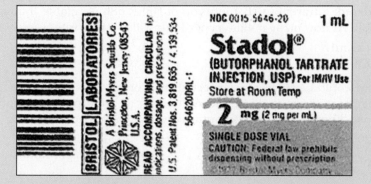

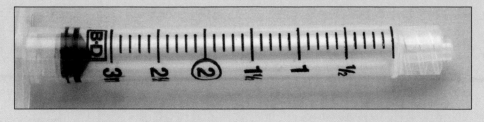

How many milliliters will you prepare, to the nearest measurable dose, on the syringe provided?

1. 0.6 mL   **3.** 1.2 mL
2. 1 mL   **4.** 1.5 mL

Did your estimate support the answer?

10 Ordered: Solu-Cortef 150 mg IM stat for a patient with a severe allergic reaction.

> Single-Dose Vial   For IV or IM use
> Contains Benzyl Alcohol as a Preservative
> See package insert for complete
> product information.
> Per 2 mL (when mixed):
> • hydrocortisone sodium succinate equiv.
>   to hydrocortisone, 250 mg. Protect
>   solution from light. Discard after 3 days.
>
> 814 070 205   Reconstituted . . . .
> The Upjohn Company
> Kalamazoo, MI 49001, USA
>
> 2 mL Act-O-Vial®   NDC 0009-0909-06
> **Solu-Cortef**®   Sterile Powder
> hydrocortisone sodium succinate
> for injection, USP
> **250 mg***

How many milliliters will you prepare?

1. 0.8 mL   **3.** 1.8 mL
2. 1.2 mL   **4.** 2.5 mL

Did your estimate support the answer?

11 Ordered: atropine sulfate 0.3 mg.

> NDC 0002-1675-01
> 20 mL   VIAL No. 419
> ® *Lilly*
> POISON
> **ATROPINE
> SULFATE**
> INJECTION, USP
> **0.4 mg
> per mL**
> CAUTION—Federal (U.S.A.) law
> prohibits dispensing without
> prescription.

How many milliliters will you prepare, to the nearest hundredth of a milliliter?

1. 0.03 mL   **3.** 0.75 mL
2. 0.04 mL   **4.** 1.33 mL

Did your estimate support the answer?

12 Ordered: intravenous (IV) infusion of D5LR q8h. Available: 1-liter bag of D5LR. At how many milliliters per hour will the flow rate be set?

1. 125 mL   **3.** 175 mL
2. 150 mL   **4.** 200 mL

13 What would be an average expected D5W or LR IV maintenance flow rate range of unmedicated isotonic solution for an adult patient in good health who will be on nothing-by-mouth (NPO) status for 1 or 2 days?

1. 200-250 mL per hour   **3.** 25-50 mL per hour
2. 75-125 mL per hour   **4.** 10-25 mL per hour

14 Ordered: 1000 mL D5W at 50 mL per hour. Available: macrodrip administration set with a drop factor of 15. What flow rate will you set?

1. 50 mL per hour

2. 50 drops per minute

3. 12.5 drops per minute

4. 13 drops per minute

15 Ordered: 250 mL D5W at 30 mL per hour. Available: microdrip pediatric administration set. What flow rate will you set?

1. 15 mL per hour

2. 30 drops per minute

3. 250 drops per minute

4. 60 drops per minute

Did your estimate support your answer?

16 Ordered: 500 mL N/S at 100 mL per hour. Available: macrodrip administration set with a drop factor of 20. What flow rate will you set?

1. 166 mL per hour

2. 166 drops per minute

3. 33 mL per hour

4. 33 drops per minute

17 What is the fastest reasonable rate of drops per minute that can be counted when using a pediatric administration set according to the text?

1. 30 drops per minute

2. 60 drops per minute

3. 90 drops per minute

4. 100 drops per minute

18 Ordered: a transfusion of 250 mL of packed red cells for a patient with anemia. What solution must be used to prime the IV line Y tubing before and after the blood is administered?

1. NS

2. D5W

3. L/R

4. D10W

19 Ordered: a transfusion for a patient. Agency policy calls for 2 mL per minute flow rate for the first 30 minutes while the patient is observed for possible adverse reactions. What flow rate in milliliters per hour will you set on an infusion pump for the first 30 minutes?

1. 30 mL per hour

2. 60 mL per hour

3. 90 mL per hour

4. 120 mL per hour

Did your estimate support your answer?

20 Ordered: a blood transfusion for a patient. Available: IV gravity device and tubing administration sets with drop factors of 10, 15, 20, and 60. Which set has the largest diameter, permitting the largest drop, and is used to administer blood?

1. DF 10

2. DF 15

3. DF 20

4. DF 60

Did your estimate support your answer?

21 Ordered: an IVPB of 40 mL to be infused over 30 minutes on an infusion pump. What will be the flow rate in milliliters per hour?

1. 30 mL per hour

2. 75 mL per hour

3. 80 mL per hour

4. 90 mL per hour

Did your estimate support your answer?

22 Ordered: an IVPB of 20 mL to be infused over 20 minutes on an infusion pump. What will be the flow rate in milliliters per hour?

1. 20 mL per hour

2. 40 mL per hour

3. 60 mL per hour

4. 80 mL per hour

Did your estimate support your answer?

23 Ordered: an IVPB of 30 mL to be infused over 30 minutes on a gravity device with microdrip tubing. What will be the flow rate?

    1. 30 mL per hour   **3.** 30 drops per minute

    2. 60 mL per hour   **4.** 60 drops per minute

Did your estimate support your answer?

24 How many grams of carbohydrate are there in an IV of 500 mL of D5NS?

    1. 25 g   **3.** 75 g

    2. 50 g   **4.** 100 g

25 How many kilocalories of carbohydrate are there in an IV of 1000 mL D5W?

    1. 1000 kcal   **3.** 200 kcal

    2. 500 kcal   **4.** 50 kcal

26 Ordered: heparin 800 units per hr IV. Available: 25,000 units of heparin in 500 mL of NS. How many milliliters per hour will deliver 800 units per hr?

    1. 4 mL per hour   **3.** 12 mL per hour

    2. 8 mL per hour   **4.** 16 mL per hour

27 Infusing: heparin IV at 10 mL per hour. Available: 25,000 units of heparin in 250 mL of NS. How many units per hour are infusing?

    1. 25 units per hour   **3.** 250 units per hour

    2. 100 units per hour   **4.** 1000 units per hour

28 Ordered: IV of Nipride (nitroprusside sodium) at 0.5 mcg/kg per min to maintain a patient's blood pressure. Available: Nipride 50 mg in 500 mL D5W. Patient weight: 70 kg.

What flow rate in milliliters per hr should be set on the IV infusion pump?

    1. 12 mL per hour   **3.** 42 mL per hour

    2. 21 mL per hour   **4.** 70 mL per hour

29 Which is the most appropriate action for the nurse to take for insulin mix orders?

    1. Check the labels of the two insulins to be sure they are compatible.

    2. Call the prescriber before preparing the insulin mix.

    3. Administer dextrose before administering the insulin mix.

    4. Be prepared to administer glucagon after administering the insulin mix.

30 Ordered: insulin glargine (Lantus) 15 units subcut at bedtime. The patient's current blood glucose (BG) is 55. The patient complains of shakiness and nervousness. What decision will the nurse make?

    1. Give the patient a diet cola and administer the insulin.

    2. Prepare and administer the insulin because it does not have a peak.

    3. Hold the insulin, follow agency and prescriber protocols, and contact the prescriber promptly because the patient is hyperglycemic.

    4. Hold the insulin, follow agency and prescriber protocols for hypoglycemic episodes, and contact the prescriber promptly.

31 Which types of insulin can be administered via the IV route?

    1. NPH and Lente

    2. Insulin glargine and insulin mixes

    3. Regular insulin and insulin aspart (Novolog)

    4. Insulin zinc suspensions and Humulin U

32 The insulin bottle label states U-100. Identify the correct meaning of U-100 on the label.

1. It refers to the total contents. There are 100 units in the bottle.
2. It refers to the concentration. There are 100 units per mL.
3. It refers to the recommended adult dose of 100 units.
4. It refers to the number of units per 100 mL.

33 Ordered: carbamazepine susp 50 mg PO 4 times daily for a 10-year-old child who is experiencing seizures. SDR for the 24-hr period for a child less than 12 years old: 10 to 20 mg per kg per day in 3 or 4 divided doses. The child weighs 44 lb. The SDR is:

1. 100-200 mg per day   **3.** 500-1000 mg per day
2. 200-400 mg per day   **4.** 998-1936 mg per day

34 Select the statement that best describes the difference between mg and m^2:

1. mg is a metric measurement of weight, and m^2 refers to micrograms
2. mg is a metric measurement of volume, and m^2 refers to lean body mass
3. mg is a metric measurement of weight, and m^2 refers to square meters of body surface area (BSA)
4. mg is a metric measurement of weight, and m^2 refers to square milligrams of weight

35 What is the risk associated with an overdose of the high-alert drugs heparin and warfarin?

1. Constipation and flatulence   **3.** Bleeding and/or hemorrhage
2. Hyperglycemic episodes   **4.** Deep vein thrombosis (DVT)

COMPREHENSIVE FINAL PRACTICE: CHAPTERS 1-13 (ANSWERS ON P. 574)

Directions: *Estimate and calculate doses using DA style equations where requested. Evaluate your answer in terms of the estimate and the equation result. If you cannot estimate the dose, estimate whether it will be more or less of unit dose supplied. Use a calculator for long division and multiplication. Label all answers.*

1 Ordered: Aricept 10 mg PO daily at bedtime for a patient with Alzheimer's disease.

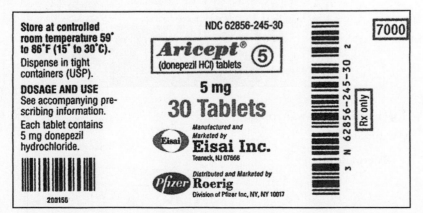

How many tablets will you administer?

a. Estimated dose:

DA equation:

b. Evaluation:

2 Ordered: alprazolam 0.5 mg PO at bedtime for a patient with high anxiety.

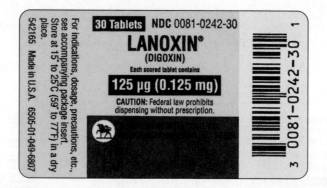

How many tablets will you administer?

a. Estimated dose:

DA equation:

b. Evaluation:

3 Ordered: digoxin 250 mcg PO daily for an adult with heart failure.

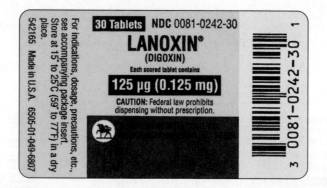

How many tablets will you administer?

a. Estimated dose:

DA equation:

b. Evaluation:

c. Which is the generic name of this medication? _____

4 Ordered: ciprofloxacin hydrochloride 1.5 g PO for a patient with a severe infection.

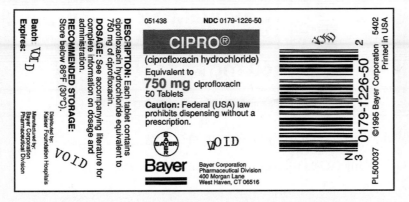

How many tablets will you administer?

a. Estimated dose:

DA equation:

b. Evaluation:

c. Which is the generic name of this medication? _____

5 Ordered: dexamethasone 500 mcg PO stat for a patient with acute allergy attack.

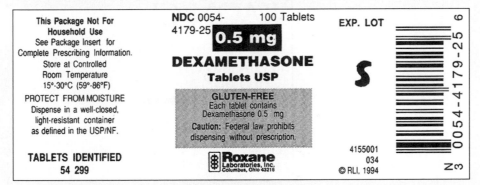

How many tablets will you administer?

a. Estimated dose:

DA equation:

b. Evaluation:

6 Ordered diltiazem sustained-release tablets 0.12 g PO daily at bedtime for a patient with hypertension.

Label A   **Label B**

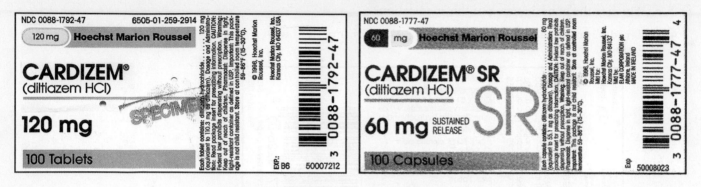

Which medication will you administer? _____

How many tablets will you administer?

a. Estimated dose:

   DA equation:

b. Evaluation:

7 Ordered: 20% potassium chloride liquid 20 mEq PO daily for a patient taking a diuretic.

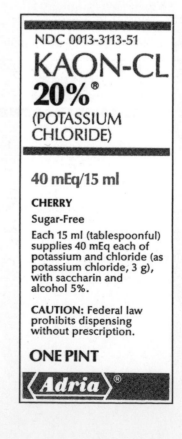

How many mL will you administer?

a. Estimated dose:

DA equation:

b. Evaluation:

Shade in the medicine cup to the nearest 5 mL. Mark the syringe at the additional amount to be added.

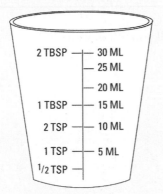

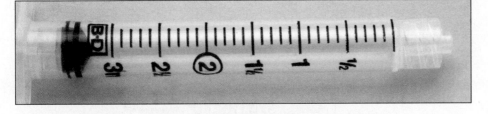

8 Ordered: codeine 45 mg PO q4-6h prn for an adult with pain.

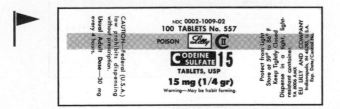

a. What is the metric unit dose available? _____

b. What is the apothecary system equivalent unit dose noted in parentheses on the label? _____

c. How many tablets will you administer?

d. Estimated dose:

DA equation:

e. Evaluation:

9 Ordered: metformin 1.5 g PO daily with breakfast for a diabetic patient.

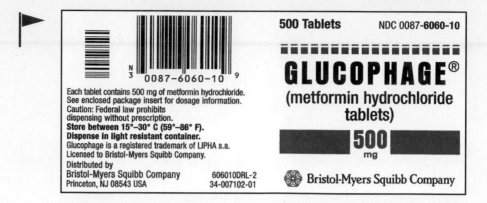

How many tablets will you administer?

a. Estimated dose:

DA equation:

b. Evaluation:

10 Ordered: levothyroxine 0.1 mg PO daily in AM for a patient who is hypothyroid.

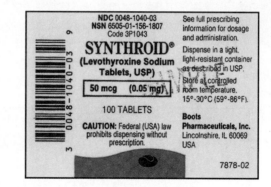

How many tablets will you administer?

a. Estimated dose:

DA equation:

b. Evaluation:

c. What is the equivalent of the dose ordered in micrograms? _____

11 Ordered: morphine sulfate 10 mg IM stat for a patient in pain.

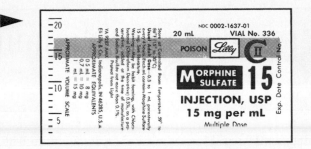

How many mL will you administer to the nearest hundredth of a mL?

a. Estimated dose:

DA equation:

b. Evaluation:

Mark the syringe to the nearest measurable amount.

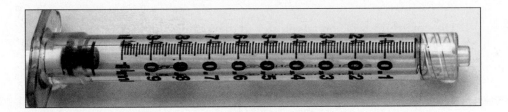

12 Ordered: furosemide 30 mg IM stat for a patient with urinary retention.

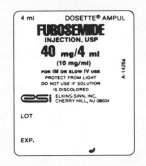

How many mL will you administer?

a. Estimated dose:

DA equation:

b. Evaluation:

Mark the syringe to the nearest measurable amount.

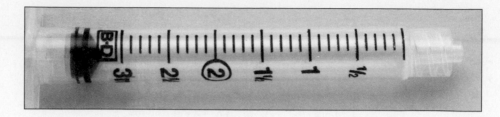

13 Ordered: digoxin 0.3 mg IM on admission for a patient in heart failure.

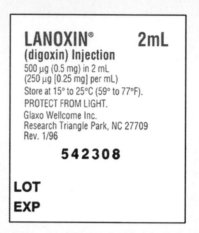

LANOXIN®   **2mL**
(digoxin) Injection
500 µg (0.5 mg) in 2 mL
(250 µg [0.25 mg] per mL)
Store at 15° to 25°C (59° to 77°F).
PROTECT FROM LIGHT.
Glaxo Wellcome Inc.
Research Triangle Park, NC 27709
Rev. 1/96

542308

LOT

EXP

How many mL will you administer to the nearest hundredth of a mL?
a. Estimated dose:

   DA equation:

b. Evaluation:

Mark the syringe to the nearest measurable amount.

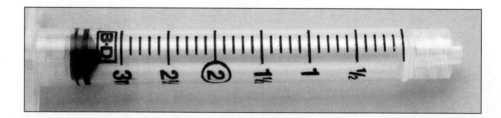

14 Ordered: hydromorphone HCl 2 mg ⎱ IM stat for a patient in pain
promethazine 20 mg ⎰

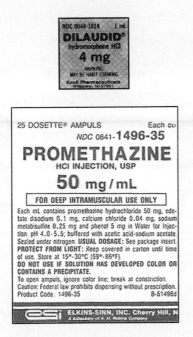

How many mL of hydromorphone will you prepare?

a. Estimated hydromorphone dose: _____

DA equation:

b. Evaluation:

How many mL of promethazine will you prepare?

c. Estimated promethazine dose: _____

DA equation:

d. Evaluation:

e. What is the total dose in mL to be administered?

Mark the syringe with the total dose to the nearest measurable amount.

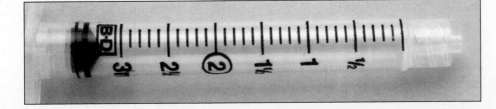

15 Ordered: Penicillin G Procaine susp 400,000 units IM stat for a patient with a skin infection.

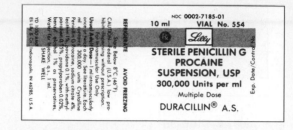

How many mL will you administer (to the nearest tenth of a mL)?

a. Estimated dose:

DA equation:

b. Evaluation:

16 Ordered: an antibiotic 600 mg IM q6h daily for a patient with a respiratory infection. Directions for reconstitution: Add 2 mL SW for injection. Each 2.5 mL will contain 1 g of antibiotic.

How many mL will you administer (to the nearest tenth of a mL)?

a. What is the concentration of the solution in mg after reconstitution for IM injection? _____

b. Estimated dose:

DA equation:

c. Evaluation:

d. What is the amount (in mL) of water displacement by the powder?

17 Ordered: Novolin regular insulin for a diabetic patient on a sliding scale tid 30 minutes ac and at bedtime. Current BGM is 300.

Using the sliding scale that follows, how many units of insulin will be administered? _____

Sliding Scale BG mg/dL	Insulin Dose (Novolin)
70 – 180	0 Units
181 – 200	2 Units
201 – 250	4 Units
251 – 300	6 Units
Over 300	Call physician

a. Mark the syringe to the nearest measurable dose:

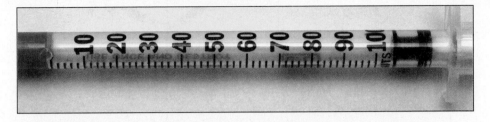

b. Is this a fast, intermediate, or long acting insulin? _____
c. Will insulin raise or lower the blood glucose level? _____

18 Ordered: Humulin R 6 units
Humulin N 20 units } subcut 30 minutes ac breakfast daily

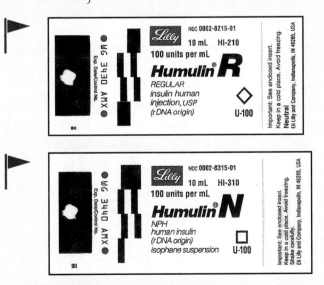

From which bottle should the insulin be withdrawn first? _____

Mark total dose on the insulin syringe provided. Place an arrow pointing to the calibration which reflects the intermediate acting insulin dose.

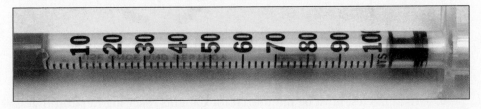

19 Ordered: insulin glargine 24 units subcut daily at bedtime.

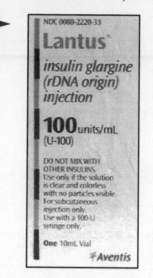

Mark the total dose on the 50 unit insulin syringe provided.*

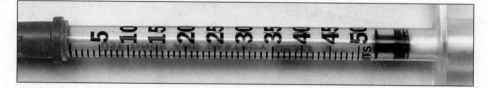

a. Is this insulin a short-, intermediate-, or long-acting insulin?

_____

b. Which is the advantage of the 50 unit 0.5 mL syringe as opposed to the 100 unit 1 mL syringe? _____

*Lo-Dose syringes are calibrated for U-100 insulin.

20 Ordered: heparin IV infusion 1000 units per hour.
Available: heparin 20,000 units in 500 mL D5/W.

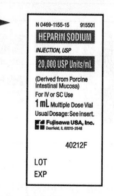

How many mL per hour will you infuse?

    DA equation:

a. Evaluation:

b. Which lab test must be monitored for patients receiving heparin therapy?

_____

21 Infusing: heparin at 30 mL per hour in an IV of D5W 250 mL containing heparin 10,000 units.

How many units per hour are infusing?

DA equation:

a. Evaluation:

b. What is the major potential adverse effect of heparin overdose?

_____

22 Infusing: regular insulin at 7 mL per hour IV.

Available: Humulin regular insulin 100 units in 100 mL of NS.

How many units per hour are infusing?

a. Estimated units per hour:

DA equation:

b. Evaluation:

c. What is the major potential adverse effect of an insulin overdose?

_____

23 Ordered: IV KCl to infuse at 10 mEq per hour for a patient with hypokalemia.

Available: 500 mL NS with 40 mEq of KCl added premixed by pharmacy.

Directions: _"Recheck serum K levels when 40 mEq of KCl have been infused."_

What flow rate will you set on the infusion pump? _____

DA equation:

a. Evaluation:

b. The IV was started at 1300 hours. At what time on the 24-hr clock would the nurse need to order and recheck a serum K level? _____

24 Ordered: IV antibiotic to be piggybacked on a primary line: 50 mL to infuse over 30 minutes.

How many mL per hour will you set the infusion pump?

a. Estimated flow rate:

DA equation:

b. Evaluation:

25 Ordered: IV antibiotic 100 mg q6h for 72 hours. Available from pharmacy: IV antibiotic solution in 30 mL of D5W to be piggybacked to a primary line. Directions: *"Infuse over 20 minutes."*

How many mL per hour will you set the infusion pump?

a. Estimated flow rate:

DA equation:

b. Evaluation:

26 Ordered: IV antibiotic 250 mg q4h for 48 hrs. Available from pharmacy: IV antibiotic solution in 20 mL to be piggybacked on a primary line: Directions: *"Infuse over 60 minutes."*

a. What flow rate will you set on a gravity microdrip device? _____
b. Estimated flow rate:

DA equation:

c. Evaluation:

27 Ordered: IV D5W of 500 mL over 4 hours. Available: A gravity device. Drop factor on the tubing: 15.

What flow rate will you set? _____

DA equation:

a. Evaluation:

28 Ordered: IV medication for a pediatric patient of 100 mg diluted to a total volume of 20 mL in NS to be administered over 30 minutes. Agency policy requires a volume control device for all medicated IVs for pediatric patients with a maximum 1 hour's worth of fluid.

Available: medication 100 mg per 2 mL.

  a. What flow rate will be set on the infusion pump for the medication administration? _____

  DA equation:

  b. What procedure must be followed (according to agency policy) before and after a medication is infused on a primary line? _____

29 Ordered: hyperalimentation (PN) continuous infusion in a central line at 60 mL per hour for a patient who has a gastrointestinal disorder. Among the contents ordered:
15% dextrose solution
4.25% amino acids

How many grams of dextrose are contained in a liter of the PN solution?*

  DA equation:

  a. Evaluation:
  b. How many approximate carbohydrate kilocalories will the dextrose provide per liter of PN solution?

  DA equation:

  c. Evaluation:

  d. How many grams of amino acids are contained in a liter of the PN solution?*

  DA equation:

---

*A calculation of 4 calories per g of CHO, 4 calories per g of amino acids, and 9 calories per gram of fat yield an approximate amount of calories.

e. Evaluation:

f. How many approximate* protein kilocalories will the amino acids provide per liter of PN solution?

DA equation:

g. Evaluation:

30 The prescriber also orders a lipid solution for the patient mentioned in problem 29: 200 mL of 20% fat emulsion to be added to the total volume once a day.

How many grams of lipid are contained in the liter?*

DA equation:

a. Evaluation:
b. How many kilocalories will each lipid solution provide?

DA equation:

c. Evaluation:

31 Ordered: Start Pitocin IV at 2 milliunits per minute for a patient in labor.
Available: Pitocin 5 units in 500 mL of D5W.
Conversion factors: 1000 milliunits = 1 unit; 60 minutes = 1 hour
At how many mL per hour will the flow rate be set?

DA equation:

a. Evaluation:

*A calculation of 4 calories per g of CHO, 4 calories per g of amino acids, and 9 calories per gram of fat yield an approximate amount of calories.

32 Ordered: Dobutamine HCl 3 mcg/kg per minute. Patient weight: 154 lb.

Available: Dobutamine 250 mg in 500 mL.

Estimated wt in kg: _____

a. Actual wt in kg: _____

DA equation:

b. Evaluation:

c. Dose ordered in mcg per minute _____

d. Dose ordered in mg per minute _____

e. At how many mL per hour will the flow rate be set (to the nearest tenth of a mL)?

DA equation:

f. Evaluation:

33 Ordered: diazepam 10 mg direct IV before endoscopy procedure.

Directions: Injection undiluted at a rate of 5 mg per minute.

Total mL to be injected: _____

a. Estimated dose: _____

DA equation:

b. Evaluation:

c. Using a 10-mL syringe, how many mL per minute will you inject?

_____

DA equation:

d. Evaluation:

e. Over how many total minutes will you inject? _____
seconds? _____

f. How many seconds per calibration will you inject? _____

34 Ordered: phenytoin oral suspension 175 mg PO daily in the AM for a child with seizures.

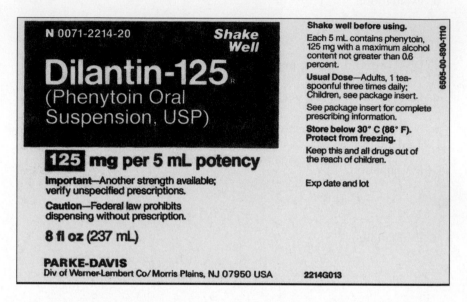

SDR child: 250 mg per m^2 per day as single dose or divided in 2 doses.

Child's BSA: 0.7 m^2

What is the safe dose for this child? _____

    DA equation:

    a. Evaluation:

    b. If safe dose ordered, how many mL will you administer?

    DA equation:

    c. Evaluation:

Shade in medicine cup to nearest measurable dose. Mark the syringe at the additional amount to be added.

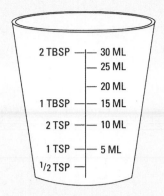

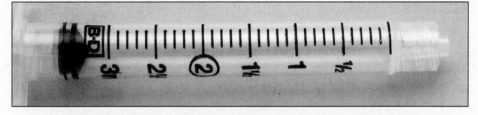

35 Ordered: Epoetin alfa 5000 units IV 3 times weekly for a pediatric cancer patient. Pt weight: 25 kg. SDR: 600 units per kg weekly.

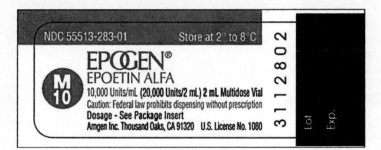

a. What is the child's wt in kg? _____

SDR for this child

DA equation:

b. Evaluation: If safe, dose in mL for this child.

DA equation:

c. Evaluation:

Essential Math Self-Assessment (p. 2)

1 greater than

2 less than

3 greater than or equal to

4 less than or equal to

5 $\geq$

6 $\dfrac{100}{1}$

7 425.

8 125

9 $\dfrac{256}{256}$

10 90

11 1, 2, 4, 8, 16

12 1, 2, 5, 10

13 15, 30, 45

14 $10 \times 10 \times 10 = 1000$

15 $3^2 = 9$

16 $\sqrt{25} = 5$

17 10

18 8

19 $\dfrac{2}{3}\ \dfrac{\text{numerator}}{\text{denominator}}$

20 a. $\dfrac{1}{10}$; **b.** $\dfrac{1}{4}$

21 $5\frac{1}{6}$

22 $\dfrac{36}{5}$

23 8; 30

24 5

25 a. $\dfrac{4}{5}$; **b.** $\dfrac{1}{25}$

26 $\frac{17}{12} = 1\frac{5}{12}\ \left(\frac{9}{12} + \frac{8}{12}\right)$

27 $\dfrac{3}{8}$

28 a. $\frac{4}{8} = \frac{1}{2}$; **b.** $\frac{3}{5}$

29 a. $\frac{9}{2} = 4\frac{1}{2}$; **b.** 16

30 a. $\dfrac{10\text{ diapers}}{1\text{ pkg}}$; **b.** $\dfrac{\$2}{1\text{ gallon}}$; **c.** $\dfrac{\$30}{1\text{ hour}}$

31 0.25; 0.13

32 $\frac{25}{100}$; $\frac{25}{1000}$

33 0.5; 0.1

34 1.34

35 0.235

36 0.23

37 0.1

38 a. $\dfrac{3}{10}$; **b.** $\dfrac{5}{10} = \dfrac{1}{2}$; **c.** $\dfrac{125}{1000} = \dfrac{1}{8}$

39 0.5

40 4

41 baseline (as in 2.4)

42 "times"—a multiplication sign $(5 \times 6 \times 3)$

43 a. 10%; **b.** 75%; **c.** 7.5%

44 50

45 60

Chapter 1

RAPID PRACTICE 1-1 (p. 7)

1 3

2 1

3 4

4 2

5 3

RAPID PRACTICE 1-2 (p. 7)

1 $<$

2 $\leq$

3 $\geq$

4 $>$

5 $\sqrt{}$

RAPID PRACTICE 1-3 (p. 9)

1 4

2 3

3 1

4 1

5 4

RAPID PRACTICE 1-4 (p. 9)

1 $\dfrac{100}{1}$

2 100.

3 125.5

4 Avoid errors. The decimal may be misread as the number one "1."

5 $\dfrac{100}{100}$

RAPID PRACTICE 1-5 (p. 11)

1 $10 \times 4 = 40$

2 2, 3, 4, 6

3 2, 4

4 12

5 5, 10, 15

RAPID PRACTICE 1-6 (p. 12)

1 5

2 2.5

3 2000

4 50

5 $\frac{1}{2}$

RAPID PRACTICE 1-7 (p. 13)

1 2

2 4

3 4

4 1

5 3

RAPID PRACTICE 1-8 (p. 13)

1 12

2 $7^2 = 7 \times 7 = 49$

3 Divisor $= \frac{1}{2}$

4 100

5 15

RAPID PRACTICE 1-9 (p. 15)

1 10×10

2 $2 \times 2 \times 2 \times 2 \times 2$

3 10^8

4 10

5 4

RAPID PRACTICE 1-10 (p. 15)

1 2
2 3
3 2

4 3
5 3

RAPID PRACTICE 1-11 (p. 16)

Number		÷ 10	÷ 100	÷ 1000	Number		× 10	× 100	× 1000
1	50	5	0.5	0.05	4	0.5	5	50	500
2	125	12.5	1.25	0.125	5	0.25	2.5	25	250
3	10	1	0.1	0.01					

RAPID PRACTICE 1-12 (p. 18)

2 $\frac{3}{1000}$

3 $\frac{25}{100}$

4 $1\frac{56}{100}$

5 $2\frac{345}{10,000}$

RAPID PRACTICE 1-13 (p. 19)

1 0.25
2 0.1
3 0.025

4 0.4
5 0.05

RAPID PRACTICE 1-14 (p. 19)

1 $\frac{8}{10}$

2 $\frac{5}{1000}$

3 $1\frac{25}{100}$

4 $\frac{25}{100}$

5 $\frac{15}{1000}$

RAPID PRACTICE 1-15 (p. 19)

1 0.5
2 0.3
3 1.32
4 0.01
5 0.6

6 0.5
7 0.006
8 0.05
9 0.5
10 1.06

RAPID PRACTICE 1-16 (p. 20)

1 **a.** 0.3
  b. 1.3
  c. 0.8
  d. 1.9
  e. 0.1

2 **a.** 0.69
  b. 3.75
  c. 0.89
  d. 2.38
  e. 0.05

3 **a.** 2
  b. 11
  c. 1
  d. 2
  e. 3

RAPID PRACTICE 1-17 (p. 21)

1 0.8
2 0.1
3 0.25

4 9.
5 0.5

RAPID PRACTICE 1-18 (p. 22)

1 $0.1\overline{)0.5} \rightarrow 1\overline{)5}$

2 $0.025\overline{)0.100} \rightarrow 25\overline{)100}$

3 $3.05\overline{)20.32} \rightarrow 305\overline{)2032}$

4 $0.25\overline{)1.00} \rightarrow 25\overline{)100}$

5 $1.2\overline{)5.06} \rightarrow 12\overline{)50.6}$

RAPID PRACTICE 1-19 (p. 23)

1 $5\overline{)20.5}$ = 4.1

2 $5\overline{)20.}$ = 4.

3 $2\overline{)3.0}$ = 1.5

4 $4\overline{)1.00}$ = 0.25

5 $250\overline{)200.}$ = 0.8

RAPID PRACTICE 1-20 (p. 25)

1 2
2 4
3 4

4 2
5 2

RAPID PRACTICE 1-21 (p. 26)

1 3
2 4
3 2

4 3
5 1

RAPID PRACTICE 1-22 (p. 27)

1 18
2 30
3 12

4 50
5 200

RAPID PRACTICE 1-23 (p. 28)

1. $\dfrac{2}{6}$

2. $\dfrac{12}{15}$

3. $\dfrac{4}{8}$

4. $\dfrac{6}{8}$

5. $\dfrac{9}{24}$

RAPID PRACTICE 1-24 (p. 28)

	LCD	Greater Fraction	Equivalent Fractions Result
2	24	$\dfrac{1}{8}$	$\dfrac{3}{24} > \dfrac{2}{24}$
3	200	$\dfrac{1}{100}$	$\dfrac{2}{200} > \dfrac{1}{200}$
4	30	$\dfrac{5}{6}$	$\dfrac{24}{30} < \dfrac{25}{30}$
5	250	$\dfrac{4}{50}$	$\dfrac{1}{250} < \dfrac{20}{250}$

RAPID PRACTICE 1-25 (p. 29)

1. 2 $\dfrac{1}{2} + \dfrac{1}{2} = \dfrac{2}{2} = 1$

2. 4 $\dfrac{2}{4} + \dfrac{1}{4} = \dfrac{3}{4}$

3. 24 $\dfrac{12}{24} + \dfrac{8}{24} = \dfrac{20}{24} = \dfrac{5}{6}$

4. 200 $\dfrac{1}{100} = \dfrac{2}{200} + \dfrac{1}{200} = \dfrac{3}{200}$

5. 12 $\dfrac{8}{12} + \dfrac{3}{12} = \dfrac{11}{12}$

RAPID PRACTICE 1-26 (p. 30)

	LCD	Answer			
1	2	$1\frac{1}{2} - \frac{1}{2} = 1$	4	8	$9\frac{10}{8} - 4\frac{5}{8} = 5\frac{5}{8}$
2	10	$\frac{6}{10} - \frac{5}{10} = \frac{1}{10}$	5	40	$\frac{1}{8} - \frac{1}{10} = \frac{5}{40} - \frac{4}{40} = \frac{1}{40}$
3	12	$\frac{14}{12} - \frac{9}{12} = \frac{5}{12}$			

RAPID PRACTICE 1-27 (p. 31)

1 $\dfrac{1}{27}$

2 $\dfrac{3}{8}$

3 $\dfrac{2}{30} = \dfrac{1}{15}$

4 $\dfrac{1}{500}$

5 $\dfrac{27}{50}$

RAPID PRACTICE 1-28 (p. 32)

1 $\dfrac{3}{8}$ $\quad\left(\dfrac{1}{\cancel{2}} \times \dfrac{\overset{3}{\cancel{6}}}{8} = \dfrac{3}{8}\right)$

2 $2\dfrac{1}{2}$ $\quad\dfrac{5}{\cancel{3}} \times \dfrac{\overset{1}{\cancel{3}}}{2} = \dfrac{5}{2} = 2\dfrac{1}{2}$

3 $2\dfrac{1}{6}$ $\quad\dfrac{13}{\cancel{5}} \times \dfrac{\overset{1}{\cancel{5}}}{6} = \dfrac{13}{6} = 2\dfrac{1}{6}$

4 $\dfrac{2}{3}$ $\quad\left(\dfrac{\overset{1}{\cancel{4}}}{5} \times \dfrac{\overset{2}{\cancel{10}}}{\underset{3}{\cancel{12}}} = \dfrac{2}{3}\right)$

5 $\dfrac{2}{5}$ $\quad\left(\dfrac{\overset{2}{\cancel{100}}}{\underset{1}{\cancel{200}}} \times \dfrac{\overset{1}{\cancel{200}}}{\underset{5}{\cancel{250}}} = \dfrac{2}{5}\right)$

RAPID PRACTICE 1-29 (p. 33)

1 $\dfrac{5}{16}$ $\quad\left(\dfrac{1}{4} \times \dfrac{5}{4} = \dfrac{5}{16}\right)$

2 $\dfrac{38}{9} = 4\dfrac{2}{9}$ $\quad\left(\dfrac{19}{\cancel{6}} \times \dfrac{\overset{2}{\cancel{4}}}{3} = \dfrac{38}{9} = 4\dfrac{2}{9}\right)$

3 $\dfrac{5}{4} = 1\dfrac{1}{4}$ $\quad\left(\dfrac{5}{2} \times \dfrac{1}{2} = \dfrac{5}{4} = 1\dfrac{1}{4}\right)$

4 $\dfrac{13}{15}$ $\quad\left(\dfrac{1}{5} \times \dfrac{13}{3} = \dfrac{13}{15}\right)$

5 $\dfrac{17}{48}$ $\quad\left(\dfrac{1}{6} \times \dfrac{17}{8} = \dfrac{17}{48}\right)$

RAPID PRACTICE 1-30 (p. 33)

1 3 $\quad\left(\dfrac{1}{\cancel{2}} \times \dfrac{\overset{3}{\cancel{6}}}{1} = \dfrac{3}{1} = 3\right)$

2 $2\dfrac{2}{3}$ $\quad\left(\dfrac{1}{3} \times \dfrac{8}{1} = \dfrac{8}{3} = 2\dfrac{2}{3}\right)$

3 $1\dfrac{3}{5}$ $\quad\left(\dfrac{2}{5} \times \dfrac{4}{1} = \dfrac{8}{5} = 1\dfrac{3}{5}\right)$

4 5 $\quad\left(\dfrac{5}{\cancel{4}} \times \dfrac{\overset{1}{\cancel{4}}}{1} = 5\right)$

5 5 $\quad\left(\dfrac{5}{\cancel{2}} \times \dfrac{\overset{1}{\cancel{2}}}{1} = 5\right)$

RAPID PRACTICE 1-31 (p. 34)

1 25% $(1 \div 4 = 25\%)$

2 75% $(3 \div 4 = 75\%)$

6 $\dfrac{1}{10}$ $\left(10\% = \dfrac{\cancel{10}}{100}\right)$

7 $\dfrac{3}{20}$ $\left(15\% = \dfrac{15}{100} = \dfrac{3}{20}\right)$

3 16.7%

4 33.3%

5 83.3%

8 $\frac{1}{2}$

9 $\frac{1}{8}$

10 $\frac{1}{4}$

RAPID PRACTICE 1-32 (p. 35)

2 0.35

3 0.75

4 0.055

5 2

6 10%

7 5%

8 12.5%

9 5.25%

10 50%

RAPID PRACTICE 1-33 (p. 36)

	Fraction	Decimal	Percentage		Fraction	Decimal	Percentage
1	$\frac{3}{10}$	0.3	30%	**4**	$\frac{1}{5}$	0.2	20%
2	$1\frac{5}{10}$	1.5	150%	**5**	$\frac{6}{10}$	0.6	60%
3	$\frac{75}{100}$	0.75	75%				

RAPID PRACTICE 1-34 (p. 37)

2 $320 \div 80 = 4$ calories per gram of carbohydrate

3 $300 \div 12 = 25$ miles per gallon

4 $6000 \div 6 = 1000$ megabytes per gigabyte

5 $960 \div 4 = 240$ mL per cup

CHAPTER 1 MULTIPLE-CHOICE REVIEW (p. 39)

1 4

    Note: Do not handwrite this symbol in medical records. It may be misinterpreted. You will see symbols in printed materials.

2 2

3 4

4 4

5 1

6 2

7 3

8 3

9 3

10 2

11 2

12 1

13 3

14 3

15 3

16 2

17 3

18 4

19 4

20 1

CHAPTER 1 FINAL PRACTICE (p. 41)

1 For children *"less than"* two

2 $\sqrt{9}$

3 greater than or equal to

4 $\dfrac{50}{1}$

5 $85.\cancel{0} = 85$

6 $500.\cancel{00} = 500$

7 $\dfrac{500}{500}$

8 $8 + 7 = 15$

9 $8 \times 7 = 56$

10 1, 2, 3, 4, 6, 12

11 2, 5, 10

12 12

13 10, 15, 20, . . .

14 $\dfrac{1}{2}$

15 $10 \times 10 \times 10 \times 10 \ (= 10,000)$

16 $12^2 = 12 \times 12 = 144$

17 $\sqrt{100} = 10$

18 10

19 8

20 $\dfrac{3}{4}$

21 Numerator = 7; Denominator = 8

22 $\dfrac{1}{100}$ (the denominator is a power of 10)

23 0.42

24 1.259 (1.25.9)

25 8030 (8.030.)

26 0.9

27 0.01

28 50

29 $\dfrac{5}{10} = \dfrac{1}{2}$

30 $\dfrac{25}{1000} = \dfrac{1}{40}$

31 0.05

32 0.232

33 3.39

34 $\dfrac{1}{8}$

35 $\dfrac{1}{15}$

36 $\dfrac{1}{100} = 1\%$

37 $6\frac{1}{4}$

38 $\dfrac{7}{6}$

39 12

40 $\dfrac{2}{3} = \dfrac{4}{6} = \dfrac{6}{9} = \dfrac{8}{12}$

41 greater than

42 4

43 $\dfrac{15}{60} = \dfrac{1}{4}$

44 $\dfrac{12}{24} + \dfrac{4}{24} + \dfrac{3}{24} = \dfrac{19}{24}$

45 $\dfrac{8}{40} - \dfrac{5}{40} = \dfrac{3}{40}$

46 $\dfrac{5}{4} \times \dfrac{17}{7} = \dfrac{85}{28} = 3\frac{1}{28}$

47 $\dfrac{2}{\cancel{3}} \times \dfrac{\overset{2}{\cancel{6}}}{1} = 4$

48 **a.** 0.01; **b.** 1%

49 $\dfrac{\$75}{50} = \$1.50$ per syringe

50 $10 \times 8 = 80$

Chapter 2

RAPID PRACTICE 2-1 (p. 44)

1 **a.** Desired answer units
  b. Quantity and units (factors to convert)
  c. Conversion factor(s)

2 Quantity is a number; unit is a dimension.

3 A conversion factor expresses equivalent amounts for two entities.

4 3 is the numerator

5 8 is the denominator

RAPID PRACTICE 2-2 (p. 48)

1 $\dfrac{12 \text{ eggs}}{1 \text{ dozen}}$

2 $\dfrac{1 \text{ km}}{0.6 \text{ miles}}$

3 $\dfrac{4 \text{ qts}}{1 \text{ gallon}}$

4 $\dfrac{60 \text{ seconds}}{1 \text{ minute}}$

5 $\dfrac{16 \text{ oz}}{1 \text{ lb}}$

➤ Note that all the starting factors in these problems are conversion factors.

RAPID PRACTICE 2-3 (p. 49)

Desired Answer Units	Starting Factors	Given Quantity Units
2 quarts:	$\dfrac{1 \text{ quart}}{4 \text{ cups}}$	$\dfrac{8 \text{ cups}}{1}$
3 yards:	$\dfrac{1 \text{ yard}}{1 \text{ meter}}$	$\dfrac{50 \text{ meters}}{1}$
4 dozen:	$\dfrac{12 \text{ dozen}}{1 \text{ gross}}$	$\dfrac{2 \text{ gross}}{1}$
5 Eurodollars:	$\dfrac{1 \text{ Eurodollar}}{\$1.40}$	$\dfrac{\$500}{1}$

Note: Note that original numbers and units to be converted do not have a denominator and are placed in the numerator position with an implied denominator of 1. This helps prevent multiplication errors.

RAPID PRACTICE 2-4 (p. 51)

1 a. Yes
b. N/A
c. Larger

2 a. No
b. $\dfrac{1 \text{ kg}}{2.2 \text{ lb}}$
c. Smaller

3 a. No
b. $\dfrac{1 \text{ L}}{1000 \text{ mL}}$
c. Smaller

4 a. Yes
b. N/A
c. Larger

5 a. Yes
b. N/A
c. Larger

RAPID PRACTICE 2-5 (p. 53)

2 hours : $\dfrac{1 \text{ hour}}{20 \text{ dollars}} \times \dfrac{500 \text{ dollars}}{1} = 25$ hours

3 megabytes : $\dfrac{1000 \text{ megabytes}}{1 \text{ gigabyte}} \times \dfrac{4 \text{ gigabytes}}{1} = 4000$ megabytes

4 gallons : $\dfrac{1 \text{ gallon}}{4 \text{ liters}} \times \dfrac{40 \text{ liters}}{1} = 10$ gallons

5 LPNs : $\dfrac{2 \text{ LPNs}}{5 \text{ CNAs}} \times \dfrac{40 \text{ CNAs}}{1} = 16$ LPNs

RAPID PRACTICE 2-6 (p. 55)

1 A cups: $\dfrac{2 \text{ cups}}{1 \text{ pint}} \times \dfrac{2 \text{ pints}}{1 \text{ quart}} \times \dfrac{5 \text{ quarts}}{1} = 20$ cups

2 B inches : $\dfrac{12 \text{ inches}}{1 \text{ foot}} \times \dfrac{3 \text{ feet}}{1 \text{ yard}} \times \dfrac{20 \text{ yards}}{1} = 720$ inches

3 B weeks : $\dfrac{4 \text{ weeks}}{1 \text{ month}} \times \dfrac{12 \text{ months}}{1 \text{ year}} \times \dfrac{4 \text{ years}}{1} = 192$ weeks

4 B mm : $\dfrac{10 \text{ mm}}{1 \text{ cm}} \times \dfrac{2.5 \text{ cm}}{1 \text{ inch}} \times \dfrac{10 \text{ inches}}{1} = 250$ mm

5 B grams : $\dfrac{1 \text{ g}}{1000 \text{ mg}} \times \dfrac{1 \text{ mg}}{1000 \text{ mcg}} \times \dfrac{\overset{4}{4000 \text{ mcg}}}{1} = \dfrac{4}{1000} = 0.004$ g

RAPID PRACTICE 2-7 (p. 57)

1 lbs : $\dfrac{2.2 \text{ lbs}}{1 \text{ kg}} \times \dfrac{80 \text{ kg}}{1} = 176$ lbs

2 pints : $\dfrac{2 \text{ pints}}{1 \text{ qt}} \times \dfrac{4 \text{ qts}}{1 \text{ gallon}} \times \dfrac{5 \text{ gallon}}{1} = 40$ pints

3 inches : $\dfrac{1 \text{ inch}}{2.5 \text{ cm}} \times \dfrac{1 \text{ cm}}{10 \text{ mm}} \times \dfrac{25 \text{ mm}}{1} = 1$ inch

4 hours : $\dfrac{1 \text{ hr}}{60 \text{ min}} \times \dfrac{1 \text{ min}}{60 \text{ sec}} \times \dfrac{7200 \text{ sec}}{1} = 2$ hours

5 capsules : $\dfrac{3 \text{ capsules}}{1 \text{ day}} \times \dfrac{7 \text{ days}}{1 \text{ week}} \times \dfrac{2 \text{ weeks}}{1} = 42$ capsules for 2 weeks

CHAPTER 2 MULTIPLE-CHOICE REVIEW (p. 57)

1 3		**6** 1	
2 1		**7** 3	
3 2		**8** 3	
4 2		**9** 1	
5 3		**10** 4	

1 a. Desired answer units
   b. Given quantity and units (factors to convert)
   c. Conversion factors

2 Eggs : $\dfrac{12 \text{ eggs}}{1 \text{ dozen}} \times \dfrac{10 \text{ dozen}}{1} = 120$ eggs

3 meters : $\dfrac{1 \text{ meter}}{1.09 \text{ yards}} \times \dfrac{30 \text{ yards}}{1} = 27.5$ meters

4 lbs : $\dfrac{2.2 \text{ lbs}}{1 \text{ Kg}} \times \dfrac{60 \text{ Kg}}{1} = 132$ lbs

5 Inches : $\dfrac{12 \text{ Inches}}{1 \text{ foot}} \times \dfrac{3 \text{ feet}}{1 \text{ yard}} \times \dfrac{50 \text{ yards}}{1} = 1800$ inches

6 mm : $\dfrac{10 \text{ mm}}{1 \text{ cm}} \times \dfrac{2.5 \text{ cm}}{1 \text{ inch}} \times \dfrac{1 \text{ inch}}{1} = 25$ mm (millimeters)

Comment: 2.5 cm is an approximate equivalent. There are 2.54 cm in an inch.

7 Km : $\dfrac{1 \text{ km}}{0.6 \text{ miles}} \times \dfrac{50 \text{ miles}}{1} = 83.3$ km

8 DVDs : $\dfrac{1 \text{ DVD}}{8 \text{ dollars}} \times \dfrac{100 \text{ dollars}}{1} = 12.5$ DVDs (12 DVDs with $4 remaining)

9 Rx : $\dfrac{1 \text{ Rx}}{50 \text{ dollars}} \times \dfrac{2000 \text{ dollars}}{1} = 40$ Rx

10 Nurses : $\dfrac{1 \text{ nurse}}{\text{Shift}} \times \dfrac{480 \text{ beds}}{12 \text{ beds}} = 40$ nurses per shift

11 Liters : $\dfrac{1 \text{ liter}}{1 \text{ qt}} \times \dfrac{4 \text{ qt}}{1 \text{ gallon}} \times \dfrac{8 \text{ gallons}}{1} = 32$ liters (L)

12 Inches : $\dfrac{12 \text{ inches}}{1 \text{ foot}} \times \dfrac{3 \text{ feet}}{1 \text{ yard}} \times \dfrac{10 \text{ yards}}{1} = 360$ inches

13 Tablespoons : $\dfrac{2 \text{ tbs}}{1 \text{ oz}} \times \dfrac{8 \text{ oz}}{1 \text{ cup}} \times \dfrac{1 \text{ cup}}{1} = 16$ tbs (tablespoons)

14 Cups : $\dfrac{2 \text{ cups}}{1 \text{ pt}} \times \dfrac{2 \text{ pt}}{1 \text{ qt}} \times \dfrac{2 \text{ qt}}{1} = 8$ cups

15 Seconds : $\dfrac{60 \text{ seconds}}{1 \text{ minute}} \times \dfrac{60 \text{ minutes}}{1 \text{ hr}} \times \dfrac{2 \text{ hrs}}{1} = 7200$ seconds

16 mL : $\dfrac{5 \text{ mL}}{1 \text{ tsp}} \times \dfrac{3 \text{ tsp}}{1 \text{ tbs}} \times \dfrac{3 \text{ tbs}}{1} = 45$ mL (milliliters)

17 $\dfrac{\text{NA}}{\text{shift}} : \dfrac{2 \text{ NA}}{1 \text{ RN}} \times \dfrac{1 \text{ RN}}{10 \text{ beds}} \times \dfrac{\overset{30}{\cancel{300 \text{ beds}}}}{1} = 60$ NA per shift

18 Inches : $\dfrac{1 \text{ inch}}{2.5 \text{ cm}} \times \dfrac{100 \text{ cm}}{1 \text{ meter}} \times \dfrac{1 \text{ meter}}{1} = 40$ inches

Note: A meter is a little longer than a yard (36 in).

19 cm : $\dfrac{2.5 \text{ cm}}{1 \text{ inch}} \times \dfrac{12 \text{ inches}}{1 \text{ ft}} \times \dfrac{1 \text{ ft}}{1} = 30$ cm (centimeters)

20 mcg : $\dfrac{1000 \text{ mcg}}{1 \text{ mg}} \times \dfrac{1000 \text{ mg}}{1 \text{ gram}} \times \dfrac{2 \text{ grams}}{1} = 2{,}000{,}000$ mcg (micrograms)

Chapter 3

RAPID PRACTICE 3-1 (p. 65)

1 gram, liter, meter
2 To avoid confusion with the number 1
3 Inconsistent capacities of household measures
4 modern metric system
5 TJC; ISMP

RAPID PRACTICE 3-2 (p. 68)

1 milli-	m	6 liter	L
2 centi-	c	7 meter	m
3 micro-	mc	8 gram	g
4 deci-	d	9 meter	
5 kilo-	k	10 milli-	

RAPID PRACTICE 3-3 (p. 69)

1 Liter, L
2 k (kilo)
3 80 milligrams per deciliter
4 mc
5 g = gram; L = liter; m = meter

RAPID PRACTICE 3-4 (p. 69)

1 4
2 2
3 1
4 2
5 3

Note: Metric unit abbreviations are not pluralized.

RAPID PRACTICE 3-5 (p. 70)

1 mg
2 mcg
3 mm
4 mL
5 kg

RAPID PRACTICE 3-6 (p. 70)

1 L = liter
2 m = meter
3 L = liter
4 g = gram
5 g = gram

RAPID PRACTICE 3-7 (p. 71)

2 175 mcg (microgram) (0.175 mg)(milligram)
3 1 mg (milligram)
4 100 mg (milligram)
5 1 g (gram)

RAPID PRACTICE 3-8 (p. 74)

1 4	**4** 1
2 1	**5** 1
3 3	

RAPID PRACTICE 3-9 (p. 76)

1 500 mg = 0.5 g	**6** 0.25 g = 250 mg
2 2000 mg = 2 g	**7** 0.6 g = 600 mg
3 250 mg = 0.25 g	**8** 0.125 g = 125 mg
4 1500 mg = 1.5 g	**9** 0.04 g = 40 mg
5 60 mg = 0.06 g	**10** 2 g = 2000 mg

RAPID PRACTICE 3-10 (p. 77)

1 mg : $\dfrac{1000 \text{ mg}}{1 \cancel{g}} \times \dfrac{1.5 \cancel{g}}{1} = 1500$ mg

2 mg : $\dfrac{1000 \text{ mg}}{1 \cancel{g}} \times \dfrac{0.15 \cancel{g}}{1} = 150$ mg

3 mg : $\dfrac{1000 \text{ mg}}{1 \cancel{g}} \times \dfrac{4 \cancel{g}}{1} = 4000$ mg

4 g : $\dfrac{1 \text{ g}}{\underset{2}{\cancel{1000 \text{ mg}}}} \times \dfrac{\overset{1}{\cancel{500 \text{ mg}}}}{1} = 0.5$ g   **Note:** Reduce large numbers to make the calculations easier.

5 g : $\dfrac{1 \text{ g}}{100\cancel{0 \text{ mg}}} \times \dfrac{6\cancel{0 \text{ mg}}}{1} = 0.06$ g

RAPID PRACTICE 3-11 (p. 78)

1 3	**4** 1
2 2	**5** 4
3 1	

RAPID PRACTICE 3-12 (p. 78)

mg	mcg	mg and g
1 5 mg	**6** 2000 mcg	**11** 1 mg
2 0.3 mg	**7** 500 mcg	**12** 5 g
3 1.5 mg	**8** 1800 mcg	**13** 400 mg
4 20 mg	**9** 150 mcg	**14** 0.6 g
5 2.5 mg	**10** 600 mcg	**15** 30 mg

RAPID PRACTICE 3-13 (p. 79)

1 centimeter	**6** L
2 milliliter	**7** m
3 milligram	**8** kg
4 millimeter	**9** km
5 microgram	**10** dL

RAPID PRACTICE 3-14 (p. 79)

1 1000 mg	**6** 1000 mL
2 1000 g	**7** 2500 mg
3 10 mm	**8** 0.5 g
4 1000 mcg	**9** 2.5 g
5 1,000,000 mcg	**10** 0.5 mg

RAPID PRACTICE 3-15 (p. 82)

1 240 mL	**4** 15 mL
2 10 mL	**5** 30 mL
3 15 mL	

CHAPTER 3 MULTIPLE-CHOICE REVIEW (p. 84)

1 1	**6** 2
2 2	**7** 4
3 3	**8** 1
4 3	**9** 2
5 1	**10** 3

CHAPTER 3 FINAL PRACTICE (p. 85)

1 **a.** meter = m   **d.** kilo- = k

   b. liter = L   **e.** centi- = c

   c. gram = g   **f.** deci- = d

                           g. milli- = m

                           h. micro- = mc

2 g : $\dfrac{1\ g}{1000\ \cancel{mg}} \times \dfrac{400\ \cancel{mg}}{1} = 0.4\ g$

3 mg : $\dfrac{1000\ mg}{1\ \cancel{g}} \times \dfrac{0.15\ \cancel{g}}{1} = 150\ mg$

Note: The first numerator, mg, matches the described answer units, mg. Only mg remains in the answer.

4 mL : $\dfrac{1000\ ml}{1\ \cancel{L}} \times \dfrac{0.25\ \cancel{L}}{1} = 250\ mL$

5 mg : $\dfrac{1\ mg}{10\cancel{0}0\ \cancel{mcg}} \times \dfrac{150\cancel{0}\ \cancel{mcg}}{1} = 1.5\ mg$

6 g : $\dfrac{1000\ g}{1\ \cancel{kg}} \times \dfrac{1.5\ \cancel{kg}}{1} = 1500\ g$

7 mg : $\dfrac{1000\ mg}{1\ \cancel{g}} \times \dfrac{0.1\ \cancel{g}}{1} = 100\ mg$

8 cm : $\dfrac{\overset{1}{\cancel{100}}\ cm}{1\ \cancel{m}} \times \dfrac{1\ \cancel{m}}{\underset{10}{\cancel{1000}\ mm}} \times \dfrac{15\ \cancel{mm}}{1} = \dfrac{15}{10} = 1.5\ cm$

Note: Notice the diagonal direction of the cancelled units.

9 mcg : $\dfrac{1000 \text{ mcg}}{1 \text{ mg}} \times \dfrac{0.2 \text{ mg}}{1} = 200$ mcg

10 g : $\dfrac{1 \text{ g}}{\underset{4}{1000 \text{ mg}}} \times \dfrac{1 \text{ mg}}{1000 \text{ mcg}} \times \dfrac{\overset{1}{250{,}000} \text{ mcg}}{1} = 0.25$ g

11 mL : $\dfrac{5 \text{ mL}}{1 \text{ tsp}} \times \dfrac{3 \text{ tsp}}{1} = 15$ mL

12 mL : $\dfrac{15 \text{ mL}}{1 \text{ tbs}} \times \dfrac{2 \text{ tbs}}{1} = 30$ mL

13 mL : $\dfrac{30 \text{ mL}}{1 \text{ oz}} \times \dfrac{1.5 \text{ oz}}{1} = 45$ mL

14 tsp : $\dfrac{3 \text{ tsp}}{1 \text{ tbs}} \times \dfrac{1 \text{ tbs}}{1} = 3$ tsp

15 tbs : $\dfrac{2 \text{ tbs}}{1 \text{ oz}} \times \dfrac{2 \text{ oz}}{1} = 4$ tbs

16 1000 g

17 2.2 lbs

18 mL : $\dfrac{1000 \text{ mL}}{1 \text{ L}} \times \dfrac{0.5 \text{ L}}{1} = 500$ mL

19 **a.** 84 mg per mL
  b. 1 mEq per mL

20 **a.** 149 mg per mL
  b. 2 mEq per mL

Note: Potassium chloride is a high-alert medication (see Appendix B).

Chapter 4

RAPID PRACTICE 4-1 (p. 91)

1 1   **4** 2
2 3   **5** 2
3 2

RAPID PRACTICE 4-2 (p. 95)

1 cap   **6** LA
2 DS   **7** XL
3 XR   **8** ENT
4 supp   **9** CD
5 tab   **10** UNG

RAPID PRACTICE 4-3 (p. 96)

1 scored tablet   **4** compound
2 cap   **5** XR; XL; SR; CD; LA
3 enteric-coated tablet; capsules

RAPID PRACTICE 4-4 (p. 97)

1 susp.
2 mixt.
3 sol.

4 elix.
5 aq.

RAPID PRACTICE 4-5 (p. 99)

1 bucc
2 SL
3 NG
4 left ear
5 GT

6 top
7 PO
8 MDI
9 vag
10 NPO

RAPID PRACTICE 4-6 (p. 104)

1 after meals
2 twice a day
3 as needed
4 without
5 immediately (and only one dose)
6 every 4 hours
7 nothing by mouth
8 before meals
9 with (as "with meals")
10 give as desired (pertaining to fluids or activity)
11 $\bar{c}$

12 prn
13 D/C (e.g., specific medication [D/C aspirin] or treatment [D/C catheter])
14 tid
15 ac
16 each, every
17 qid
18 q2h
19 $\bar{s}$
20 q12h

RAPID PRACTICE 4-7 (p. 104)

1 T = tricycle; B = bicycle
   (3 wheels)   (2 wheels)
2 PRN
3 q4h = 6 times a day
4 **a.** Give "Tears No More" 2 (two) drops in each eye twice a day as needed for itching or burning
   b. Give Mylanta antacid 1 (one) ounce three times a day before meals
   c. Pharmacy
5 4; 6

RAPID PRACTICE 4-8 (p. 105)

1	susp	11	cheek (to be dissolved, not swallowed)
2	elix	12	as desired (for fluids, activity)
3	sol	13	metered dose inhaler
4	fld	14	two times daily
5	fld ext	15	intradermal
6	prn	16	as needed; when necessary
7	NPO	17	nothing by mouth
8	IM	18	intravenous piggyback*
9	stat	19	Give medication when X-ray calls for the patient.
10	top	20	every 6 hours

*Do not use the abbreviation IVP for medication routes. IVP is an IV renal function test.

RAPID PRACTICE 4-9 (p. 105)

1	sublingual	11	oral, by mouth
2	solution	12	gastrostomy tube
3	intramuscular	13	before meals
4	double strength	14	every night at bedtime
5	every hour	15	after meals
6	elixir	16	as needed, when necessary
7	every six hours	17	two times daily
8	nasogastic tube	18	every eight hours
9	every four hours	19	three times daily
10	nothing by mouth	20	immediately (for only one dose)

RAPID PRACTICE 4-10 (p. 107)

1	3	4	1
2	3	5	4
3	2		

RAPID PRACTICE 4-11 (p. 113)

1. **a.** Sinemet
   b. 2 (it is a compound drug)
   c. carbidopa 10 mg, levodopa 100 mg
2. **a.** lorazepam
   b. 100 tab
   c. 0.5 mg
3. **a.** multiple dose vial
   b. 400 mcg per mL
   c. 0.4 mg per mL
4. **a.** potassium chloride
   b. 40 mEq per 15 mL
5. **a.** Elixir
   b. 20 mg per 5 mL
   c. 14%

RAPID PRACTICE 4-12 (p. 116)

2 a. capsules
  b. 250 mg per capsule
  c. 0.5 g
  d. 1000 mg = 1 gram
  e. 1.5 g or 1500 mg (q8h = 3 times in 24 hrs)
  f. 0.5 g = 0.500. = 500 mg

3 a. mL
  b. 125 mg per 5 mL
  c. 0.25 g
  d. 1000 mg = 1 g
  e. 1 g (0.25 g × 4 doses) = 1 gram per day
  f. 0.250 g = 250 mg

4 a. mL
  b. 15 mg per mL
  c. intramuscular
  d. immediately
  e. intramuscular, subcutaneous, intravenous

5 a. loracarbef
  b. Suspension
  c. 200 mg per 5 mL—label B (0.2 g = 200 mg)
  d. 0.2 g
  e. 1000 mg = 1 gram

RAPID PRACTICE 4-13 (p. 120)

1 with = $\bar{c}$; without = $\bar{s}$
2 the prescriber
3 medication errors due to misinterpretation, forgetting, not hearing, etc.
4 Prepare and mix medications together; deliver immediately by intramuscular route.
5 They may look like other numbers such as 1 and 0.

RAPID PRACTICE 4-14 (p. 124)

1 penicillin; ASA (aspirin)
2 1800
3 Humalog
4 Lasix. Document the clarification. Report to nurse supervisor.
5 2400
6 NKDA–No
7 losartan (Cozaar). Blood pressure assessment is needed.
8 acetaminophen
9 Consult prescriber and document.
10 every 4 hours

RAPID PRACTICE 4-15 (p. 127)

1 d
2 a
3 e
4 b
5 c
6 g
7 f

CHAPTER 4 MULTIPLE-CHOICE REVIEW (p. 128)

1	1	**11**	2
2	2	**12**	2 (scored tablet)
3	3	**13**	2
4	4	**14**	1
5	2	**15**	3
6	1	**16**	2
7	3	**17**	2
8	2	**18**	3
9	4	**19**	1
10	2	**20**	1

CHAPTER 4 FINAL PRACTICE (p. 133)

1 immediately

2 every hour

3 as needed

4 intravenously

5 nothing by mouth

6 by mouth

7 total parenteral nutrition

8 nasogastric

9 intravenously

10 subcutaneously

11 nasogastric

12 by mouth

13 every 2 hours

14 as desired

15 intramuscularly every 4 hours as needed

16 suppositories

17 by mouth

18 elixirs and suspensions two times daily

19 without

20 sublingually

21 right patient

22 right drug

23 right dose

24 right time

25 right route

26 right documentation

27 right to refuse

28 2 capsules

$$\frac{\text{capsules}}{\text{dose}} : \frac{1 \text{ capsule}}{\overset{1}{\underset{}{\cancel{50 \text{ mg}}}}} \times \frac{\overset{20}{\cancel{1000 \text{ mg}}}}{1 \text{ g}} \times \frac{0.1 \text{ g}}{\text{dose}} = \frac{2 \text{ capsules}}{\text{dose}}$$

29 a. the ordered dose; the unit dose concentration
b. one or more conversion formulas

30 a. ERY-TAB
b. 0.5 g × 2 = 1 g per day or 1000 mg per day
c. 250 mg per tablet
d. 2 tablets per dose

$$\frac{\text{tab}}{\text{dose}} : \frac{1 \text{ tab}}{\underset{1}{\cancel{250 \text{ mg}}}} \times \frac{\overset{4}{\cancel{1000 \text{ mg}}}}{1 \cancel{\text{ g}}} \times \frac{0.5 \cancel{\text{ g}}}{\text{dose}} = \frac{2 \text{ tabs}}{\text{dose}}$$

Chapter 5

RAPID PRACTICE 5-1 (p. 136)

1 True
2 True
3 True

4 False
5 True

RAPID PRACTICE 5-2 (p. 136)

1 2 tablets
2 1.5 tablets
3 2 capsules
4 0.5 tablet
5 2 tablets

6 2 tablets
7 0.5 tablet
8 2 capsules
9 2.5 tablets
10 0.5 tablet

RAPID PRACTICE 5-3 (p. 137)

2 a. 1000 mg = 1 gram
b. 2 tablets (250 = 2 × 125)
c. 2 tablets per dose

$$\frac{\text{tablet}}{\text{dose}} : \frac{1 \text{ tablet}}{\cancel{125 \text{ mg}}} \times \frac{\overset{2}{\cancel{250 \text{ mg}}}}{\text{dose}} = \frac{2 \text{ tablets}}{\text{dose}}$$

d. Equation is balanced. Answer equals estimate.

3 a. No conversion formula needed
b. 2 tablets (0.1 = 2 × 0.5)
c. 2 tablets per dose

$$\frac{\text{tablet}}{\text{dose}} : \frac{1 \text{ tablet}}{\underset{1}{\cancel{0.05 \text{ g}}}} \times \frac{\overset{2}{\cancel{0.1 \text{ g}}}}{\text{dose}} = \frac{2 \text{ tablets}}{\text{dose}}$$

d. Equation is balanced. Answer equals estimate.

4 a. No conversion formula needed
b. $1\frac{1}{2}$ tablets ($75 = 1\frac{1}{2} \times 50$)
c. 1.5 tablets per dose

$$\frac{\text{tablet}}{\text{dose}} : \frac{1 \text{ tablet}}{\underset{2}{\cancel{50 \text{ mcg}}}} \times \frac{\overset{3}{\cancel{75 \text{ mcg}}}}{\text{dose}} = \frac{1.5 \text{ tablets}}{\text{dose}}$$

d. Equation is balanced. Answer equals estimate.

5 a. No conversion formula needed

b. 2 tablets ($20 = 2 \times 10$)

c. 2 tablets per dose

$$\frac{\text{tab}}{\text{dose}} : \frac{1 \text{ tab}}{\cancel{10 \text{ mEq}}_{1}} \times \frac{\cancel{20 \text{ mEq}}^{2}}{\text{dose}} = \frac{2 \text{ tabs}}{\text{dose}}$$

d. Equation is balanced. Answer equals estimate.

6 a. 1000 mg = 1 gram

b. 0.2 g = 200 mg; 2 capsules ($200 = 2 \times 100$)

c. 2 capsules per dose

$$\frac{\text{capsule}}{\text{dose}} : \frac{1 \text{ capsule}}{\cancel{100 \text{ mg}}_{1}} \times \frac{\cancel{1000 \text{ mg}}^{10}}{1 \cancel{g}} \times \frac{0.2 \cancel{g}}{\text{dose}} = \frac{2 \text{ capsules}}{\text{dose}}$$

d. Equation is balanced. Answer equals estimate.

7 a. 1000 mg = 1 g

b. 250 mg = 0.25 g; 1 capsule

c. 1 capsule per dose

$$\frac{\text{capsule}}{\text{dose}} : \frac{1 \text{ capsule}}{0.25 \cancel{g}} \times \frac{1 \cancel{g}}{\cancel{1000 \text{ mg}}_{4}} \times \frac{\cancel{250 \text{ mg}}^{1}}{\text{dose}} = \frac{1}{1} = \frac{1 \text{ capsule}}{\text{dose}}$$

d. Equation is balanced. Answer equals estimate.

8 a. 1000 mg = 1 g

b. $0.25 = 2 \times 0.125$; 2 capsules

c. 2 capsules per dose

$$\frac{\text{capsule}}{\text{dose}} : \frac{1 \text{ capsule}}{\cancel{125 \text{ mg}}_{1}} \times \frac{\cancel{1000 \text{ mg}}^{8}}{1 \cancel{g}} \times \frac{0.25 \cancel{g}}{\text{dose}} = \frac{2 \text{ capsules}}{\text{dose}}$$

d. Equation is balanced. Answer equals estimate.

9 a. 1000 mcg = 1 mg

b. 0.175 mg = 175 mcg = $\frac{1}{2}$ of 350 mcg = $\frac{1}{2}$ tablet

c. 0.5 tablet per dose

$$\frac{\text{tab}}{\text{dose}} : \frac{1 \text{ tab}}{350 \cancel{\text{mcg}}} \times \frac{1000 \cancel{\text{mcg}}}{1 \cancel{\text{mg}}} \times \frac{0.175 \cancel{\text{mg}}}{\text{dose}} = \frac{175}{350} = \frac{0.5 \text{ tab}}{\text{dose}}$$

d. Equation is balanced. Answer equals estimate.

Note: If you use a calculator to multiply larger numbers, verify the result by reentering the factors a second time.

10 a. 1000 mcg = 1 mg

b. 0.1 mg = 100 mcg = 2×50 mcg; 2 tablets

c. 2 tablets ($100 = 50 \times 2$)

$$\frac{\text{tab}}{\text{dose}} : \frac{1 \text{ tablet}}{\cancel{50 \text{ mcg}}_{1}} \times \frac{\cancel{1000 \text{ mcg}}^{20}}{1 \cancel{\text{mg}}} \times \frac{0.1 \cancel{\text{mg}}}{\text{dose}} = \frac{2 \text{ tablets}}{\text{dose}}$$

d. Equation is balanced. Answer equals estimate.

RAPID PRACTICE 5-4 (p. 140)

2 100 mg   100,000 mcg

3 80 mg   0.08 g

| 4 | 25 mg | 0.025 g |
| 5 | 300 mg | 0.3 g |

RAPID PRACTICE 5-5 (p. 141)

No.	Decimal Place	Answer
2	3	0.2 mg
3	3	500 mcg
4	6	0.015 g
5	6	4000 mcg
6	3	2.2 g
7	3	0.35 mg
8	6	0.05 g
9	3	50 mg
10	3	0.5 g

RAPID PRACTICE 5-6 (p. 141)

1 a. 60 mg = 30 mg × 2
b. 2 tablets per dose

$$\frac{tab}{dose} : \frac{1\ tab}{\cancel{30\ mg}} \times \frac{\cancel{60\ mg}}{dose} = \frac{2\ tablets}{dose}$$

c. Equation is balanced. Estimate equals answer.

2 a. 1 mg = 2 × 0.5 mg
b. 2 tablets per dose

$$\frac{tab}{dose} : \frac{1\ tab}{\cancel{0.5\ mg}} \times \frac{\cancel{1\ mg}}{dose} = \frac{2\ tablets}{dose}$$

c. Equation is balanced. Estimate equals answer.

3 a. 0.25 g = 250 mg
b. 1 tablet per dose

$$\frac{tab}{dose} : \frac{1\ tab}{\underset{1}{\cancel{250\ mg}}} \times \frac{\overset{4}{\cancel{1000\ mg}}}{1\ \cancel{g}} \times \frac{0.25\ \cancel{g}}{dose} = \frac{1\ tablet}{dose}$$

c. Equation is balanced. Estimate equals answer.

4 a. 0.1 g = 100 mg; 50 × 2 = 100
b. 2 tablets per dose

$$\frac{tab}{dose} : \frac{1\ tab}{\underset{1}{\cancel{50\ mg}}} \times \frac{\overset{20}{\cancel{1000\ mg}}}{1\ \cancel{g}} \times \frac{0.1\ \cancel{g}}{dose} = \frac{2\ tablets}{dose}$$

c. Equation is balanced. Estimate equals answer.

5 a. 15 mg = 7.5 mg × 2 tabs
b. 2 tablets per dose

$$\frac{tab}{dose} : \frac{1\ tab}{\underset{1}{\cancel{7.5\ mg}}} \times \frac{\overset{2}{\cancel{15\ mg}}}{dose} = \frac{2\ tablets}{dose}$$

c. Equation is balanced. Estimate equals answer.

RAPID PRACTICE 5-7 (p. 143)

1 a. 0.25 mg × 2 = 0.5 mg; 2 tablets

$$\frac{tab}{dose} : \frac{1 \text{ tab}}{\underset{1}{\cancel{0.25 \text{ mg}}}} \times \frac{\overset{2}{\cancel{0.5 \text{ mg}}}}{dose} = \frac{2 \text{ tablets}}{dose}$$

b. Equation is balanced. Answer equals estimate.

2 a. 0.5 g = 500 mg; 500 mg × 2 = 1000 mg; 2 tablets

$$\frac{tab}{dose} : \frac{1 \text{ tablet}}{0.5 \text{ g}} \times \frac{1 \text{ g}}{\cancel{1000 \text{ mg}}} \times \frac{\cancel{1000 \text{ mg}}}{dose} = \frac{1}{0.5} = \frac{2 \text{ tablets}}{dose}$$

b. Equation is balanced. Answer equals estimate.

3 a. 5 mg = 2.5 mg × 2 tablets

$$\frac{tab}{dose} : \frac{1 \text{ tab}}{\underset{1}{\cancel{2.5 \text{ mg}}}} \times \frac{\overset{2}{\cancel{5 \text{ mg}}}}{dose} = \frac{2 \text{ tablets}}{dose}$$

b. Equation is balanced. Answer equals estimate.

4 a. 0.3 g = 300 mg; 3 capsules

$$\frac{cap}{dose} : \frac{1 \text{ cap}}{\underset{1}{\cancel{100 \text{ mg}}}} \times \frac{\overset{10}{\cancel{1000 \text{ mg}}}}{1 \text{ g}} \times \frac{0.3 \text{ g}}{dose} = \frac{3 \text{ capsules}}{dose}$$

b. Equation is balanced. Answer equals estimate.

5 a. Would select label A—The order does not state SR (sustained release).
b. 0.12 g = 120 mg; 1 tablet

$$\frac{tab}{dose} : \frac{1 \text{ tab}}{120 \text{ mg}} \times \frac{1000 \text{ mg}}{1 \text{ g}} \times \frac{0.12 \text{ g}}{dose} = \frac{120}{120} = \frac{1 \text{ tablet}}{dose}$$

c. Equation is balanced. Answer equals estimate.

RAPID PRACTICE 5-8 (p. 146)

2 5000 mcg = 5 mg   more   2 mL
3 0.1 g = 100 mg   less   0.3 mL
4 750 mg = 0.75 g   more   1.5 mL
5 200 mg = 0.2 g   more   2 mL

RAPID PRACTICE 5-9 (p. 149)

1 a. (0.2 g = 200 mg) Give 10 mL (2 × the unit dose supplied)

$$\frac{mL}{dose} : \frac{5 \text{ mL}}{\underset{1}{\cancel{100 \text{ mg}}}} \times \frac{\overset{10}{\cancel{1000 \text{ mg}}}}{1 \text{ g}} \times \frac{0.2 \text{ g}}{dose} = \frac{10 \text{ mL}}{dose}$$

b. The estimate supports the answer. The equation is balanced.
2 a. Give about $1\frac{1}{2}$ times the 5 mL supplied

$$\frac{mL}{dose} : \frac{5 \text{ mL}}{\cancel{5 \text{ mg}}} \times \frac{8 \text{ mg}}{dose} = \frac{8 \text{ mL}}{dose}$$

b. Equation is balanced. Estimate supports answer.

3 a. Give slightly more than 5 mL (15 mg is more than 12.5 mg)

$$\frac{mL}{dose} : \frac{5\ mL}{12.5\ \text{mg}} \times \frac{15\ \text{mg}}{dose} = \frac{75}{12.5} = \frac{6\ mL}{dose}$$

b. Equation is balanced. Estimate supports answer.

4 a. Give half the dose per mL supplied ($\frac{1}{2}$ of 1 mL).

$$\frac{mL}{dose} : \frac{1\ mL}{\underset{2}{\cancel{50\ \text{mcg}}}} \times \frac{\overset{1}{\cancel{25\ \text{mcg}}}}{dose} = \frac{1}{2} = \frac{0.5\ mL}{dose}$$

b. Equation is balanced. Estimate supports answer.

5 a. Give about $1\frac{1}{2} \times 5$ mL (7.5 mL).

$$\frac{mL}{dose} : \frac{5\ mL}{\underset{2}{\cancel{4\ \text{mg}}}} \times \frac{\overset{3}{\cancel{6\ \text{mg}}}}{dose} = \frac{15}{2} = \frac{7.5\ mL}{dose}$$

b. Equation is balanced. Estimate supports answer.

RAPID PRACTICE 5-10 (p. 153)

	Amount to Prepare	Place in Cup	Place in Syringe	Syringe Size
1	6.5 mL	5	1.5	3
2	14 mL	10	4	5
3	9 mL	5	4	5
4	17 mL	15	2	3
5	27.4 mL	25	2.4	3

RAPID PRACTICE 5-11 (p. 154)

1 a. Give $1\frac{1}{2}$ times the available unit dose of 1 mL or 1.5 mL

$$\frac{mL}{dose} : \frac{1\ mL}{\underset{2}{\cancel{50\ \text{mg}}}} \times \frac{\overset{3}{\cancel{75\ \text{mg}}}}{dose} = \frac{1.5\ mL}{dose}$$

b. Equation is balanced. Estimate equals answer.

2 a. Give 4×5 mL (20 mL).

$$\frac{mL}{dose} : \frac{\cancel{5}\ mL}{\cancel{5}\ \text{mg}} \times \frac{20\ \cancel{\text{mg}}}{dose} = \frac{20\ mL}{dose}$$

b. Equation is balanced. Answer equals estimate.

3 a. Give slightly more than 4 mL.

$$\frac{mL}{dose} : \frac{2\ mL}{\underset{3}{\cancel{15\ \text{mg}}}} \times \frac{\overset{7}{\cancel{35\ \text{mg}}}}{dose} = \frac{14}{3} = \frac{4.7\ mL}{dose}$$

b. Equation is balanced. Estimate supports answer.

4 a. Give more than 8 mL but less than 16 mL.

$$\frac{mL}{dose} : \frac{8\ mL}{\underset{3}{\cancel{75\ \text{mg}}}} \times \frac{\overset{5}{\cancel{125\ \text{mg}}}}{dose} = \frac{40}{3} = \frac{13.3\ mL}{dose}$$

b. Equation is balanced. Estimate supports answer.

5 a. Give slightly less than 20 mL.

$$\frac{mL}{dose} : \frac{10\ mL}{\underset{5}{\cancel{25\ mg}}} \times \overset{9}{\cancel{45\ mg}} = \frac{90}{5} = \frac{18\ mL}{dose}$$

b. Equation is balanced. Estimate supports answer.

RAPID PRACTICE 5-12 (p. 155)

1 a. Give slightly more than 5 mL.

$$\frac{mL}{dose} : \frac{5\ mL}{\underset{4}{\cancel{20\ mg}}} \times \overset{5}{\cancel{25\ mg}} = \frac{25}{4} = 6.25,\ \text{rounded to}\ \frac{6.3\ mL}{dose}$$

b. Equation is balanced. Estimate supports answer.

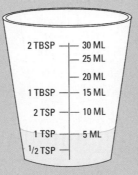

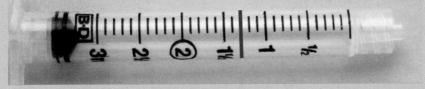

2 a. Give less than 15 mL but more than 7.5 mL.

$$\frac{mL}{dose} : \frac{15\ mL}{\underset{8}{\cancel{40\ mEq}}} \times \overset{5}{\cancel{25\ mEq}} = \frac{75}{8} = 9.37,\ \text{rounded to}\ \frac{9.4\ mL}{dose}$$

b. Equation is balanced. Estimate supports answer.

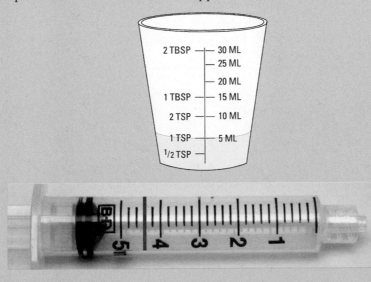

3 a. Give about $\dfrac{3}{4}$ of a mL

$$\dfrac{\text{mL}}{\text{dose}} : \dfrac{\text{mL}}{1 \ \cancel{\text{mg}}} \times \dfrac{0.75 \ \cancel{\text{mg}}}{\text{dose}} = \dfrac{0.75 \ \text{mL}}{\text{dose}} \text{ from dropper provided}$$

b. Equation is balanced. The answer is the same as the estimate.

4 a. 0.5 g = 500 mg. Give about about $2\dfrac{1}{2}$ times the 5 mL unit dose (slightly more than 10 mL).

$$\dfrac{\text{mL}}{\text{dose}} : \dfrac{5 \ \text{mL}}{\underset{1}{\cancel{200 \ \text{mg}}}} \times \dfrac{\overset{5}{\cancel{1000 \ \text{mg}}}}{1 \ \cancel{\text{g}}} \times \dfrac{0.5 \ \cancel{\text{g}}}{\text{dose}} = \dfrac{12.5 \ \text{mL}}{\text{dose}}$$

b. The estimate supports the answer. The equation is balanced.

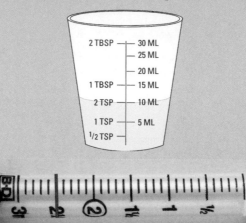

5 a. 0.6 g = 600 mg; Give about 2 × the unit dose of 5 mL

$$\dfrac{\text{mL}}{\text{dose}} : \dfrac{5 \ \text{mL}}{\cancel{300 \ \text{mg}}} \times \dfrac{\cancel{1000 \ \text{mg}}}{1 \ \cancel{\text{g}}} \times \dfrac{0.6 \ \cancel{\text{g}}}{\text{dose}} = \dfrac{30}{3} = \dfrac{10 \ \text{mL}}{\text{dose}}$$

b. The answer equals the estimate. The equation is balanced.

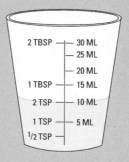

RAPID PRACTICE 5-13 (p. 161)

	SDR	Patient's Weight (lb)	Estimated Weight (kg) to the Nearest Whole Number	Actual Weight (kg) to the Nearest Tenth	Total SDR to Nearest Tenth
2	0.2-0.5 g per kg per day	44	22	20	0.2 × 20 = 4 g per day 0.5 × 20 = 10 g per day SDR = 4-10 g per day
3	0.25-1.5 mg per kg per day	150	75	68.2	0.25 × 68.2 = 17.1 mg per day 1.5 × 68.2 = 102.3 mg per day SDR = 17.1-102.3 mg per day

506 **ANSWER KEYS**

	SDR	Patient's Weight (lb)	Estimated Weight (kg) to the Nearest Whole Number	Actual Weight (kg) to the Nearest Tenth	Total SDR to Nearest Tenth
4	2-5 mcg per kg per day	180	90	81.8	$2 \times 81.8 = 163.6$ mcg per day $5 \times 81.8 = 409$ mcg per day SDR = 163.6-409 mcg per day
5	10-20 mg per kg per day in 3 divided doses	200	100	90.9	$10 \times 90.9 = 909$ mg per day $20 \times 90.9 = 1818$ mg per day SDR = 909-1818 mg per day

RAPID PRACTICE 5-14 (p. 162)

2 a. Estimated weight in kg = 80 kg; actual weight in kg = 72.7 kg
 b. SDR low, $1 \times 72.7 = 72.7$ mg per day; SDR high, $2 \times 72.7 = 145.4$ mg per day*
 c. 50 mg $\times$ 6 = 300 mg
 d. No. The ordered dose exceeds the high safe dose.
 e. Hold medication and clarify promptly with prescriber.

3 a. Estimated weight in kg = 60 kg; actual weight in kg = 54.5 kg
 b. SDR low, $2 \times 54.5 = 109$ mg per day; SDR high, $4 \times 54.5 = 218$ mg per day
 c. 50 mg $\times$ 4 = 200 mg
 d. Yes
 e. Order within SDR and safe to give.

4 a. Estimated weight in kg = 50 kg; actual weight in kg = 45.5 kg
 b. SDR low, $10 \times 45.5 = 455$ mg per day; SDR high, $20 \times 45.5 = 910$ mg per day
 c. 250 mg $\times$ 3 = 750 mg (0.25 g = 250 mg)
 d. Yes
 e. Order within SDR and safe to give.

5 a. Estimated weight in kg = 30 kg; actual weight in kg = 27.3 kg
 b. SDR low, $5 \times 27.3 = 136.5$ mg per day; SDR high, $10 \times 27.3 = 273$ mg per day
 c. 25 mg $\times$ 2 = 50 mg
 d. No. The ordered dose is significantly less than the low safe dose.
 e. Hold medication and clarify promptly with prescriber.

*SDR is usually seen in printed drug literature with a slash for "per." Do not use slashes in patient records. Estimated kg weight can prevent major math errors. Follow up with verification of actual DA weight.

RAPID PRACTICE 5-15 (p. 164)

2 a. 300 mg per 5 mL (**Tip:** Examine orders and labels carefully!)
 b. Yes. Order is within SDR.
 c. Give 2 times the unit dose volume of 5 mL (10 mL).
 d. 10 mL per dose

$$\frac{mL}{dose} = \frac{5\ mL}{300\ \cancel{mg}} \times \frac{1000\ \cancel{mg}}{1\ \cancel{g}} \times \frac{0.6\ \cancel{g}}{dose} = \frac{30}{3} = \frac{10\ mL}{dose}$$

e. Equation is balanced. Estimate supports answer.

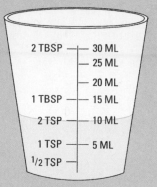

3 a. 1 mg per 5 mL
   b. Yes. Order is within SDR.
   c. Give two times dose per volume supplied: 10 mL
   d. 10 mL per dose

$$\frac{mL}{dose} : \frac{5\ mL}{1\ \text{mg}} \times \frac{2\ \text{mg}}{dose} = \frac{10\ mL}{dose}$$

e. Equation is balanced. Estimate supports answer.

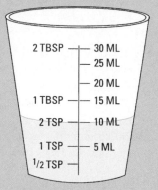

4 a. 40 mEq per 15 mL
   b. Yes. Order is within SDR.
   c. Give slightly more than 15 mL
   d. 16.9 mL

$$\frac{mL}{dose} : \frac{15\ mL}{\underset{8}{40\ \text{mEq}}} \times \frac{\overset{9}{45\ \text{mEq}}}{dose} = \frac{135}{8} = \frac{16.9\ mL}{dose}$$

e. Equation is balanced. Estimate supports answer.

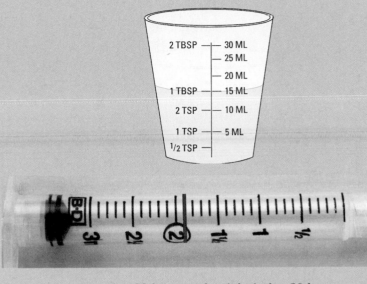

5 Estimated weight in kg: 22 kg; actual weight in kg: 20 kg

   a. 100 mg per 15 mL

   b. No. Order is not within SDR. Hold and contact prescriber promptly.

$$\frac{mg}{day} : \frac{3\ mg}{\cancel{kg} \times day} \times \frac{20\ \cancel{kg}}{1} = 60 \text{ mg per day low safe dose}$$

$$\frac{mg}{day} : \frac{6\ mg}{\cancel{kg} \times day} \times \frac{20\ \cancel{kg}}{1} = 120 \text{ mg per day high safe dose}$$

   c. N/A

   d. N/A

   e. N/A

CHAPTER 5 MULTIPLE-CHOICE REVIEW (p. 169)

1	2	**6**	3
2	1	**7**	4
3	2	**8**	1
4	4	**9**	4
5	1	**10**	3

CHAPTER 5 FINAL PRACTICE (p. 170)

1 **a.** SDR 325-650 mg q4h up to 12 tablets per day or 2-3 tablets (325-975 mg)
     q6h up to 12 tablets in 24 hr.
     Order: 0.65 g (625 mg) 6 times a day (12 tablets)

   b. Safe to give

   c. 2; more

   d. Will give 2 tabs (325 mg mEq × 2 = 650 mg)

$$\frac{tab}{dose} = \frac{1\ tab}{325\ \cancel{mg}} \times \frac{1000\ \cancel{mg}}{1\ \cancel{g}} \times \frac{0.65\ \cancel{g}}{dose} = \frac{2\ tablets}{dose}$$

   e. Equation is balanced. Answer equals estimate.

2 **a.** SDR: 325-650 mg q4-6h up to 4 g (4000 mg) daily.
     Order: 0.65 g (650 mg 4× daily = 2600 mg [2.6 g] daily)

   b. Safe to give

   c. 2 × 10.15 mL (2 × 325 mg) (about 20 mL)

   d. 20.3 mL

$$\frac{mL}{dose} : \frac{10.15\ mL}{325\ \cancel{mg}} \times \frac{1000\ \cancel{mg}}{1\ \cancel{g}} \times \frac{0.65\ \cancel{g}}{dose} = \frac{6597.5}{325} = \frac{20.3\ mL}{dose}$$

e. Equation is balanced. Answer equals estimate.

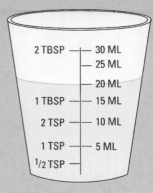

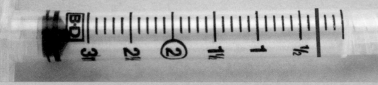

3 a. SDR 60 mg daily.
   Order: 0.06 g (60 mg) × 2 = 120 mg ordered daily
   b. Unsafe. Order exceeds SDR. Hold medication. Call prescriber promptly.
   c. N/A
   d. N/A
   e. N/A

4 a. SDR: 20-40 mEq per day.
   Order: 30 mEq per day.
   b. Safe to give
   c. Give less than dose per volume supplied of 15 mL (about 12 mL).
   d. 11.3 mL

$$\frac{mL}{dose} : \frac{15\ mL}{\underset{4}{\cancel{40\ mEq}}} \times \frac{\overset{3}{\cancel{30\ mEq}}}{dose} = \frac{45}{4} = 11.25,\ rounded\ to\ \frac{11.3\ mL}{dose}$$

e. Equation is balanced. Estimate supports answer.

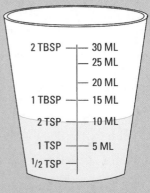

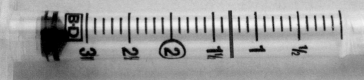

5 a. SDR: 10 mg × 50 kg = 500 mg low safe daily dose. 15 mg × 50 kg = 750 mg high safe daily dose.

Order: 300 mg bid (600 mg per day)

b. Safe to give

c. Estimate: slightly more than 5 mL unit dose

d. 6 mL

$$\frac{mL}{dose} : \frac{5\ mL}{\underset{5}{\cancel{250\ mg}}} \times \frac{\overset{6}{\cancel{300}}\ \cancel{mg}}{dose} = \frac{30}{5} = \frac{6\ mL}{dose}$$

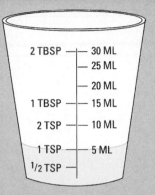

e. Equation is balanced. Estimate equals answer.

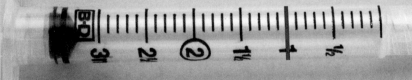

6 a. SDR 100-300 mg per day in divided doses or at bedtime.

Order: 0.09 g (90 mg) × 2 doses = 180 mg per day.

b. Safe to give

c. 3 tablets (0.09 g ordered = 90 mg); 30 mg × 3 = 3 tablets (90 mg).

d. 3 tablets

$$\frac{tab}{dose} : \frac{1\ tab}{30\ \cancel{mg}} \times \frac{1000\ \cancel{mg}}{1\ \cancel{g}} \times \frac{0.09\ \cancel{g}}{dose} = \frac{90}{30} = \frac{3\ tabs}{dose}$$

e. Equation is balanced. Estimate equals answer.

Note: Recheck orders for doses exceeding 1 or 2 tablets. In this case the patient diagnosis and the current drug literature support the administration of 90 mg.

7 a. SDR: 200 mg bid to start.

Order: 0.2 g (200 mg) bid.

b. Safe to give

c. 2 tablets = 100 mg × 2 = 200 mg = 2 tablets

d. 2 tablets

$$\frac{tab}{dose} : \frac{1\ tab}{100\ \cancel{mg}} \times \frac{1000\ \cancel{mg}}{1\ \cancel{g}} \times \frac{0.2\ \cancel{g}}{1} = \frac{2\ tabs}{dose}$$

e. Equation is balanced. Estimate equals answer.

8 a. SDR maintenance: 75-125 mcg daily.

Order: 0.1 mg = 100 mcg daily.

b. Safe to give

c. 2 tablets ($0.05 \times 2 = 0.1$)

d. 2 tablets

$$\frac{tab}{dose} : \frac{1\ tab}{\underset{1}{\cancel{0.05\ mg}}} \times \frac{\overset{2}{\cancel{0.1\ mg}}}{1} = \frac{2\ tabs}{dose}$$

e. Equation is balanced. Estimate equals answer.

9 a. SDR: 8-16 mg sol 1 hr pre op

Order: 14 mg 1 hr preoperatively

b. Safe to give

c. 4×5 mL = 20 mL

d. 17.5 mL

$$\frac{mL}{dose} : \frac{5\ mL}{\underset{2}{\cancel{4\ mg}}} \times \frac{\overset{7}{\cancel{14\ mg}}}{dose} = \frac{35}{2} = \frac{17.5\ mL}{dose}$$

e. Equation is balanced. Estimate supports answer.

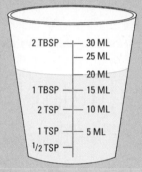

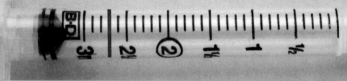

10 a. SDR: 125-250 mg q6-8h.

Order: 0.25 g (250 mg) q8h.

b. Safe to give

c. 1 tablet (0.25 g = 250 mg)

d. 1 tablet

$$\frac{tab}{dose} : \frac{1\ tab}{\underset{1}{\cancel{250\ mg}}} \times \frac{\overset{4}{\cancel{1000\ mg}}}{1\ \cancel{g}} \times \frac{0.25\ \cancel{g}}{dose} = \frac{1\ tab}{dose}$$

e. Equation is balanced. Estimate equals answer.

Chapter 6

RAPID PRACTICE 6-1 (p. 179)

1 calibrations

2 intradermal; 1 mL

3 parenteral

4 gauge

5 smaller

RAPID PRACTICE 6-2 (p. 183)

1 20 mL

2 5

3 1 mL

4-5

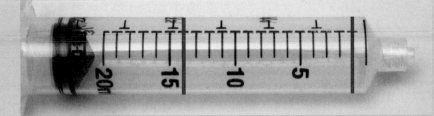

6 10 mL

7 5

8 0.2 mL

9-10

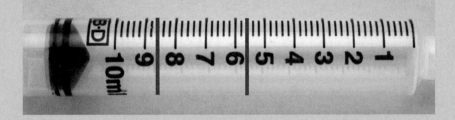

RAPID PRACTICE 6-3 (p. 184)

1 5 mL

2 5

3 0.2 mL

4-5

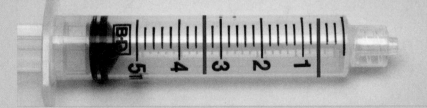

Note: There are also 5-mL syringes with 10 calibrations per mL.

6 1 mL

7 10

8 0.01 mL

9-10

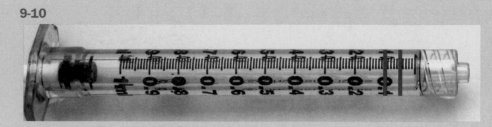

Note: Pay special attention to the decimal place when preparing small doses.

RAPID PRACTICE 6-4 (p. 185)

1 3 mL

2 0.1 mL

3

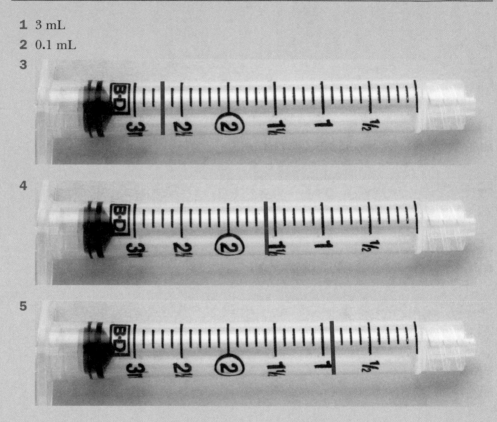

4

5

RAPID PRACTICE 6-5 (p. 186)

	Ordered Dose	Syringe Size (in mL)		Ordered Dose	Syringe Size (in mL)
1	2.8 mL	3	**6**	9.6 mL	10
2	3.2 mL	5	**7**	12.6 mL	20
3	6.4 mL	10	**8**	0.6 mL	1
4	0.08 mL	1	**9**	1.5 mL	3
5	1.7 mL	3	**10**	0.1 mL	1

In some clinical situations a larger syringe may be selected.

RAPID PRACTICE 6-6 (p. 187)

1 The volume of medication to be administered

4 3 mL; 2.9 mL

2 No. Check agency and state policies.

5 5 mL; 3.2 mL

3 1 mL

RAPID PRACTICE 6-7 (p. 194)

1 a. 5 mL
b. 5
c. 0.2 mL
d. 3.6 mL

4 a. 10 mL
b. 5
c. 0.2 mL
d. 5.8 mL

2 a. 1 mL
b. 10
c. 0.01 mL
d. 0.45 mL

5 a. 20 mL
b. 1
c. 1 mL
d. 18 mL

3 a. 3 mL
b. 10
c. 0.1 mL
d. 1.3 mL

RAPID PRACTICE 6-8 (p. 195)

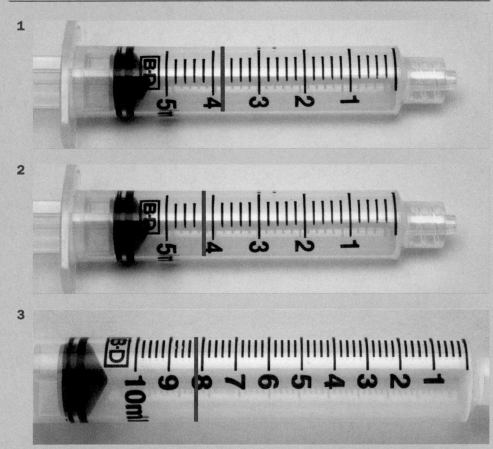

4

5

RAPID PRACTICE 6-9 (p. 196)

1

2

3

4

5

RAPID PRACTICE 6-10 (p. 197)

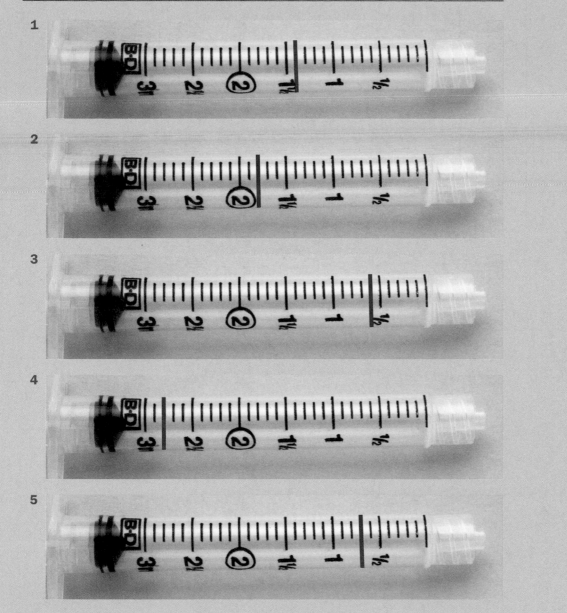

CHAPTER 6 MULTIPLE-CHOICE REVIEW (p. 199)

1	1	6	3
2	2	7	1
3	2	8	1
4	1	9	1
5	1	10	3

CHAPTER 6 FINAL PRACTICE (p. 200)

1 **a.** more
  b. give twice unit dose (2 mL)

$$\frac{mL}{dose} : \frac{mL}{\underset{1}{\cancel{100\ mg}}} \times \overset{2}{\cancel{200\ mg}} = \frac{2\ mL}{dose}$$

c. Equation is balanced. Estimate supports answer.

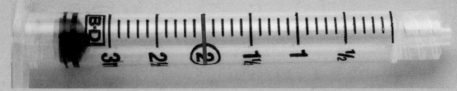

2 a. less

b. give half of unit dose. (0.5 mL)

$$\frac{mL}{dose} : \frac{mL}{\underset{2}{\cancel{30\ mg}}} \times \overset{1}{\cancel{15\ mg}} = \frac{0.5\ mL}{dose}$$

c. Equation is balanced. Estimate supports answer.

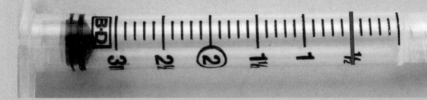

3 a. more (about 6 times the unit dose, or 6-7 mL)

b. 6.4 mL

$$\frac{mL}{dose} : \frac{mL}{50\ \cancel{mg}} \times \frac{320\ \cancel{mg}}{dose} = \frac{6.4\ mL}{dose}$$

c. Equation is balanced. Estimate supports answer.

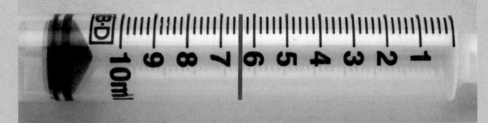

4 a. more than 1 mL, less than 2 mL

b. 1.1 mL

$$\frac{mL}{dose} : \frac{mL}{75\ \cancel{mg}} \times \frac{80\ \cancel{mg}}{dose} = 1.066,\ \text{rounded to } \frac{1.1\ mL}{dose}$$

c. Equation is balanced. Estimate supports answer

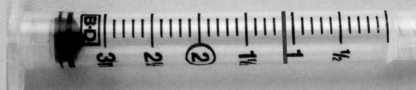

5 a. more (order is 5 times unit dose concentration, or about 5 mL)
b. 5 mL

$$\frac{mL}{dose} : \frac{mL}{\underset{1}{\cancel{10\ mg}}} \times \overset{5}{\cancel{50\ mg}} = \frac{5\ mL}{dose}$$

c. Equation is balanced. Estimate supports answer.

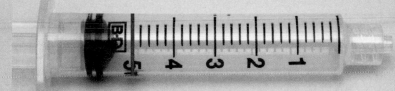

6 a. less than 1 mL
b. 0.8 mL

$$\frac{mL}{dose} : \frac{1\ mL}{\underset{5}{\cancel{50\ mg}}} \times \overset{4}{\cancel{40\ mg}} = \frac{0.8\ mL}{dose}$$

c. Equation is balanced. Estimate supports answer.

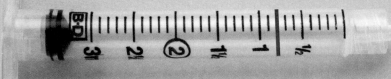

7 a. more (about 12 mL)
b. 12 mL per dose

$$\frac{mL}{dose} : \frac{mL}{\underset{1}{\cancel{10\ mg}}} \times \overset{12}{\cancel{120\ mg}} = \frac{12\ mL}{dose}$$

c. Equation is balanced. Estimate supports answer.

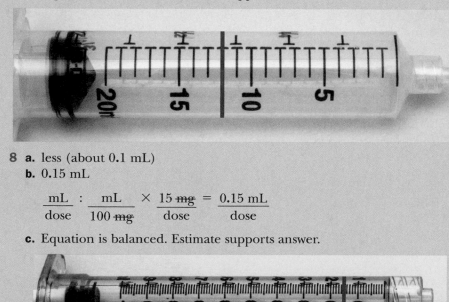

8 a. less (about 0.1 mL)
b. 0.15 mL

$$\frac{mL}{dose} : \frac{mL}{100\ \cancel{mg}} \times 15\ \cancel{mg} = \frac{0.15\ mL}{dose}$$

c. Equation is balanced. Estimate supports answer.

9 **a.** Total mL volume of the order
   b. After calculating dose

10 **a.** Never recap used needles. Use sharps container promptly for used needles per agency policies.
   b. Hepatitis B and C and AIDS

Chapter 7

RAPID PRACTICE 7-1 (p. 205)

1 2   **4** 1
2 4   **5** 2
3 2

RAPID PRACTICE 7-2 (p. 208)

1 a. Oral suspension syrup
  b. doxycyline calcium
  c. 50 mg per 5 mL
  d. Multidose
  e. 473 mL
  f. store below 86 °F in a light-resistant container

2 a. Oral suspension when reconstituted from powder
  b. Water
  c. 78 mL
  d. Tap until all powder flows freely. Add $\frac{1}{3}$ of 78 mL (24 mL). After shaking vigorously, add remaining $\frac{2}{3}$ (52 mL) and shake vigorously.
  e. 125 mg per 5 mL
  f. 250-500 mg every 8 hrs
  g. 20-40 mg per kg per day in divided doses every 8 hours, depending on age, weight, or infection severity.
  h. Multidose
  i. Discard suspension after 14 days

3 a. oral suspension when reconstituted from powder
  b. 39 mL of water
  c. 50 mL
  d. 200 mg per 5 mL
  e. Refrigeration preferable but not required.
  f. Shake well before using.
  g. Discard suspension after 14 days.

4 a. Vancocin HCl
  b. vancomycin hydrochloride
  c. Oral
  d. 1 g
  e. 250 mg per 5 mL

5 a. 4 mL
  b. 2 mL
  c. In a location at room temperature

1 a. 36 mL water divided in 2 portions

b. More than 5 mL

c. 12 mL

$$\dfrac{\text{mL}}{\text{dose}} \;:\; \dfrac{5\ \text{mL}}{\underset{1}{\cancel{125\ \text{mg}}}} \times \dfrac{\overset{8}{\cancel{1000\ \text{mg}}}}{1\ \text{g}} \times \dfrac{0.3\ \cancel{\text{g}}}{\text{dose}} = \dfrac{12\ \text{mL}}{\text{dose}}$$

d. The estimate supports the answer. Only mL remain. The equation is balanced.

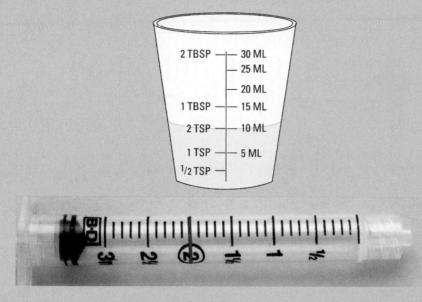

2 a. Add 60 mL water followed by 30 mL of water for a total of 90 mL.

b. Estimate will give more than 2 times unit dose of 5 mL (0.25 g = 250 mg).

c. 10 mL

$$\dfrac{\text{mL}}{\text{dose}} \;:\; \dfrac{5\ \text{mL}}{\underset{1}{\cancel{125\ \text{mg}}}} \times \dfrac{\overset{8}{\cancel{1000\ \text{mg}}}}{1\ \cancel{\text{g}}} \times \dfrac{0.25\ \cancel{\text{g}}}{\text{dose}} = \dfrac{10\ \text{mL}}{\text{dose}}$$

d. Equation is balanced. Estimate supports answer

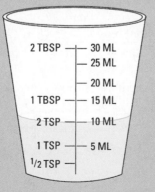

A syringe is not needed.

3 a. More than 5 mL (0.2 g = 200 mg)

b. 8 mL

$$\dfrac{\text{mL}}{\text{dose}} \;:\; \dfrac{5\ \text{mL}}{\underset{1}{\cancel{125\ \text{mg}}}} \times \dfrac{\overset{8}{\cancel{1000\ \text{mg}}}}{1\ \text{g}} \times \dfrac{0.2\ \cancel{\text{g}}}{\text{dose}} = \dfrac{8\ \text{mL}}{\text{dose}}$$

c. Equation in balanced. Estimate supports answer

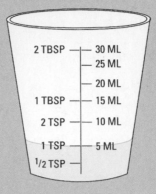

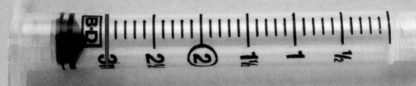

4 a. 24 mL distilled or purified water
b. More than 1 mL or 3 times more ($10 \times 3 = 30$)
c. 3 mL

$$\frac{mL}{dose} : \frac{1\ mL}{\underset{1}{\cancel{10\ mg}}} \times \frac{\overset{100}{\cancel{1000\ mg}}}{1\ \cancel{g}} \times \frac{0.03\ \cancel{g}}{dose} = \frac{3\ mL}{dose}$$

d. Equation is balanced. Estimate supports answer

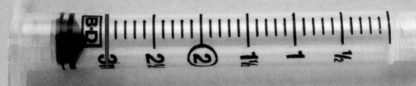

5 a. 105 mL of water in 2 portions
b. same ($0.25\ g = 250\ mg$)
c. 5 mL

$$\frac{mL}{dose} : \frac{5\ mL}{\underset{1}{\cancel{250\ mg}}} \times \frac{\overset{4}{\cancel{1000\ mg}}}{1\ \cancel{g}} \times \frac{0.25\ \cancel{g}}{dose} = \frac{5\ mL}{dose}$$

d. Equation is balanced. Estimate supports answer

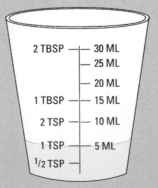

522   **ANSWER KEYS**

2 a. 4 mL (0.1 g = 100 mg) (know your metric equivalents)
  b. 100 mg per mL
  c. 1 mL (100 mg = 0.1 g)

3 a. 2 mL (0.25 g = 250 mg)
  b. 250 mg per mL
  c. 1 mL (250 mg = 0.25 g)

4 a. 2 mL (0.3 g = 300 mg)
  b. 250 mg per mL
  c. 1.2 mL (300 mg is more than 250 mg)

$$\frac{mL}{dose} : \frac{1\ mL}{\underset{1}{\cancel{250\ mg}}} \times \frac{\overset{4}{\cancel{1000\ mg}}}{1\ g} \times \frac{0.3\ g}{dose} = 4 \times 0.3 = \frac{1.2\ mL}{dose}$$

  d. Equation is balanced. Estimate supports answer.

5 a. 12 mL
  b. 50 mg per mL
  c. 10 mL

$$\frac{mL}{dose} : \frac{1\ mL}{\underset{1}{\cancel{50\ mg}}} \times \frac{\overset{20}{\cancel{1000\ mg}}}{1\ g} \times \frac{0.5\ g}{dose} = \frac{10\ mL}{dose}$$

  d. Equation is balanced. Estimate supports answer.

2 a. Sterile water for injection
  b. 2.7 mL
  c. 250 mg per 1.5 mL
  d. 200 mg is less than 250 mg; estimated dose less than 1.5 mL.
  e. 1.2 mL

$$\frac{mL}{dose} : \frac{1.5\ mL}{\underset{5}{\cancel{250\ mg}}} \times \frac{\overset{4}{\cancel{200\ mg}}}{dose} = \frac{1.2\ mL}{dose}$$

  f. Equation is balanced. Estimate supports answer.

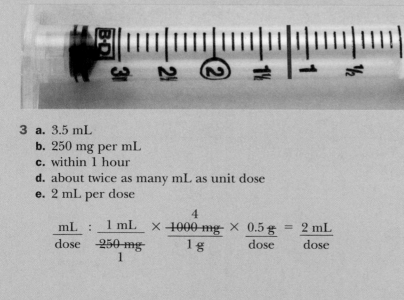

3 a. 3.5 mL
  b. 250 mg per mL
  c. within 1 hour
  d. about twice as many mL as unit dose
  e. 2 mL per dose

$$\frac{mL}{dose} : \frac{1\ mL}{\underset{1}{\cancel{250\ mg}}} \times \frac{\overset{4}{\cancel{1000\ mg}}}{1\ g} \times \frac{0.5\ g}{dose} = \frac{2\ mL}{dose}$$

f. Estimate supports answer. Equation is balanced.

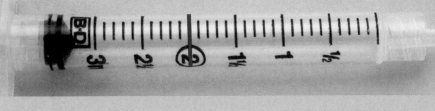

4 **a.** Sterile water
   b. Slightly more
   c. more than 1 mL

$$\frac{mL}{dose} : \frac{mL}{\cancel{400\ mg}} \times \frac{\cancel{1000\ mg}}{1\ \cancel{g}} \times \frac{0.5\ \cancel{g}}{dose} = \frac{5}{4} = 1.25\ mL, \text{rounded to} \quad \frac{1.3\ mL}{dose}$$

d. Equation is balanced. Estimate supports answer.

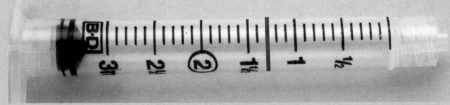

5 **a.** 1.8 mL
   b. less
   c. 1.4 mL

$$\frac{mL}{dose} : \frac{1\ mL}{\underset{5}{\cancel{250,000\ units}}} \times \frac{\overset{8}{\cancel{400,000\ units}}}{dose} = 1.37, \text{rounded to} \frac{1.4\ mL}{dose}$$

d. Equation is balanced. Estimate supports answer.

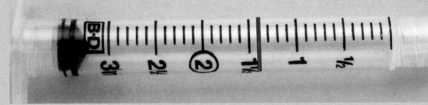

RAPID PRACTICE 7-6 (p. 226)

	Fractional Strength	Ratio	Percent	Amount Active Ingredient	Amount Diluent Inactive Ingredient
2	$\frac{1}{2}$	1:1	50%	30 mL	30 mL
3	$\frac{3}{4}$	3:1	75%	750 mL	250 mL
4	$\frac{1}{5}$	1:4	20%	48 mL	192 mL
5	$\frac{1}{10}$	1:9	10%	5 mL	45 mL

1	3	**6**	1
2	4	**7**	2
3	1	**8**	1
4	2	**9**	2
5	1	**10**	3

CHAPTER 7 FINAL PRACTICE (p. 227)

1 a. slightly more than 10 mL
   b. 12 mL

$$\frac{mL}{dose} : \frac{5\ mL}{\cancel{125\ mg}_1} \times \frac{\overset{8}{\cancel{1000\ mg}}}{1\ g} \times \frac{0.3\ \cancel{g}}{dose} = \frac{12\ mL}{dose}$$

   c. Equation is balanced. Estimate supports answer.

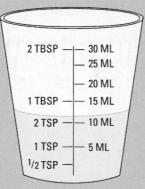

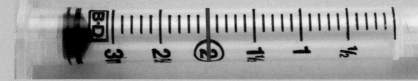

2 a. less than 5 mL (0.2 g = 200 mg)
   b. 4 mL

$$\frac{mL}{dose} : \frac{5\ mL}{\cancel{250\ mg}_1} \times \frac{\overset{4}{\cancel{1000\ mg}}}{1\ g} \times \frac{0.2\ \cancel{g}}{dose} = \frac{4\ mL}{dose}$$

   c. Equation is balanced. Estimate supports answer.

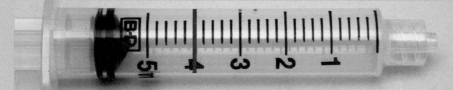

   Note: A medicine cup is not appropriate for an amount less than 5 mL.

3 a. B. 350 mg per mL is closer to dose needed with less volume.
   b. More than 1 mL (0.45 g = 450 mg)

Estimate: more than unit dose

$$\text{DA} \; \frac{\text{mL}}{\text{dose}} \; : \; \frac{1 \text{ mL}}{\underset{7}{\cancel{350}} \text{ mg}} \times \frac{\overset{20}{\cancel{1000 \text{ mg}}}}{1 \text{ g}} \times \frac{0.45 \text{ g}}{\text{dose}} = \frac{1.28 \text{ mL}}{\text{dose}} = \frac{1.3 \text{ mL}}{\text{dose}}$$

c. Estimate supports answer. The equation is balanced

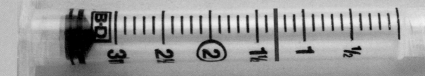

4 a. 280 mg per mL
 b. more
 c. near 3 mL
 d. 2.67, rounded to 2.7 mL

$$\frac{\text{mL}}{\text{dose}} \; : \; \frac{1 \text{ mL}}{250 \text{ mg}} \times \frac{750 \text{ mg}}{\text{dose}} = 2.67, \text{ rounded to } \frac{2.7 \text{ mL}}{\text{dose}}$$

e. Estimate supports answer. Equation is balanced.

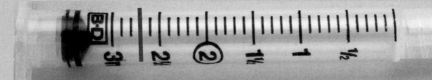

5 a. slightly more than 5 mL
 b. 6 mL

$$\frac{\text{mL}}{\text{dose}} \; : \; \frac{5 \text{ mL}}{\underset{1}{\cancel{125}} \text{ mg}} \times \frac{\overset{8}{\cancel{1000 \text{ mg}}}}{1 \text{ g}} \times \frac{0.15 \text{ g}}{1} = \frac{6 \text{ mL}}{\text{dose}}$$

c. Equation is balanced. Estimate supports answer.

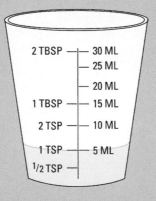

6 a. 1:3

   b. $\frac{25}{100} = \frac{1}{4}$

   c. mL : 200 mL × 0.25 = 50 mL (or 200 mL × $\frac{1}{4}$ = 50 mL Ensure)

   d. 200 mL − 50 mL = 150 mL water

7 a. 33%

   b. 1:2

   c. mL : 30 mL × 0.33 = 9.9 mL (or 30 × $\frac{1}{3}$ = 10 mL formula)

   d. 30 mL − 10 mL = 20 mL diluent of SW

8 a. 50%

   b. $\frac{1}{2}$

   c. mL : 30 mL × 0.5 = 15 mL (or 30 × $\frac{1}{2}$ = 15 mL formula)

   d. 30 mL − 15 mL = 15 mL diluent of SW

9 a. Less (1% × $\frac{1}{100}$) (0.9% = $\frac{0.9}{100}$)

   b. 0.9 g solute

   c. 9 g

$$\frac{g}{solute} : \frac{0.9 \text{ g solute}}{\cancel{100 \text{ mL}}_{1}} \times \frac{\cancel{1000 \text{ mL}}^{10}}{1} = 9 \text{ g solute}$$

10 a. 1:1

   b. 25 mL

   c. 25 mL (25 + 25 = 50 mL)

Chapter 8

RAPID PRACTICE 8-1 (p. 235)

1 1		**4** 4	
2 2		**5** 3	
3 3			

RAPID PRACTICE 8-2 (p. 239)

1 a. 250 mg per mL

   b. 0.45 g = 450 mg. Give almost 2 mL.

   c. 1.8 mL

$$\frac{mL}{dose} : \frac{1 \text{ mL}}{\cancel{250 \text{ mg}}_{1}} \times \frac{\cancel{1000 \text{ mg}}^{4}}{1 \text{ g}} \times \frac{0.45 \text{ g}}{dose} = \frac{1.8 \text{ mL}}{dose}$$

   d. Equation is balanced. Estimate supports answer.

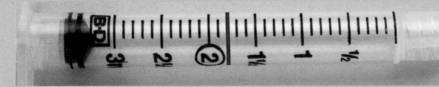

2 a. 10 mg per 2 mL
b. between 1 and 2 mL
c. 1.2 mL

$$\frac{mL}{dose} : \frac{2\ mL}{\overset{}{\underset{5}{\cancel{10}}\ mg}} \times \frac{\overset{3}{\cancel{6}}\ mg}{dose} = \frac{1.2\ mL}{dose}$$

d. Equation is balanced. Estimate supports answer.

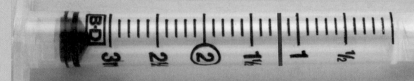

3 a. 15 mg per mL
b. give slightly more than 0.5 mL
c. 0.6 mL

$$\frac{mL}{dose} : \frac{1\ mL}{\underset{5}{\cancel{15\ mg}}} \times \frac{\overset{3}{\cancel{9\ mg}}}{dose} = \frac{3}{5} = \frac{0.6\ mL}{dose}$$

d. Equation is balanced. Estimate supports answer.

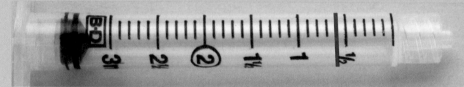

4 a. 4 mg per mL
b. give one half or 0.5 mL
c. 0.5 mL

$$\frac{mL}{dose} : \frac{1\ mL}{\underset{2}{\cancel{4\ mg}}} \times \frac{\overset{1}{\cancel{2\ mg}}}{dose} = \frac{1}{2} = \frac{0.5\ mL}{dose}$$

d. Equation is balanced. Estimate supports answer.

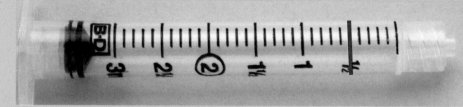

5 a. 0.5 mg per 2 mL

b. 0.125 mg is $\frac{1}{4}$ of 0.5 mg. Give $\frac{1}{4}$ of 2 mL or 0.5 mL.

c. 0.5 mL

$$\frac{mL}{dose} : \frac{\overset{4}{\cancel{2}} \text{ mL}}{\underset{1}{\cancel{0.5 \text{ mg}}}} \times \frac{0.125 \cancel{\text{ mg}}}{dose} = \frac{0.5 \text{ mL}}{dose}$$

d. Equation is balanced. Estimate supports answer.

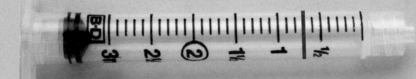

RAPID PRACTICE 8-3 (p. 242)

1 a. give less than 1 mL (0.02 g = 20 mg)

b. 0.7 mL

$$\frac{mL}{dose} : \frac{1 \text{ mL}}{30 \cancel{\text{ mg}}} \times \frac{1000 \cancel{\text{ mg}}}{1 \cancel{\text{ g}}} \times \frac{0.02 \cancel{\text{ g}}}{dose} = \frac{2}{3} = 0.66, \text{ rounded to } \frac{0.7 \text{ mL}}{dose}$$

c. Equation is balanced. Estimate supports answer.

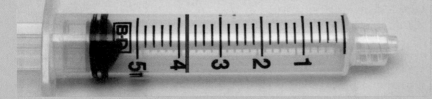

2 a. give slightly less than 4 mL

b. 3.5 mL

$$\frac{mL}{dose} : \frac{\overset{1}{4} \text{ mL}}{\underset{10}{\cancel{40 \text{ mg}}}} \times \frac{38 \cancel{\text{ mg}}}{dose} = \frac{38}{10} = \frac{3.8 \text{ mL}}{dose}$$

c. Equation is balanced. Estimate supports answer.

d. 0.2 mL

3 a. Give more than 2 mL. 2 vials will be needed.
   b. 2.4 mL

$$\frac{mL}{dose} : \frac{2\ mL}{\underset{1}{\cancel{250\ mg}}} \times \frac{\overset{4}{\cancel{1000\ mg}}}{1\ \cancel{g}} \times \frac{0.3\ \cancel{g}}{dose} = \frac{2.4\ mL}{dose}$$

   c. Equation is balanced. Estimate supports answer.

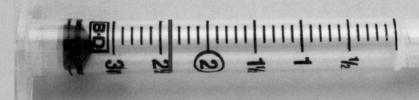

4 a. give less than 1 mL
   b. 0.75 mL

$$\frac{mL}{dose} : \frac{1\ mL}{0.4\ \cancel{mg}} \times \frac{0.3\ \cancel{mg}}{dose} = \frac{0.75\ mL}{dose}$$

   c. Equation is balanced. Estimate supports answer.

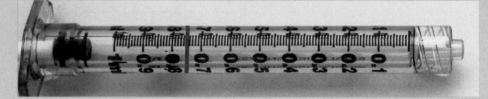

5

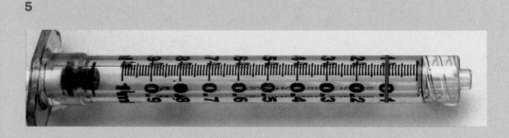

RAPID PRACTICE 8-4 (p. 246)

2 a. Give less than half of 1 mL.
   b. 0.4 mL

$$\frac{mL}{dose} : \frac{1\ mL}{4\ \cancel{mg}} \times \frac{1.5\ \cancel{mg}}{dose} = 0.37,\ \text{rounded to}\ \frac{0.4\ mL}{dose}\ \text{Dilaudid}$$

   c. Equation is balanced. Estimate supports answer.
   d. 1 mL
   e. 1 mL

$$\frac{mL}{dose} : \frac{1\ mL}{\cancel{0.4\ mg}} \times \frac{\cancel{0.4\ mg}}{dose} = \frac{1\ mL}{dose}\ \text{Atropine}$$

   f. Equation is balanced. Estimate supports answer.
   g.   0.4 Dilaudid
        + 1.0 Atropine
        ―――――――――――
        1.4 mL Total Volume

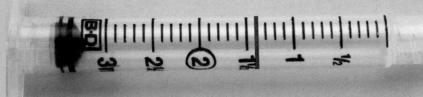

3 a. Prepare slightly less than 1 mL.
  b. 0.8 mL

$$\frac{mL}{dose} : \frac{1\ mL}{\overset{}{\underset{5}{\cancel{10\ mg}}}} \times \overset{4}{\cancel{8\ mg}} = \frac{0.8\ mL}{dose}\ \text{Morphine}$$

  c. Equation is balanced. Estimate supports DA equation.
  d. Prepare more than 1 mL.
  e. 1.5 mL

$$\frac{mL}{dose} : \frac{1\ mL}{\overset{}{\underset{2}{\cancel{0.4\ mg}}}} \times \overset{3}{\cancel{0.6\ mg}} = \frac{1.5\ mL}{dose}\ \text{Atropine}$$

  f. Equation is balanced. Estimate supports DA equation.
  g. 0.8 mL Morphine
     + 1.5 mL Atropine
     ―――――――――――
      2.3 mL Total Volume

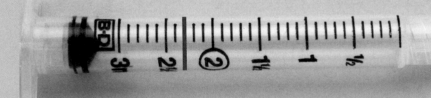

4 a. Prepare less than 1 mL.
  b. $\dfrac{mL}{dose} : \dfrac{1\ mL}{4\ \cancel{mg}} \times \dfrac{3\ \cancel{mg}}{dose} = 0.75\ mL$, rounded to $\dfrac{0.8\ mL}{dose}$ Dilaudid
  c. Equation is balanced. Estimate supports answer.
  d. Prepare less than 1 mL.
  e. $\dfrac{mL}{dose} : \dfrac{1\ mL}{\underset{5}{\cancel{50}}\ mg} \times \overset{1}{\cancel{10}}\ mg = \dfrac{1}{5} = \dfrac{0.2\ mL}{dose}$

  f. Equation is balanced. Estimate supports answer.
  g. 0.8 mL Dilaudid
     + 0.2 mL Promethazine
     ―――――――――――――
      1.0 mL Total Volume

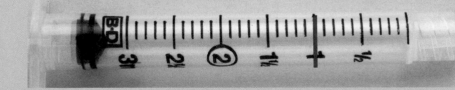

5 a. Prepare less than 1 mL.
   b. 0.8 mL

$$\frac{mL}{dose} \; : \; \frac{1 \; mL}{\underset{5}{\cancel{15 \; mg}}} \times \overset{4}{\cancel{12 \; mg}} = \frac{0.8 \; mL}{dose} \; Morphine$$

   c. Equation is balanced. Estimate supports answer.
   d. Prepare less than 1 mL.
   e. 0.8 mL

$$\frac{mL}{dose} \; : \; \frac{1 \; mL}{0.4 \; \cancel{mg}} \times \frac{0.3 \; mg}{dose} = 0.75, \text{ rounded to } \frac{0.8 \; mL}{dose} \; Atropine$$

   f. Equation is balanced. Estimate supports answer.
   g.   0.8 mL Morphine

   $\underline{+ \; 0.8 \; mL \; Atropine}$

        1.6 mL Total Volume

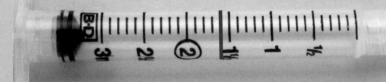

CHAPTER 8 MULTIPLE-CHOICE REVIEW (p. 252)

1 4 (1 mL Staclol + 0.4 mL Promethazine)   **6** 2
2 2   **7** 3
3 3   **8** 4
4 1   **9** 1
5 3   **10** 4 (**Note:** This applies to IV
                                                         fluids and medications also.)

CHAPTER 8 FINAL PRACTICE (p. 253)

1 a. less than 1 mL
   b. 0.7 mL

$$\frac{mL}{dose} \; : \; \frac{1 \; mL}{\underset{3}{\cancel{15 \; mg}}} \times \overset{2}{\cancel{10 \; mg}} = 0.66, \text{ rounded to } \frac{0.7 \; mL}{dose} \; Morphine$$

   Equation is balanced. Estimate supports answer.
   c. half of one mL
   d. 0.5 mL

$$\frac{mL}{dose} \; : \; \frac{1 \; mL}{\underset{2}{\cancel{400 \; mcg}}} \times \overset{1}{\cancel{200 \; mcg}} = \frac{0.5 \; mL}{dose} \; Atropine$$

   Equation is balanced. Estimate supports answer.

e.   0.7 mL Morphine

+ 0.5 mL Atropine

1.2 mL Total Volume

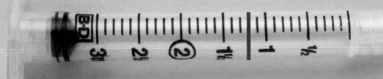

2 a. less than 1 mL

b. 0.7 mL

$$\frac{mL}{dose} : \frac{1\ mL}{10\ \cancel{mg}} \times \frac{7\ \cancel{mg}}{dose} = \frac{0.7\ mL}{dose}\ \ \text{Morphine}$$

Equation is balanced. Estimate supports answer.

c. less than $\frac{1}{2}$ mL

d. 0.4 mL

$$\frac{mL}{dose} : \frac{1\ mL}{\underset{5}{\cancel{50\ mg}}} \times \frac{\overset{2}{\cancel{20\ mg}}}{dose} = \frac{0.4\ mL}{dose}\ \ \text{Promethazine}$$

Equation is balanced. Estimate supports answer.

e.   0.7 mL Morphine

+ 0.4 mL Promethazine

1.1 mL Total Volume

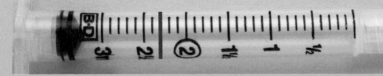

3 a. Slightly less than 1 mL

b. 0.8 mL

$$\frac{mL}{dose} : \frac{1\ mL}{\underset{5}{\cancel{15\ mg}}} \times \frac{\overset{4}{\cancel{12\ mg}}}{dose} = \frac{4}{5} = \frac{0.8\ mL}{dose}$$

Equation is balanced. Estimate supports answer.

c. $\frac{3}{4}$ of 2 mL or 1.5 mL

d. 1.5 mL

$$\frac{mL}{dose} : \frac{2\ mL}{0.4\ \cancel{mg}} \times \frac{0.3\ \cancel{mg}}{dose} = \frac{0.6}{0.4} = \frac{1.5\ mL}{dose}$$

Equation is balanced. Estimate supports answer.

e. 1.5 + 0.8 = 2.3 mL total

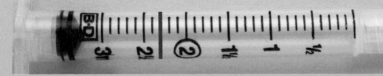

4 a. less than 1 mL (about $\frac{1}{3}$ of 1 mL)

   b. 0.3 mL

$$\frac{mL}{dose} : \frac{1\ mL}{\underset{3}{\cancel{30\ mg}}} \times \overset{1}{\cancel{10\ mg}} = \frac{0.33\ mL}{dose}\ \text{on a 1 mL syringe}$$

Equation is balanced. Estimate supports answer.

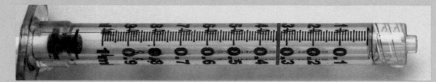

5 a. 2 g = 2000 mg

   b. 6.6 mL

   c. 250 mg per mL

   d. between 1-2 mL (0.14 g = 400 mg)

   e. 1.6 mL

$$\frac{mL}{dose} : \frac{1\ mL}{\underset{1}{\cancel{250\ mg}}} \times \overset{4}{\cancel{1000\ mg}} \times \frac{0.4\ \cancel{g}}{dose} = \frac{1.6\ mL}{dose}$$

Equation is balanced. Estimate supports answer.

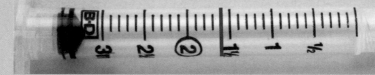

6 a. 1 g = 1000 mg

   b. 3.5 mL

   c. 250 mg per mL

   d. more than 0.5 mL (0.2 g = 200 mg)

   e. 0.8 mL

$$\frac{mL}{dose} : \frac{1\ mL}{\underset{1}{\cancel{250\ mg}}} \times \overset{4}{\cancel{1000\ mg}} \times \frac{0.2\ \cancel{g}}{dose} = \frac{0.8\ mL}{dose}$$

Equation is balanced. Estimate supports answer.

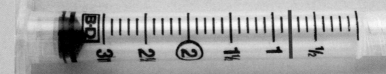

7 a. 120 mg

   b. 1 mL SW for injection

   c. 120 mg per mL

   d. Slightly less than 1 mL (0.1 g = 100 mg)

   e. 0.8 mL

$$\frac{mL}{dose} : \frac{1\ mL}{\cancel{120\ mg}} \times \frac{1000\ \cancel{mg}}{1\ \cancel{g}} \times \frac{0.1\ \cancel{g}}{dose} = \frac{10}{12} = \frac{5}{6} = 0.83\ mL,\ \text{rounded to}\ \underline{0.8\ mL}\ \text{for this syringe dose}$$

Equation is balanced. Estimate supports answer.

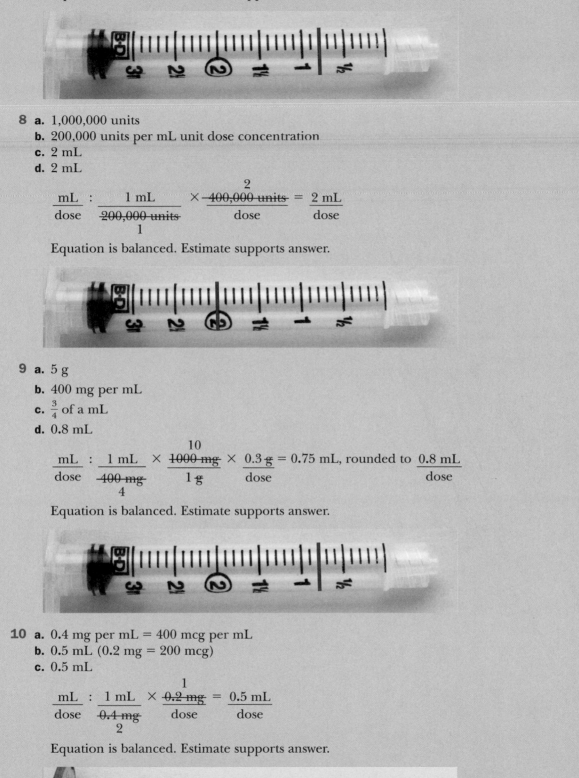

8 a. 1,000,000 units
  b. 200,000 units per mL unit dose concentration
  c. 2 mL
  d. 2 mL

$$\frac{mL}{dose} : \frac{1\ mL}{\underset{1}{\cancel{200,000\ units}}} \times \frac{\overset{2}{\cancel{400,000\ units}}}{dose} = \frac{2\ mL}{dose}$$

Equation is balanced. Estimate supports answer.

9 a. 5 g
  b. 400 mg per mL
  c. $\frac{3}{4}$ of a mL
  d. 0.8 mL

$$\frac{mL}{dose} : \frac{1\ mL}{\underset{4}{\cancel{400\ mg}}} \times \frac{\overset{10}{\cancel{1000\ mg}}}{1\ \cancel{g}} \times \frac{0.3\ \cancel{g}}{dose} = 0.75\ mL,\ rounded\ to\ \frac{0.8\ mL}{dose}$$

Equation is balanced. Estimate supports answer.

10 a. 0.4 mg per mL = 400 mcg per mL
  b. 0.5 mL (0.2 mg = 200 mcg)
  c. 0.5 mL

$$\frac{mL}{dose} : \frac{1\ mL}{\underset{2}{\cancel{0.4\ mg}}} \times \frac{\overset{1}{\cancel{0.2\ mg}}}{dose} = \frac{0.5\ mL}{dose}$$

Equation is balanced. Estimate supports answer.

Chapter 9

RAPID PRACTICE 9-1 (p. 264)

1 A continuous IV infuses without interruption. It does not have a stop date or time. Intermittent IVs are delivered at intervals; they do not continue indefinitely.

2 A primary line is the main IV line. A secondary line connects to ports on the primary tubing line for additional medications and solutions to be added.

3 **a.** DF refers to the number of drops per mL delivered through IV tubing, on gravity infusion equipment.
   b. A microdrip (pediatric) set delivers the smallest drops (60 drops per mL).

4 Nonvolumetric EID are gravity dependent. Volumetric pumps are not gravity dependent. They deliver fluids under positive pressure.

5 mL per hr

RAPID PRACTICE 9-2 (p. 266)

1 3		**4** 1	
2 2		**5** 3	
3 2			

RAPID PRACTICE 9-3 (p. 270)

	Order	Abbreviation(s) for Solution	Flow Rate (mL per hr)	Time to Infuse (hr and min if applicable)
1	Infuse 500 mL normal saline over 6 hr	NS	83	6 hr
2	1000 mL 5% dextrose in water at 125 mL per hr	D5W 5DW	125	8 hr
3	1 L lactated Ringer's q10h	LRS RLS	100	10 hr
4	250 mL half-strength normal saline q4h	0.45% NaCl Sol $\frac{1}{2}$ NS $\frac{1}{2}$ strength NS	63	4 hr
5	500 mL 5% dextrose in lactated Ringer's at 40 mL per hr	D5 L/R D5 R/L D5 RLS	40	12 hr, 30 min

RAPID PRACTICE 9-4 (p. 277)

2 **a.** 83 mL per hr (1000 ÷ 12)

b. 28 drops per min

$$\frac{\text{drops}}{\text{minute}} : \frac{\overset{1}{\cancel{20}} \text{ drops}}{1 \text{ } \cancel{mL}} \times \frac{1000 \text{ } \cancel{mL}}{12 \text{ } \cancel{hr}} \times \frac{1 \text{ } \cancel{hr}}{\underset{3}{\cancel{60} \text{ min}}} = \frac{1000}{36} = 27.7, \text{ rounded to } 28 \text{ drops per minute}$$

c. Equation is balanced. Only drops per min remain. Min had to be entered in a conversion formula in the denominator to match the desired answer.

Note: You have a choice of substituting the $\frac{83\ mL}{hr}$ for $\frac{1000\ mL}{12\ hr}$.

3 a. 75 mL per hr

b. 13 drops per min

$$\frac{drops}{min} : \frac{\overset{1}{\cancel{10}}\ drops}{1\ \cancel{mL}} \times \frac{75\ \cancel{mL}}{1\ \cancel{hr}} \times \frac{1\ \cancel{hr}}{\underset{6}{\cancel{60}}\ min} = \frac{75}{6} = 12.5,\ \text{rounded to}\ 13\ \text{drops per minute}$$

c. Equation is balanced. Only drops per min remain.

4 a. 83 mL per hr

$$\frac{mL}{hr} : \frac{500\ mL}{6\ hr} = 83.3,\ \text{rounded to 83 mL per hr}$$

b. 28 drops per min

$$\frac{drops}{minute} : \frac{\overset{1}{\cancel{20}}\ drops}{1\ \cancel{mL}} \times \frac{500\ \cancel{mL}}{6\ \cancel{hr}} \times \frac{1\ \cancel{hr}}{\underset{3}{\cancel{60}}\ min} = \frac{500}{18} = 27.7,\ \text{rounded to}\ 28\ \text{drops per minute}$$

c. Equation is balanced. Only drops per min remain.

Note: $\frac{83\ mL}{1\ hr}$ could have been substituted for $\frac{500\ mL}{6\ hr}$ in the equation.

5 a. 10 hours; 100 ÷ 10 = 10 hr duration

b. 10 drops per min

$$\frac{drops}{minute} : \frac{\cancel{60}\ drops}{1\ \cancel{mL}} \times \frac{10\ \cancel{mL}}{1\ \cancel{hr}} \times \frac{1\ \cancel{hr}}{\cancel{60}\ min} = 10\ \text{drops per minute}$$

c. Equation is balanced. Only drops per min remain.

Note: Note that the 60 DF and 60 min cancel each other so that mL per hr (10) = drops per min (10).

RAPID PRACTICE 9-5 (p. 279)

1 75 mL per hr

$$\frac{mL}{hr} : \frac{600\ mL}{8\ hr} = 75\ \text{mL per hr}$$

2 a. 25 mL per hr will equal 25 drops per min because the DF is 60.

b. 25 drops per min

$$\frac{drops}{min} : \frac{\cancel{60}\ drops}{1\ \cancel{mL}} \times \frac{25\ \cancel{mL}}{1\ \cancel{hr}} \times \frac{1\ \cancel{hr}}{\cancel{60}\ min} = 25\ \text{drops per minute}$$

c. Equation is balanced. Estimate equals answer.

3 a. 13 drops per min

$$\frac{drops}{min} : \frac{\overset{1}{\cancel{10}}\ drops}{1\ \cancel{mL}} \times \frac{80\ \cancel{mL}}{1\ \cancel{hr}} \times \frac{1\ \cancel{hr}}{\underset{6}{\cancel{60}}\ min} = \frac{80}{6} = 13\ \text{drops per minute}$$

b. Equation is balanced. Only drops per minute remain.

c. Yes. 13 drops per minute can be counted.

4 a. 6 drops per min

$$\text{drops} : \frac{\overset{1}{\cancel{15}} \text{ drops}}{\text{min}} \times \frac{25 \text{ mL}}{1 \text{ mL}} \times \frac{1 \text{ hr}}{\underset{4}{\cancel{60}} \text{ min}} = \frac{25}{4} = 6.25, \text{ rounded to 6 drops per minute}$$

b. Equation is balanced. Only drops per minute remain.
c. Yes. 6 drops per minute can be counted.

> **Note:** It is a very slow rate. The site may coagulate.

5 a. 33 drops per min

$$\text{drops} : \frac{\overset{1}{\cancel{20}} \text{ drop}}{\text{min}} \times \frac{100 \text{ mL}}{1 \text{ mL}} \times \frac{1 \text{ hr}}{\underset{3}{\cancel{60}} \text{ min}} = \frac{100}{3} = 33.3, \text{ rounded to 33 drops per minute}$$

b. Equation is balanced. Only drops per minute remain.
c. Yes. 33 drops per minute can be counted.

RAPID PRACTICE 9-6 (p. 280)

1 a. 10 drops per min because DF is 60.
 b. Microdrip
 c. A needle-like projection delivers the small drops for the microdrip (pediatric) tubing.

2 a. 17 drops per min

$$\text{drops} : \frac{\overset{1}{\cancel{10}} \text{ drops}}{\text{min}} \times \frac{100 \text{ mL}}{1 \text{ mL}} \times \frac{1 \text{ hr}}{\underset{6}{\cancel{60}} \text{ min}} = \frac{100}{6} = 16.6, \text{ rounded to 17 drops per min}$$

b. Equation is balanced. Only drops per min remain. Note that 1 hr = 60 min is often the last entry in DF equations.

3 a. 31 drops per min

$$\text{drops} : \frac{\overset{1}{\cancel{15}} \text{ drops}}{\text{minute}} \times \frac{125 \text{ mL}}{1 \text{ mL}} \times \frac{1 \text{ hr}}{\underset{4}{\cancel{60}} \text{ min}} = \frac{125}{4} = 31 \text{ drops per min}$$

b. Equation is balanced. Only drops per min remain.

4 a. 25 drops per min

$$\text{drops} : \frac{\overset{1}{\cancel{20}} \text{ drops}}{\text{min}} \times \frac{75 \text{ mL}}{1 \text{ mL}} \times \frac{1 \text{ hr}}{\underset{3}{\cancel{60}} \text{ min}} = \frac{75}{3} = 25 \text{ drops per min}$$

b. Equation is balanced. Only drops per min remain.

5 a. 20 drops per min

$$\text{drops} : \frac{\overset{1}{\cancel{10}} \text{ drops}}{\text{minute}} \times \frac{120 \text{ mL}}{1 \text{ mL}} \times \frac{1 \text{ hr}}{\underset{6}{\cancel{60}} \text{ min}} = \frac{120}{6} = 20 \text{ drops per min}$$

b. Equation is balanced. Only drops per min remain.

RAPID PRACTICE 9-7 (p. 281)

1 a. 21 drops per min

$$\text{drops} : \frac{\overset{1}{\cancel{10}} \text{ drops}}{\text{minute}} \times \frac{125 \text{ mL}}{1 \text{ mL}} \times \frac{1 \text{ hr}}{\underset{6}{\cancel{60}} \text{ min}} = 20.8, \text{ rounded to 21 drops per min}$$

b. Equation is balanced. Only drops per min remain.

2 a. 13 drops per min

$$\frac{\text{drops}}{\text{minute}} : \frac{\overset{1}{\cancel{15} \text{ drops}}}{1 \text{ } \cancel{mL}} \times \frac{50 \text{ } \cancel{mL}}{1 \text{ } \cancel{hr}} \times \frac{1 \text{ } \cancel{hr}}{\underset{4}{\cancel{60} \text{ min}}} = 12.5, \text{ rounded to 13 drops per min}$$

b. Equation is balanced. Only drops per min remain.

3 a. 17 drops per min

$$\frac{\text{drops}}{\text{minute}} : \frac{\overset{1}{\cancel{20} \text{ drops}}}{1 \text{ } \cancel{mL}} \times \frac{50 \text{ } \cancel{mL}}{1 \text{ } \cancel{hr}} \times \frac{1 \text{ } \cancel{hr}}{\underset{3}{\cancel{60} \text{ min}}} = \frac{50}{3} = 16.6, \text{ rounded to } 17 \text{ drops per min}$$

b. Equation is balanced. Only drops per min remain.

4 a. 13 drops per min

$$\frac{\text{drops}}{\text{minute}} : \frac{\overset{1}{\cancel{10} \text{ drops}}}{1 \text{ } \cancel{mL}} \times \frac{75 \text{ } \cancel{mL}}{1 \text{ } \cancel{hr}} \times \frac{1 \text{ } \cancel{hr}}{\underset{6}{\cancel{60} \text{ min}}} = \frac{75}{6} = 12.5, \text{ rounded to } 13 \text{ drops per min}$$

b. Equation is balanced. Only drops per min remain.

5 a. 40 drops per min

$$\frac{\text{drops}}{\text{min}} : \frac{\cancel{60} \text{ drops}}{1 \text{ } \cancel{mL}} \times \frac{40 \text{ } \cancel{mL}}{1 \text{ } \cancel{hr}} \times \frac{1 \text{ } \cancel{hr}}{\cancel{60} \text{ min}} = 40 \text{ drops per min}$$

b. Equation is balanced. Only drops per min remain.

RAPID PRACTICE 9-8 (p. 285)

2 a. 160 mL per hr (80 × 2)

$$\frac{mL}{hr} : \frac{80 \text{ mL}}{\underset{1}{\cancel{30} \text{ min}}} \times \frac{\overset{2}{\cancel{60} \text{ min}}}{1 \text{ hr}} = 160 \text{ mL per hr}$$

b. Equation is balanced. Estimate equals answer.

3 a. 3 × 50 = 150 mL per hr

$$\frac{mL}{hr} : \frac{50 \text{ mL}}{\underset{1}{\cancel{20} \text{ min}}} \times \frac{\overset{3}{\cancel{60} \text{ min}}}{1 \text{ hr}} = 150 \text{ mL per hr}$$

b. Equation is balanced. Estimate equals answer.

4 a. 30 × 3 = 90 mL per hr

$$\frac{mL}{hr} : \frac{30 \text{ mL}}{\underset{1}{\cancel{20} \text{ min}}} \times \frac{\overset{3}{\cancel{60} \text{ min}}}{1 \text{ hr}} = 90 \text{ mL per hr}$$

b. Equation is balanced. Estimate equals answer.

5 a. 25 mL × 2 = 50 mL per hr

$$\frac{mL}{hr} : \frac{25 \text{ mL}}{\underset{1}{\cancel{30} \text{ min}}} \times \frac{\overset{2}{\cancel{60} \text{ min}}}{1 \text{ hr}} = 50 \text{ mL per hr}$$

b. Equation is balanced. Estimate equals answer.

RAPID PRACTICE 9-9 (p. 286)

1 a. 150 mL per hr (50 × 3) (20 min periods)
  b. 25 drops per minute

$$\frac{drops}{minute} : \frac{\overset{1}{\cancel{10}} \, drops}{1 \, \cancel{mL}} \times \frac{50 \, \cancel{mL}}{\underset{2}{\cancel{20}} \, min} = 25 \text{ drops per minute}$$

  c. Equation is balanced. Only drops per minute remain.

2 a. 100 × 2 (30 min periods) = 200 mL per hr
  b. 50 drops per minute

$$\frac{drops}{minute} : \frac{\overset{1}{\cancel{15}} \, drops}{1 \, \cancel{mL}} \times \frac{100 \, \cancel{mL}}{\underset{2}{\cancel{30}} \, min} = 50 \text{ drops per minute}$$

  c. Equation is balanced. Only drops per minute remain.

3 a. 75 mL per hr
  b. 25 drops per min

$$\frac{drops}{minute} : \frac{\overset{1}{\cancel{20}} \, drops}{1 \, \cancel{mL}} \times \frac{75 \, \cancel{mL}}{\underset{3}{\cancel{60}} \, min} = \frac{75}{3} = 25 \text{ drops per minute}$$

  c. Equation is balanced. Only drops per minute remain.

4 a. 60 mL per hr (30 min × 2) with microdrip mL per hr = 60 drops per minute
  b. 60 drops per minute

$$\frac{drops}{minute} : \frac{\overset{2}{\cancel{60}} \, drops}{1 \, \cancel{mL}} \times \frac{30 \, \cancel{mL}}{\underset{1}{\cancel{30}} \, min} = 60 \text{ drops per minute}$$

  c. Equation is balanced. Only drops per minute remain.

5 a. 150 mL per hr (50 × 3) (three 20-min periods = 1 hr)
  b. 25 drops per minute

$$\frac{drops}{minute} : \frac{\overset{1}{\cancel{10}} \, drops}{1 \, \cancel{mL}} \times \frac{50 \, \cancel{mL}}{\underset{2}{\cancel{20}} \, min} = 25 \text{ drops per minute}$$

  c. Equation is balanced. Only drops per minute remain.

RAPID PRACTICE 9-10 (p. 288)

Order	Estimated Flow Rate	DA
2 30-mL anticancer medication to infuse in 20 min on EID	90 mL per hr (three 20-min volumes in 60 min per 1 hr)	$\dfrac{mL}{hr} : \dfrac{30 \, mL}{\underset{1}{\cancel{20}} \, \cancel{min}} \times \dfrac{\overset{3}{\cancel{60}} \, \cancel{min}}{1 \, hr} = 90 \text{ mL per hr}$
3 20-mL antibiotic solution to infuse in 30 min on Gravity Device DF60	40 ml per hr (20 mL × 2) (2 × 30 min = 60 min)	$\dfrac{drops}{min} : \dfrac{\overset{2}{\cancel{60}} \, drops}{1 \, \cancel{mL}} \times \dfrac{20 \, \cancel{mL}}{\underset{1}{\cancel{30}} \, min} = 40 \text{ drops per minute}$ $\left(DF \, 60 \, \dfrac{drops}{min} = \dfrac{mL}{hr} \right)$

Order	Estimated Flow Rate	DA
4 60-mL antibiotic solution to infuse in 40 min on EID	90 mL per hr (half the rate of a 20-min order) (180 ÷ 2)	$\dfrac{mL}{hr} : \dfrac{60\ mL}{\underset{2}{\cancel{40\ min}}} \times \dfrac{\overset{3}{\cancel{60\ min}}}{1\ hr} = \dfrac{180}{2} = 90\ mL\ per\ hr$
5 25-mL antibiotic solution in 20 min on Gravity Infusion Device DF20	75 mL per hr (3-20 min periods in 60 minutes)	$\dfrac{drops}{min} : \dfrac{\cancel{20}\ drops}{1\ mL} \times \dfrac{25\ \cancel{mL}}{\cancel{20}\ min} = 25\ drops\ per\ minute$

RAPID PRACTICE 9-11 (p. 288)

Order	Equipment Available	Continuous or Intermittent	Flow Rate Equation (Label Answer)
1 1000 mL D5W q10h	IV administration set DF 10	Continuous	$\dfrac{drops}{min} : \dfrac{\cancel{10}\ drops}{1\ \cancel{mL}} \times \dfrac{1000\ \cancel{mL}}{\cancel{10}\ \cancel{hr}} \times \dfrac{1\ \cancel{hr}}{60\ min} = \dfrac{1000}{60}$ $= 17\ drops\ per\ minute$
2 50 mL antibiotic solution to infuse over 20 minutes	Volumetric pump	Intermittent	$\dfrac{mL}{hr} : \dfrac{50\ mL}{\underset{1}{\cancel{20\ min}}} \times \dfrac{\overset{3}{\cancel{60\ min}}}{1\ hr} = 150\ mL\ per\ hr$
3 250 mL D5W over 4 hours	Electronic rate controller	Intermittent	$\dfrac{mL}{hr} : \dfrac{250\ mL}{4\ hr} = 62.5,\ rounded\ to\ 63\ mL\ per\ hr$
4 500 mL NS q6h	IV administration set DF 15	Continuous	$\dfrac{drops}{min} : \dfrac{\overset{1}{\cancel{15}}\ drops}{1\ \cancel{mL}} \times \dfrac{500\ \cancel{mL}}{6\ \cancel{hr}} \times \dfrac{1\ \cancel{hr}}{\underset{4}{\cancel{60}}\ min} = \dfrac{500}{24}$ $= 20.8,\ rounded\ to\ 21\ drops\ per\ minute$
5 30 mL antibiotic solution to infuse over 30 minutes	Pediatric micro-drip administration set	Intermittent	$\dfrac{drops}{min} : \dfrac{60\ drops}{1\ \cancel{mL}} \times \dfrac{\cancel{30}\ \cancel{mL}}{\cancel{30}\ min} = 60\ drops\ per\ minute$

RAPID PRACTICE 9-12 (p. 292)

Drop Count/Time	Drops per min (Mental Calculation)	Administration Set DF	Flow Rate Equation
2 8 drops per 30 s	16	10	$\dfrac{mL}{hr} : \dfrac{1\ mL}{\underset{1}{\cancel{10}\ drops}} \times \dfrac{16\ \cancel{drops}}{1\ \cancel{min}} \times \dfrac{\overset{6}{\cancel{60}\ \cancel{min}}}{1\ hr} = 96\ mL\ per\ hr$
3 6 drops per 15 s	24	60	$\dfrac{mL}{hr} : \dfrac{1\ mL}{\cancel{60}\ drops} \times \dfrac{24\ \cancel{drops}}{1\ \cancel{min}} \times \dfrac{\cancel{60}\ \cancel{min}}{1\ hr} = 24\ mL\ per\ hr$
4 12 drops per 30 s	24	15	$\dfrac{mL}{hr} : \dfrac{1\ mL}{\underset{1}{\cancel{15}\ drops}} \times \dfrac{24\ \cancel{drops}}{1\ \cancel{min}} \times \dfrac{\overset{4}{\cancel{60}\ \cancel{min}}}{1\ hr} = 96\ mL\ per\ hr$
5 15 drops per 30 s	30	60	$\dfrac{mL}{hr} : \dfrac{1\ mL}{\cancel{60}\ drops} \times \dfrac{30\ \cancel{drops}}{1\ \cancel{min}} \times \dfrac{\cancel{60}\ \cancel{min}}{1\ hr} = 30\ mL\ per\ hr$

RAPID PRACTICE 9-13 (p. 293)

1 2

2 4

3 3

4 2

5 3

RAPID PRACTICE 9-14 (p. 294)

1 a. macrodrip

b. 150 mL per hr

c. 38 drops per min

$$\frac{drops}{minute} : \frac{\overset{1}{\cancel{15}}\ drops}{1\ \cancel{mL}} \times \frac{150\ \cancel{mL}}{1\ \cancel{hr}} \times \frac{1\ \cancel{hr}}{60\ min} = 37.5,\ \text{rounded to 38 drops per minute}$$

d. Equation is balanced. Only drops per minute remain.

e. 6 hr 42 min infusion duration time

$$hr : \frac{1\ hr}{\underset{3}{\cancel{150\ mL}}} \times \overset{20}{\cancel{1000\ mL}} = 6.66,\ \text{rounded to 6.7 hr}$$

$$min : \frac{60\ min}{1\ \cancel{hr}} \times 0.7\ \cancel{hrs} = 42\ \text{minutes}$$

2 a. microdrip

b. 50 drops per min

$$\frac{drops}{minute} : \frac{\cancel{60}\ drops}{1\ \cancel{mL}} \times \frac{500\ \cancel{mL}}{10\ \cancel{hr}} \times \frac{1\ \cancel{hr}}{\cancel{60}\ min} = \frac{500}{10} = 50\ \text{drops per minute}$$

c. Equation is balanced. Only drops per minute remain.

3 a. macrodrip

b. 21 drops per min

$$\frac{drops}{minute} : \frac{\overset{1}{\cancel{10}}\ drops}{1\ \cancel{mL}} \times \frac{1000\ \cancel{mL}}{8\ \cancel{hr}} \times \frac{1\ \cancel{hr}}{\underset{6}{\cancel{60}}\ min} = \frac{1000}{48} = 20.8,\ \text{rounded to 21 drops per minute}$$

c. Equation is balanced. Only drops per minute remain.

4 a. microdrip

b. 40 drops per min

$$\frac{drops}{minute} : \frac{\overset{1}{\cancel{60}}\ drops}{1\ \cancel{mL}} \times \frac{40\ \cancel{mL}}{\underset{1}{\cancel{60}}\ min} = 40\ \text{drops per minute}$$

c. Equation is balanced. Only drops per minute remain.

5 a. macrodrip

b. 17 drops per min

$$\frac{drops}{minute} : \frac{\overset{1}{\cancel{10}}\ drops}{1\ \cancel{mL}} \times \frac{100\ \cancel{mL}}{\underset{6}{\cancel{60}}\ min} = \frac{100}{6} = 17\ \text{drops per minute}$$

c. Equation is balanced. Only drops per minute remain.

RAPID PRACTICE 9-15 (p. 297)

1 a. 21 drops per min

$$\frac{\text{drops}}{\text{minute}} : \overset{1}{\cancel{15}} \text{ drops} \times \frac{\overset{250}{\cancel{1000} \text{ mL}}}{12 \text{ } \cancel{hr}} \times \frac{1 \text{ } \cancel{hr}}{\underset{\underset{1}{4}}{\cancel{60}} \text{ min}} = \frac{250}{12} = 20.8, \text{ rounded to } 21 \text{ drops per minute}$$

b. Equation is balanced. Only drops per minute remain.

2 a. 125 mL per hr

$$\frac{\text{mL}}{\text{hr}} : \frac{500}{4} = 125 \text{ mL per hr}$$

b. Equation is balanced. Only mL per hr remain.

3 a. 125 mL per hr

$$\frac{\text{mL}}{\text{hr}} : \frac{1000 \text{ mL}}{8 \text{ hr}} = 125 \text{ mL per hr}$$

b. Equation is balanced. Only mL per hr remain.

Note: mL per hr can be dialed on a dial-a-flow device.

4 a. 14 drops per min

$$\frac{\text{drops}}{\text{min}} : \overset{1}{\cancel{20}} \text{ drops} \times \frac{250 \text{ } \cancel{mL}}{6 \text{ } \cancel{hr}} \times \frac{1 \text{ } \cancel{hr}}{\underset{3}{\cancel{60}} \text{ min}} = \frac{250}{18} = 13.6, \text{ rounded to } 14 \text{ drops per minute}$$

b. Equation is balanced. Only mL per hr remain.

5 a. 42 drops per min

$$\frac{\text{drops}}{\text{min}} : \overset{1}{\cancel{60}} \text{ drops} \times \frac{1000 \text{ } \cancel{mL}}{24 \text{ } \cancel{hr}} \times \frac{1 \text{ } \cancel{hr}}{\underset{1}{\cancel{60}} \text{ min}} = \frac{1000}{24} = 41.6, \text{ rounded to } 42 \text{ drops per minute}$$

b. Equation is balanced. Only drops per minute remain.

Note: With 60 DF and a continuous IV, mL per hr = drops per minute.

RAPID PRACTICE 9-16 (p. 299)

2 a. 75 grams Dextrose

$$\text{g Dextrose} : \frac{5 \text{ g}}{\underset{1}{\cancel{100} \text{ mL}}} \times \frac{\overset{15}{\cancel{1500} \text{ mL}}}{1} = 75 \text{ g Dextrose}$$

b. Equation is balanced. Only grams remain.

3 a. 13.5 g NaCL

$$\text{g NaCl} : \frac{0.9 \text{ g}}{\underset{1}{\cancel{100} \text{ mL}}} \times \frac{\overset{15}{\cancel{1500} \text{ mL}}}{1} = 13.5 \text{ g NaCL}$$

b. Equation is balanced. Only grams remain.

4 a. 200 g Dextrose

$$\text{g Dextrose}: \frac{10\text{ g}}{\cancel{100\text{ mL}}_1} \times \frac{\cancel{2000\text{ mL}}^{20}}{1} = 200\text{ g Dextrose}$$

b. Equation is balanced. Only g remain.

5 a. 2.25 g NaCL

$$\text{g NaCL}: \frac{0.45\text{ g}}{\cancel{100\text{ mL}}_1} \times \frac{\cancel{500\text{ mL}}^{5}}{1} = 2.25\text{ g NaCl}$$

b. Equation is balanced. Only g remain.
Remember: NS contains slightly less than 1% NaCl. Watch the decimal.

RAPID PRACTICE 9-17 (p. 307)

2 a. 10 hr
   b. 7 hr
   c. 900 mL; 700 mL (100 mL × 7 hr)
   d. ahead
   e. 3 hr; 100 mL
   f. 33 mL per hr (100 ÷ 3)

3 a. 5 hr (250 ÷ 50)
   b. 2 hr
   c. 50 mL; 100 mL (50 mL × 2 hr)
   d. behind
   e. 3 hr; 200 mL
   f. 67 mL per hr (200 ÷ 3)

4 a. 4 hr
   b. 2 hr
   c. 400 mL; 250 mL
   d. ahead
   e. 2 hr; 100 mL
   f. 50 mL per hr (100 ÷ 2)

5 a. 10 hr
   b. 2 hr
   c. 50 mL; 50 mL
   d. on time
   e. 8 hr; 200 mL
   f. Continue at 25 mL per hr. No adjustment is needed.

CHAPTER 9 MULTIPLE-CHOICE REVIEW (p. 308)

1 2   **6** 1
2 3   **7** 3
3 1   **8** 3
4 3   **9** 2
5 2   **10** 4 (100 g per 100 mL)

1 Fluid and electrolyte maintenance, replacement of prior losses, and administration of medications and nutrients

2 0.9% NaCl, D5W, L/R (RLS) (R/L)

3 secondary

4 The tubing delivers a drop factor of 10 drops per mL.

5 **a.** 60 drops per mL
   b. 60 drops per min (60 mL per hr)

6 **a.** 2.25 g NaCL

$$\text{g NaCL}: \dfrac{0.9\text{ g}}{\underset{2}{\cancel{100\text{ mL}}}} \times \dfrac{\overset{5}{\cancel{250\text{ mL}}}}{1} = \dfrac{4.5}{2} = 2.25\text{ g NaCL}$$

   b. Equation is balanced.
   c. 10 drops per minute

$$\dfrac{\text{drops}}{\text{minute}}: \dfrac{\overset{1}{\cancel{10}\text{ drops}}}{1\ \cancel{\text{mL}}} \times \dfrac{250\ \cancel{\text{mL}}}{4\ \cancel{\text{hr}}} \times \dfrac{1\ \cancel{\text{hr}}}{\underset{6}{\cancel{60}}\text{ min}} = \dfrac{250}{24} = 10.4,\ \text{rounded to } 10 \text{ drops per minute}$$

   d. Equation is balanced. Only drops per minute remain.

7 **a.** 5 hr
   b. 225 mL

$$\dfrac{50\text{ mL}}{1\ \cancel{\text{hr}}} \times 4.5\ \cancel{\text{hr}} = 225\text{ mL}$$

8 **a.** 63 mL per hr

$$\dfrac{\text{mL}}{\text{hr}}: \dfrac{500\text{ mL}}{8\text{ hr}} = 62.5 \rightarrow 63\text{ mL per hr}$$

   b. 1200 + 7.5 hr = 1930 hr

9 Ensure that the primary IV is flowing at its ordered rate.

10 Cardiac arrest (a sentinel event)

11 120 mL per hr

$$\dfrac{\text{mL}}{\text{hour}}: \dfrac{2\text{ mL}}{1\ \cancel{\text{min}}} \times \dfrac{60\ \cancel{\text{min}}}{1\text{ hr}} = 120\text{ mL per hr}$$

12 **a.**

$$\dfrac{\text{drops}}{\text{minute}}: \dfrac{\overset{1}{\cancel{10}\text{ drops}}}{1\ \cancel{\text{mL}}} \times \dfrac{\overset{125}{\cancel{250\text{ mL}}}}{\underset{1}{\cancel{2\text{ hr}}}} \times \dfrac{1\ \cancel{\text{hr}}}{\underset{6}{\cancel{60}}\text{ min}} = \dfrac{125}{6} = 20.8,\ \text{rounded to } 21 \text{ drops per minute}$$

   b. Equation is balanced. Only drops per minute remain.
   Note: Equation can be simplified by substituting mL per hr for total mL per total hours.

13 **a.**

$$\dfrac{\text{drops}}{\text{min}}: \dfrac{\overset{1}{\cancel{15}\text{ drops}}}{1\ \cancel{\text{mL}}} \times \dfrac{3000\ \cancel{\text{mL}}}{24\ \cancel{\text{hr}}} \times \dfrac{1\ \cancel{\text{hr}}}{\underset{4}{\cancel{60}}\text{ min}} = 31.25,\ \text{rounded to } 31 \text{ drops per minute}$$

   b. Equation is balanced. Only drops per minute remain.

14 a. $\dfrac{\text{drops}}{\text{min}} : \dfrac{\overset{1}{\cancel{20}} \text{drops}}{1 \, \cancel{\text{mL}}} \times \dfrac{500 \, \cancel{\text{mL}}}{8 \, \cancel{\text{hr}}} \times \dfrac{1 \, \cancel{\text{hr}}}{\underset{3}{60} \, \text{min}} = 20.8$, rounded to 21 drops per minute

b. Equation is balanced. Only drops per minute remain.

15 a. 25 g Dextrose

$$\text{g Dextrose} : \dfrac{50 \, \text{g}}{\underset{2}{\cancel{100 \, \text{mL}}}} \times \dfrac{\overset{1}{\cancel{50 \, \text{mL}}}}{1} = 25 \text{ g Dextrose}$$

b. Equation is balanced. Only g remain.

16 a. Volume-control burette device

b. 1-2 hr worth of ordered fluid. Refer to agency policy.

17 a. 600 mL

b. 1800 hr

c. 6 hours

d. 800 ÷ 6 = 133.3 mL per hour

18 100 mL per hr (50 × 2)

19 a. 60 drops per min (20 × 3)

$$\dfrac{\text{mL}}{\text{hr}} : \dfrac{\overset{3}{\cancel{60}} \text{drops}}{1 \, \cancel{\text{mL}}} \times \dfrac{20 \, \cancel{\text{mL}}}{\underset{1}{\cancel{20}} \, \text{min}} = 60 \text{ drops per minute}$$

b. Equation is balanced. Only drops per minute remain.

20 Agency policies; reason for the delay (equipment/site patency/position); whether the solution is medicated; patient condition; amount of deficit; amount of time remaining in IV schedule

Chapter 10

RAPID PRACTICE 10-1 (p. 314)

1 2   **4** 1

2 3   **5** 4

3 3

RAPID PRACTICE 10-2 (p. 314)

2 a. 120 ÷ 60 = 2 mL per min

$$\dfrac{\text{mL}}{\text{min}} : \dfrac{\overset{2}{\cancel{120}} \, \text{mL}}{1 \, \cancel{\text{hr}}} \times \dfrac{1 \, \cancel{\text{hr}}}{\underset{1}{60} \, \text{min}} = 2 \text{ mL per minute}$$

b. Estimate equals answer.

3 a. 4 mg × 60 = 240 mg per hr

$$\dfrac{\text{mg}}{\text{hr}} : \dfrac{4 \, \text{mg}}{1 \, \cancel{\text{min}}} \times \dfrac{60 \, \cancel{\text{min}}}{1\text{hr}} = 240 \text{ mg per hr}$$

b. Estimate equals answer.

4 a. 60 ÷ 60 = 1 mg per min

$$\dfrac{\text{mg}}{\text{min}} : \dfrac{\overset{1}{\cancel{60}} \, \text{mg}}{1 \, \cancel{\text{hr}}} \times \dfrac{1 \, \cancel{\text{hr}}}{\underset{1}{60} \, \text{min}} = 1 \text{ mg per minute}$$

b. Estimate equals answer.

5 a. 2 mg × 10 kg = 20 mg per minute

$$\frac{mg}{min} : \frac{2\ mg}{1\ \cancel{kg}} \times \frac{10\ \cancel{kg}}{1\ min} = 20\ mg\ per\ min;\ 2\ mg \times 10\ kg = 20\ mg\ per\ minute$$

b. Estimate equals answer.

c. 20 mg × 60 min = 1200 mg per hr

$$\frac{mg}{hour} : \frac{2\ mg}{1\ \cancel{kg} \times \cancel{min}} \times \frac{10\ \cancel{kg}}{1} \times \frac{60\ \cancel{min}}{1\ hr} = \frac{1200\ mg}{hr}$$

d. Estimate equals answer.

Remember: Units following "per" need to be in the denominator of equations; e.g., mL per hr ($\frac{mL}{hr}$) and mg per minute ($\frac{mg}{minute}$). The answer can be in fraction form ($\frac{mg}{hr}$) *or* written out (mg per hr).

RAPID PRACTICE 10-3 (p. 317)

1 a. 120 mL per hr

$$\frac{mL}{hr} : \frac{\cancel{1000}\ mL}{\cancel{1000}\ \cancel{mg}} \times \frac{2\ \cancel{mg}}{1\ \cancel{min}} \times \frac{60\ \cancel{min}}{1\ hr} = \frac{120\ mL}{hr}$$

b. Equation is balanced. Only mL per hr remain. Note that mL must be entered in the first numerator, and hr must be entered in a denominator in the equation.

2 a. 120 mL per hr

$$\frac{mL}{hr} : \frac{\overset{2}{\cancel{1000}}\ mL}{\underset{1}{\cancel{500}\ \cancel{mg}}} \times \frac{1\ \cancel{mg}}{1\ \cancel{min}} \times \frac{60\ \cancel{min}}{1\ hr} = \frac{120\ mL}{hr}$$

b. Equation is balanced. Only mL per hr remain.

3 a. 15 mL per hr

$$\frac{mL}{hr} : \frac{\overset{1}{\cancel{250}}\ mL}{\underset{\underset{1}{\cancel{2}}}{\cancel{500}\ \cancel{mg}}} \times \frac{0.5\ \cancel{mg}}{1\ \cancel{min}} \times \frac{\overset{30}{\cancel{60}\ \cancel{min}}}{1\ hr} = \frac{15\ mL}{hr}$$

b. Equation is balanced. Only mL per hr remain.

4 a. 12 mL per hr

$$\frac{mL}{hr} : \frac{\overset{1}{\cancel{100}}\ mL}{\underset{1}{\cancel{100}\ \cancel{mg}}} \times \frac{0.2\ \cancel{mg}}{1\ \cancel{min}} \times \frac{60\ \cancel{min}}{1\ hr} = \frac{12\ mL}{hr}$$

b. Equation is balanced. Only mL per hr remain.

5 a. 96 mL per hr

$$\frac{mL}{hr} : \frac{\overset{4}{\cancel{1000}}\ mL}{\underset{1}{\cancel{250}\ \cancel{mg}}} \times \frac{0.4\ \cancel{mg}}{1\ \cancel{min}} \times \frac{60\ \cancel{min}}{1\ hr} = \frac{96\ mL}{hr}$$

Note: 1 L = 1000 mL.

b. Equation is balanced. Only mL per hr remain.

2 a. 45 mL per hr

$$\frac{mL}{hr} : \frac{\overset{1}{\cancel{100}}\, mL}{\cancel{10}\, \cancel{mg}} \times \frac{1\, \cancel{mg}}{\underset{\underset{1}{10}}{\cancel{1000}\, \cancel{mcg}}} \times \frac{75\, \cancel{mcg}}{1\, \cancel{min}} \times \frac{\overset{6}{\cancel{60}}\, \cancel{min}}{1\, hr} = \frac{450}{10} = \frac{45\, mL}{hr}$$

b. Equation is balanced. Only mL per hr remain.

3 a. 60 mL per hr

$$\frac{mL}{hr} : \frac{\overset{1}{\cancel{200}}\, mL}{1\, \cancel{g}} \times \frac{1\, \cancel{g}}{\underset{5}{\cancel{1000}}\, \cancel{mg}} \times \frac{5\, \cancel{mg}}{1\, \cancel{min}} \times \frac{60\, \cancel{min}}{1\, hr} = \frac{300}{5} = \frac{60\, mL}{hr}$$

b. Equation is balanced. Only mL per hr remain.

4 a. 6 mL per hr

$$\frac{mL}{hr} : \frac{\overset{1}{\cancel{250}}\, mL}{\underset{2}{\cancel{500}}\, \cancel{mg}} \times \frac{1\, \cancel{mg}}{\underset{5}{\cancel{1000}}\, \cancel{mcg}} \times \frac{\overset{1}{\cancel{200}}\, \cancel{mcg}}{1\, \cancel{min}} \times \frac{60\, \cancel{min}}{1\, hr} = \frac{60}{10} = \frac{6\, mL}{hr}$$

b. Equation is balanced. Only mL per hr remain.

5 a. 9 mL per hr

$$\frac{mL}{hr} : \frac{\overset{1}{\cancel{200}}\, mL}{2\, \cancel{g}} \times \frac{1\, \cancel{g}}{\underset{5}{\cancel{1000}}\, \cancel{mg}} \times \frac{1.5\, \cancel{mg}}{1\, \cancel{minute}} \times \frac{60\, \cancel{min}}{1\, hr} = \frac{90}{10} = \frac{9\, mL}{hr}$$

b. Equation is balanced. Only mL per hr remain.

RAPID PRACTICE 10-5 (p. 322)

2 20 mL per hr

a. $$\frac{mL}{hr} : \frac{\overset{1}{\cancel{250}}\, mL}{\underset{\underset{1}{\cancel{2}}}{\cancel{500}\, \cancel{mg}}} \times \frac{0.5\, \cancel{mg}}{1\, \cancel{kg} \times hr} \times \frac{\overset{40}{\cancel{80}\, \cancel{kg}}}{1} = \frac{20\, mL}{hr}$$

b. Equation is balanced. Only mL per hr remain.

3 60 mL per hr

a. $$\frac{mL}{hr} : \frac{\overset{1}{\cancel{250}}\, mL}{1\, \cancel{mg}} \times \frac{1\, \cancel{mg}}{\underset{\underset{1}{\cancel{4}}}{\cancel{1000}\, \cancel{mcg}}} \times \frac{0.1\, \cancel{mcg}}{\cancel{kg} \times \cancel{min}} \times \frac{\overset{10}{\cancel{40}\, \cancel{kg}}}{1} \times \frac{60\, \cancel{min}}{1\, hr} = \frac{60\, mL}{hr}$$

b. Equation is balanced. Only mL per hr remain.

4 15.8 mL per hr

a. $\dfrac{\text{mL}}{\text{hr}} : \dfrac{500 \text{ mL}}{400 \text{ mg}} \times \dfrac{1 \text{ mg}}{1000 \text{ mcg}} \times \dfrac{3 \text{ mcg}}{\text{kg} \times \text{min}} \times \dfrac{70 \text{ kg}}{1} \times \dfrac{60 \text{ min}}{1 \text{ hr}} = 15.75,$ rounded to $\dfrac{15.8 \text{ mL}}{\text{hr}}$

b. Equation is balanced. Only mL per hr remain.

5 7.5 mL per hr

a. $\dfrac{\text{mL}}{\text{hr}} : \dfrac{\overset{1}{1000} \text{ mL}}{1 \text{ g}} \times \dfrac{1 \text{ g}}{\underset{1}{1000 \text{ mg}}} \times \dfrac{2 \text{ mg}}{\text{min}} \times \dfrac{60 \text{ min}}{1 \text{ hr}} = \dfrac{120 \text{ mL}}{\text{hr}}$

b. Equation is balanced. Only mL per hr remain.

RAPID PRACTICE 10-6 (p. 325)

1 a. 7.5 mL per hr

$\dfrac{\text{mL}}{\text{hr}} : \dfrac{\overset{5}{250} \text{ mL}}{\underset{4}{200} \text{ mg}} \times \dfrac{0.1 \text{ mg}}{1 \text{ min}} \times \dfrac{\overset{15}{60} \text{ min}}{1 \text{ hr}} = \dfrac{7.5 \text{ mL}}{\text{hr}}$

b. Equation is balanced. Only mL per hr remain.

2 a. 120 mL per hr

$\dfrac{\text{mL}}{\text{hr}} : \dfrac{2 \text{ mL}}{1 \text{ min}} \times \dfrac{60 \text{ min}}{1 \text{ hr}} = \dfrac{120 \text{ mL}}{\text{hr}}$

b. Equation is balanced. Only mL per hr remain.

c. No, the microdrip flow rate (DF 60) in drops per minute = the mL per hr rate. A rate greater than 60 drops per minute is too difficult to count.

3 a. 75 mL per hr

$\dfrac{\text{mL}}{\text{hr}} : \dfrac{\overset{1}{250} \text{ mL}}{1 \text{ g}} \times \dfrac{1 \text{ g}}{\underset{4}{1000 \text{ mg}}} \times \dfrac{5 \text{ mg}}{1 \text{ min}} \times \dfrac{\overset{15}{60} \text{ min}}{1 \text{ hr}} = \dfrac{75 \text{ mL}}{\text{hr}}$

b. Equation is balanced. Only mL per hr remain.

4 a. 352 mcg

$\dfrac{\text{mcg}}{\text{min}} : \dfrac{8 \text{ mcg}}{1 \text{ kg}} \times \dfrac{44 \text{ kg}}{1 \text{ min}} = \dfrac{352 \text{ mcg}}{\text{minute}}$ per initial dose

b. 42.2 mL per hr

$\dfrac{\text{mL}}{\text{hr}} : \dfrac{\overset{1}{1000 \text{ mL}}}{500 \text{ mg}} \times \dfrac{1 \text{ mg}}{\underset{1}{1000 \text{ mcg}}} \times \dfrac{8 \text{ mcg}}{1 \text{ kg} \times \text{min}} \times \dfrac{44 \text{ kg}}{1} \times \dfrac{60 \text{ min}}{1 \text{ hr}} = \dfrac{2112}{50}$

$= \dfrac{42.2 \text{ mL}}{\text{hr}}$ initial flow rate

c. Equation is balanced. Only mL per hr remain.

Note: Remember to enter calculations twice for verification.

5 a. 440 mcg

$$\text{mcg}:\ \frac{10\ \text{mcg}}{1\ \cancel{\text{kg}}}\ \times\ \frac{44\ \cancel{\text{kg}}}{1\ \text{min}}\ =\ \frac{440\ \text{mcg}}{\text{minute}}$$

b. 52.8 mL per hr

$$\frac{\text{mL}}{\text{hr}}:\ \frac{\cancel{1000\ \text{mL}}}{500\ \text{mg}}\ \times\ \frac{1\ \cancel{\text{mg}}}{\underset{1}{\cancel{1000\ \text{mcg}}}}\ \times\ \frac{10\ \cancel{\text{mcg}}}{1\ \cancel{\text{kg}}\ \times\ \cancel{\text{min}}}\ \times\ \frac{44\ \cancel{\text{kg}}}{1}\ \times\ \frac{\cancel{60\ \text{min}}}{1\ \text{hr}}$$

$$=\ \frac{\cancel{2640}}{\cancel{50}}\ =\ \frac{52.8\ \text{mL}}{\text{hr}}$$

Note: Experienced nurses mentally convert 1 L to 1000 mL.

c. Equation is balanced. Only mL per hr remain.

RAPID PRACTICE 10-7 (p. 328)

2 a. 0.25 mg per mL

b. 125 mcg per minute

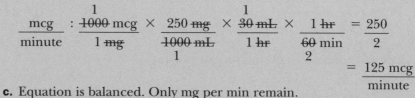

$$\frac{\text{mcg}}{\text{minute}}:\ \overset{1}{\cancel{1000}}\ \text{mcg}\ \times\ \frac{250\ \cancel{\text{mg}}}{\underset{1}{\cancel{1000\ \text{mL}}}}\ \times\ \frac{\overset{1}{\cancel{30\ \text{mL}}}}{1\ \cancel{\text{hr}}}\ \times\ \frac{1\ \cancel{\text{hr}}}{\underset{2}{\cancel{60}}\ \text{min}}\ =\ \frac{250}{2}$$

$$=\ \frac{125\ \text{mcg}}{\text{minute}}$$

c. Equation is balanced. Only mg per min remain.

Note: The mcg to mg conversion formula were entered first because mcg were needed in the first numerator.

3 a. 2 mg per mL (500 mg per 250 mL)

b. 0.83 mg per minute

$$\frac{\text{mg}}{\text{min}}:\ \frac{\overset{2}{\cancel{500}}\ \text{mg}}{\underset{1}{\cancel{250\ \text{mL}}}}\ \times\ \frac{\overset{5}{\cancel{25\ \text{mL}}}}{1\ \cancel{\text{hr}}}\ \times\ \frac{1\ \cancel{\text{hr}}}{\underset{12}{\cancel{60}}\ \text{min}}\ =\ 0.83\ \text{mg per minute}$$

c. Equation is balanced. Only mg per minute remain.

4 a. 4 mg per mL (1000 mg per 250 mL)

b. 0.67 mg per minute

$$\frac{\text{mg}}{\text{minute}}:\ \overset{4}{\cancel{1000}}\ \text{mg}\ \times\ \frac{1\ \cancel{\text{g}}}{\underset{1}{\cancel{250\ \text{mL}}}}\ \times\ \frac{\overset{1}{\cancel{10\ \text{mL}}}}{\cancel{\text{hr}}}\ \times\ \frac{1\ \cancel{\text{hr}}}{\underset{6}{\cancel{60}}\ \text{min}}\ =\ \frac{4}{6}\ =\ 0.666,\ \text{rounded}$$
to 0.67 mg per minute

c. Equation is balanced. Only mg per min remain.

Note: The mg to g conversion formula were first because mg were needed in the first numerator.

5 a. 1 mg per mL (500 mg per 500 mL)

b. 0.2 mg per minute

$$\frac{\text{mg}}{\text{min}}:\ \frac{\overset{1}{\cancel{500}}\ \text{mg}}{\underset{1}{\cancel{500\ \text{mL}}}}\ \times\ \frac{\overset{1}{\cancel{12\ \text{mL}}}}{1\ \cancel{\text{hr}}}\ \times\ \frac{1\ \cancel{\text{hr}}}{\underset{5}{\cancel{60}}\ \text{min}}\ =\ \frac{1}{5}\ =\ \frac{0.2\ \text{mg}}{\text{minute}}$$

c. Equation is balanced. Only mg per min remain.

1 a. 2 mL

$$\frac{mL}{dose} : \frac{1\ mL}{\underset{1}{\cancel{0.4\ mg}}} \times \frac{\overset{2}{\cancel{0.8\ mg}}}{dose} = \frac{2\ mL}{dose}$$

b. 5 mL
c. 1 minute
d. 5 mL per min
e. 25 calibrations for 5 mL in a 10-mL syringe
f. 60 seconds (= 1 minute)
g. 2.4 seconds per calibration

$$\frac{seconds}{calibration} : \frac{60}{25} = 2.4\ \text{seconds per calibration}$$

h. Equation is balanced. Only seconds per calibration remain.

2 a. 2 mL

$$\frac{mL}{dose} : \frac{1\ mL}{\underset{1}{\cancel{5\ mg}}} \times \frac{\overset{2}{\cancel{10\ mg}}}{dose} = \frac{2\ mL}{dose}$$

b. N/A; 2 mL undiluted is total amount
c. 2 minutes
d. 1 mL per min (5 mg per min)
e. 10 calibrations for 2 mL on a 10-mL syringe
f. 120 seconds
g. 12 seconds per calibration

$$\frac{seconds}{calibration} : \frac{120}{10} = \frac{12\ seconds}{calibration}$$

h. Equation is balanced. Only seconds per calibration remain.

3 a. 0.8 mL

$$\frac{mL}{dose} : \frac{1\ mL}{\underset{4}{\cancel{120\ mg}}} \times \overset{3}{\cancel{90\ mg}} = 0.75, \text{rounded to } \frac{0.8\ mL}{dose}$$

b. 3 mL
c. 3 minutes
d. 1 mL per min
e. 15 calibrations on a 10-mL syringe
f. 180 seconds (3 minutes)
g. 12 seconds per calibration

$$\frac{seconds}{calibration} : \frac{180}{15} = \frac{12\ seconds}{calibration}$$

h. Equation is balanced. Only seconds per calibration remain.

4 a. 0.8 mL

$$\frac{mL}{dose} : \frac{1\ mL}{\underset{5}{\cancel{75\ mg}}} \times \frac{\overset{4}{\cancel{60\ mg}}}{dose} = \frac{0.8\ mL}{dose}$$

b. 5 mL
c. 5 minutes

d. 1 mL per min

e. 25 calibrations

5 a. 4 mL

b. N/A

c. 10 minutes (4 mg per min)

d. 0.4 mL per min

e. 20 calibrations in 10-mL syringe

f. 600 (10 × 60) seconds

g. 30 seconds per calibration

$$\frac{\text{seconds}}{\text{calibration}} : \frac{600}{20} = \frac{30 \text{ seconds}}{\text{calibration}}$$

h. Equation is balanced. Only seconds per calibration remain.

CHAPTER 10 MULTIPLE-CHOICE REVIEW (p. 340)

1 4

$$(2 \text{ mL} \times 60 \text{ min per hr}) \left(\frac{2 \text{ mL}}{1 \text{ min}} \times \frac{60 \text{ min}}{1 \text{ hr}} = \frac{120 \text{ mL}}{\text{hr}} \right)$$

2 4

$$\frac{\text{mL}}{\text{hr}} : \frac{500 \text{ mL}}{\overset{}{\underset{4}{40 \text{ mEq}}}} \times \frac{\overset{1}{10 \text{ mEq}}}{1 \text{ hr}} - \frac{500}{4} = \frac{125 \text{ mL}}{\text{hr}}$$

3 1

$$\frac{\text{mg}}{\text{mL}} : \frac{\overset{4}{1000} \text{ mg (1 g)}}{\underset{1}{250}} \text{ mg} = \frac{4 \text{ mg}}{\text{mL}}$$

4 4

$$\text{g Dextrose} : \frac{25 \text{ g}}{\underset{1}{100 \text{ mL}}} \times \frac{\overset{10}{1000 \text{ mL}}}{1} = 250 \text{ g Dextrose}$$

$$\text{kcal} : \frac{4 \text{ kcal}}{1 \text{ g}} \times \frac{250 \text{ g}}{1} = 1000 \text{ kcal Dextrose}$$

5 2

$$\frac{\text{drops}}{\text{min}} : \frac{60 \text{ drops}}{1 \text{ mL}} \times \frac{\overset{1}{30 \text{ mL}}}{\underset{1}{30} \text{ min}} = \frac{60 \text{ drops}}{\text{minute}}$$

6 1

The diluted volume is used for the calculation: 5 mL in 5 minutes = 1 mL in 1 minute

7 4

8 2

$$\frac{500 \text{ mL remaining}}{3 \text{ hr remaining}} = \frac{167 \text{ mL}}{\text{hr}}$$

9 3

1 mg for each mL is the most concentrated solution.

10 2

$$\frac{mg}{hr} : \frac{\overset{1}{\cancel{500}}\ mg}{\underset{2}{\cancel{1000}\ mL}} \times \frac{10\ \cancel{mL}}{1\ hr} = \frac{10}{2} = \frac{5\ mg}{hr}$$

CHAPTER 10 FINAL PRACTICE (p. 341)

1 a. 3 mL

$$\frac{mL}{dose} : \frac{4\ mL}{\underset{4}{\cancel{40}\ mg}} \times \overset{3}{\cancel{30}\ mg} = \frac{12}{4} = \frac{3\ mL}{dose}$$

b. 15 calibrations

c. 450 seconds

$$seconds = \frac{\overset{15}{\cancel{60}}\ sec}{1\ \cancel{min}} \times \frac{1\ \cancel{min}}{\underset{1}{\cancel{4}\ mg}} \times \frac{30\ \cancel{mg}}{1} = 15 \times 30 = 450\ seconds$$

d. 30 seconds per calibration

$$\frac{seconds}{calibration} : \frac{450\ seconds}{15\ calibrations} = \frac{30\ seconds}{calibration}$$

2 a. 11.3 mL per hr

$$\frac{mL}{hr} : \frac{\overset{1}{\cancel{250}\ mL}}{\underset{2}{\cancel{500}\ mg}} \times \frac{0.3\ mg}{kg \times hr} \times \frac{75\ \cancel{kg}}{1} = \frac{22.5}{2} = 11.25,\ rounded\ to\ \frac{11.3\ mL}{hr}$$

Equation is balanced. Only mg per hr and mL per hr remain.

b. 15 mL per hr

$$\frac{mL}{hr} : \frac{\overset{1}{\cancel{250}}}{\underset{2}{\cancel{500}\ mg}} \times \frac{0.4\ \cancel{mg}}{kg \times hr} \times \frac{75\ \cancel{kg}}{1} = \frac{30}{2} = \frac{15\ mL}{hr}$$

Equation is balanced. Only mg per hr and mL per hr remain.

3 a. 0.2 mg per mL

$$\frac{mg}{mL} : \frac{50\ mg}{\underset{1}{\cancel{250}\ mL}} = \frac{1}{5} = \frac{0.2\ mg}{mL}\ concentration$$

Equation is balanced. Only mg per mL remain.

b. 5.4 mL per hr

$$\frac{mL}{hr} : \frac{\overset{5}{\cancel{250}\ mg}}{\underset{1}{\cancel{50}\ mg}} \times \frac{0.3\ \cancel{mcg}}{kg \times \cancel{min}} \times \frac{1\ \cancel{mg}}{\cancel{1000}\ \cancel{mcg}} \times \frac{60\ kg}{1} \times \frac{60\ \cancel{min}}{1\ hr} = \frac{54}{10} =$$

$$5.4\ mL\ per\ hr$$

Equations are balanced. Only mcg per min and mL per hr remain.

4 a. 0.5 mg per mL

$$\frac{\text{mg}}{\text{mL}} : \frac{250 \text{ mg}}{500 \text{ mL}} = 0.5 \text{ mg per mL}$$

b. 19 mL per hr

$$\frac{\text{mL}}{\text{hr}} : \frac{\overset{1}{\cancel{500}} \text{ mL}}{250 \text{ mg}} \times \frac{1 \text{ mg}}{\underset{\underset{1}{2}}{\cancel{1000 \text{ mcg}}}} \times \frac{2.5 \text{ mcg}}{\text{kg} \times \text{min}} \times \frac{64 \text{ kg}}{1} \times \frac{30 \text{ min}}{1 \text{ hr}} = \frac{19.2 \text{ mL}}{\text{hr}}$$

Equation is balanced. Only mL per hr remain

5 125 mL per hr

$$\frac{\text{mL}}{\text{hr}} : \frac{500 \text{ mL}}{\underset{4}{\cancel{40 \text{ mEq}}}} \times \frac{\overset{1}{\cancel{10 \text{ mEq}}}}{1 \text{ hr}} = \frac{125 \text{ mL}}{\text{hr}}$$

6 a. 15 mg per hr

$$\frac{\text{mg}}{\text{hr}} : \frac{1 \text{ mg}}{1000 \text{ mcg}} \times \frac{3 \text{ mcg}}{\text{kg} \times \text{min}} \times \frac{82 \text{ kg}}{1} \times \frac{60 \text{ min}}{1 \text{ hr}} = \frac{14,760}{1000}$$

$$= 14.76, \text{ rounded to } \frac{15 \text{ mg}}{\text{hr}}$$

b. 18.5 mL per hr

$$\frac{\text{mL}}{\text{hr}} : \frac{\overset{\overset{1}{\cancel{5}}}{\cancel{250}} \text{ mL}}{\underset{4}{\cancel{200 \text{ mg}}}} \times \frac{1 \text{ mg}}{\underset{200}{\cancel{1000 \text{ mcg}}}} \times \frac{3 \text{ mcg}}{\text{kg} \times \text{min}} \times \frac{82 \text{ kg}}{1} \times \frac{60 \text{ min}}{1 \text{ hr}} = \frac{1476}{80}$$

$$= 18.45, \text{ rounded to } \frac{18.5 \text{ mL}}{\text{hr}}$$

Note: The nurse assesses the patient, contacts the prescriber, obtains an order to adjust the flow rate gradually to the ordered rate, and documents the incident.

7 a. 2.5 mL

$$\frac{\text{mL}}{\text{dose}} : \frac{1 \text{ mL}}{0.4 \text{ mg}} \times \frac{1 \text{ mg}}{\text{dose}} = \frac{2.5 \text{ mL}}{\text{dose}}$$

b. 6 sec per mL

$$\frac{\text{seconds}}{\text{mL}} : \frac{60 \text{ s}}{10 \text{ mL}} = \frac{6 \text{ s}}{\text{mL}}$$

8 a. 5 mL (ampules)

$$\frac{\text{mL}}{\text{dose}} : \frac{1 \text{ mL}}{0.4 \text{ mg}} \times \frac{2 \text{ mg}}{\text{dose}} = \frac{5 \text{ mL}}{\text{dose}}$$

b. 8 mL per hr

$$\frac{\text{mL}}{\text{hr}} : \frac{\overset{250}{\cancel{500 \text{ mL}}}}{\cancel{2 \text{ mg}}} \times \frac{0.03 \text{ mg}}{1 \text{ hr}} = \frac{7.5 \text{ mL}}{\text{hr}}$$

9 a. 8 mL

$$\frac{\text{mL}}{\text{dose}} : \frac{1 \text{ mL}}{\underset{1}{\cancel{500 \text{ mg}}}} \times \frac{\overset{2}{\cancel{1000 \text{ mg}}}}{1 \text{ g}} \times \frac{4 \text{ g}}{\text{dose}} = \frac{8 \text{ mL}}{\text{dose}}$$

b. 150 mL per hr

$$\frac{mL}{hr} : \frac{2.5\ mL}{1\ \cancel{min}} \times \frac{60\ \cancel{min}}{1\ hr} = \frac{150\ mL}{hr}$$

c. 4 g : 4000 mg

$$\frac{mg}{min} : \frac{4000\ mg}{250\ mL} \times \frac{2.5\ mL}{1\ min} = \frac{1000}{25} = \frac{40\ mg}{minute}$$

Note: mg is the approved abbreviation for milligram. Do not abbreviate magnesium.

10 a. yes

b. 125 mL per hr

$$\frac{mL}{hr} : \frac{\overset{25}{\cancel{1000}}\ mL}{\underset{1}{\cancel{40}\ \cancel{mEq}}} \times \frac{5\ \cancel{mEq}}{hr} = \frac{125\ mL}{hr}$$

c. 8 hr

$$hr : \frac{1\ hr}{\underset{1}{\cancel{125}\ \cancel{mL}}} \times \frac{\overset{8}{\cancel{1000}\ \cancel{mL}}}{1} = 8\ hr$$

Chapter 11

RAPID PRACTICE 11-1 (p. 353)

1 Stat BG—immediate, current level

FBS (fasting blood sugar)—level of blood sugar after fasting for at least 8 hours

2-hour postprandial—level 2 hours after a meal

fructosomine—average level over past 2 weeks

HbA1c (glycosylated hemoglobin)—average level over past 2 to 3 months

2 SMBG

3 70-100 mg per dL (the normal FBS level varies slightly)

4 Insulin is a hormone lowers blood glucose levels by facilitating entry into muscle cells and other storage sites—insulin helps glucose get into cells

5 Insulin shock—urgent *hypoglycemic* condition treated with glucose and other therapies

DKA—urgent *hyperglycemic* condition treated with insulin and other therapies.

---

*Potassium chloride is a common additive to IV solutions. Concentrated KCL can cause arrhythmias and cardiac arrest if given undiluted. After dilution, the IV bag must be gently rotated several times before hanging to ensure that the Potassium is dispersed *throughout* the bag. It is preferably administered via an infusion pump. It *must be administered* via an infusion pump in stronger concentrations. Notify the prescriber if by chance the infusion is administered at a rate that exceed the order. A timed tape is helpful for monitoring volume infused even when a pump is being used.

RAPID PRACTICE 11-2 (p. 359)

1 Humalog (insulin lispro), Novolog (insulin aspart)
2 a. 100 units per mL
  b. 1000 units (100 units × 10 mL)
3 Dextrose (glucose)
4 Diet products do not contain dextrose.
5 a. Novolin R; **c.** Humulin R

RAPID PRACTICE 11-3 (p. 361)

1 Two injections per day, one AM and one PM.
2 No.
3 100 units per mL
4 Cloudy
5 There is potential for overlapping duration. They are trying to avoid a hypo-glycemic episode during sleep

RAPID PRACTICE 11-4 (p. 363)

1 Insulin glargine
2 They have relatively flat action. They do not have a peak.
3 No. They contain additives.
4 100 units per mL
5 No.

RAPID PRACTICE 11-5 (p. 367)

1 16 units
2 22 units
3
4
5

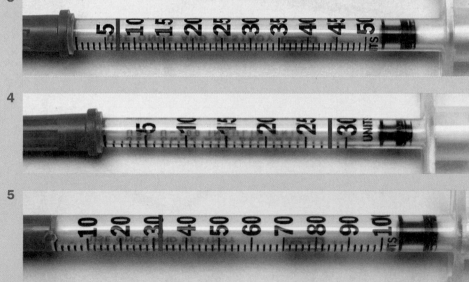

1

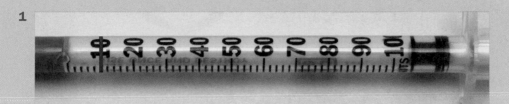

2 Give 12 units Humulin R subcut. Recheck BG in 1 hr.

3 Call physician immediately. Draw plasma BG.

4 To verify the accuracy of the fingerstick BG before instituting more aggressive treatment.

5 Hold insulin (0 units).

RAPID PRACTICE 11-7 (p. 372)

2 a. intermediate

　b. suspension

　c. Yes. Some manufacturers recommend *gentle shaking*. Others recommend *rolling the vial*. Read the directions on the product.

　d. 6 to12 hr

　e. subcut

　f.

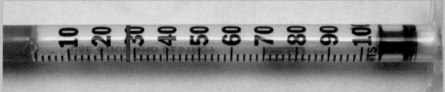

3 a. 30 minutes

　b. $2\frac{1}{2}$ to 5 hr

　c. 8 hr

　d.

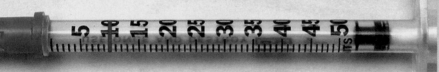

4 a. 1000 units

　b. rapid

　c. 100 units per mL

5 a. subcutaneous

　b.

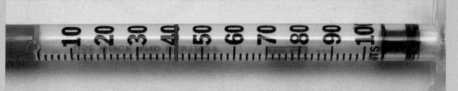

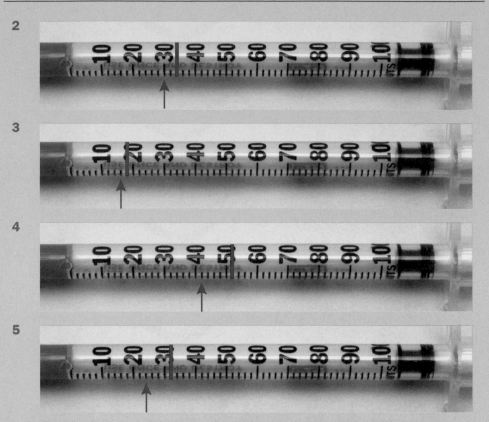

➤ Assess patient mental status, vision, and hand-eye coordination if self-administration will be needed at home.

RAPID PRACTICE 11-9 (p. 382)

1 a. 3 mL per hr, because concentration is 1:1.
  b. 3 mL per hr

$$\frac{mL}{hr} : \frac{\overset{1}{\cancel{100}}\,mL}{\underset{1}{\cancel{100\ units}}} \times \frac{3\ \cancel{units}}{1\ hr} = \frac{3\ mL}{hr}$$

  c. Equation is balanced. Estimate equals answer.

  Note: A "U" for units can be misread as a zero (0).

2 a. 8 mL per hr, because concentration is 1 unit : 2 mL.
  b. 8 mL per hr

$$\frac{mL}{hr} : \frac{\overset{2}{\cancel{100}}\,mL}{\underset{1}{\cancel{50\ units}}} \times \frac{4\ \cancel{units}}{1\ hr} = \frac{8\ mL}{hr}$$

  c. Equation is balanced. Estimate equals answer.

3 a. 12 mL per hr, because concentration is 1:2.
  b. 12 mL per hr

$$\frac{mL}{hr} : \frac{\overset{2}{\cancel{100}}\,mL}{\underset{1}{\cancel{50\ units}}} \times \frac{6\ \cancel{units}}{1\ hr} = \frac{12\ mL}{hr}$$

  c. Evaluation: Equation is balanced. Estimate equals answer.

4 a. 6 mL per hr (half of original order)

b. 6 mL per hr

$$\frac{mL}{hr} : \frac{\overset{2}{\cancel{100}} \text{ mL}}{\underset{1}{\cancel{50 \text{ units}}}} \times \frac{3 \text{ \cancel{units}}}{hr} = \frac{6 \text{ mL}}{hr}$$

c. 6 mL per hr is 50% of original 12 mL ordered. Estimate supports answer.

5 a. 4 mL per hr, because concentration is 1 unit : 2 mL.

b. 4 mL per hr

$$\frac{mL}{hr} : \frac{\overset{2}{\cancel{100}} \text{ mL}}{\underset{1}{\cancel{50 \text{ units}}}} \times \frac{2 \text{ \cancel{units}}}{1 \text{ hr}} = \frac{4 \text{ mL}}{hr} \text{ ordered flow rate}$$

c. Flow rate is incorrect. It is half the ordered rate.

d. Assess current BG level. Consult with prescriber for flow rate order changes. Document. Check agency policy about an incident report.

RAPID PRACTICE 11-10 (p. 383)

1 a. Regular insulins insulin aspart (Novolog) and insulin glulisine (Apidra)

b. clear

2 short- and intermediate-acting

3 a. 100 units per mL and 500 units per mL

b. U-100 is the most commonly used.

4 No.

5 a. The intermediate-acting insulin is usually the larger dose.

b. It is a modified product to cover a longer duration.

CHAPTER 11 MULTIPLE-CHOICE REVIEW (p. 386)

1 4

Note: If a short-acting insulin is needed, it can be given separately.

2 2

3 1

4 4

5 3

6 4

7 3

Note: This helps prevent hypoglycemic episodes during sleep.

8 1

9 2

10 3

CHAPTER 11 FINAL PRACTICE (p. 387)

1 a. 100 units per mL

b. Regular insulin must be withdrawn first to protect it from contamination from an intermediate-acting insulin.

c. Contamination would alter (lengthen) the action of the regular insulin.

2

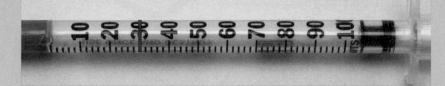

(The choice of syringe in the text is a 100 unit insulin syringe.)

3 a. Humulin R insulin to prevent the regular insulin from contamination by the product.

b.

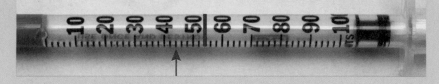

The nurse must focus so as not to confuse the doses.

4 a. Novolin R

b.

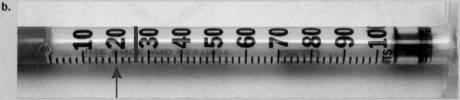

5 a. Insulin lispro is rapid acting.

b.

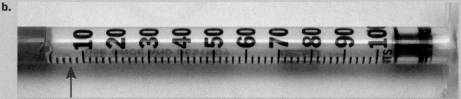

6 a. 1 unit per mL

$$\frac{\text{units}}{\text{mL}} : \frac{\overset{1}{\cancel{100}}\text{ units}}{\underset{1}{\cancel{100}}\text{ mL}} = \frac{1\text{ unit}}{\text{mL}}$$

b. 5 mL per hr of a 1:1 solution (for 5 units per hr)

$$\frac{\text{mL}}{\text{hr}} : \frac{\overset{1}{\cancel{100}}\text{ mL}}{\underset{1}{\cancel{100}\text{ units}}} \times \frac{5\text{ }\cancel{\text{units}}}{\text{hr}} = \frac{5\text{ mL}}{\text{hr}}$$

c. Estimate equals answer.

d. Yes. Insulin solutions for IV administration should be administered on an infusion pump on a separate line.

7 a. 4 mL per hr to deliver $\dfrac{4\text{ units}}{\text{hr}}$

b. $\dfrac{\text{mL}}{\text{hr}} : \dfrac{\overset{1}{\cancel{100}}\text{ mL}}{\underset{1}{\cancel{100}\text{ units}}} \times \dfrac{4\text{ }\cancel{\text{units}}}{1\text{ hr}} = \dfrac{4\text{ mL}}{\text{hr}}$

c. Estimate equals answer

560   **ANSWER KEYS**

8 a. 50 g

$$\text{g glucose}: \frac{5\text{ g}}{\cancel{100\text{ mL}}} \times \frac{\cancel{1000\text{ mL}}^{10}}{1} = 50\text{ g glucose}$$

b. Equation is balanced. Only g remain.

9 a. $\frac{1}{2}$ of 4 mL per hr = 2 mL per hr

50% = 0.5 or $\frac{1}{2}$

$$\frac{\text{mL}}{\text{hr}} : \frac{\cancel{4}^{2}\text{ mL}}{\text{hr}} \times \frac{1}{\cancel{2}_{1}} = \frac{2\text{ mL}}{\text{hr}}$$

b. Estimate equals answer.

10 a. Short-, intermediate-, and long-acting commerical preparations

Note: Endogenous insulin refers to insulin produced by the individual's own beta cells. Exogenous and endogenous insulin can be differentiated by a C peptide assay test.

b. Glucose, followed by a complex carbohydrate

Chapter 12

RAPID PRACTICE 12-1 (p. 396)

1	4	**4**	1
2	1	**5**	3
3	1		

RAPID PRACTICE 12-2 (p. 396)

1	3	**4**	3
2	4	**5**	3
3	4		

RAPID PRACTICE 12-3 (p. 398)

1 a

2 23-29 seconds (2 × 11.5 seconds and 2.5 × 11.5 seconds)

3 a

4 a. 2

b. 0.2 mL

$$\frac{\text{mL}}{\text{dose}} : \frac{1\text{ mL}}{\cancel{10\text{ mg}}_{5}} \times \frac{\cancel{2\text{ mg}}^{1}}{\text{dose}} = \frac{0.2\text{ mL}}{\text{dose}}$$

Equation is balanced. Only mL remain.

5 a. one half tablet using a pill cutter

b. 2.5 mg

RAPID PRACTICE 12-4 (p. 403)

1 1 mL

2 10 units per mL

3 maintain patency of venous access devices

4 SASH includes Heparin in addition to saline

5 10,000 units per mL

6 1:1000 (one part drug per 1000 mL)

7 10,000 units per mL

➤ Understanding questions 5, 6, and 7 is critical for patient safety.

8 bleeding or hemorrhage

9 20,000 to 40,000 units

10 of possible adverse interactions

RAPID PRACTICE 12-5 (p. 406)

1 Thrombocytopenia predisposes to bleeding. The addition of heparin would increase the risk.

2 a. 10 mL per hr

$$\frac{mL}{hr} : \frac{\overset{1}{\cancel{250}}\ mL}{\underset{\underset{1}{\cancel{100}}}{\cancel{25{,}000}\ \text{units}}} \times \frac{\overset{10}{\cancel{1000}\ \text{units}}}{1} = \frac{10\ mL}{hr}$$

b. Equation is balanced. Only mL per hr remains.

3 a. 45 to 75 seconds $(1.5 \times 30 = 45\ \text{seconds})\,(2.5 \times 30 = 75\ \text{seconds})$
b. Yes
c. No. Between 45 and 75, no adjustment is necessary.
d. N/A

4 a. 45 to 75 seconds
b. No
c. Yes. The units per hr need to be reduced by 1 unit per kg per hr.
d. 80 units per hr

$$\frac{\text{units}}{hr} : \frac{1\ \text{unit}}{1\ \cancel{kg}} \times \frac{80\ \cancel{kg}}{hr} = 80\ \text{units reduction per hour}$$

$$1000\ \text{units} - 80\ \text{units} = 920\ \text{units rounded to}\ \frac{900\ \text{units}}{hr}$$

e. Yes
f. 9 mL per hr

$$\frac{mL}{hr} : \frac{\overset{1}{\cancel{250}}\ mL}{\underset{\underset{1}{\cancel{100}}}{\cancel{25{,}000}\ \text{units}}} \times \frac{\overset{9}{\cancel{900}\ \text{units}}}{1} = \frac{9\ mL}{hr}$$

5 a. 1600

$$\frac{\text{units}}{hr} : \frac{\overset{50}{\cancel{12{,}500}}\ \text{units}}{\underset{1}{\cancel{250}\ \cancel{mL}}} \times \frac{32\ \cancel{mL}}{hr} = \frac{1600\ \text{units}}{hr}$$

b. Flow rate is correct.
c. Yes $(1600 \times 24 = 38{,}400\ \text{units in } 24\ \text{hr})$.

1 a. 1100 units per hr (1080, rounded to 1100)
 b. 22 mL per hr

$$\frac{mL}{hr} : \frac{\overset{1}{\cancel{500}} \, mL}{\underset{50}{\cancel{25,000} \, \cancel{units}}} \times \frac{1100 \, \cancel{units}}{1} = \frac{22 \, mL}{hr}$$

 c. Equation is balanced. Only mL per hr remains.

2 a. bleeding
 b. 1100 units (1080, rounded to 1100)
 c. 550 units
 d. 5.5 mg

$$mg : \frac{1 \, mg}{\underset{1}{\cancel{100 \, units}}} \times \frac{\overset{5.5}{\cancel{550 \, units}}}{1} = 5.5 \, mg \text{ protamine sulfate}$$

 e. Equation is balanced. Only mg remain.

3 a. 0.6 mL

$$\frac{mL}{dose} : \frac{1 \, mL}{10 \, mg} \times \frac{5.5 \, mg}{1} = 0.55 \, mL, \text{ rounded to } \frac{0.6 \, mL}{dose}$$

 b. Equation is balanced. Only mL remain.

4 a. half of 0.2 mL = 0.1 mL

 b. $$\frac{mL}{dose} : \frac{0.2 \, mL}{\underset{2}{\cancel{5000 \, units}}} \times \frac{\overset{1}{\cancel{2500 \, units}}}{dose} = \frac{0.2}{2} = \frac{0.1 \, mL}{dose}$$

 c. Equation is balanced. Estimate supports answer.

5 a. 55 (110 ÷ 2)

$$kg : \frac{1 \, kg}{\underset{1}{\cancel{2.2 \, lb}}} \times \frac{\overset{50}{\cancel{110 \, lb}}}{1} = 50 \, kg$$

 b. Equation is balanced. Estimate supports answer.
 c. 4000 units

$$units : \frac{80 \, units}{1 \, \cancel{kg}} \times 50 \, \cancel{kg} = 4000 \, units$$

 d. Equation is balanced. Only units remain.
 e. less than 1 mL

$$\frac{mL}{dose} : \frac{0.2 \, mL}{\underset{5}{\cancel{5000 \, units}}} \times \overset{4}{\cancel{4000 \, units}} = \frac{0.8}{5} = \frac{0.16 \, mL}{dose}$$

 Note: Whether you give 0.16 or 0.2 mL depends on the calibration of the available syringe and agency and prescriber protocols.

 f. Equation is balanced. Estimate supports answer.

CHAPTER 12 MULTIPLE-CHOICE REVIEW (p. 411)

1	4	**4**	1
2	1	**5**	2
3	3	**6**	1

CHAPTER 12 FINAL PRACTICE (p. 412)

1 a. Lower it

b. Keep all the unused dosages (prescriptions) stored separately from the current dose strength.

2 a. 2000 units per hr. The infusion rate is correct.

$$\frac{\text{units}}{\text{hr}} : \frac{\overset{100}{\cancel{25{,}000}}\text{ units}}{\underset{1}{\cancel{250\text{ mL}}}} \times \frac{20\text{ }\cancel{\text{mL}}}{\text{hr}} = \frac{2000\text{ units}}{\text{hr}}$$

b. The equation is balanced. The ordered units per hr are being infused.

3 a. 1300 units per hr

$$\frac{18\text{ units}}{1\text{ }\cancel{\text{kg}}} \times \frac{70\text{ }\cancel{\text{kg}}}{1\text{ hr}} = 1260\text{, rounded to 1300 units per hr}$$

b. Equation is balanced. Only units per hr remains.

c. 26 mL per hr

$$\frac{\text{mL}}{\text{hr}} : \frac{\overset{1}{\cancel{500}}\text{ mL}}{\underset{50}{\cancel{25{,}000}\text{ units}}} \times \frac{1300\text{ }\cancel{\text{units}}}{1} = 26\text{ mL per hr}$$

d. Equation is balanced. Only mL per hr remains.

4 a. IV rate is too slow and needs to be adjusted to 30 mL per hr. Assess patient. Document. Check agency policy for IV rate adjustments. Contact prescriber.

$$\frac{\text{mL}}{\text{hr}} : \frac{\overset{1}{\cancel{500}}\text{ mL}}{\underset{\underset{1}{50}}{\cancel{25{,}000}\text{ units}}} \times \frac{\overset{30}{\cancel{1500}\text{ units}}}{1\text{ hr}} = \frac{30\text{ mL}}{\text{hr}}$$

b. Equation is balanced. Only mL per hr remain.

5 a. LMWH

b. 0.3 mL

$$\frac{\text{mL}}{\text{dose}} : \frac{0.4\text{ mL}}{\underset{4}{\cancel{40\text{ mg}}}} \times \frac{\overset{3}{\cancel{30\text{ mg}}}}{\text{dose}} = \frac{1.2}{4} = \frac{0.3\text{ mL}}{\text{dose}}$$

c. Equation is balanced. Only mL remain.

6 a. 10 mL per hr

$$\frac{\text{mL}}{\text{hr}} : \frac{\overset{1}{\cancel{250}}\text{ mL}}{\underset{\underset{1}{100}}{\cancel{25{,}000}\text{ units}}} \times \frac{\overset{10}{\cancel{1000}\text{ units}}}{\text{hr}} = \frac{10\text{ mL}}{\text{hr}}$$

b. Equation is balanced. Only mL per hr remains.

c. The aPTT is too low at 40 seconds. Rate needs to be increased by 3 units per kg per hr

d. 200 units increase per hr

$$\frac{\text{units}}{\text{hr}} : \frac{3\text{ units}}{1\text{ }\cancel{\text{kg}}} \times \frac{70\text{ }\cancel{\text{kg}}}{1\text{ hr}} = 210\text{ units per hr increase needed}$$
(rounded to 200 units increase per hr)

e. Equation is balanced. Only units per hr remains.

f. 12 mL per hr

$$\frac{mL}{hr} : \frac{\overset{1}{\cancel{250}} \, mL}{\underset{\underset{1}{\cancel{100}}}{\cancel{25,000} \, units}} \times \frac{\overset{12}{\cancel{1200} \, units}}{hr} = \frac{12 \, mL}{hr}$$

g. Equation is balanced. Only mL per hr remains. Flow rate needs to be increased to 12 mL per hr.

7 a. No adjustment is needed.

 b. N/A

8 a. 2000 units per hr

$$\frac{units}{hr} : \frac{\overset{50}{\cancel{25,000}} \, units}{\underset{1}{\cancel{500} \, mL}} \times \frac{40 \, \cancel{mL}}{1 \, hr} = \frac{2000 \, units}{hr}$$

 b. Equation is balanced. Only units per hr remains.

 c. No. 48,000 units for 24 hours (2000 units × 24) exceeds recommendations for up to 40,000 units per 24 hr. Contact prescriber promptly about the order and document the response.

9 a. 24 mL per hr

$$\frac{mL}{hr} : \frac{\overset{1}{\cancel{500}} \, mL}{\underset{50}{\cancel{25,000} \, units}} \times \frac{\overset{12}{\cancel{1200} \, units}}{hr} = \frac{1200}{50} = \frac{24 \, mL}{hr}$$

 b. Monitor for bleeding

10 a. "Delayed coagulation," "delayed clotting time," an effect of anticoagulants

 b. It is a high-risk drug with potential for serious adverse effects of bleeding and hemorrhage. An infusion pump delivers a controlled rate.

Chapter 13

RAPID PRACTICE 13-1 (p. 419)

1 Fractional

2 SDR

3 mg per kg

4 mg per kg; mcg per kg; g per kg, mg per m^2; mcg per m^2

5 m^2 (square meters)

RAPID PRACTICE 13-2 (p. 421)

1 1000 mcg = 1 mg

2 Adult—once a day at bedtime; child—every 6 hours

3 Child with postoperative pain: 0.04 mg per kg per hr; child with chronic cancer pain: 2.6 mg per kg per hr

4 Child over 10 years—12 mcg per kg; premature infant—25 mcg per kg

Note: As the weight and age groups increase, the number of mcg per kg decreases for the drug schedule.

5 Contact prescriber.

RAPID PRACTICE 13-3 (p. 422)

1 a. 12 ÷ 2 = approximately 6 kg

  b. 5.5 kg

    lb : $\dfrac{1 \text{ lb}}{16 \text{ oz}} \times 3 \text{ oz} = \dfrac{3}{16} = 0.18$, rounded to 0.2 lb

    0.2 lb + 12 lb = 12.2 lb

    kg : $\dfrac{1 \text{ kg}}{2.2 \text{ lb}} \times 12.2 \text{ lb} = 5.5$ kg

  c. Estimate supports answer. Equation is balanced.

2 a. 20 ÷ 2 = approximately 10 kg

  b. 9.3 kg

    lb : $\dfrac{1 \text{ lb}}{16 \text{ oz}} \times \dfrac{6 \text{ oz}}{1} = 0.375$, rounded to 0.4 lb

    kg : $\dfrac{1 \text{ kg}}{2.2 \text{ lb}} \times \dfrac{20.4 \text{ lb}}{1} = 9.3$ kg

  c. Estimate supports answer. Equation is balanced.

3 a. 4 ÷ 2 = approximately 2 kg

  b. 2 kg

    lb : $\dfrac{1 \text{ lb}}{16 \text{ oz}} \times \dfrac{8 \text{ oz}}{1} = 0.5$ lb

    kg : $\dfrac{1 \text{ kg}}{2.2 \text{ lb}} \times \dfrac{4.5 \text{ lb}}{1} = 2.04$, rounded to 2 kg

  c. Equation is balanced. Estimate supports answer.

4 a. 25 ÷ 2 = approximately 12.5 kg

  b. 11.6 kg

    lb : $\dfrac{1 \text{ lb}}{16 \text{ oz}} \times 9 \text{ oz} = \dfrac{9}{16} = 0.56$, rounded to 0.6 lb

    kg : $\dfrac{1 \text{ kg}}{2.2 \text{ lb}} \times 25.6 \text{ lb} = 11.63$, rounded to 11.6 kg

  c. Equation is balanced. Estimate supports answer.

5 a. 18 ÷ 2 = approximately 9 kg

  b. 8.5 kg

    lb : $\dfrac{1 \text{ lb}}{16 \text{ oz}} \times \dfrac{12 \text{ oz}}{1} = 0.75$, rounded 0.8 lb

    kg : $\dfrac{1 \text{ kg}}{2.2 \text{ lb}} \times \dfrac{18.8 \text{ lb}}{1} = 8.54$, rounded to 8.5 kg

  c. Equation is balanced. Equation supports answer.

RAPID PRACTICE 13-4 (p. 424)

1 a. (66 lb ÷ 2); 33 kg; kg = $\dfrac{1 \text{ kg}}{2.2 \text{ lb}} \times 66 \text{ lb} = 30$ kg

  b. SDR: 300-600 mcg per hr

    $\dfrac{\text{mcg}}{\text{hr}} : \dfrac{10 \text{ mcg}}{1 \text{ kg} \times \text{hr}} \times \dfrac{30 \text{ kg}}{1} = 300$ mcg per hr low safe dose

566   ANSWER KEYS

$$\text{mcg}: \frac{20 \text{ mcg}}{1 \text{ kg} \times \text{hr}} \times \frac{30 \text{ kg}}{1} = 600 \text{ mcg per hr high safe dose}$$

   c. Dose ordered 500 mcg per hr is within SDR. Safe to give.

2 a. 6 kg (12 ÷ 2); $\text{kg}: \frac{1 \text{ kg}}{2.2 \text{ lb}} \times \frac{12 \text{ lb}}{1} = 5.45$, rounded to 5.5 kg actual weight

   Note: kg are usually calculated to the nearest tenth.

   b. SDR 1100-2750 mcg per day

$$\frac{\text{mcg}}{\text{day}}: \frac{200 \text{ mcg}}{1 \text{ kg} \times \text{day}} \times \frac{5.5 \text{ kg}}{1} = 1100 \text{ mcg per day low safe dose}$$

$$\frac{\text{mcg}}{\text{day}}: \frac{500 \text{ mcg}}{1 \text{ kg} \times \text{day}} \times \frac{5.5 \text{ kg}}{1} = 2750 \text{ mcg per day high safe dose}$$

   c. Hold and contact prescriber promptly. Overdose. Order is 15,000 mcg per day.

3 a. SDR: 1-1.5 g in four divided doses
   b. Ordered 250 mg × 4 = 1000 mg = 1 g per day
   c. Safe to give. Order is within SDR.

4 a. 22 ÷ 2 = 11 kg; actual weight: 10 kg

$$\text{kg}: \frac{1 \text{ kg}}{2.2 \text{ lb}} \times \frac{22 \text{ lb}}{1} = 10 \text{ kg}$$

   b. SDR: 5000-8000 mcg per day in 4-6 divided doses

$$\frac{\text{mcg}}{\text{day}}: \frac{500 \text{ mcg}}{1 \text{ kg} \times \text{day}} \times \frac{10 \text{ kg}}{1} = 5000 \text{ mcg per day low safe dose}$$

$$\frac{\text{mcg}}{\text{day}}: \frac{800 \text{ mcg}}{1 \text{ kg} \times \text{day}} \times \frac{10 \text{ kg}}{1} = 8000 \text{ mcg per day high safe dose}$$

   c. Safe to give (2 mg = 2000 mcg). Order is 2 mg four times a day (or 8000 mcg per day).

5 a. 10 kg; actual weight: 9.2 kg

$$\text{lb}: \frac{1 \text{ lb}}{\underset{4}{16 \text{ oz}}} \times \frac{\overset{1}{4 \text{ oz}}}{1} = 0.25, \text{ rounded to 0.3 lb} = \frac{1}{4} = 0.25 \text{ lb}$$

$$\text{kg}: \frac{1 \text{ kg}}{2.2 \text{ lb}} \times \frac{20.3 \text{ lb}}{1} = \frac{20.3}{2.2} = 9.2 \text{ kg}$$

   b. SDR = 9.2-27.6 mg per day. 9.2 mg per day low safe dose

$$\text{SDR}: \frac{\text{mg}}{\text{day}}: \frac{3 \text{ mg}}{\text{kg}} \times \frac{9.2 \text{ kg}}{1} = 27.6 \text{ mg per day high safe dose}$$

   c. Hold and contact prescriber promptly. Ordered dose of 35 mg exceeds SDR.

RAPID PRACTICE 13-5 (p. 427)

1 a. 0.27 m²

   b. $\text{units}: \frac{20,000 \text{ units}}{1 \text{ m}^2} \times \frac{0.27 \text{ m}^2}{\text{dose}} = 5400 \text{ units every 24 hr}$

   c. Safe to give. The order is within in SDR (5400 ÷ 24 = 225 units per hr).

2 a. 0.6 m²

   b. 0.9-1.2 mg

$$\frac{\text{mg}}{\text{week}}: \frac{1.5 \text{ mg}}{1 \text{ m}^2 \times \text{week}} \times \frac{0.6 \text{ m}^2}{1} = 0.9 \text{ mg low safe dose once a week}$$

$$\frac{mg}{week} : \frac{2\ mg}{1\ \cancel{m^2} \times week} \times \frac{0.6\ \cancel{m^2}}{1} = 1.2\ mg\ high\ safe\ dose\ once\ a\ week$$

    c. Safe to give. The order is within SDR.

3 a. 1.10 m²

    b. $\dfrac{mg}{dose} : \dfrac{3.3\ mg}{1\ \cancel{m^2}} \times \dfrac{1.10\ \cancel{m^2}}{dose} = 3.6\ mg\ safe\ daily\ dose$

    c. Unsafe order. Overdose. Call prescriber promptly. Document.

4 a. BSA is not needed. The SDR is not based on m² of BSA.

    b. 100-125 mg every 8 hr

$$\frac{mg}{dose} : \frac{2\ mg}{1\ \cancel{kg}} \times \frac{50\ \cancel{kg}}{dose} = 100\ mg\ low\ safe\ dose$$

$$\frac{mg}{dose} : \frac{2.5\ mg}{1\ \cancel{kg}} \times \frac{50\ \cancel{kg}}{dose} = 125\ mg\ high\ safe\ dose$$

    c. Order is safe. It is within SDR.

5 a. B.S.A is not needed. The SDR is not based on m² of BSA.

    b. 5-25 mcg per min

$$\frac{mcg}{min} : \frac{1\ mcg}{1\ \cancel{kg} \times min} \times \frac{5\ \cancel{kg}}{1} = 5\ mcg\ per\ min\ low\ safe\ dose$$

$$\frac{mcg}{min} : \frac{5\ mcg}{1\ \cancel{kg} \times min} \times \frac{5\ \cancel{kg}}{1} = 25\ mcg\ per\ min\ high\ safe\ dose$$

    c. Safe to give. The order is within SDR.

RAPID PRACTICE 13-6 (p. 430)

1 a. 410-820 mg per day.

$$kg : \frac{1\ kg}{2.2\ \cancel{lb}} \times \frac{36\ \cancel{lb}}{1} = 16.36,\ rounded\ to\ 16.4\ kg$$

$$\frac{mg}{day} : \frac{25\ mg}{1\ \cancel{kg} \times day} \times \frac{16.4\ \cancel{kg}}{1} = 410\ mg\ low\ safe\ dose\ per\ day$$

$$\frac{mg}{day} : \frac{50\ mg}{1\ \cancel{kg} \times day} \times \frac{16.4\ \cancel{kg}}{1} = 820\ mg\ high\ safe\ dose\ per\ day$$

    b. Safe to give. Order of 150 mg 4 × daily is within SDR.

    c. $\dfrac{mg}{container} : \dfrac{125\ mg}{\cancel{5\ mL}} \times \dfrac{\overset{12}{\cancel{60\ mL}}}{container} = 1500\ mg\ total\ in\ container$

    d. Add 36 mL in 2 portions; shake well after each addition.

    e. 6 mL

$$\frac{mL}{dose} : \frac{\overset{1}{\cancel{5\ mL}}}{\underset{\underset{1}{25}}{\cancel{125\ mg}}} \times \frac{\overset{6}{\cancel{150\ mg}}}{dose} = \frac{6\ mL}{dose}$$

2 a. $SDR : \dfrac{10\ mg}{1\ \cancel{m^2}} \times \dfrac{1.10\ \cancel{m^2}}{dose} = 11\ mg\ safe\ dose$

    b. Hold and clarify promptly. Ordered dose exceeds safe dose recommendation.

    c. N/A

    d. N/A

3 a. SDR : 15 mg per kg per day

44 lb ÷ 2.2 = 20 kg

$$\frac{mg}{day} : \frac{15\ mg}{1\ \cancel{kg} \times day} \times \frac{20\ \cancel{kg}}{1} = 300\ mg\ per\ day\ divided\ into\ two\ 150\ mg\ doses$$

b. Safe to give

c. Reconstitute with 55 mL of water in two portions. Shake after each addition.

d. 6 mL

$$\frac{mL}{dose} : \frac{5\ mL}{\underset{5}{\cancel{125\ mg}}} \times \overset{6}{\cancel{150\ mg}} = \frac{30}{5} = \frac{6\ mL}{dose}$$

4 a. 0.12-0.24 mg per day

$$\frac{mg}{day} : \frac{0.006\ mg}{1\ \cancel{kg} \times day} \times \frac{18\ \cancel{kg}}{1} = 0.1\ mg\ low\ safe\ dose\ per\ day$$

$$\frac{mg}{day} : \frac{0.012\ mg}{1\ \cancel{kg} \times day} \times \frac{18\ \cancel{kg}}{1} = 0.2\ mg\ high\ safe\ dose\ per\ day$$

b. Order of 0.1 mg bid is within safe dose range and frequency.

c. 2 mL (2 × 0.05 = 0.1 mg)

$$\frac{mL}{dose} : \frac{1\ mL}{0.05\ \cancel{mg}} \times \frac{0.1\ \cancel{mg}}{dose} = \frac{0.1}{0.05} = \frac{2\ mL}{dose}$$

d. 50 mcg per mL

Note: Microgram is abbreviated μg on the label. Use mcg in your written records.

5 a. 18.2 mg safe total daily dose

20 lb = 9.1 kg

$$\frac{mg}{day} : \frac{2\ mg}{1\ \cancel{kg} \times day} \times \frac{9.1\ \cancel{kg}}{1} = 18.2\ mg\ per\ day$$

b. Hold. Order exceeds daily safe dose.

c. N/A

RAPID PRACTICE 13-7 (p. 435)

1 a. 0.2 mg

$$\frac{mg}{dose} : \frac{0.01\ mg}{1\ \cancel{kg}} \times \frac{22.9\ \cancel{kg}}{dose} = 0.229,\ rounded\ to\ 0.2\ mg\ per\ dose$$

b. Safe to give

c. 0.5 mL

$$\frac{mL}{dose} : \frac{1\ mL}{\underset{2}{\cancel{0.4\ mg}}} \times \overset{1}{\cancel{0.2\ mg}} = \frac{0.5\ mL}{dose}$$

d. Equation is balanced. Only mL remain.

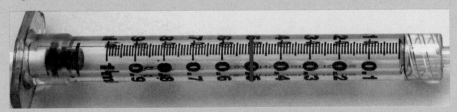

2 a. SDR for this child 2-5 mg once a week

b. Safe to give. Order is within SDR.

c. Give 0.4 mL.

$$\frac{mL}{dose} : \frac{1\ mL}{\underset{5}{\cancel{10\ mg}}} \times \frac{\overset{2}{\cancel{4\ mg}}}{dose} = 0.4\ mL\ per\ dose$$

d. Estimate of less than 0.5 mL supports answer. Equation is balanced.

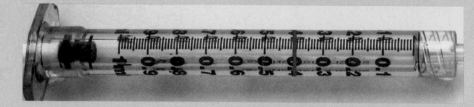

3 a. 2-4 units

b. Safe to give; within safe dose range.

c.

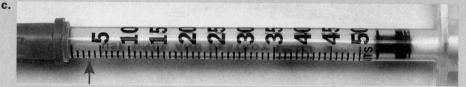

d. Yes. Bedtime snacks needed for long-acting, intermediate, and evening insulin administration to avoid hypoglycemic events during sleep.

4 a. 0.3-0.9 mg per dose

$$kg : \frac{1\ kg}{2.2\ \cancel{lb}} \times \frac{66\ \cancel{lb}}{1} = 30\ kg$$

$30 \times 0.01 = 0.3\ mg;\ 30 \times 0.03 = 0.9\ mg$

b. Hold and clarify promptly with prescriber. Overdose ordered.

c. If the drug were safe to give, Adrenalin (upper label) 1:1000 is the correct concentration for this order.

d. The 1:1000 solution is 10 times more concentrated than 1:10,000.

e. N/A

5 a.

$$kg : \frac{1\ kg}{2.2\ \cancel{lb}} \times \frac{44\ \cancel{lb}}{1} = 20\ kg$$

$$\frac{mg}{dose} : \frac{0.5\ mg}{1\ \cancel{kg} \times dose} \times \frac{20\ \cancel{kg}}{1} = \frac{10\ mg}{dose}$$

b. Safe to give

c. 0.33 mL

$$\frac{mL}{dose} : \frac{mL}{\underset{3}{\cancel{30\ mg}}} \times \frac{\overset{1}{\cancel{10\ mg}}}{dose} = \frac{0.33\ mL}{dose}$$

d. Equation is balanced. Only mL remain.

e. Grain (gr) is an outdated apothecary unit of measurement. Use mg.

RAPID PRACTICE 13-8 (p. 443)

2 a. $20 - 10 = 10$ mL diluent

b. 10 mL

c. 40 mL per hr

$$\frac{mL}{hr} : \frac{20\ mL}{\underset{1}{\cancel{30\ min}}} \times \frac{\overset{2}{\cancel{60\ min}}}{1\ hr} = \frac{40\ mL}{hr}$$

570   ANSWER KEYS

d. Equation is balanced. Only $\dfrac{\text{mL}}{\text{hr}}$ remain.

3 a. $50 - 25 = 25$ mL

  b. 25 mL

  c. 50 drops per min (drops per min = mL per hr on a microdrip set)

4 a. $30 - 15 = 15$ mL

  b. 15 mL

  c. 90 mL per hr will deliver 30 mL in 20 min. (There are three 20-minute periods in 1 hr).

5 a. 3 mL

  b. 30 drops per min

$$\frac{\text{drops}}{\text{min}} : \frac{\overset{2}{\cancel{60}}\,\text{drops}}{1\,\cancel{\text{mL}}} \times \frac{15\,\cancel{\text{mL}}}{\underset{1}{\cancel{30}}\,\text{min}} = \frac{30\,\text{drops}}{\text{minute}}$$

  c. Only drops per min remain to be infused when the minutes are less than 1 hr; mL will not equal drops per minute.

RAPID PRACTICE 13-9 (p. 445)

1 a. $5\,\text{mcg} \times 60\,\text{min} = 300$ mcg per hr

  b. 10 mg = 10,000 mcg (1000 mcg = 1 mg)

  c. 40 mcg per mL

$$\frac{\text{mcg}}{\text{mL}} : \frac{10,000\,\text{mcg}}{250\,\text{mL}} = \frac{40\,\text{mcg}}{\text{mL}}$$

  d. Equation is balanced. Only mcg per mL remains.

  e. 8 mL per hr

$$\frac{\text{mL}}{\text{hr}} : \frac{\overset{1}{\cancel{250}}\,\text{mL}}{\underset{1}{\cancel{10}}\,\text{mg}} \times \frac{1\,\cancel{\text{mg}}}{\underset{4}{\cancel{1000}}\,\cancel{\text{mcg}}} \times \frac{5\,\cancel{\text{mcg}}}{1\,\cancel{\text{min}}} \times \frac{\overset{6}{\cancel{60}}\,\cancel{\text{min}}}{1\,\text{hr}} = \frac{15}{2} = 7.5,\ \text{rounded to}\ 8\ \text{mL per hr}$$

  f. Equation is balanced. Only mL per hr remains.

2 a. 16 mL (8 mL × 2 hr)

  b. 12 mL per hr

$$\frac{\text{mL}}{\text{hr}} : \frac{\overset{1}{\cancel{250}}\,\text{mL}}{\underset{1}{\cancel{10}}\,\text{mg}} \times \frac{1\,\cancel{\text{mg}}}{\underset{4}{\cancel{1000}}\,\cancel{\text{mcg}}} \times \frac{\overset{2}{\cancel{8}}\,\cancel{\text{mcg}}}{1\,\cancel{\text{min}}} \times \frac{\overset{6}{\cancel{60}}\,\cancel{\text{min}}}{1\,\text{hr}} = 12\ \text{mL per hr}$$

  c. Equation is balanced. Only mL per hr remain.

  Note: It should be estimated that the flow rate would be increased from 8 mL per hr in problem 1, but not doubled.

3 a. SDR: 4.5-18 mg per dose $(0.5 \times 9)(2 \times 9)$

  b. Hold and contact prescriber immediately. Dose ordered exceeds the SDR by 7 mg.

  c. N/A

  d. N/A

4 a. SDR:

$$\frac{3\,\text{mEq}}{1\,\cancel{\text{kg}}} \times \frac{8\,\cancel{\text{kg}}}{1} = 24\ \text{mEq q24h for this baby}$$

  b. $\dfrac{\text{mEq}}{\text{day}} : \dfrac{0.1\,\text{mEq}}{1\,\cancel{\text{kg}} \times \cancel{\text{hr}}} \times \dfrac{8\,\cancel{\text{kg}}}{1} \times \dfrac{24\,\cancel{\text{hr}}}{1\,\text{day}} = 19.2$ mEq per day ordered

c. Order is within SDR. Safe to give.

d. 8 mL per hr

$$\frac{mL}{hr} : \frac{\overset{10}{\cancel{100}} \text{ mL}}{\underset{1}{\cancel{10 \text{ mEq}}}} \times \frac{0.1 \text{ } \cancel{mEq}}{1 \text{ } \cancel{kg} \times hr} \times \frac{8 \text{ } \cancel{kg}}{1} = 8 \text{ mL per hr}$$

e. Equation is balanced. Only mL per hr remains.

5 a. 6.6 kg

$$\frac{1 \text{ kg}}{2.2 \text{ } \cancel{lb}} \times \frac{14.5 \text{ } \cancel{lb}}{1} = 6.6 \text{ kg}$$

Note: Remember to change oz (8) to lb (0.5) before solving equation.

b. SDR: 6.6-19.8 mg (1 × 6.6) (3 × 6.6)

c. Hold and clarify promptly with prescriber. Ordered dose of 50 mg exceeds SDR.

d. N/A

e. N/A

CHAPTER 13 MULTIPLE-CHOICE REVIEW (p. 447)

1 4 (essential foods)   **6** 1

2 3   **7** 2

3 2   **8** 4

4 3   **9** 2 (pediatric [microdrip] set)

5 1 (Check agency polices.)   **10** 2

CHAPTER 13 FINAL PRACTICE (p. 449)

1 a. 5 mL (1 teaspoon)

b. popsicle

2 a. 760 mg to 1520 mg per day divided in 2 doses

b. Hold and clarify promptly with prescriber. A 2000 g per day order is an overdose and exceeds the required frequency.

c. N/A

d. N/A

3 a. 60 mg per day

$$\frac{mg}{day} : \frac{100 \text{ mg}}{1 \text{ m}^2 \times day} \times \frac{0.6 \text{ m}^2}{1} = \frac{60 \text{ mg}}{day}$$

b. Hold and clarify promptly with prescriber. Order is greater than SDR.

c. N/A

d. N/A

4 a. 2.5 mL

$$mL : \frac{1 \text{ mL}}{\underset{2}{\cancel{100,000 \text{ units}}}} \times \frac{\overset{5}{\cancel{250,000 \text{ units}}}}{dose} = 2.5 \text{ mL total dose}$$

b. Order is safe.

c. Needleless syringe or calibrated dropper

d. Place 1.25 mL on each side in the mouth of the child.

5 a. Label B, infant preparation; enclosed dropper

b. Yes, it is safe. 1.6 mL

c. 32 mg per mL (160 mg per 5 mL); measuring cup

d. 80 mg per 0.8 mL; equal to 100 mg per mL

e. The infant preparation is much more concentrated. This reduces the volume of mL for the infant.

6 a. 20 to 40 mg every 4 to 6 hours

$$\text{mg}: \frac{0.5 \text{ mg}}{1 \text{ kg}} \times \frac{40 \text{ kg}}{1} = 20 \text{ mg low safe dose q4-6h}$$

$$\frac{\text{mg}}{\text{dose}}: \frac{1 \text{ mg}}{1 \text{ kg} \times \text{dose}} \times \frac{40 \text{ kg}}{1} = 40 \text{ mg high safe dose}$$

b. Safe to give; within SDR.

c. Will give less than 1 mL.

d. 0.67 mL

$$\frac{\text{mL}}{\text{dose}}: \frac{1 \text{ mL}}{\overset{}{\underset{3}{30 \text{ mg}}}} \times \frac{\overset{2}{20 \text{ mg}}}{\text{dose}} = 0.67 \text{ mL (a 1 mL syringe is calibrated in hundredths)}$$

e. Equation is balanced. Estimate supports answer.

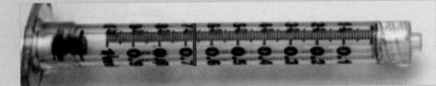

7 a. $\text{kg} = \dfrac{1 \text{ kg}}{2.2 \text{ lb}} \times \dfrac{42 \text{ lb}}{1} = 19.1 \text{ kg}$

b. 9.6-19.1 mEq per IV dose

$$\frac{\text{mEq}}{\text{dose}}: \frac{0.5 \text{ mEq}}{\text{kg} \times \text{dose}} \times \frac{19.1 \text{ kg}}{1} = 9.55 \text{ mEq rounded to 9.6 mEq low safe dose}$$

$$\frac{\text{mEq}}{\text{dose}}: \frac{1 \text{ mEq}}{\text{kg} \times \text{dose}} \times \frac{19.1 \text{ kg}}{1} = 19.1 \text{ mEq high safe dose}$$

c. 30 mEq per dose

d. Overdose. Obtain new orders promptly from prescriber.

e. N/A

f. N/A

8 a. $\text{kg}: \dfrac{1 \text{ kg}}{2.2 \text{ lb}} \times \dfrac{44 \text{ lb}}{1} = 20 \text{ kg}$

b. SDR: 0.2-0.6 mg (200-600 mcg)

0.2-0.6 mg (200-600 mcg)

0.01 × 20 = 0.2 mg low safe

0.03 × 20 = 0.6 mg high and safe dose

c. 500 mcg

d. Safe to give; within SDR.

e. more than 1 mL

f. 1.3 mL

$$\frac{\text{mL}}{\text{dose}}: \frac{\text{mL}}{\overset{}{\underset{4}{400 \text{ mcg}}}} \times \frac{\overset{5}{500 \text{ mcg}}}{1} = 1.25 \text{ mL, rounded to 1.3 mL per dose}$$

g. Equation is balanced. Only mL remain.

9 a. SDR: $\dfrac{40 \text{ mg}}{1 \text{ kg} \times \text{day}} \times \dfrac{35 \text{ kg}}{1} = 1400$ mg per day

   b. Hold medication and contact prescriber promptly. Order exceeds SDR for dose and frequency. Order of 3 g exceeds SDR for dose and frequency.

   c. N/A

10 a. 11.1 kg

   24 lb 6 oz = 24.4 lb

   6 oz ÷ 16 = 0.38, rounded to 0.4 lb

   kg : $\dfrac{1 \text{ kg}}{2.2 \text{ lb}} \times \dfrac{24.4 \text{ lb}}{1} = 11.09$, rounded to 11.1 kg

   b. 83.3 mcg − 133.2 mcg ÷ 2

   11.1 × 7.5 = 83.3 mcg (0.08 mg ÷ 2 = 0.04 mg)

   11.1 × 12 = 133.2 mcg (0.13 mg ÷ 2 = 0.07 mg)

   c. 0.5 mg

   d. Hold. Overdose. Contact prescriber promptly

   e. N/A

Multiple-Choice Final Review: Chapters 1-13 (p. 456)

1	3	19	4
2	4	20	1
3	2	21	3
4	4	22	3
5	3	23	4
6	4	24	1 (5 g per 100 mL)
7	3	25	3 (5 g per 100 mL)
8	4	26	4
9	1	27	4
10	2	28	2
11	3	29	1
12	1	30	4
13	2	31	3
14	4	32	2
15	2	33	2
16	4	34	3
17	2	35	3
18	1		

Comprehensive Final Practice: Chapters 1-13 (p. 461)

1 a. 2 tabs (5 × 2 = 10 mg)

$$\dfrac{\text{tab}}{\text{dose}} : \dfrac{1}{\overset{}{\underset{1}{8}}} \times \dfrac{\overset{2}{\cancel{10}}}{\text{dose}} = 2 \text{ tabs}$$

b. $\dfrac{\text{tab}}{\text{dose}} : \dfrac{1 \text{ tab}}{\overset{}{\underset{1}{5} \text{ mg}}} \times \dfrac{\overset{2}{\cancel{10}} \text{ mg}}{\text{dose}} = 2 \text{ tabs per dose}$

2 a. 2 tabs (0.25 × 2 = 0.5)

$$\frac{\text{tab}}{\text{dose}} : \frac{1 \text{ tab}}{\underset{1}{\cancel{0.25 \text{ mg}}}} \times \frac{\overset{2}{\cancel{0.5 \text{ mg}}}}{\text{dose}} = 2 \text{ tabs}$$

b. Estimate supports answer.

3 a. 2 tabs (0.125 × 2 = 0.25 mg = 250 mcg)

$$\frac{\text{tab}}{\text{dose}} : \frac{1 \text{ tab}}{\underset{1}{\cancel{125 \text{ mcg}}}} \times \frac{\overset{2}{\cancel{250 \text{ mcg}}}}{\text{dose}} = \frac{2 \text{ tabs}}{\text{dose}}$$

b. Estimate supports answer.

c. digoxin

4 a. 2 tabs

$$\frac{\text{tab}}{\text{dose}} : \frac{1 \text{ tab}}{\underset{3}{\cancel{750 \text{ mg}}}} \times \frac{\overset{4}{\cancel{1000 \text{ mg}}}}{1 \cancel{\text{ g}}} \times \frac{1.5 \cancel{\text{ g}}}{\text{dose}} = \frac{6}{3} = \frac{2 \text{ tabs}}{\text{dose}}$$

b. Estimate supports answer.

c. ciprofloxacin hydrochloride

5 a. 1 tab

$$\frac{\text{tab}}{\text{dose}} : \frac{1 \text{ tab}}{0.5 \cancel{\text{ mg}}} \times \frac{1 \cancel{\text{ mg}}}{\underset{2}{\cancel{1000 \text{ mcg}}}} \times \frac{\overset{1}{\cancel{500 \text{ mcg}}}}{\text{dose}} = \frac{1 \text{ tab}}{\text{dose}}$$

b. Estimate supports answer.

6 Label B, Cardizem SR

a. 2 tabs

$$\frac{\text{tab}}{\text{dose}} : \frac{1 \text{ tab}}{60 \cancel{\text{ mg}}} \times \frac{1000 \cancel{\text{ mg}}}{1 \cancel{\text{ g}}} \times \frac{0.12 \cancel{\text{ g}}}{\text{dose}} = \frac{120}{60} = \frac{2 \text{ tabs}}{\text{dose}}$$

b. Equation is balanced. Answer equals estimate.

7 a. $\frac{1}{2}$ of 40 = 20; $\frac{1}{2}$ of 15 mL = 7.5 mL

$$\frac{\text{mL}}{\text{dose}} : \frac{15 \text{ mL}}{\underset{2}{\cancel{40 \text{ mEq}}}} \times \frac{\overset{1}{\cancel{20 \text{ mEq}}}}{\text{dose}} = \frac{15}{2} = \frac{7.5 \text{ mL}}{\text{dose}} \; \begin{array}{l}(5 \text{ mL in cup, 2.5 mL in} \\ \text{syringe})\end{array}$$

b. Estimate supports answer.

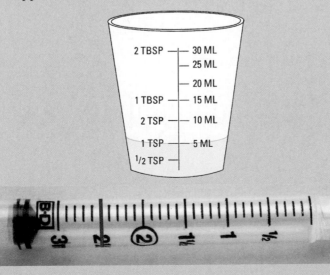

8 a. 15 mg per tab*

   b. $(\frac{1}{4}$ gr$)$

   c. $45 \div 15 = 3$ tabs

   d. $\dfrac{\text{tab}}{\text{dose}} : \dfrac{1 \text{ tab}}{\underset{1}{\cancel{15 \text{ mg}}}} \times \dfrac{\overset{3}{\cancel{45 \text{ mg}}}}{\text{dose}} = \dfrac{3 \text{ tab}}{\text{dose}}$

   e. Estimate supports answer. Recheck orders for more than 1-2 tablets.
     *Use the metric dose.

9 a. 1.5 g $= 1500$ mg $\div 500$ mg $= 3$ tabs*

    $\dfrac{\text{tab}}{\text{dose}} : \dfrac{1 \text{ tab}}{\underset{1}{\cancel{500 \text{ mg}}}} \times \dfrac{\overset{2}{\cancel{1000 \text{ mg}}}}{1 \text{ g}} \times \dfrac{1.5 \text{ g}}{\text{dose}} = \dfrac{3 \text{ tabs}}{\text{dose}}$

   b. Estimate supports answer.
     *Recheck dose order and amount when it exceeds two times the unit dose.

10 a. 100 mcg $\div 50$ mcg $= 2$ tabs

    $\dfrac{\text{tab}}{\text{dose}} : \dfrac{1 \text{ tab}}{\underset{1}{\cancel{50 \text{ mcg}}}} \times \dfrac{\overset{20}{\cancel{1000 \text{ mcg}}}}{1 \text{ mg}} \times \dfrac{0.1 \text{ mg}}{\text{dose}} = 20 \times 0.1 = \dfrac{2 \text{ tab}}{\text{dose}}$

   b. Estimate supports answer.
   c. 0.1 mg $= 100$ mcg

11 a. Give less than 1 mL.

    $\dfrac{\text{mL}}{\text{dose}} : \dfrac{1 \text{ mL}}{\underset{3}{\cancel{15 \text{ mg}}}} \times \dfrac{\overset{2}{\cancel{10 \text{ mg}}}}{\text{dose}} = \dfrac{0.67 \text{ mL}}{\text{dose}}$

   b. Estimate supports answer.

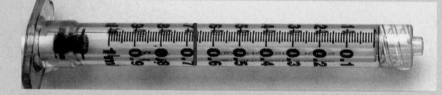

12 a. Give less than 4 mL, about one quarter less.

    $\dfrac{\text{mL}}{\text{dose}} : \dfrac{4 \text{ mL}}{\underset{4}{\cancel{40 \text{ mg}}}} \times \dfrac{\overset{3}{\cancel{30 \text{ mg}}}}{\text{dose}} = \dfrac{12}{4} = \dfrac{3 \text{ mL}}{\text{dose}}$

   b. Estimate supports answer.

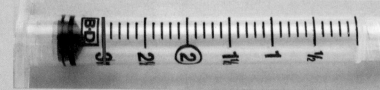

13 a. Give less than 2 mL.

    $\dfrac{\text{mL}}{\text{dose}} : \dfrac{2 \text{ mL}}{0.5 \text{ mg}} \times \dfrac{0.3 \text{ mg}}{\text{dose}} = \dfrac{0.6}{0.5} = \dfrac{1.2 \text{ mL}}{\text{dose}}$

576   **ANSWER KEYS**

b. Estimate supports answer.

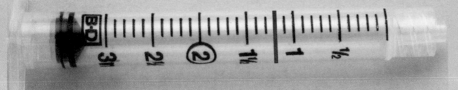

14 a. about 0.5 mL

$$\frac{mL}{dose} : \frac{1\ mL}{\underset{2}{\cancel{4\ mg}}} \times \overset{1}{\cancel{2\ mg}} = \frac{1}{2} = \frac{0.5\ mL}{dose}\ \text{Hydromorphone}$$

b. Estimate supports answer.

c. less than $\frac{1}{2}$ mL

$$\frac{mL}{dose} : \frac{mL}{\underset{5}{\cancel{50\ mg}}} \times \overset{2}{\cancel{20\ mg}} = \frac{0.4\ mL}{dose}\ \text{Promethazine}$$

d. Estimate supports answer.

e. 0.5 + 0.4 = 0.9 mL

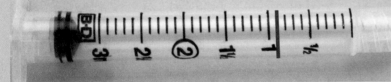

15 a. Will give slightly more than 1 mL

$$\frac{mL}{dose} : \frac{1\ mL}{\underset{3}{\cancel{300,000\ units}}} \times \overset{4}{\cancel{400,000\ units}} \frac{4}{3} = \frac{1.3\ mL}{dose}$$

b. Estimate supports answer.

16 a. Concentration after dilution is 1 g per 2.5 mL.

b. Give less than 2.5 mL.

$$\frac{mL}{dose} : \overset{0.5}{\cancel{2.5\ mL}} \times \frac{1\ \cancel{g}}{\underset{1}{\cancel{1000\ mg}}} \times \overset{3}{\cancel{600\ mg}} = \frac{1.5\ mL}{dose}$$

c. Estimate supports answer.

d. 0.5 mL (2.5 mL − 2 mL SW = 0.5 mL)

17 6 units Novolin regular insulin*

a.

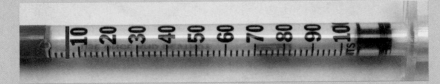

b. fast acting

c. lower

*Note that it would be easier to visualize units on a Lo-Dose insulin syringe (see problem 19 on the next page).

18 Humulin R, the fast-acting clear insulin

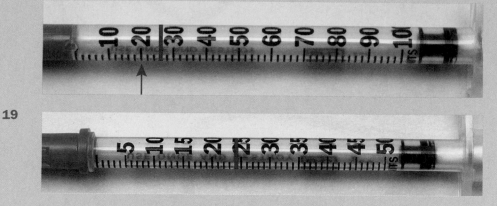

19

a. long acting (up to 24 hours)
b. A 50-unit syringe permits easier visualization and more accurate measurement of insulin doses of 50 units or less. It is calibrated for U-100 insulin (100 units per mL).

20 25 mL per hr

$$\frac{mL}{hr} : \frac{500 \text{ mL}}{\underset{20}{\cancel{20,000 \text{ units}}}} \times \frac{\overset{1}{\cancel{1000 \text{ units}}}}{1 \text{ hr}} = \frac{50\cancel{0}}{2\cancel{0}} = \frac{25 \text{ mL}}{hr}$$

a. Equation is balanced. Only mL per hr remains.
b. The aPTT must be monitored.

21 1200 units per hr

$$\frac{units}{hr} : \frac{\overset{40}{\cancel{10,000}} \text{ units}}{\underset{1}{\cancel{250 \text{ mL}}}} \times \frac{30 \text{ }\cancel{mL}}{1 \text{ hr}} = \frac{1200 \text{ units}}{hr}$$

a. Equation is balanced. Only units per hr remains.
b. hemorrhage

22 a. 7 units per hr (100 units per 100 mL is a 1:1 solution)

$$\frac{units}{hr} : \frac{\overset{1}{\cancel{100}} \text{ units}}{\underset{1}{\cancel{100 \text{ mL}}}} \times \frac{7 \text{ }\cancel{mL}}{hr} = \frac{7 \text{ units}}{hr}$$

b. Equation is balanced. Only mL per hr remains.
c. hypoglycemia

23 125 mL per hr

$$\frac{mL}{hr} : \frac{\overset{125}{\cancel{500}} \text{ mL}}{\underset{\underset{1}{4}}{\cancel{40 \text{ mEq}}}} \text{ KCl} \times \frac{\overset{1}{\cancel{10 \text{ mEq}}}}{1 \text{ hr}} = \frac{125 \text{ ml}}{hr}$$

a. Equation is balanced. Only mL per hr remains.
b. 1300 + 4 hr = 1700 hr. At 1700 the nurse needs to recheck serum K level.

$$hr : \frac{1 \text{ hr}}{10 \text{ }\cancel{mEq}} \times 40 \text{ }\cancel{mEq} = 4 \text{ hr}$$

578 A N S W E R   K E Y S

24 a. 100 mL per hr (30 min × 2 = 60 min; 50 × 2 = 100 mL per hr)

$$\frac{mL}{hr} : \frac{50\ mL}{\overset{1}{\cancel{30\ min}}} \times \frac{\overset{2}{\cancel{60\ min}}}{1\ hr} = \frac{100\ mL}{hr}$$

b. Equation is balanced. Estimate supports answer.

25 a. 90 mL per hr (there are 3 20-minute periods in an hour)

$$\frac{mL}{hr} : \frac{30\ mL}{\underset{1}{\cancel{20\ min}}} \times \frac{\overset{3}{\cancel{60\ min}}}{1\ hr} = \frac{90\ mL}{hr}$$

b. Estimate supports answer.

26 a. 20 drops per min with a DF60 set = 20 mL per hr
b. 20 drops per min

$$\frac{drops}{min} : \frac{\overset{1}{\cancel{60}}\ drops}{1\ \cancel{mL}} \times \frac{20\ \cancel{mL}}{\underset{1}{\cancel{60}}\ min} = \frac{20\ drops}{minute}$$

c. Estimate supports answer.

27 31 drops per min

$$\frac{drops}{min} : \frac{\overset{1}{\cancel{15}}\ drops}{1\ \cancel{mL}} \times \frac{\overset{125}{\cancel{500\ mL}}}{\underset{1}{\cancel{4\ hr}}} \times \frac{1\ \cancel{hr}}{\underset{4}{\cancel{60}}\ min} = \frac{125}{4} = 31.25,\ rounded\ to\ \frac{31\ drops}{minute}$$

a. Equation is balanced. Only drops per min remains.

28 a. 40 mL per hr using 2 mL of medication and 18 mL of diluent

$$\frac{mL}{hr} : \frac{20\ mL}{\underset{1}{\cancel{30\ min}}} \times \frac{\overset{2}{\cancel{60\ min}}}{1\ hr} = \frac{40\ mL}{hr}$$

b. The volume control device must be flushed with a compatible solution according to agency policies and manufacturer's recommendations.

29 150 g Dextrose

$$g\ Dextrose : \frac{15\ g}{\underset{1}{\cancel{100\ mL}}} \times \overset{10}{\cancel{1000\ mL}} = 150\ g\ of\ Dextrose$$

a. Equation is balanced. Only g remain.
b. 600 kcal CHO

$$kcal : \frac{4\ kcal}{1\ \cancel{g}} \times \frac{150\ \cancel{g}}{1} = 600\ kcal\ CHO$$

c. Equation is balanced. Only kcal remain.
d. 42.5 g amino acids

$$g\ amino\ acids : \frac{4.25\ g}{\underset{1}{\cancel{100\ mL}}} \times \frac{\overset{10}{\cancel{1000\ mL}}}{1} = 42.5\ g\ of\ amino\ acids$$

e. Equation is balanced. Only amino acids remain.

f. kcal amino acids : $\dfrac{4 \text{ kcal}}{1 \text{ \cancel{g}}} \times \dfrac{42.5 \text{ \cancel{g}}}{1} = 170$ kcal amino acids

g. Equation is balanced. Only kcal remain.

30 40 g lipids

g Lipid : $\dfrac{20 \text{ g}}{\underset{1}{\cancel{100 \text{ mL}}}} \times \dfrac{\overset{2}{\cancel{200 \text{ mL}}}}{1} = 40$ g lipids

a. Equation is balanced. Only g remain.

b. 360 kcal lipids

kcal lipids : $\dfrac{9 \text{ kcal}}{1 \text{ \cancel{g}}} \times 40 \text{ \cancel{g}} = 360$ kcal lipids

c. Equation is balanced. Only kcal remain.

31 12 mL per hr

$\dfrac{\text{mL}}{\text{hr}} : \dfrac{\overset{1}{\cancel{500}} \text{ mL}}{5 \text{ \cancel{units}}} \times \dfrac{1 \text{ \cancel{unit}}}{\underset{\frac{2}{1}}{\cancel{1000 \text{ milliunits}}}} \times \dfrac{\overset{1}{\cancel{2} \text{ \cancel{milliunits}}}}{1 \text{ \cancel{min}}} \times \dfrac{60 \text{ \cancel{min}}}{1 \text{ hr}} = \dfrac{12 \text{ mL}}{\text{hr}}$

a. Equation is balanced. Only mL per hr remains.

Note: "milli" means $\frac{1}{1000}$.

32 77 kg (154 lb ÷ 2)

a. 70 kg

$\dfrac{1 \text{ kg}}{2.2 \text{ \cancel{lb}}} \times \dfrac{154 \text{ \cancel{lb}}}{1} = 70$ kg

b. Only kg remain. Estimate supports answer.

c. $\dfrac{\text{mcg}}{\text{min}} : \dfrac{3 \text{ mcg}}{1 \text{ \cancel{kg}}} \times \dfrac{70 \text{ \cancel{kg}}}{1} = \dfrac{210 \text{ mcg}}{\text{minute}}$

d. $\dfrac{\text{mg}}{\text{min}} : 0.21$ mg per min (210 ÷ 1000)

e. $\dfrac{\text{mL}}{\text{hr}} : \dfrac{\overset{2}{\cancel{500}} \text{ mL}}{\underset{1}{\cancel{250 \text{ mg}}}} \times \dfrac{1 \text{ \cancel{mg}}}{1000 \text{ \cancel{mcg}}} \times \dfrac{210 \text{ \cancel{mcg}}}{1 \text{ \cancel{min}}} \times \dfrac{60 \text{ \cancel{min}}}{1 \text{ hr}} = \dfrac{25{,}200}{1000} = \dfrac{25.2 \text{ mL}}{\text{hour}}$

f. Equation is balanced. Only mL per hr remains.

33 a. 2 mL (5 mg × 2 = 10 mg)

$\dfrac{\text{mL}}{\text{dose}} : \dfrac{1 \text{ mL}}{\underset{1}{\cancel{5 \text{ mg}}}} \times \dfrac{\overset{2}{\cancel{10 \text{ mg}}}}{\text{dose}} = \dfrac{2 \text{ mL}}{\text{dose}}$

b. Equation is balanced. Only mL remain.

c. $\dfrac{\text{mL}}{\text{min}} : \dfrac{\overset{1}{\cancel{2}} \text{ mL}}{\underset{\frac{2}{1}}{\cancel{10 \text{ mg}}}} \times \dfrac{\overset{1}{\cancel{5 \text{ mg}}}}{1 \text{ min}} = \dfrac{1 \text{ mL}}{\text{minute}}$

d. Equation is balanced. Only mL per minute remain.

e. Total minutes = 2 ($\dfrac{1 \text{ min}}{\underset{1}{\cancel{5 \text{ mg}}}} \times \dfrac{\overset{2}{\cancel{10 \text{ mg}}}}{1} = 2$ min)

Total seconds = 120 ($\dfrac{60 \text{ sec}}{1 \text{ min}}$ × $\dfrac{2 \text{ min}}{1}$ = 120 sec)

f. $\dfrac{\text{seconds}}{\text{calibration}}$: $\dfrac{120 \text{ sec}}{10 \text{ calibrations}}$ = $\dfrac{12 \text{ sec}}{\text{calibration}}$

34 175 mg per day

$\dfrac{\text{mg}}{\text{day}}$: $\dfrac{250 \text{ mg}}{\text{mg} \times \text{day}}$ × $\dfrac{0.7 \text{ m}^2}{\text{dose}}$ = 175 mg per day safe dose

a. Equation is balanced. Only mg remain.

b. 7 mL

$\dfrac{\text{mL}}{\text{dose}}$: $\dfrac{5 \text{ mL}}{\underset{5}{\cancel{125 \text{ mg}}}}$ × $\dfrac{\overset{7}{\cancel{175 \text{ mg}}}}{1}$ = $\dfrac{35}{5}$ = $\dfrac{7 \text{ mL}}{\text{dose}}$

c. Equation is balanced. Only mL remain.

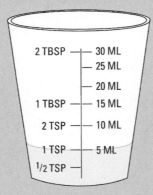

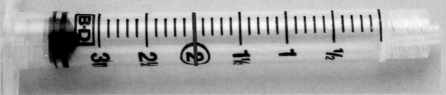

35 a. 25 kg

b. SDR:

$\dfrac{\text{units}}{\text{week}}$: $\dfrac{600 \text{ units}}{1 \cancel{\text{kg}} \times \text{week}}$ × $\dfrac{25 \cancel{\text{kg}}}{1}$ = 15,000 units per week

c. Safe order

$\dfrac{\text{mL}}{\text{dose}}$: $\dfrac{\overset{1}{\cancel{2}} \text{ mL}}{\underset{10}{\cancel{20,000 \text{ units}}}}$ × $\dfrac{\cancel{5,000 \text{ units}}}{\text{dose}}$ = 0.5 mL per dose

Apothecary System Measurements

The old, imprecise apothecary system has mostly been phased out. It has been replaced with simpler metric measurements in most health care literature, physician orders, patient records, and medication labels in order to reduce medication errors. Only a few countries in the world have not completely "metrified." Celsius temperatures, liters of gas and milk, milligrams and grams of medication, and kilograms of weight are the norm in most countries of the world.

The grains (gr) of the apothecary system (originally meant to indicate a grain of sand) have been confused with the metric gram (g; 15 gr = 1 g), resulting in medication errors. Grains are used for apothecary solid medication forms such as powders, tablets, and capsules. Whereas the metric system uses only one base measurement for liquids (the liter), the apothecary system uses several unit descriptors.

The change to the metric system has been recommended by all the major national agencies dealing with patient safety. If you come across an unfamiliar abbreviation or term (such as gr., minim, or dram), consult the pharmacy and/or the prescriber.

Use metric, but recognize apothecary!

Metric-Apothecary Conversion Clock

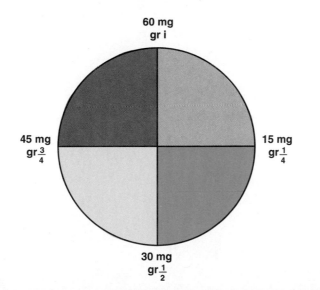

Metric, Household, and Apothecary Liquid Equivalents*

Metric	Household	Apothecary
1 mL		15-16 minims*
5 mL	1 teaspoon (tsp)	1 dram*
15 mL	1 tablespoon (tbs) (½ ounce) (oz)	4 drams* (oz ss)
30 mL	2 tablespoons (1 oz)	8 drams (oz i)
240 mL	1 measuring cup (8 oz)	8 oz (oz viii)
500 mL	1 pint (pt) (16 oz)	1 pint (16 oz)
1000 mL (1 liter)	1 quart (qt) (32 oz)	1 quart (32 oz)
4 liters	1 gallon (gal) (4 quarts)	1 gallon (4 quarts)

Note: These equivalents are approximate.
*Minims and drams are no longer used in medication orders in the United States.

Comparison of Metric and Apothecary Weights

Metric	Apothecary
1000 g = 1 kg	2.2 lb
1000 mg = 1 g	15 grains (gr $\overline{xv}$)
60 mg	gr †
30 mg	gr $\frac{1}{2}$ or $\overline{ss}$
0.6 mg	gr $\frac{1}{100}$
0.4 mg	gr $\frac{1}{150}$
0.3 mg	gr $\frac{1}{200}$

➤ Please refer to the TJC and ISMP lists on pp. 101-103.

➤ Consult a pharmacist or the prescriber for all unfamiliar medication-related measurements that you encounter.

ISMP's List of High-Alert Medications

High-alert medications are drugs that bear a heightened risk of causing significant patient harm when they are used in error. Although mistakes may or may not be more common with these drugs, the consequences of an error are clearly more devastating to patients. We hope you will use this list to determine which medications require special safeguards to reduce the risk of errors. This may include strategies like improving access to information about these drugs; limiting access to high-alert medications; using auxiliary labels and automated alerts; standardizing the ordering, storage, preparation, and administration of these products; and employing redundancies such as automated or independent double-checks when necessary. (Note: Manual independent double-checks are not always the optimal error-reduction strategy and may not be practical for all of the medications on the list.)

Classes/Categories of Medications
adrenergic agonists, IV (e.g., epinephrine, phenylephrine, norepinephrine)
adrenergic antagonists, IV (e.g., propranolol, metoprolol, labetalol)
anesthetic agents, general, inhaled and IV (e.g., propofol, ketamine)
antiarrhythmics, IV (e.g., lidocaine, amiodarone)
antithrombotic agents (anticoagulants), including warfarin, low-molecular-weight heparin, IV unfractionated heparin, Factor Xa inhibitors (fondaparinux), direct thrombin inhibitors (e.g., argatroban, lepirudin, bivalirudin), thrombolytics (e.g., alteplase, reteplase, tenecteplase), and glycoprotein IIb/IIIa inhibitors (e.g., eptifibatide)
cardioplegic solutions
chemotherapeutic agents, parenteral and oral
dextrose, hypertonic, 20% or greater
dialysis solutions, peritoneal and hemodialysis
epidural or intrathecal medications
hypoglycemics, oral
inotropic medications, IV (e.g., digoxin, milrinone)
liposomal forms of drugs (e.g., liposomal amphotericin B)
moderate sedation agents, IV (e.g., midazolam)
moderate sedation agents, oral, for children (e.g., chloral hydrate)
narcotics/opiates, IV, transdermal, and oral (including liquid concentrates, immediate and sustained-release formulations)
neuromuscular blocking agents (e.g., succinylcholine, rocuronium, vecuronium)
radiocontrast agents, IV
total parenteral nutrition solutions

Specific Medications
colchicine injection*
epoprostenol (Flolan), IV
insulin, subcutaneous and IV
magnesium sulfate injection
methotrexate, oral, non-oncologic use
opium tincture
oxytocin, IV
nitroprusside sodium for injection
potassium chloride for injection concentrate
potassium phosphates injection
promethazine, IV
sodium chloride for injection, hypertonic (greater than 0.9% concentration)
sterile water for injection, inhalation, and irrigation (excluding pour bottles) in containers of 100 mL or more

Although colchicine injection should no longer be used, it will remain on the list until shipments of unapproved colchicine injection cease in August 2008. For details, please visit: www.fda.gov/bbs/topics/ NEWS/2008/EW01791.html.

Background
Based on error reports submitted to the USP-ISMP Medication Errors Reporting Program, reports of harmful errors in the literature, and input from practitioners and safety experts, ISMP created and periodically updates a list of potential high-alert medications. During February-April 2007, 770 practitioners responded to an ISMP survey designed to identify which medications were most frequently considered high-alert drugs by individuals and organizations. Further, to assure relevance and completeness, the clinical staff at ISMP, members of our advisory board, and safety experts throughout the US were asked to review the potential list. This list of drugs and drug categories reflects the collective thinking of all who provided input.

5-Minute Sample Verbal Communication Hand-off Report

A hand-off report is the transfer and acceptance of patient care responsibilities through effective communication between caregivers at shift change or for transfer between units, agencies, or to home, to ensure patient safety. Many errors, *including medication errors,* have been attributed to inadequate hand-off communication. The highlighted areas in the sample report presented here pertain to key medication-related information. Additional information would be given for discharge communication to home, including accompanying written materials about all medications and treatments and when to make appointments for checkups. Whereas only major medication issues are verbally reported for a shift change, complete medication resolution must be provided in writing for all physical patient transfers. Check agency procedures and forms for hand-off communication and medication resolution.

Situation: Nurse giving report to next caregiver at shift change on a medical-surgical unit

(Sex, Age, Mental/Emotional Status, Main Diagnoses, Dates of Admission and Transfers, Additional Diagnoses, Allergies)

"Mr. G. is a 73-year-old, moderately hard-of-hearing, alert, oriented × 3 (to person, time, and place), cooperative English-speaking male in no acute distress, admitted to ICU with uncontrolled hypertension and acute bronchitis on the 3rd of October and transferred to our unit on the 6th. He also has chronic prostatitis, mild anemia, an artificial hip replacement as of a year ago that requires use of a cane for stability, and occasional asthmatic episodes controlled with an inhaler. He is allergic to penicillin and aspirin, reacting with hives and wheezing as well as diarrhea from penicillin, and is a fairly reliable historian. He lives with his daughter, so it's best to include her in all teaching, particularly because of the hearing loss.

(Vital Signs)

His vitals signs are all stable today.

(Meds: Med Changes, Meds Due, Related Orders)

He had a central line removed before transfer here. His main medications are an intravenous antibiotic piggyback (IVPB) every 6 hr for 24 more hr for his bronchitis. His next one is due soon at 1700 hr. He is on digoxin every morning and two new blood pressure meds, one a diuretic in the morning and the other an ace inhibitor in the evening. His blood pressure needs to be recorded each shift and after any complaint of weakness or extreme fatigue. Notify the attending physician if the systolic pressure exceeds 170. Make sure his inhaler is within reach and record his use.

(Labs)

His white blood count is still elevated at 13,000 but has been improving steadily. He is NPO after midnight for fasting blood work and also has a lung function test scheduled in the morning. His other labs are within normal limits. Hold the diuretic in the morning until the labs are completed.

(Treatments)

The discontinued central line site needs to be assessed once a day. He is receiving respiratory therapy every morning beween 0800 and 0900 hr and wants to bathe before they come.

(Nutrition/Intake and Output)

He is now tolerating a regular diet well but needs encouragement to drink more fluids. Since he started on the diuretic, he self-limits fluids to try to reduce urination. The fluid intake and urinary output is to be recorded until discharge. Notify the attending physician if the intake or output drops below 1000 mL per day.

(Activity Level: Mobility)

He does need assistance and encouragement getting in and out of bed but does not need assistance walking as long as he has the cane. The doctor wants him to be out of bed most of the day if possible. Bedrails are up at bedtime and a urinal within reach at all times because of the diuretic and urinary frequency.

(Other Needs/Discharge Planning)

His discharge is tentatively planned for next Monday, so special emphasis needs to be given to teaching Mr. G about the new medication regime and need for fluids and activity. He lives with his daughter, who visits after work daily. Be sure to include her in all teaching and discharge because the day shift doesn't see her often. A main issue is that he is unhappy about having to take "new pills," so we've already started reinforcing the importance of compliance with him and the daughter. Be sure to get feedback because he does not always mention that he did not hear everything.

Note: Although this seems like a lot of information, the nurse who cares for the patient for a full shift and who has *established a sequential format* for the reporting information can communicate this information verbally on each assigned patient with ease. It helps to keep a checklist on hand with abbreviated cues (see the sample boldfaced subheadings) to ensure the verbal hand-off report covers all the major areas. The receiving nurse refers to the written record for further details. There are many potential variations for reporting; for example, fasting could be included under Nutrition/Intake and Output instead of Labs.

Index

Page numbers followed by *b, t,* or *f* indicate boxes, tables, or figures, respectively.

589

Metric Equivalents

Weight	Length
1000 mcg (microgram) = 1 mg (milligram)	10 mm (millimeter) = 1 cm (centimeter)
1000 mg = 1 g (gram)	100 cm = 1 m (meter)
1000 g = 1 kg (kilogram)	1000 mm = 1 m
Pound to Kilogram Conversion	**Volume**
2.2 lb = 1 kg	1000 mL (milliliter) = 1 L (liter)
Household to Metric Length Equivalent	
1 inch = 2.54 cm	
39.37 inches = 1 m	

Temperature Conversions: Celsius (C) and Fahrenheit (F)

0° C (freezing) = 32° F   100° C (boiling) = 212° F   37° C = 98.6° F

To convert Fahrenheit to Celsius: **To convert Celsius to Fahrenheit:**

1. Subtract 32   1. Multiply by 1.8
2. Divide by 1.8   2. Add 32